T0185840

Cancer Drug Discovery and Development

Series Editor
Beverly A. Teicher
Bethesda, MD, USA

The Cancer Drug Discovery and Development series (Beverly A Teicher, series editor) is the definitive book series in cancer research and oncology, providing comprehensive coverage of specific topics and the field. Volumes cover the process of drug discovery, preclinical models in cancer research, specific drug target groups and experimental and approved therapeutic agents. The volumes are current and timely, anticipating areas where experimental agents are reaching FDA approval. Each volume is edited by an expert in the field covered and chapters are authored by renowned scientists and physicians in their fields of interest.

More information about this series at http://www.springer.com/series/7625

Henning Willers • Iris Eke

Editors

Molecular Targeted Radiosensitizers

Opportunities and Challenges

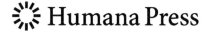 Humana Press

Editors
Henning Willers
Department of Radiation Oncology
Massachusetts General Hospital
Harvard Medical School
Boston, MA, USA

Iris Eke
Department of Radiation Oncology
Stanford University School of Medicine
Stanford, CA, USA

ISSN 2196-9906   ISSN 2196-9914   (electronic)
Cancer Drug Discovery and Development
ISBN 978-3-030-49703-3   ISBN 978-3-030-49701-9   (eBook)
https://doi.org/10.1007/978-3-030-49701-9

This Humana imprint is published by the registered company Springer Nature Switzerland AG
The registered company address is: Gewerbestrasse 11, 6330 Cham, Switzerland

Preface

It has been almost an entire century since Dr. Hermann Holthusen of Hamburg, Germany, correctly surmised that the relationship between the probability of tumor control and the total dose of radiation delivered can be described by a sigmoid data fit on linear scales (Strahlentherapie 57, 254–69, 1936). Similarly, the probability of normal tissue complications with increasing dose follows a sigmoid dose–response relationship. Achieving nearly 100% tumor control while having a very low likelihood of severe complications remains the quintessential goal of curative radiation therapy. Because the maximum dose of radiation that can be safely delivered is limited by the radiation tolerance of the normal tissues and organs surrounding the tumor, there has been a longstanding interest in combining radiation with drugs that can increase radiation-mediated tumor cell kill but without substantially increasing normal tissue toxicity. However, treatment combinations of radiation with biological sensitizers or enhancers have had very limited clinical success to date. The challenges to successful clinical translation of these agents have served as motivation for this volume. Here, we provide a comprehensive review by experts in the field of key preclinical research components required to identify effective and safe radiosensitizing drugs. We sincerely hope that ultimately this text will help harness the tremendous opportunities that these drugs offer to increase the likelihood of uncomplicated cures in our cancer patients.

We are indebted to all authors for their hard work contributing outstanding reviews, despite their busy schedules! It has been a true pleasure to compile the chapters and assemble what we believe is a uniquely comprehensive and timely overview of this exciting and fast-moving field that the readers will enjoy.

We could not have tackled the task of editing this book without the teachings of many mentors and educators in our field, including Michael Baumann, Hans-Peter Beck Bornholdt, Norm Coleman, Nils Cordes, Kathy Held, Simon Powell, and Herman Suit. A special thanks also goes to Jeff Settleman and the Dana-Farber/Harvard Cancer Center SPORE in Lung Cancer for inspiring the application of precision oncology concepts to the study of radiation/drug combinations more than 10 years ago.

We are also intensely grateful for the love and support of our families. Without their tolerance for after-hours and weekend work, this project would not have come to fruition.

Lastly, we are deeply motivated and inspired by our patients—whose lives we saved and whose lives we lost. Biological advances in radiation therapy that will extend lives or achieve new cures cannot arrive soon enough.

Boston, MA, USA   Henning Willers
Stanford, CA, USA   Iris Eke

Contents

Contributors

Mohamed E. Abazeed Department of Radiation Oncology, Northwestern Memorial Hospital, Northwestern University, Chicago, IL, USA

Bryan G. Allen Department of Radiation Oncology, Free Radical and Radiation Biology Program, Holden Comprehensive Cancer Center, University of Iowa, Carver College of Medicine, Iowa City, IA, USA

Michael Baumann German Cancer Research Center (DKFZ), Heidelberg, Germany

OncoRay—National Center for Radiation Research in Oncology, Faculty of Medicine and University Hospital Carl Gustav Carus, Technische Universität Dresden, Helmholtz-Zentrum Dresden—Rossendorf, Dresden, Germany

Department of Radiotherapy and Radiation Oncology, Faculty of Medicine and University Hospital Carl Gustav Carus, Technische Universität Dresden, Dresden, Germany

Michael S. Binkley Department of Radiation Oncology, Stanford University School of Medicine, Stanford, CA, USA

Elizabeth Bowler Department of Oncology, Oxford Institute for Radiation Oncology, University of Oxford, Oxford, UK

Kevin A. Camphausen Radiation Oncology Branch, Center for Cancer Research, National Cancer Institute, Bethesda, MD, USA

Jessica A. Castrillon Department of Translational Hematology Oncology Research, Cleveland Clinic, Cleveland, OH, USA

Deborah E. Citrin Radiation Oncology Branch, Center for Cancer Research, National Cancer Institute, Bethesda, MD, USA

Nils Cordes OncoRay—National Center for Radiation Research in Oncology, Technische Universität Dresden, Dresden, Germany

Sara Sofia Deville OncoRay—National Center for Radiation Research in Oncology, Technische Universität Dresden, Dresden, Germany

Maximilian Diehn Department of Radiation Oncology, Stanford University School of Medicine, Stanford, CA, USA

Nadja Ebert German Cancer Research Center (DKFZ), Heidelberg, Germany

OncoRay—National Center for Radiation Research in Oncology, Faculty of Medicine and University Hospital Carl Gustav Carus, Technische Universität Dresden, Helmholtz-Zentrum Dresden—Rossendorf, Dresden, Germany

Iris Eke Department of Radiation Oncology, Stanford University School of Medicine, Stanford, CA, USA

John Floberg Department of Human Oncology, University of Wisconsin School of Medicine and Public Health, Milwaukee, WI, USA

Warren Floyd Department of Radiation Oncology, Duke University Medical Center, Durham, NC, USA

Priyanka Gopal Department of Radiation Oncology, Northwestern Memorial Hospital, Northwestern University, Chicago, IL, USA

Ester M. Hammond Department of Oncology, Oxford Institute for Radiation Oncology, University of Oxford, Oxford, UK

Geoff S. Higgins Department of Oncology, Oxford Institute for Radiation Oncology, University of Oxford, Oxford, UK

Jonathon E. Himes Department of Radiation Oncology, Duke University Medical Center, Durham, NC, USA

Rakesh K. Jain Edwin L. Steele Laboratories, Department of Radiation Oncology, Massachusetts General Hospital and Harvard Medical School, Boston, MA, USA

David G. Kirsch Department of Radiation Oncology, Duke University Medical Center, Durham, NC, USA

Hsuan-Cheng Kuo Department of Radiation Oncology, Duke University Medical Center, Durham, NC, USA

Ina Kurth German Cancer Research Center (DKFZ), Heidelberg, Germany

Theodore S. Lawrence Department of Radiation Oncology, University of Michigan Medical School, Ann Arbor, MI, USA

Jonathan E. Leeman Department of Radiation Oncology, Dana Farber Cancer Institute/Brigham and Women's Hospital, Boston, MA, USA

Steven H. Lin Division of Radiation Oncology, Department of Radiation Oncology, MD Anderson Cancer Center, Houston, TX, USA

John D. Martin NanoCarrier Co. Ltd., Kashiwa, Chiba, Japan

Matthew T. McMillan Department of Radiation Oncology, University of Michigan Medical School, Ann Arbor, MI, USA

Meredith A. Morgan Department of Radiation Oncology, University of Michigan Medical School, Ann Arbor, MI, USA

Rutulkumar Patel Department of Radiation Oncology, Duke University Medical Center, Durham, NC, USA

Michael Petronek Department of Radiation Oncology, Free Radical and Radiation Biology Program, University of Iowa, Iowa City, IA, USA

Rashmi Ramachandran Department of Radiation Oncology, Washington University School of Medicine, Saint Louis, MO, USA

Karolin Schneider German Cancer Research Center (DKFZ), Heidelberg, Germany

Jonathan D. Schoenfeld Department of Radiation Oncology, Dana Farber Cancer Institute/Brigham and Women's Hospital, Boston, MA, USA

Julie K. Schwarz Department of Radiation Oncology, Washington University School of Medicine, Saint Louis, MO, USA

Alvin J. Siteman Cancer Center, Washington University School of Medicine, Saint Louis, MO, USA

Department of Cell Biology and Physiology, Washington University School of Medicine, Saint Louis, MO, USA

Michael Skwarski Department of Oncology, Oxford Institute for Radiation Oncology, University of Oxford, Oxford, UK

Anne Vehlow National Center for Tumor Diseases Dresden, Dresden, Germany

OncoRay—National Center for Radiation Research in Oncology, Technische Universität Dresden, Dresden, Germany

Daniel Wahl Department of Radiation Oncology, University of Michigan, Ann Arbor, MI, USA

Yifan Wang Division of Radiation Oncology, Department of Radiation Oncology, MD Anderson Cancer Center, Houston, TX, USA

Henning Willers Department of Radiation Oncology, Massachusetts General Hospital, Harvard Medical School, Boston, MA, USA

Joseph D. Wilson Department of Oncology, Oxford Institute for Radiation Oncology, University of Oxford, Oxford, UK

Rui Ye Division of Radiation Oncology, Department of Radiation Oncology, MD Anderson Cancer Center, Houston, TX, USA

Chapter 1
Introduction to Molecular Targeted Radiosensitizers: Opportunities and Challenges

Henning Willers and Iris Eke

Abstract The practice of radiation oncology is currently primarily based on precise technical delivery of highly conformal, image-guided radiation treatments. The precision medicine revolution has provided radiation oncologists with tremendous opportunities to enhance the anti-tumor effects of radiation therapy, potentially with less normal tissue toxicity than traditional chemotherapeutic radiosensitizers. However, a large body of preclinical research and clinical investigations on radiosensitizers has not yet translated into any meaningful number of FDA-approved combinations of radiation with targeted radiosensitizers ± chemotherapy. There exist distinct challenges to clinical translation of radiation/drug combinations that the field is only beginning to appreciate. These considerations have served as motivation for this book, which provides a comprehensive review by experts in the field of key preclinical research components required to identify effective and safe (chemo-)radiosensitizing drugs. Readers will be provided with a detailed and timely insight into the framework of targeted radiosensitizer research coupled with recent developments in immuno-oncology. Ultimately, this book will support the identification of appropriately validated and biomarker-directed targeted drug/radiation combinations that will have a higher likelihood than in the past to be incorporated into standard management of human cancers. These developments, coupled with the increasing technical power of radiation therapy to safely increase local control for many solid tumors, are expected to improve survival outcomes and cure rates for our patients.

H. Willers (✉)
Department of Radiation Oncology, Massachusetts General Hospital, Harvard Medical School, Boston, MA, USA
e-mail: hwillers@mgh.harvard.edu

I. Eke
Department of Radiation Oncology, Stanford University School of Medicine, Stanford, CA, USA
e-mail: iris.eke@stanford.edu

© Springer Nature Switzerland AG 2020
H. Willers, I. Eke (eds.), *Molecular Targeted Radiosensitizers*, Cancer Drug Discovery and Development, https://doi.org/10.1007/978-3-030-49701-9_1

1

Keywords Biomarkers · Cancer stem cells · Clonogenic survival assays · Hallmarks of cancer · Molecular targeted radiosensitizers · Molecular targets · Preclinical models · Radiosensitization · Tumor heterogeneity

1 Opportunities for Targeted Radiosensitizers

Radiation therapy is an important treatment modality that is given to over 50% of cancer patients at some time during the course of their disease (Bristow et al. 2018). The goal of curative radiation therapy is to sterilize all cancer stem cells (CSC) or CSC-like cells that could give rise to a local tumor recurrence while limiting injury to normal tissues around the tumor and to the patient (Willers et al. 2019). Curative radiation is often combined with surgery or/and chemotherapy depending on cancer type, tumor stage, and other factors. In clinical settings where cure is not possible, radiation can provide palliation or extend progression-free survival in conjunction with systemic therapies. However, in many patients, the dose of radiation that can be safely administered is insufficient to achieve high rates of local tumor control and cure. In others, normal tissue injury may be a concern even at moderate doses. Ideally, in these settings, radiation would be combined with drugs that can enhance its tumoricidal effects (local or even abscopal) but without or only little added toxicity (Bristow et al. 2018; Baumann et al. 2016; Kirsch et al. 2018; Lin et al. 2013b).

1.1 Molecular Targeted Drugs

Over the past two decades, cancer therapy has been revolutionized by personalized (or precision) medicine, with prominent examples being the use of small molecule inhibitors against chronic myeloid leukemia driven by the BCR-ABL fusion protein or non-small cell lung cancer (NSCLC) cancers with oncogenic mutations in the epidermal growth factor receptor (EGFR) (Cohen et al. 2002; Lynch et al. 2004). Molecular targeted therapy can be defined as blocking a target that controls biological processes critical to the initiation and maintenance of cancer. Ideally, the target should be measurable in the clinic and measurement of the target should correlate with clinical benefit following administration of the targeted therapy (Sledge Jr. 2005). The arrival of targeted therapies has enabled oncologists to try to turn incurable cancers into chronic disease, or to at least achieve significant prolongations of progression-free survival (Chong and Janne 2013).

Importantly, many of the cellular pathways that promote tumor growth and survival may also play a role in response to treatment with ionizing radiation, suggesting that their pharmacological inhibition could cause tumor radiosensitization (Bristow et al. 2018). For example, while EGFR signaling may drive tumor growth in the small subset of NSCLC patients whose tumors harbor activating mutations in its tyrosine kinase domain, wild-type EGFR is expressed in the majority of lung and

	Precision Medicine	Precision *Radiation* Medicine
Endpoint	Response	Tumor control (kill all CSCs)
Intent	Chronic disease	Cure
Selectivity	Drug effective in a few	Radiosensitizer ideally effective in most tumors (similar to radiation effect)
Mechanism	Drug targets tumor dependence	• Radiosensitizing mechanism of action may be different from drug alone effect • Ideally not toxic by itself
Target	• Single drug target • Increasing use of drug combos	• Radiation has multiple effects • Sensitizer may need to hit >1 target or a central mechanism (DNA repair)
Biomarkers	Required for drug effect	• Understudied • To identify radioresistant tumors, or/and predict radiosensitization

Fig. 1.1 Comparison of precision medicine concepts in medical oncology vs radiation oncology aka precision radiation medicine. *CSCs* cancer stem cells

other cancers where it potentially can modulate responses to radiation (Baumann et al. 2007). However, targeting EGFR for radiosensitization has only been successful in an unselected population of patients with head and neck squamous cell carcinomas treated without chemotherapy and has failed in other clinical settings (Bonner et al. 2006; Bradley et al. 2020; Gillison et al. 2019; Ang et al. 2014).

Important differences in the utility of targeted drugs in mono-therapy versus their use as radiosensitizer likely exist and are summarized in Fig. 1.1. Traditionally, radiosensitizers have been regarded as effective in unselected patients, similar to the concept of combining radiation with chemotherapy. However, it appears increasingly possible that this "one-size-fits-all" approach is not viable in the clinic and that targeted agents only radiosensitize subsets of tumors, which would require predictive biomarkers to identify those patients who are most likely to benefit. Alternatively, biomarkers may be employed to identify radioresistant or radiosensitive strata of patients. The use of targeted agents with chemoradiation, which could be associated with increased toxicity, may only be justified in patients with radioresistant disease.

1.2 Predictive Biomarkers

Molecular targeted drugs can produce dramatic clinical responses in subsets of patients with disseminated cancer. The discovery of these agents has been concurrent with the characterization of the molecular genetic changes in an individual's tumor that can play a critical role in determining the clinical response to a particular drug. Human cancers vary enormously in their somatic genetic alterations, and it is becoming widely accepted that these genetic differences, even in tumors with the same basic histological features, are the important determinants of response to these targeted drugs. The genomic characterization of human cancers that has been fueled by the successes of targeted drugs now also provides a basis for a more rational, biologically informed use of radiation therapy, with or without the addition of targeted radiosensitizers (Hall et al. 2018; Eke et al. 2016b; Kamran and Mouw 2018).

Analogous to the concept of precision medicine, "precision radiation medicine" may thus leverage genomic information derived from human cancers or preclinical tumor models to identify subsets that are sensitive to specific radiation/drug combinations, or radiation alone. Genomic biomarkers of radiosensitization may include oncogenic driver mutations, as increasingly found in for example lung cancers, or passenger mutations that do not affect tumor cell growth/survival in the absence of radiation exposure but that become important determinants of survival once cells suffer radiation damage. This remains a vastly understudied area, particularly in comparison with recent advances in matching drug-alone sensitivities to oncogenic driver mutations. Furthermore, as we are acquiring a deeper understanding of the hallmarks of cancer and how they may differ across individual tumors and patients, we will be in a better position to identify molecular targets for tumor radiosensitization (Fig. 1.2) (Willers et al. 2019). Importantly, many of the hallmarks of cancer are intimately linked to effects of radiation, examples being the impact of DNA repair alterations on radiosensitivity and the role of local immune escape on radiation response (Boss et al. 2014).

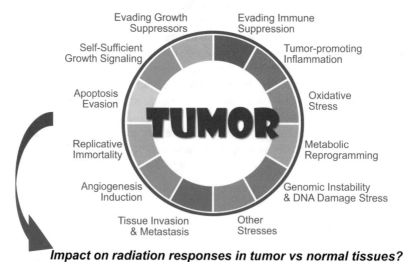

Fig. 1.2 How do the hallmarks of cancer impact tumor response to radiation treatment? (Redrawn from Willers et al. (2019))

1.3 Targeted Radiosensitizers and Immunotherapy

As we have firmly entered the era of immuno-oncology, what does this mean for the preclinical and clinical development of targeted radiosensitizers? In the future, immunotherapy rather than targeted radiosensitizers may be used to enhance tumor control and cures in many patients with solid tumors. However, it can be assumed that immunotherapy will not be of benefit in all cancer patients so that targeted radiosensitizers will retain their importance in at least subsets of patients. In addition, increasing evidence suggests that targeted radiosensitizers, particular DNA repair inhibitors, can modulate the immune response (Zhang et al. 2019; Konstantinopoulos et al. 2019; Vendetti et al. 2018). This opens up an exciting area for investigation into novel radiation/drug regimens. Lastly, immune checkpoint inhibitors may themselves have radiosensitizing properties (Azad et al. 2017; Deng et al. 2014; Crittenden et al. 2018).

Taken together, combining molecular targeted and immuno-modulating agents with radiation continues to show great promise both to radiosensitize tumors and to maximize protection of normal tissues. For many promising targeted agents and immune checkpoint inhibitors, one of their greatest impacts in oncology could ultimately rest in their combination with established treatment modalities such as radiation with/without chemotherapy to further cure and survival rates (Bristow et al. 2018).

2 Challenges for Targeted Radiosensitizers

Preclinical and clinical drug development with radiation therapy has been considered of critical importance to cancer research (Lawrence et al. 2013; Colevas et al. 2003; Harrington et al. 2011; Katz et al. 2009; Bristow et al. 2018). However, a large body of preclinical radiation/drug studies has not translated into an adequate number of successful radiation trials (Lawrence et al. 2013; Morris and Harari 2014). In fact, cetuximab remains to this date the only molecular targeted agent approved by the U.S. Food and Drug Administration—for use with radiation therapy in head and neck cancers (Bonner et al. 2006). A number of reasons likely exist, many of which have been discussed (Higgins et al. 2015; Lawrence et al. 2013; Lin et al. 2013b; Morris and Harari 2014; Coleman et al. 2016; Stone et al. 2016). Here, we wish to highlight what could be some of the most pressing challenges to the identification of successful radiation/drug combinations for the clinic.

2.1 Reproducibility of Preclinical Radiation Data

Preclinical evaluation of radiation effects is challenging due to the need to measure loss of replicative tumor cell potential, integrate concurrent chemotherapy which is the standard-of-care in many cancer types, and model the impact of the tumor microenvironment (Morgan et al. 2014). Furthermore, radiosensitizing drug effects in clonogenic survival assays (CSA) are often small with dose enhancement factors much below 2. This stands in contrast to the effects of targeted drugs on in vitro measures of tumor response, i.e., a reduction in cell number/viability, which is often pronounced (Barretina et al. 2012; Garnett et al. 2012).

These challenges are compounded by shortcomings in the design and reporting of radiation/drug experiments according to a recent review of 125 publications by Stone and colleagues (Stone et al. 2016). The authors described a large number of instances in which experimental studies contained inadequate or unclear information (222 problems in 104 in vitro studies and 109 problems in 51 in vivo experiments). These issues could hamper efforts to replicate or compare the data and weaken the evidence for any subsequent clinical trials. Areas needing improvement include:

1. Authentication of cell lines and testing for pathogens such as mycoplasma
2. Sufficient information on drug source, storage, vehicle, preparation, concentrations, etc.
3. Description of radiation source, irradiation setup, dosimetry, and other factors, including traceability of output verification of X-ray tube to National Standards
4. Information on in vitro and in vivo drug administration schedules, including exact timing and relationship to irradiation, and the underlying rationale
5. Proper conduct of CSA
6. Information on number of independent biological repeats performed
7. Inclusion of full data set in supplement if representative data are shown
8. Appropriate statistical analysis of results in consultation with a statistician
9. Blinded counting of colonies and outcome assessments wherever possible
10. For mouse experiments, detailed descriptions that include tumor size at start of treatment, whether treatment was started when tumors reached a given size or at a given time after implantation. Tumors should be sufficiently large at the start of treatment to have biological properties of established tumors and to facilitate accurate measurement. Information on tumor transplantation procedure, site, method and frequency of measurement, etc.

The authors stressed that preclinical radiation/drug studies should meet standards of design, execution, and interpretation, and report necessary information to ensure high quality and reproducibility of studies. These improvements may provide a more robust basis for prioritizing drugs for clinical radiation therapy trials and for the design of such trials.

2.2   Modeling of Clinically Relevant Intertumoral Heterogeneity

Established cancer cell lines remain critically important for mechanistic studies of radiation/drug interactions, target validation, and in vivo confirmation as xenografts. Traditionally, radiation/drug combinations have been studied in limited numbers of cell lines (Kleiman et al. 2013; Lin et al. 2014; Carmichael et al. 1987; Wang et al. 2001; Lally et al. 2007). However, any radiosensitizing effects in one or a few cell lines may not be representative of efficacy in an unselected larger number of genetically heterogeneous tumors, which may only be revealed when the agent under study has entered clinical trials. Historically, the choice of targeted radiosensitizers has conformed to a "one-size-fits-all" philosophy, but it is becoming increasingly possible that radiosensitizing effects are tumor genotype-dependent, which would require predictive biomarkers for appropriate patient selection (Lin et al. 2013a; Das et al. 2010; Liu et al. 2015; Willers and Hong 2015; Wang et al. 2018). Therefore, an appropriate number of human cancer-derived cell lines, for a given tumor type, may need to mirror the number of cell lines used in previous drug-alone screens, i.e., dozens per cancer type, given our emerging knowledge of the considerable genetic heterogeneity of tumors even within the same cancer type and histology (Cancer Genome Atlas Research Network 2012; Imielinski et al. 2012; Neve et al. 2006; Sos et al. 2009; Garnett et al. 2012; Barretina et al. 2012; Iorio et al. 2016). A larger number of cell lines would be needed to identify potential associations of radiosensitization with genomic alterations that have a low but still clinically relevant frequency of, for instance, 10–15% in the population.

The CSA has been considered the gold standard for assessing the cell-inactivating effects of radiation in vitro (Puck and Marcus 1956; Katz et al. 2008; Kahn et al. 2012). However, CSAs are not ideal for the kind of high-throughput screens that are needed to match diverse genomic tumor profiles with radiation/drug sensitivities owing to the frequently poor colony-forming ability of human cancer cell lines and the time it takes to conduct these assays. Short-term cell viability/survival assays, on the other hand, are historically not considered to provide appropriate surrogate endpoints of clonogenic survival (Lin et al. 2014; Brown and Wouters 1999; Brown and Wilson 2003). However, plate formats have been successfully tested and provide an opportunity for examining larger numbers of genomically characterized cancer cell lines and targeted drugs than have been historically pursued (Yard et al. 2016; Liu et al. 2015; Wang et al. 2014; Lin et al. 2014; Eke et al. 2016a). More work is required to validate these different approaches.

2.3 Integration of Experimental Approaches

Coleman and colleagues recently outlined a bench-to-bedside workflow to identify the most promising radiation/drug combinations for clinical testing (Coleman et al. 2016). This workflow involves an initial unbiased screening of cancer cell lines with radiation/drug combinations, followed by refinement and validation of "hits," after which tumor efficacy and treatment toxicity are assessed in appropriate animal models. An adapted preclinical workflow is shown in Fig. 1.3 and discussed below. Preclinical development of radiation/drug combos in such a manner is expected to be resource-intensive and time-consuming and requires integration of synergistic preclinical tumor models and capabilities of several institutions (e.g., NCI FOA PAR-16-111).

2.3.1   In Vitro Screening

As discussed above, initial testing of radiation/drug combinations may employ an appropriate number of authenticated cancer cell lines whose genomic and phenotypic characteristics are representative of the tumor type being studied. Treatment of one or a few cell lines with radiosensitizing agents likely produces biased results that will not translate into a more diverse tumor population. Drugs need to be given at multiple concentrations that are achievable in patients and have no or little toxicity by itself. Consideration should be given to pursuing more physiologic in vitro culturing conditions that better resemble in vivo tumor growth (such as use of 3D growth formats, extracellular matrix, physiologic oxygen concentrations, patient-derived cell line models and co-cultures). Initial investigations of immunotherapies or targeted drugs that interact with the tumor microenvironment have to be conducted in appropriate in vivo models such as genetically engineered mouse models (GEMM) (Castle et al. 2017) or perhaps in ex vivo systems (Jenkins et al. 2018).

2.3.2   In Vitro Validation

Screening results should be confirmed with CSA whenever possible. Additional assays may consider CSC-like cells that are relevant for radioresistance, for example, through the use of tumor spheres. In vitro validation may also include assessing the impact of concurrently administered chemotherapeutics on radiosensitizing drug effects although laboratory modeling of clinically relevant dosing and timing of chemotherapies is not trivial. The inclusion of patient-derived tumor models is recommended if the initial screen was done on established cancer cell lines. For other tasks, see Fig. 1.3. In general, this step narrows down the number of compounds that will undergo more expensive and time-consuming animal testing.

2.3.3   In Vivo Testing

Initial tumor models may be xenografts derived from genomically characterized cell lines used in the in vitro investigation or appropriate PDX models. Assessment of efficacy in murine models should consider treatments that are clinically relevant, including fractionated radiation and standard-of-care chemoradiation regimens. This approach provides initial assessments of drug efficacy, mechanistic insight as well as pharmacokinetic/pharmacodynamic measures. However, results from tumor growth delay assays may not always be consistent with the results of local control (TCD50) assays (Gurtner et al. 2011; Krause et al. 2006). TCD50 assays are performed much less commonly than growth delay assays because of the larger number of animals required and higher cost (Coleman et al. 2016). Nevertheless, before clinical trials with curative endpoints are initiated, TCD50 assays, which better reflect CSC inactivation, should be considered to reduce the chance of a negative trial. Additional animal models such as GEMMs harboring a natural tumor micro-

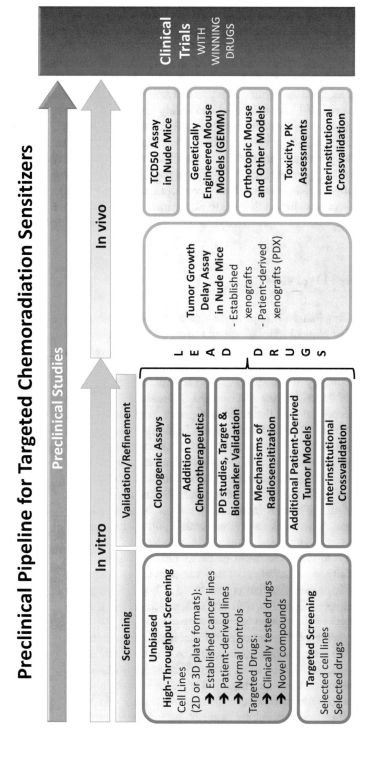

Fig. 1.3 Proposed preclinical pipeline for identifying "winning" targeted chemoradiosensitizers. (Inspired by Coleman et al. (2016))

environment and an intact immune system are also important components within the preclinical pipeline before bringing radiation/drug combos into the clinic (see Fig. 1.3).

The above considerations have served as motivation for this book, which provides a comprehensive review by experts in the field of key preclinical research components required to identify effective and safe (chemo-)radiosensitizing drugs. Readers are provided with a detailed and timely insight into the framework of targeted radiosensitizer research coupled with recent developments in immuno-oncology. Ultimately, this volume will support the identification of appropriately validated, and potentially biomarker-directed, targeted drug/radiation combinations that will have a higher likelihood than in the past to be incorporated into standard management of human cancers. These developments, coupled with the increasing technical power of radiation therapy to safely increase local control for many solid tumors, are expected to improve survival outcomes and cure rates for our patients.

3 Chapter Overview

Citrin and Camphausen (Chap. 2) provide a comprehensive review on the unique challenges that clinical translation and testing of targeted radiosensitizers present. These include how to best sequence agents and radiation, establishing biomarkers of efficacy, and integration into the current standard of care which includes cytotoxic chemotherapy in many settings. The authors conclude that an expanding knowledge of the underlying mechanisms of resistance and recurrence after radiation therapy coupled with the growing capacity to molecularly profile tumors provide great hope for future progress in this field. Abazeed and colleagues (Chap. 3) introduce the readers to preclinical studies of radiation responses and targeted sensitizers. They focus on the review our emerging knowledge of tumor and normal tissue genomics and their impact on the outcomes after radiation therapy (i.e., the "radiogenome"). They emphasize that given this knowledge population-based estimates of treatment effects increasingly cannot be justified. Critically, genomic tumor and patient features have considerable potential to serve as predictive biomarkers that can guide the clinical development of targeted radiosensitizers. Because targeted radiosensitizers or chemoradiosensitizers are expected to have particular utility in the treatment of radioresistant cancers, we summarize clinically relevant mechanisms of radiation resistance (Chap. 4). Of particular interest are tumor mutations in *KEAP1* as well as *KRAS*, which define an emerging area of need for intensification of radiation-based treatment regimens.

Starting a series of chapters on preclinical models for the study of targeted radiosensitizers, Lin and colleagues (Chap. 5) provide a comprehensive overview of preclinical strategies for testing of targeted radiosensitizers with a focus on clonogenic and non-clonogenic screening assays. They also review published guidelines and recommendations for the conduct of these studies. Three-dimensional (3D) cell cultures are well suited to model the extracellular matrix of tumors and provide more physiological treatment responses than traditional 2D cell cultures, as reviewed by Cordes and colleagues (Chap. 6). In particular, radioresistance and the effects of radiosensitizing agents are effectively captured by 3D tumor models, which comprise an important level of investigation before moving drug testing into animals. Baumann and colleagues (Chap. 7) discuss the conduct of radiation and radiation/drug studies in different mouse models. While every model has advantages and disadvantages, the use of genomically defined heterotopic xenograft tumor models facilitates testing of clinically relevant radiation dose fractionation schedules and assessments of local tumor control. Kirsch and colleagues (Chap. 8) review the advantages of genetically engineered mouse models for the study of targeted radiosensitizers as well as radiation biology in general. These include preservation of the natural tumor microenvironment, ability to assess clinically relevant normal tissue injury, precise temporal and spatial control of genetic alterations that may affect radiation/drug responses, and lastly, the presence of an intact immune system.

Moving on to clinically promising therapeutic targets, Morgan and colleagues (Chap. 9) provide an in-depth review of clinically relevant small molecule inhibitors directed against kinases in the cellular DNA damage response (DDR). Of special interest is the recently recognized link of DDR targets to immuno-modulation which creates opportunities for novel radiation/drug regimens. The promise of targeting altered cellular metabolism, a hallmark of cancer, is comprehensively addressed by Schwarz, Allen, and colleagues (Chap. 10). Preclinical and clinical evidence supports the combined use of a number of metabolically targeted agents with radiation therapy, including those that affect nucleotide metabolism, glutaminolysis, oxidative stress, or iron metabolism. Hammond and colleagues (Chap. 11) provide an overview of tumor hypoxia, long known to limit the effectiveness of radiation therapy. Novel therapeutic approaches are emerging that include targeting oxidative metabolism in tumors. The authors emphasize the need for clinical development of hypoxia biomarkers without which patients most likely to benefit cannot be selected for hypoxia-targeted treatment strategies. Jain and Martin (Chap. 12) describe pioneering work on the effects that the altered tumor microenvironment has on cancer therapy outcomes including radiation. Novel approaches to inhibit tumor angiogenesis and desmoplasia can normalize the tumor microenvironment towards alleviating hypoxia and reversing radioresistance. The authors stress the need for appropriate preclinical models and imaging tools to identify optimal combinations of radiation with anti-angiogenic treatments, mechanotherapeutics, chemotherapy, and immune checkpoint inhibitors in the context of TME normalization. Lastly, Leeman and Schoenfeld (Chap. 13) provide an overview of the rapidly expanding field of radiation combined with immune checkpoint inhibitors, both with regard to enhancing local tumor control and eliciting abscopal effects. Because molecular targeted agents are being increasingly recognized as having immuno-modulatory effects, additional opportunities, as well as challenges, exist for multi-modality approaches that employ radiation and systemic combinations of chemotherapy, targeted agents, and/or checkpoint inhibitors.

References

Ang KK, Zhang Q, Rosenthal DI, Nguyen-Tan PF, Sherman EJ, Weber RS, Galvin JM, Bonner JA, Harris J, El-Naggar AK, Gillison ML, Jordan RC, Konski AA, Thorstad WL, Trotti A, Beitler JJ, Garden AS, Spanos WJ, Yom SS, Axelrod RS (2014) Randomized phase III trial of concurrent accelerated radiation plus cisplatin with or without cetuximab for stage III to IV head and neck carcinoma: RTOG 0522. J Clin Oncol 32(27):2940–2950. https://doi.org/10.1200/JCO.2013.53.5633

Azad A, Yin Lim S, D'Costa Z, Jones K, Diana A, Sansom OJ, Kruger P, Liu S, McKenna WG, Dushek O, Muschel RJ, Fokas E (2017) PD-L1 blockade enhances response of pancreatic ductal adenocarcinoma to radiotherapy. EMBO Mol Med 9(2):167–180. https://doi.org/10.15252/emmm.201606674

Barretina J, Caponigro G, Stransky N, Venkatesan K, Margolin AA, Kim S, Wilson CJ, Lehar J, Kryukov GV, Sonkin D, Reddy A, Liu M, Murray L, Berger MF, Monahan JE, Morais P, Meltzer J, Korejwa A, Jane-Valbuena J, Mapa FA, Thibault J, Bric-Furlong E, Raman P, Shipway A, Engels IH, Cheng J, Yu GK, Yu J, Aspesi P Jr, de Silva M, Jagtap K, Jones MD, Wang L, Hatton C, Palescandolo E, Gupta S, Mahan S, Sougnez C, Onofrio RC, Liefeld T, MacConaill L, Winckler W, Reich M, Li N, Mesirov JP, Gabriel SB, Getz G, Ardlie K, Chan V, Myer VE, Weber BL, Porter J, Warmuth M, Finan P, Harris JL, Meyerson M, Golub TR, Morrissey MP, Sellers WR, Schlegel R, Garraway LA (2012) The cancer cell line encyclopedia enables predictive modelling of anticancer drug sensitivity. Nature 483(7391):603–607

Baumann M, Krause M, Dikomey E, Dittmann K, Dorr W, Kasten-Pisula U, Rodemann HP (2007) EGFR-targeted anti-cancer drugs in radiotherapy: preclinical evaluation of mechanisms. Radiother Oncol 83(3):238–248

Baumann M, Krause M, Overgaard J, Debus J, Bentzen SM, Daartz J, Richter C, Zips D, Bortfeld T (2016) Radiation oncology in the era of precision medicine. Nat Rev Cancer 16(4):234–249. https://doi.org/10.1038/nrc.2016.18

Bonner JA, Harari PM, Giralt J, Azarnia N, Shin DM, Cohen RB, Jones CU, Sur R, Raben D, Jassem J, Ove R, Kies MS, Baselga J, Youssoufian H, Amellal N, Rowinsky EK, Ang KK (2006) Radiotherapy plus cetuximab for squamous-cell carcinoma of the head and neck. N Engl J Med 354(6):567–578. https://doi.org/10.1056/NEJMoa053422

Boss MK, Bristow R, Dewhirst MW (2014) Linking the history of radiation biology to the hallmarks of cancer. Radiat Res 181(6):561–577. https://doi.org/10.1667/RR13675.1

Bradley JD, Hu C, Komaki RR, Masters GA, Blumenschein GR, Schild SE, Bogart JA, Forster KM, Magliocco AM, Kavadi VS, Narayan S, Iyengar P, Robinson CG, Wynn RB, Koprowski CD, Olson MR, Meng J, Paulus R, Curran WJ Jr, Choy H (2020) Long-term results of NRG oncology RTOG 0617: standard- versus high-dose chemoradiotherapy with or without cetuximab for unresectable stage III non-small-cell lung cancer. J Clin Oncol 38(7):706–714. https://doi.org/10.1200/JCO.19.01162

Bristow RG, Alexander B, Baumann M, Bratman SV, Brown JM, Camphausen K, Choyke P, Citrin D, Contessa JN, Dicker A, Kirsch DG, Krause M, Le QT, Milosevic M, Morris ZS, Sarkaria JN, Sondel PM, Tran PT, Wilson GD, Willers H, Wong RKS, Harari PM (2018) Combining precision radiotherapy with molecular targeting and immunomodulatory agents: a guideline by the American Society for Radiation Oncology. Lancet Oncol 19(5):e240–e251. https://doi.org/10.1016/S1470-2045(18)30096-2

Brown JM, Wilson G (2003) Apoptosis genes and resistance to cancer therapy: what does the experimental and clinical data tell us? Cancer Biol Ther 2(5):477–490

Brown JM, Wouters BG (1999) Apoptosis, p53, and tumor cell sensitivity to anticancer agents. Cancer Res 59(7):1391–1399

Cancer Genome Atlas Research Network (2012) Comprehensive genomic characterization of squamous cell lung cancers. Nature 489(7417):519–525

Carmichael J, DeGraff WG, Gazdar AF, Minna JD, Mitchell JB (1987) Evaluation of a tetrazolium-based semiautomated colorimetric assay: assessment of radiosensitivity. Cancer Res 47(4):943–946

Castle KD, Chen M, Wisdom AJ, Kirsch DG (2017) Genetically engineered mouse models for studying radiation biology. Transl Cancer Res 6(Suppl 5):S900–S913. https://doi.org/10.21037/tcr.2017.06.19

Chong CR, Janne PA (2013) The quest to overcome resistance to EGFR-targeted therapies in cancer. Nat Med 19(11):1389–1400. https://doi.org/10.1038/nm.3388

Cohen MH, Williams G, Johnson JR, Duan J, Gobburu J, Rahman A, Benson K, Leighton J, Kim SK, Wood R, Rothmann M, Chen G, Khin Maung U, Staten AM, Pazdur R (2002) Approval summary for imatinib mesylate capsules in the treatment of chronic myelogenous leukemia. Clin Cancer Res 8(5):935–942

Coleman CN, Higgins GS, Brown JM, Baumann M, Kirsch DG, Willers H, Prasanna PG, Dewhirst MW, Bernhard EJ, Ahmed MM (2016) Improving the predictive value of preclinical studies in support of radiotherapy clinical trials. Clin Cancer Res 22(13):3138–3147. https://doi.org/10.1158/1078-0432.CCR-16-0069

Colevas AD, Brown JM, Hahn S, Mitchell J, Camphausen K, Coleman CN (2003) Development of investigational radiation modifiers. J Natl Cancer Inst 95(9):646–651

Crittenden MR, Zebertavage L, Kramer G, Bambina S, Friedman D, Troesch V, Blair T, Baird JR, Alice A, Gough MJ (2018) Tumor cure by radiation therapy and checkpoint inhibitors depends on pre-existing immunity. Sci Rep 8(1):7012. https://doi.org/10.1038/s41598-018-25482-w

Das AK, Bell MH, Nirodi CS, Story MD, Minna JD (2010) Radiogenomics predicting tumor responses to radiotherapy in lung cancer. Semin Radiat Oncol 20(3):149–155

Deng L, Liang H, Burnette B, Beckett M, Darga T, Weichselbaum RR, Fu YX (2014) Irradiation and anti-PD-L1 treatment synergistically promote antitumor immunity in mice. J Clin Invest 124(2):687–695. https://doi.org/10.1172/JCI67313

Eke I, Hehlgans S, Sandfort V, Cordes N (2016a) 3D matrix-based cell cultures: automated analysis of tumor cell survival and proliferation. Int J Oncol 48(1):313–321. https://doi.org/10.3892/ijo.2015.3230

Eke I, Makinde AY, Aryankalayil MJ, Ahmed MM, Coleman CN (2016b) Comprehensive molecular tumor profiling in radiation oncology: how it could be used for precision medicine. Cancer Lett 382(1):118–126. https://doi.org/10.1016/j.canlet.2016.01.041

Garnett MJ, Edelman EJ, Heidorn SJ, Greenman CD, Dastur A, Lau KW, Greninger P, Thompson IR, Luo X, Soares J, Liu Q, Iorio F, Surdez D, Chen L, Milano RJ, Bignell GR, Tam AT, Davies H, Stevenson JA, Barthorpe S, Lutz SR, Kogera F, Lawrence K, McLaren-Douglas A, Mitropoulos X, Mironenko T, Thi H, Richardson L, Zhou W, Jewitt F, Zhang T, O'Brien P, Boisvert JL, Price S, Hur W, Yang W, Deng X, Butler A, Choi HG, Chang JW, Baselga J, Stamenkovic I, Engelman JA, Sharma SV, Delattre O, Saez-Rodiguez J, Gray NS, Settleman J, Futreal PA, Haber DA, Stratton MR, Ramaswamy S, McDermott U, Benes CH (2012) Systematic identification of genomic markers of drug sensitivity in cancer cells. Nature 483(7391):570–575

Gillison ML, Trotti AM, Harris J, Eisbruch A, Harari PM, Adelstein DJ, Sturgis EM, Burtness B, Ridge JA, Ringash J, Galvin J, Yao M, Koyfman SA, Blakaj DM, Razaq MA, Colevas AD, Beitler JJ, Jones CU, Dunlap NE, Seaward SA, Spencer S, Galloway TJ, Phan J, Dignam JJ, Le QT (2019) Radiotherapy plus cetuximab or cisplatin in human papillomavirus-positive oropharyngeal cancer (NRG oncology RTOG 1016): a randomised, multicentre, non-inferiority trial. Lancet 393(10166):40–50. https://doi.org/10.1016/S0140-6736(18)32779-X

Gurtner K, Deuse Y, Butof R, Schaal K, Eicheler W, Oertel R, Grenman R, Thames H, Yaromina A, Baumann M, Krause M (2011) Diverse effects of combined radiotherapy and EGFR inhibition with antibodies or TK inhibitors on local tumour control and correlation with EGFR gene expression. Radiother Oncol 99(3):323–330. https://doi.org/10.1016/j.radonc.2011.05.035

Hall WA, Bergom C, Thompson RF, Baschnagel AM, Vijayakumar S, Willers H, Li A, Schultz CJ, Wilson GD, West CML, Capala J, Coleman CN, Torres-Roca JF, Weidhaas J, Feng FY (2018) Precision oncology and genomically guided radiation therapy, a report from the ASTRO/AAPM/NCI precision medicine conference. Int J Radiat Oncol Biol Phys 101(2):274–284

Harrington KJ, Billingham LJ, Brunner TB, Burnet NG, Chan CS, Hoskin P, Mackay RI, Maughan TS, Macdougall J, McKenna WG, Nutting CM, Oliver A, Plummer R, Stratford IJ, Illidge T (2011) Guidelines for preclinical and early phase clinical assessment of novel radiosensitisers. Br J Cancer 105(5):628–639

Higgins GS, O'Cathail SM, Muschel RJ, McKenna WG (2015) Drug radiotherapy combinations: review of previous failures and reasons for future optimism. Cancer Treat Rev 41(2):105–113. https://doi.org/10.1016/j.ctrv.2014.12.012

Imielinski M, Berger AH, Hammerman PS, Hernandez B, Pugh TJ, Hodis E, Cho J, Suh J, Capelletti M, Sivachenko A, Sougnez C, Auclair D, Lawrence MS, Stojanov P, Cibulskis K, Choi K, de Waal L, Sharifnia T, Brooks A, Greulich H, Banerji S, Zander T, Seidel D, Leenders F, Ansen S, Ludwig C, Engel-Riedel W, Stoelben E, Wolf J, Goparju C, Thompson K, Winckler W, Kwiatkowski D, Johnson BE, Janne PA, Miller VA, Pao W, Travis WD, Pass HI, Gabriel SB, Lander ES, Thomas RK, Garraway LA, Getz G, Meyerson M (2012) Mapping the hallmarks of lung adenocarcinoma with massively parallel sequencing. Cell 150(6):1107–1120

Iorio F, Knijnenburg TA, Vis DJ, Bignell GR, Menden MP, Schubert M, Aben N, Goncalves E, Barthorpe S, Lightfoot H, Cokelaer T, Greninger P, van Dyk E, Chang H, de Silva H, Heyn H, Deng X, Egan RK, Liu Q, Mironenko T, Mitropoulos X, Richardson L, Wang J, Zhang T, Moran S, Sayols S, Soleimani M, Tamborero D, Lopez-Bigas N, Ross-Macdonald P, Esteller M, Gray NS, Haber DA, Stratton MR, Benes CH, Wessels LF, Saez-Rodriguez J, McDermott U, Garnett MJ (2016) A landscape of Pharmacogenomic interactions in cancer. Cell 166(3):740–754. https://doi.org/10.1016/j.cell.2016.06.017

Jenkins RW, Aref AR, Lizotte PH, Ivanova E, Stinson S, Zhou CW, Bowden M, Deng J, Liu H, Miao D, He MX, Walker W, Zhang G, Tian T, Cheng C, Wei Z, Palakurthi S, Bittinger M, Vitzthum H, Kim JW, Merlino A, Quinn M, Venkataramani C, Kaplan JA, Portell A, Gokhale PC, Phillips B, Smart A, Rotem A, Jones RE, Keogh L, Anguiano M, Stapleton L, Jia Z, Barzily-Rokni M, Canadas I, Thai TC, Hammond MR, Vlahos R, Wang ES, Zhang H, Li S, Hanna GJ, Huang W, Hoang MP, Piris A, Eliane JP, Stemmer-Rachamimov AO, Cameron L, Su MJ, Shah P, Izar B, Thakuria M, LeBoeuf NR, Rabinowits G, Gunda V, Parangi S, Cleary JM, Miller BC, Kitajima S, Thummalapalli R, Miao B, Barbie TU, Sivathanu V, Wong J, Richards WG, Bueno R, Yoon CH, Miret J, Herlyn M, Garraway LA, Van Allen EM, Freeman GJ, Kirschmeier PT, Lorch JH, Ott PA, Hodi FS, Flaherty KT, Kamm RD, Boland GM, Wong KK, Dornan D, Paweletz CP, Barbie DA (2018) Ex vivo profiling of PD-1 blockade using organotypic tumor spheroids. Cancer Discov 8(2):196–215. https://doi.org/10.1158/2159-8290.CD-17-0833

Kahn J, Tofilon PJ, Camphausen K (2012) Preclinical models in radiation oncology. Radiat Oncol 7:223

Kamran SC, Mouw KW (2018) Applying precision oncology principles in radiation oncology. JCO Precis Oncol 1–23. https://doi.org/10.1200/PO.18.00034

Katz D, Ito E, Lau KS, Mocanu JD, Bastianutto C, Schimmer AD, Liu FF (2008) Increased efficiency for performing colony formation assays in 96-well plates: novel applications to combination therapies and high-throughput screening. Biotechniques 44(2):ix–xiv

Katz D, Ito E, Liu FF (2009) On the path to seeking novel radiosensitizers. Int J Radiat Oncol Biol Phys 73(4):988–996

Kirsch DG, Diehn M, Kesarwala AH, Maity A, Morgan MA, Schwarz JK, Bristow R, Demaria S, Eke I, Griffin RJ, Haas-Kogan D, Higgins GS, Kimmelman AC, Kimple RJ, Lombaert IM, Ma L, Marples B, Pajonk F, Park CC, Schaue D, Tran PT, Willers H, Wouters BG, Bernhard EJ (2018) The future of radiobiology. J Natl Cancer Inst 110(4):329–340. https://doi.org/10.1093/jnci/djx231

Kleiman LB, Krebs AM, Kim SY, Hong TS, Haigis KM (2013) Comparative analysis of radiosensitizers for K-RAS mutant rectal cancers. PLoS One 8(12):e82982

Konstantinopoulos PA, Waggoner S, Vidal GA, Mita M, Moroney JW, Holloway R, Van Le L, Sachdev JC, Chapman-Davis E, Colon-Otero G, Penson RT, Matulonis UA, Kim YB, Moore KN, Swisher EM, Farkkila A, D'Andrea A, Stringer-Reasor E, Wang J, Buerstatte N, Arora S, Graham JR, Bobilev D, Dezube BJ, Munster P (2019) Single-arm phases 1 and 2 trial of Niraparib in combination with Pembrolizumab in patients with recurrent platinum-resistant ovarian carcinoma. JAMA Oncol 5:1141. https://doi.org/10.1001/jamaoncol.2019.1048

Krause M, Zips D, Thames HD, Kummermehr J, Baumann M (2006) Preclinical evaluation of molecular-targeted anticancer agents for radiotherapy. Radiother Oncol 80(2):112–122

Lally BE, Geiger GA, Kridel S, Arcury-Quandt AE, Robbins ME, Kock ND, Wheeler K, Peddi P, Georgakilas A, Kao GD, Koumenis C (2007) Identification and biological evaluation of a novel and potent small molecule radiation sensitizer via an unbiased screen of a chemical library. Cancer Res 67(18):8791–8799

Lawrence YR, Vikram B, Dignam JJ, Chakravarti A, Machtay M, Freidlin B, Takebe N, Curran WJ Jr, Bentzen SM, Okunieff P, Coleman CN, Dicker AP (2013) NCI-RTOG translational program strategic guidelines for the early-stage development of radiosensitizers. J Natl Cancer Inst 105(1):11–24

Lin SH, George TJ, Ben-Josef E, Bradley J, Choe KS, Edelman MJ, Guha C, Krishnan S, Lawrence TS, Le QT, Lu B, Mehta M, Peereboom D, Sarkaria J, Seong J, Wang D, Welliver MX, Coleman CN, Vikram B, Yoo S, Chung CH (2013a) Opportunities and challenges in the era of molecularly targeted agents and radiation therapy. J Natl Cancer Inst 105(10):686–693

Lin SH, George TJ, Ben-Josef E, Bradley J, Choe KS, Edelman MJ, Guha C, Krishnan S, Lawrence TS, Le QT, Lu B, Mehta M, Peereboom D, Sarkaria J, Seong J, Wang D, Welliver MX, Coleman CN, Vikram B, Yoo S, Chung CH, Participants on Workshop for Preclinical and Clinical Development of Radiosensitizers; National Cancer Institute (2013b) Opportunities and challenges in the era of molecularly targeted agents and radiation therapy. J Natl Cancer Inst 105(10):686–693. https://doi.org/10.1093/jnci/djt055

Lin SH, Zhang J, Giri U, Stephan C, Sobieski M, Zhong L, Mason KA, Molkentine J, Thames HD, Yoo SS, Heymach JV (2014) A high content clonogenic survival drug screen identifies MEK inhibitors as potent radiation sensitizers for KRAS mutant non-small-cell lung cancer. J Thorac Oncol 9(7):965–973

Liu Q, Wang M, Kern AM, Khaled S, Han J, Yeap BY, Hong TS, Settleman J, Benes CH, Held KD, Efstathiou JA, Willers H (2015) Adapting a drug screening platform to discover associations of molecular targeted radiosensitizers with genomic biomarkers. Mol Cancer Res 13:713–720

Lynch TJ, Bell DW, Sordella R, Gurubhagavatula S, Okimoto RA, Brannigan BW, Harris PL, Haserlat SM, Supko JG, Haluska FG, Louis DN, Christiani DC, Settleman J, Haber DA (2004) Activating mutations in the epidermal growth factor receptor underlying responsiveness of non-small-cell lung cancer to gefitinib. N Engl J Med 350(21):2129–2139

Morgan MA, Parsels LA, Maybaum J, Lawrence TS (2014) Improving the efficacy of chemoradiation with targeted agents. Cancer Discov 4(3):280–291. https://doi.org/10.1158/2159-8290. CD-13-0337

Morris ZS, Harari PM (2014) Interaction of radiation therapy with molecular targeted agents. J Clin Oncol 32(26):2886–2893. https://doi.org/10.1200/JCO.2014.55.1366

Neve RM, Chin K, Fridlyand J, Yeh J, Baehner FL, Fevr T, Clark L, Bayani N, Coppe JP, Tong F, Speed T, Spellman PT, DeVries S, Lapuk A, Wang NJ, Kuo WL, Stilwell JL, Pinkel D, Albertson DG, Waldman FM, McCormick F, Dickson RB, Johnson MD, Lippman M, Ethier S, Gazdar A, Gray JW (2006) A collection of breast cancer cell lines for the study of functionally distinct cancer subtypes. Cancer Cell 10(6):515–527

Puck TT, Marcus PI (1956) Action of x-rays on mammalian cells. J Exp Med 103(5):653–666

Sledge GW Jr (2005) What is targeted therapy? J Clin Oncol 23(8):1614–1615. https://doi.org/10.1200/JCO.2005.01.016

Sos ML, Michel K, Zander T, Weiss J, Frommolt P, Peifer M, Li D, Ullrich R, Koker M, Fischer F, Shimamura T, Rauh D, Mermel C, Fischer S, Stuckrath I, Heynck S, Beroukhim R, Lin W, Winckler W, Shah K, LaFramboise T, Moriarty WF, Hanna M, Tolosi L, Rahnenfuhrer J, Verhaak R, Chiang D, Getz G, Hellmich M, Wolf J, Girard L, Peyton M, Weir BA, Chen TH, Greulich H, Barretina J, Shapiro GI, Garraway LA, Gazdar AF, Minna JD, Meyerson M, Wong KK, Thomas RK (2009) Predicting drug susceptibility of non-small cell lung cancers based on genetic lesions. J Clin Invest 119(6):1727–1740

Stone HB, Bernhard EJ, Coleman CN, Deye J, Capala J, Mitchell JB, Brown JM (2016) Preclinical data on efficacy of 10 drug-radiation combinations: evaluations, concerns, and recommendations. Transl Oncol 9(1):46–56. https://doi.org/10.1016/j.tranon.2016.01.002

Vendetti FP, Karukonda P, Clump DA, Teo T, Lalonde R, Nugent K, Ballew M, Kiesel BF, Beumer JH, Sarkar SN, Conrads TP, O'Connor MJ, Ferris RL, Tran PT, Delgoffe GM, Bakkenist CJ (2018) ATR kinase inhibitor AZD6738 potentiates CD8+ T cell-dependent antitumor activity following radiation. J Clin Invest 128(9):3926–3940. https://doi.org/10.1172/JCI96519

Wang Y, Li J, Booher RN, Kraker A, Lawrence T, Leopold WR, Sun Y (2001) Radiosensitization of p53 mutant cells by PD0166285, a novel G(2) checkpoint abrogator. Cancer Res 61(22):8211–8217

Wang M, Kern AM, Hulskotter M, Greninger P, Singh A, Pan Y, Chowdhury D, Krause M, Baumann M, Benes CH, Efstathiou JA, Settleman J, Willers H (2014) EGFR-mediated chromatin condensation protects KRAS-mutant cancer cells against ionizing radiation. Cancer Res 74(10):2825–2834

Wang Y, Li N, Jiang W, Deng W, Ye R, Xu C, Qiao Y, Sharma A, Zhang M, Hung MC, Lin SH (2018) Mutant LKB1 confers enhanced radiosensitization in combination with Trametinib in KRAS-mutant non-small cell lung cancer. Clin Cancer Res 24(22):5744–5756. https://doi.org/10.1158/1078-0432.CCR-18-1489

Willers H, Hong TS (2015) Towards an integrated understanding of epidermal growth factor receptor biology for radiation therapy: integrins enter. J Natl Cancer Inst 107(2):dju440

Willers H, Keane FK, Kamran SC (2019) Toward a new framework for clinical radiation biology. Hematol Oncol Clin North Am 33(6):929–945. https://doi.org/10.1016/j.hoc.2019.07.001

Yard BD, Adams DJ, Chie EK, Tamayo P, Battaglia JS, Gopal P, Rogacki K, Pearson BE, Phillips J, Raymond DP, Pennell NA, Almeida F, Cheah JH, Clemons PA, Shamji A, Peacock CD, Schreiber SL, Hammerman PS, Abazeed ME (2016) A genetic basis for the variation in the vulnerability of cancer to DNA damage. Nat Commun 7:11428. https://doi.org/10.1038/ncomms11428

Zhang Q, Green MD, Lang X, Lazarus J, Parsels JD, Wei S, Parsels LA, Shi J, Ramnath N, Wahl DR, Pasca di Magliano M, Frankel TL, Kryczek I, Lei YL, Lawrence TS, Zou W, Morgan MA (2019) Inhibition of ATM increases interferon signaling and sensitizes pancreatic cancer to immune checkpoint blockade therapy. Cancer Res 79(15):3940–3951. https://doi.org/10.1158/0008-5472.CAN-19-0761

Chapter 2
Translating Targeted Radiosensitizers into the Clinic

Deborah E. Citrin and Kevin A. Camphausen

Abstract Radiation therapy is commonly used in the curative treatment of cancer. Despite recent progress in the techniques of radiation delivery and treatment, local recurrence after radiation remains a pressing clinical concern. A growing capacity to molecularly profile tumors, coupled with the development of biologics and small molecules that target aspects of signal transduction crucial to tumor cell survival after irradiation, has led to the identification of a number of agents that have radiation sensitizing efficacy in preclinical models. Developing clinical trials to evaluate the efficacy of radiosensitizers integrated with the current standard of care presents many challenges. Herein, we review aspects of clinical trial development with radiation therapy regimens integrating radiosensitizers.

Keywords Biomarkers · Cetuximab · Chemoradiation · Clinical translation · Clinical trial · EGFR · Head and neck squamous cell carcinoma · Normal tissue toxicity · Radiation therapy · Radiosensitizers · Radiosensitization · Therapeutic ratio

1 Introduction

Radiation therapy is commonly used in the definitive and palliative therapy of cancer patients, with as many as 50% of patients receiving it at some point in the course of their disease. Enhancements in imaging, radiation treatment technology, and integration of highly conformal and ablative radiation regimens have reduced side effects and improved the local and regional cure rates for patients with numerous types of cancers. Although radiation therapy used as a single agent can lead to cure in some

D. E. Citrin (✉) · K. A. Camphausen
Radiation Oncology Branch, Center for Cancer Research, National Cancer Institute, Bethesda, MD, USA
e-mail: citrind@mail.nih.gov

© Springer Nature Switzerland AG 2020
H. Willers, I. Eke (eds.), *Molecular Targeted Radiosensitizers*, Cancer Drug Discovery and Development, https://doi.org/10.1007/978-3-030-49701-9_2

settings, efforts to improve rates of disease control locally and distantly have also led to the delivery of sensitizing chemotherapy during the course of radiation for some cancers. Improvements in survival and local control have been realized with this approach (Keys et al. 1999; Morris et al. 1999; Rose et al. 1999; Herskovic et al. 1992; Stupp et al. 2005; Pignon et al. 2009; Calais et al. 1999; Curran Jr. et al. 2011), and combined modality regimens with radiation and sensitizing chemotherapy are now considered to be the standard of care for a number of disease sites, such as squamous cell carcinoma of the head and neck (HNSCC), lung cancers, gastrointestinal malignancies, and several central nervous system tumors.

Although definitive radiation or chemoradiation regimens are potentially curative, many patients with locally advanced cancers treated with chemoradiation continue to experience local failure. In some settings, radiation dose escalation has offered enhanced cancer control and survival (Kuban et al. 2008), while in others, the toxicity of escalation has outweighed any benefits of this approach (Bradley et al. 2015; Minsky et al. 2002). The continued observation of local recurrence despite delivery of maximally tolerable radiation dose with or without sensitizing chemotherapy suggests that alternative approaches must be explored.

Over the past two decades, the oncology field has been revolutionized by efforts to identify agents capable of targeting specific molecular pathways known to play a role in cancer cell growth, metastasis, and immune evasion. Simultaneously, advances in genomics and molecular interrogation have begun to offer the opportunity for personalized approaches for therapy targeted to the specific molecular subtype, genomic phenotype, or mutational profile of a tumor. The development of these molecularly targeted agents and the growth of molecular and genomic phenotyping tools has presented a tremendous opportunity for the field of radiation oncology, as many of these agents have been found to function as radiation modifiers in preclinical studies.

Although a substantial and growing list of agents have been described as radiosensitizers, the effective translation of these agents into the clinic has lagged. This deficiency is best illustrated by the paucity of FDA-approved radiosensitizers, and the continued reliance on cytotoxic chemotherapy as the preferred method to radiosensitize tumors. This review will focus on major obstacles, opportunities, and considerations for the clinical translation of radiosensitizers and discuss methods for addressing these obstacles.

2 Clinical Translation: Disease-Related Factors

The dose of radiation that can be safely delivered to a tumor and electively treated regions is usually derived by a critical evaluation of the therapeutic index. The dose is often chosen that will provide the highest chance of local control at an acceptable level of toxicity to surrounding normal structures. Rarely is local control achieved in all patients with this approach. The use of a radiosensitizer makes logical sense if

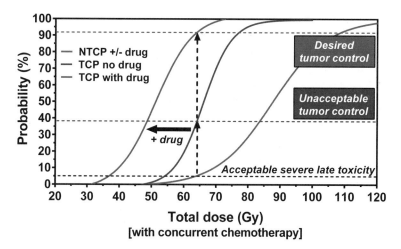

Fig. 2.1 Tumor control probability (TCP) and normal tissue complication probability (NTCP) with and without systemic drug therapy at different total radiation doses

local control is limited with the current standard approach or if the current standard approach results in excessive toxicity. If the radiosensitizer is selective to tumor tissue, the combination would increase the effective dose of radiation while minimizing the increased risk to adjacent normal tissues, favorably altering the therapeutic ratio (Fig. 2.1). In the setting of the candidate radiosensitizer demonstrating single agent activity in the disease of choice or when the investigational agent is anticipated to alter physiology or microenvironment, the effect of a sensitizer may not be purely related to an enhancement of radiation dose equivalent. Ideally, investigational radiosensitizers would be tested at sites where local failure is common.

For situations in which local control is not difficult to achieve with doses of radiation that result in appreciable normal tissue toxicity, the introduction of a radiosensitizer could be appropriate with the goal of de-escalating radiation. In this situation, the sensitizer should have a clear preference for tumor tissue and the expected composite toxicity of the reduced dose radiation and the investigational agent should not exceed that of the standard dose radiation.

3   Clinical Translation: Choice of Agent and Biomarkers

The optimal radiosensitizer would have the ability to selectively sensitize tumor tissue while having minimal impact on normal tissue response to radiation. In reality, most agents evaluated as radiosensitizers have at least some amount of single agent efficacy and single agent toxicity, and thus are more appropriately categorized as radiation modifiers. Chemotherapy agents currently used as radiosensitizers are in fact radiation modifiers based on these characteristics. The recent development of agents targeting signal transduction pathways, the tumor microenvironment, and other pathways specific to tumors may provide agents that fit the definition of radiosensitizer much more closely due to minimal single agent activity, tumor selectivity, and the possibility for reduced toxicity.

Another consideration in designing clinical trials testing candidate radiosensitizing agents relates to the integration into the current standard of care for the specific type of cancer of interest. It is important that there is a lack of negative interactions in terms of efficacy with the current standard chemotherapy and that there is no or minimal overlapping toxicity with the current standard chemotherapy if the radiosensitizer will be added to an established regimen. Unless these criteria are met, the addition of the new agent to a concurrent chemoradiation regimen may result in a prohibitively toxic or less efficacious regimen.

Perhaps most importantly, the target of the sensitizer of interest should be expressed or inducible in the tumor type in which the agent will be tested. Further, pharmacokinetic and pharmacodynamic studies should demonstrate that the dosing of the radiosensitizing agent chosen for clinical translation is capable of inhibiting the target of interest at a time in which radiotherapy will be delivered. Clear and convincing preclinical studies identifying imaging, tissue based, or circulating biomarkers predictive of radiosensitizing efficacy of the agent and signaling downstream of the target are useful in this regard if there is substantial variability in target expression within a histology or tumor type based on molecular phenotype, tumor genotype, or tumor physiology. Although the primary endpoint of phase I trials is to establish tolerable dosing regimens, evaluation of biomarkers identified in preclinical studies is often included as exploratory endpoints so that preliminary correlation of biomarker presence with response can be made. Thus, phase I trials are not powered to conclusively demonstrate the capacity of a biomarker to predict for efficacy; however, they may provide a hint of utility.

In phase II trials, these same biomarkers may be included as exploratory (correlative), integrated, or integral depending on the strength of the evidence of usefulness in phase I trials. Integrated biomarkers are measured in all patients but are not used for medical decision-making. Thus, integrated biomarkers are testing a hypothesis about how the biomarker relates to the endpoints of the trial. In contrast, integral biomarkers are critical to the conduct of the trial and are used to determine eligibility, stratification, or treatment assignment. Because integral markers are used for medical decision-making, there are numerous considerations for their use in clinical trials, including analytical validation of the assay, clinical validation of the assay, clinical utility of the assay, conduct of the assay in a CLIA-certified laboratory, and possible need for an investigational device exception (IDE) from the FDA (reviewed in (Schilsky et al. 2012)).

4 Clinical Translation: Considerations Relating to the Current Standard of Care

One of the major challenges in clinical translation of radiosensitizers relates to the integration of the new agent into an established standard of care. A variety of characteristics of the agent to be tested, the patient population to be tested, and the current standard of care for the disease in question should be taken into account in the development of these agents. In several tumor types and stages, combined chemotherapy and radiation is standard of care because the combination of the two agents provides increased local control, survival, or both compared to the use of radiation alone. Unfortunately, the current standard chemoradiation regimens often have sizable toxicity rates for some disease sites, such as HNSCC. Potentially increasing the toxicity of these regimens by adding in another agent may result in decreased quality of life, functional impairment, morbidity necessitating treatment breaks or delays, the need for medical intervention, or mortality when evaluated in an investigational setting or extrapolated to a broader subset of patients (Fig. 2.2).

An example of this phenomenon is the integration of cetuximab into chemoradiation for anal cancer. In the ECOG-ACRIN E3205 trial, cetuximab was integrated into a cisplatin, 5-fluorouracil (5-FU), radiation regimen for immunocompetent patients with Stage I-III squamous cell carcinoma of the anal canal. Although the addition of cetuximab in this study was found to reduce local failure relative to historical controls, Grade 4 toxicity occurred in 32% of participants, and Grade 5 toxicities (death) in 5% (Garg et al. 2017). A simultaneously reported AIDS Malignancy Consortium trial that integrated cetuximab with radiation, 5-FU, and cisplatin in patients with HIV infection and anal carcinoma demonstrated reduced locoregional

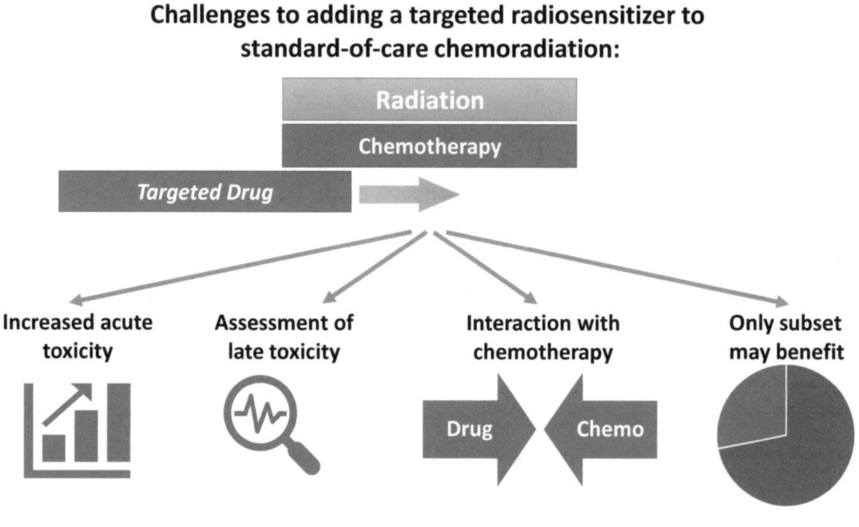

Challenges to adding a targeted radiosensitizer to standard-of-care chemoradiation:

Radiation

Chemotherapy

Targeted Drug

Increased acute toxicity

Assessment of late toxicity

Interaction with chemotherapy

Drug   Chemo

Only subset may benefit

Fig. 2.2 Schematic of how targeted therapy can interfere with standard-of-care chemoradiation

failure compared to historical controls with 26% Grade 4 toxicity and 4% treatment-related deaths (Sparano et al. 2017). Thus, despite evidence of improvement in local control with the addition of cetuximab in these trials, the rate of high-grade toxicity results in a regimen that is at or above the limit of acceptable toxicity (Glynne-Jones and Harrison 2017). In a similar fashion, in the setting of concurrent cisplatin and accelerated radiation therapy for oropharynx cancers and in lung cancers, the addition of cetuximab was found to increase the need for treatment breaks and increase acute toxicity without an observed benefit in regard to local control or survival (Ang et al. 2014; Bradley et al. 2015).

Thus, in a situation in which the current standard chemoradiation regimen is at the limits for acceptable toxicity, the options for adding a radiosensitizer become either lowering the sensitizing chemotherapy intensity, using an alternate chemotherapy, or omitting the sensitizing chemotherapy altogether. Lowering chemotherapy dose or intensity is an option if there is evidence that these reduced intensity dosing regimens are efficacious in this setting. However, in the absence of these data, patients are exposed to the toxicity of the chemotherapy, albeit possibly reduced, with the prospect of no added benefit over radiation therapy alone with the addition of the sensitizer. Although sensitizing chemotherapy is often given at doses that are considered less than that which has systemic efficacy, in some cases, the lack of systemic exposure to chemotherapy for the duration of radiation therapy is also a consideration with this approach.

Omission of chemotherapy from established regimens when integrating a potential radiosensitizer in a clinical trial is a controversial concept. The development of the current standard of care for regimens including chemoradiation has typically progressed through phase I trials to phase III trials such that the current standard of care represents the maximum tolerated dose (MTD) of the chemotherapy and radiation combination. Because adding an additional agent to an established standard regimen may have overlapping toxicities, particularly if it is effective at sensitizing (local toxicities), it can be expected that adding this agent to a combination that is already delivered at the MTD may be excessively toxic or at least limit the delivery of the investigational agent to the extent that it has minimal or no efficacy.

Omitting the sensitizing chemotherapy allows testing of the new agent with the ability to more accurately distinguish toxicities and activity attributable to the investigational agent, however may not provide adequate treatment if there is no sufficient sensitizing effect with the investigational agent. In addition, patients exposed to the lower doses of the agent in a phase I trial might be considered to be receiving, in the worst case, a regimen similar to radiation alone which is not considered as effective as the current standard of care. In addition, similar concerns exist about lack of systemic therapy if the investigational agent has no single agent efficacy. For tumors in which a potentially curative standard of care that includes chemotherapy and radiation exists, this is unlikely to be an acceptable approach without extensive efficacy data from other trials combining radiation with the agent in settings where concurrent chemotherapy with radiation is not the current standard.

When developing clinical trials integrating a candidate radiosensitizer into a standard chemoradiation regimens, the potential pharmacokinetic and pharmacodynamic interactions of the two agents must be considered (Fig. 2.2). If prior studies have not demonstrated the tolerability and pharmacokinetic effects of combining the chemotherapy and investigational agent, and any interaction is anticipated, these studies must be integrated into the planned trial. For example, a standard chemotherapy may alter the metabolism of the investigational agent or decrease/alter the target of the investigational agent resulting in decreased efficacy. Alternatively, the targeted agent could result in changes that decrease the efficacy of chemotherapy. For example, if the targeted agent is known to induce a quiescent state in tumor cells (G0 or G1 cell cycle arrest), this could potentially alter the sensitivity of the cells to chemotherapeutics that rely on tumor cell cycling. An example of a negative interaction with simultaneous use of a targeted agent and chemotherapy has been demonstrated preclinically and in clinical trials for epidermal growth factor receptor (EGFR) tyrosine kinase inhibitors combined with chemotherapy (reviewed in (Davies et al. 2006)). Any interaction such as these would result in the possibility of increased toxicity with no therapeutic gain or decreased efficacy when the investigational agent is added. In the setting in which these interactions are identified in preclinical studies, the options for clinical development would include testing the agent in a tumor site that allows a different chemotherapy that does not interact, or to omit the chemotherapy.

Finally, translational endpoints may be more difficult to interpret when multiple agents are used in combination with radiation. This becomes especially problematic if agents target pathways that may be modified by both chemotherapy and radiation, as it may be difficult to distinguish the relative contribution of each agent on the observed effect on tumor response and biomarkers. In the setting of a pathway that is activated in a specific tumor type, a lead in phase may be employed, in which the investigational agent alone is tested in the absence of radiation ± chemotherapy for a short period of time to allow pharmacodynamic assessments.

5   Phase I Trials of Radiosensitizers: Trial Design

Phase I trials of chemotherapeutic combinations or targeted agents in combination with chemotherapy have traditionally been designed to assess the safety of a combination, to determine the optimal dose of the investigational agent for further testing, and to identify toxicities associated with the combination. When radiation therapy or chemoradiation is the backbone to which the investigational agent is to be added, there are numerous considerations to trial design that uniquely apply to this context (Harrington et al. 2011).

When an investigational agent is tested in combination with an established chemotherapy regimen in phase I trials, the new agent is often combined in escalating doses with the established agent at a fixed dose in a cohort of patients with a variety of tumor types. This allows an appreciation of toxicity and tolerability of each dose level, which should not vary based on the histology of the tumor or the location of the tumor in the body. When an agent is added to a radiation regimen, in contrast, it is highly likely that the site of the body being irradiated may alter the tolerability of the combination regimen, as there is a risk of more severe local reactions if the agent sensitizes normal tissue to any degree. Thus, while the systemic toxicities may be similar when the investigational agent is added to similar chemoradiation regimens, the local toxicities may vary based on the degree to which the in-field normal tissues are sensitized.

Recently, there has been interest in developing phase I trials of radiosensitizers in combination with radiation for palliation. Part of the interest in this approach has been to minimize the risk of a severe toxicity in a patient being treated with definitive therapy resulting in a treatment interruption or discontinuation. This method results in the capacity to test an agent combined with radiation in the absence of concurrent chemotherapy. An additional benefit of this approach is the capacity to evaluate for signals of efficacy in a mixed group of tumor histologies although given the small numbers of patients included in each dose level, this is usually preliminary evidence. Similarly, preliminary signals suggested of unexpectedly severe toxicity in certain sites of the body may also be evident. The limitations of this approach include the possibility that the tolerated dose may be higher when radiation occurs at one body site versus another, which may be obscured by this design. In addition, most patients will not be able to be followed for late toxicity as they will proceed on to other systemic therapies or will be unavailable for long-term follow-up due to disease progression.

In phase I trials, testing combinations of chemotherapeutic agents and/or targeted agents, dose-limiting toxicity is generally assessed during the first cycle(s) of therapy, during active treatment, or for several weeks after treatment is concluded. When radiation is delivered as a component of a definitive or palliative therapy, this assessment should, at a minimum, include the entire course of radiation and the time in which acute toxicity should resolve. Thus, in patients receiving a 6- to 7-week course of radiation, an additional period of time, such as 4 weeks, must be added to allow for resolution of toxicities before assessment can be complete. This requires as much as 12 weeks including treatment and assessment of the last patient before escalation can proceed, resulting in pauses in accrual until this time has passed without untoward toxicity.

One method to avoid this pause in accrual is to evaluate multiple agents simultaneously in different arms in the same patient population, in a fashion similar to a platform trial (Berry et al. 2015). By accruing to multiple arms simultaneously, there is always a trial option during periods of pause for escalation of one agent. An example of such an approach is the "intertwined trial design" used to test two different investigational agents when combined with chemoradiation for the treatment of rectal cancer prior to surgery. Each agent was combined with standard therapy, and while accrual for one agent was paused to allow assessment of toxicity before escalating further, the other agent could be tested, allowing efficient accrual (Marti et al. 2019).

An additional challenge in trial design for radiation/drug combinations is how to best capture late toxicity related to the treatment, which may take months to years to manifest (Fig. 2.2). Therefore, requiring full assessment of late toxicities prior to dose escalation is not feasible due to the length of time required after completion of accrual at a specific drug dose to assess these toxicities and to allow progression to the next dose level. Thus, one consideration in designing phase I trials combining radiation with investigational agents is how best to include late toxicity assessment in a fashion that can inform dose escalation and minimize risk yet still allow a reasonable pace of accrual.

This challenge has been addressed in several different ways, including using trial designs that diverge from the classic dose escalation format. One possibility is to limit assessment of dose-limiting toxicities to those that are acute, while collecting data on late toxicities as they arise. Criteria to halt escalation based on observed late toxicities can be added to the escalation rules. However, it is probable that the dose may have been escalated far beyond the level at which the patient exhibiting the severe late toxicity was treated. This simplifies the process of dose escalation and speeds accrual but presents a risk of observing unexpectedly severe late toxicities.

Additional methods to incorporate late toxicity include the time to event continual reassessment model, which may be particularly well suited to radiation/drug combinations (Normolle and Lawrence 2006). In this model, trials are open to accrual continuously. The largest acceptable probability of toxicity is defined, and as events occur, estimates of probability of toxicity are recalculated, allowing a selection of a target dose. One concern with his approach is that the observed incidence of toxicity may increase over time, resulting in changes in probability estimates that allow substantial accrual at levels with higher than acceptable toxicity in the setting of rapid accrual. Additionally, the Bayesian dose finding methods used to incorporate late follow-up requires robust statistical support in an ongoing fashion to continuously re-estimate the probability of toxicity (Polley 2011). In contrast, the method reduces the number of patients accrued as subtherapeutic doses (Polley 2011).

6 Phase I Trials of Radiosensitizers: Methods of Escalation

There are numerous methods to integrate agents into an established radiation or chemoradiation therapy regimen for escalation purposes. The classic method of dose escalation of the investigational agent allows the current standard therapy to serve as the backbone to which the investigational agent is added. One concern with this approach is that if toxicity is observed early in the treatment course, the patient may not complete the regimen with proven efficacy or may complete it with a delay if a treatment break is required. This design often mimics phase I trials that have already incorporated the agent with the chemotherapy that is part of the regimen, so may reduce the need for pharmacokinetic studies. The design also maximizes exposure to the investigational agent during the radiation treatment.

Similarly, exposure to the investigational agent can be increased by increasing the proportion of the overall treatment during which the investigational agent is given. This may be a useful design if the anticipated effective dose is likely to cause at least moderate toxicity. This approach may also reduce the likelihood that definitive treatment would be interrupted or discontinued prematurely. Escalation of the duration would begin with the investigational agent for the first or the last portion of treatment with progressively increasing duration of exposure using the same drug dose.

A third hybrid model could be envisioned in which the duration is first escalated, followed by the dose of the investigational agent. These sorts of approaches are likely to minimize risk to the patients in terms of early discontinuation of treatment or treatment breaks, but may result in the need for larger numbers of participants.

A major consideration for developing radiation combinations trials incorporating radiosensitizers is defining the appropriate starting dose of the investigational agent. If prior trials combining the chemotherapy of interest have identified an acceptable dose of combined therapy, a similar, or slightly reduced dose may be chosen. In many cases, the chemotherapy dosing used for chemoradiation combinations may be different than those utilized for systemic therapy regimens, and these data may not exist. Simultaneously, care must be taken to avoid an unexpected severe toxicity if the agent is effective as a sensitizer of both normal and tumor tissue. Incorporation of a lead in phase of the investigational agent alone in combination with chemotherapy (if it is part of the backbone) with pharmacodynamic assessments will provide valuable evidence of target engagement at the dose delivered.

7   Phase II Trials of Radiosensitizers

The conduct of phase II trials of novel radiosensitizers may present different challenges than those associated with phase I trials. As the goal of phase II trials is typically to describe efficacy and to identify regimens for testing in randomized phase III trials, the endpoints chosen are paramount. Well-designed phase II trial endpoints may provide a greater capacity to predict eventual success in randomized trials. For example, the improved survival that was demonstrated with the addition of temozolomide to radiation in patients with glioblastoma multiforme (GBM) phase II trial (Stupp et al. 2002) was later confirmed in a large phase III trial (Stupp et al. 2005). Comparatively, phase II studies of bevacizumab had shown improved outcomes only in the setting of recurrent GBM (Kreisl et al. 2009), with phase II studies failing to demonstrate evidence of improved overall survival in newly diagnosed patients (Lai et al. 2011). Consequently, two large randomized phase III trials found that while bevacizumab improved progression-free survival in the newly diagnosed setting, this did not translate into an overall survival benefit (Chinot et al. 2014; Gilbert et al. 2014). Thus, the efficacy of regimens demonstrated in phase II trials might be able to predict phase III success.

As phase II trials serve as a method of selecting agents for further study in phase III trials, challenges in selecting agents from phase II trials for further study often relate to comparing trials in regards to outcome, as endpoints may not be consistently reported across trials. For example, even when similar groups of patients are accrued, endpoints of phase II trials may include overall survival, progression-free survival, or local control. Further, these endpoints may be reported at a specific timepoint or as a median. Thus, although direct comparisons cannot be made across separate trials, consistency of outcome measures in a specific disease setting would allow an opportunity to select the highest performing regimens for further study.

Because phase I trials may only enroll small numbers of patients at each dose level, or in some cases may include a small expansion at the MTD, another challenge in the development of phase II trials of radiosensitizers is that additional or less common toxicities may only become evident when phase II trials are conducted, as they enroll larger numbers of subjects and may have relaxed inclusion criteria compared to phase I trials. Careful recording of these toxicities is critical in determining if the combination is reasonable to consider for phase III testing, and to determine if there is evidence that specific comorbidities may predict for unreasonable toxicity.

Similar to disease outcome endpoints, toxicity reporting across phase II trials of radiosensitizers often lacks consistency. As previously noted, most trials of radiosensitizers only report acute toxicities, but even these can be challenging to compare across trials. Reporting can include cumulative rates, worst grade experienced, and raw numbers of events versus number of patients with the event. In some cases, the worst grade of toxicity may not change, but the toxicity may occur sooner or last longer, impacting the tolerability of the regimen or introducing unplanned treatment breaks. Reporting such aspects of toxicity are critical to the assessment of tolerability of the regimen.

In summary, if the outcomes of overall survival, progression-free survival, and local control are reported in addition to both acute and late toxicities for every phase II radiosensitizer trial, more effective phase III trials can be planned and executed.

8 Normal Tissue Toxicity Assessments in Clinical Trials of Radiosensitizers

One of the greatest challenges in toxicity assessment in trials of radiosensitizers is attribution of expected radiation toxicities. Often, trials are written in a fashion that expected radiation toxicities are not attributed to the investigational agents. However, if the agent functions as a radiosensitizer of normal tissue to any degree, expected radiation toxicities may occur at a greater rate, with greater severity, or longer duration. As many phase II studies add the sensitizer to the current standard of care chemoradiation regimen, it is important to note the number of delays, dose reductions, or discontinuations of components of the standard of care with the addition of the new agent. In a patient cohort expected to have a reasonable chance of local control and favorable rates of survival, it may be unethical to continue to use an agent that prevents the patient from obtaining uninterrupted standard therapy.

Although phase I trials invariably incorporate toxicity assessments, and these assessments are collected in phase II and phase II trials, these are generally collected as physician-defined adverse events using standardized criteria. Commonly used toxicity scoring criteria were designed for use in a diverse set of interventions, and thus may be challenging to use for scoring radiation-related toxicities. Further, there has been growing appreciation within the clinical research community of the importance of patient-reported measures (Basch 2010; Basch et al. 2014; Dueck et al. 2015; Movsas et al. 2011), which are generally not incorporated as an escalation criteria in phase I trials.

As described above, continued evaluation of clinical trial participants beyond the acute toxicity window and for months to years after treatment with ongoing adverse event assessment is critical to understanding the toxicity of radiosensitizer combinations. The importance of this element has been demonstrated with trials of concurrent chemotherapy (Machtay et al. 2008). Although resource intense, the inclusion of long-term assessment of trial participants allows a more accurate estimation of regimen toxicity.

9 Radiosensitizer Example: Cetuximab

It is informative to review the clinical development and current status of cetuximab, which strikingly remains the only FDA-approved targeted radiosensitizer to date. Cetuximab is a chimeric monoclonal antibody that binds to and inhibits EGFR, a growth factor receptor frequently upregulated or mutated in cancer such as squamous cell carcinomas of the head and neck and non-small cell lung cancer. The EGFR/RAS/MAPK pathway is known to enhance tumor cell proliferation, survival, and DNA repair (Cuneo et al. 2015) (Fig. 2.3). Further, the pathway is rapidly activated by radiation and has been suggested as a contributor to radiation-induced

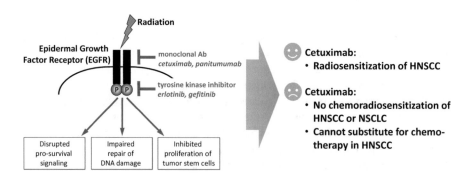

Fig. 2.3 Epidermal growth factor receptor (EGFR) regulates critical cell functions such as cellular survival, DNA repair, and proliferation and can be targeted with antibodies or tyrosine kinase inhibitors. In squamous cell carcinoma of the head and neck (HNSCC), positive results have been obtained in combination with radiation therapy alone, but not as an addition to chemoradiation or as a substitute for chemotherapy

accelerated repopulation (Schmidt-Ullrich et al. 1997). A large body of preclinical work has demonstrated that inhibiting EGFR signaling is capable of enhancing radiosensitivity (Wang et al. 2011; Raben et al. 2005; Milas et al. 2004; Nasu et al. 2001).

Initial clinical translation of cetuximab was promising, which led to the conduct of a landmark phase III clinical trial by Bonner et al. (Bonner et al. 2006; Bonner et al. 2010). This trial demonstrated an overall survival benefit with the addition of cetuximab to radiation versus radiation alone in patients with locoregionally advanced HNSCC. Similarly, a survival benefit was demonstrated when cisplatin-based chemotherapy was combined with radiation compared to radiation alone (Pignon et al. 2000, 2009), solidifying that approach as standard of care and raising the question of how to integrate cetuximab into chemoradiation treatment regimens.

With the known advantage of both chemotherapy and cetuximab combined with radiation, later trials tested the combination of cetuximab and cisplatin with radiation therapy in HNSCC. These studies have demonstrated an increase in acute toxicities with the addition of cetuximab without evidence of a survival benefit (Ang et al. 2014). The remaining question of the equivalence of cetuximab and cisplatin as radiosensitizers in HNSCC was addressed by a small randomized trial that suggested inferiority of cetuximab relative to cisplatin when combined with radiation in patients with locoregionally advanced disease (Magrini et al. 2016). Two recently reported large randomized trials addressed this question more definitively. In the De-ESCALaTE Human Papilloma Virus (HPV trial), patients with low-risk HPV-positive oropharyngeal cancer were randomized to receipt of cisplatin versus cetuximab with radiation. Patients treated with cetuximab were demonstrated to have higher rates of local recurrence and lower overall survival (Mehanna et al. 2019). In the recently reported RTOG 1016 trial, patients with HPV-positive oropharyngeal cancer were randomized to radiation with concurrent cisplatin versus cetuximab. Patients treated with cetuximab had significantly lower rates of locoregional control and overall survival compared to cisplatin (Gillison et al. 2019). As noted previously in this chapter, the addition of cetuximab to other chemoradiation combinations has resulted in increased toxicity, in most cases without evidence for enhanced local control or survival compared to the chemoradiation backbone (Ang et al. 2014; Bradley et al. 2015; Garg et al. 2017; Mehanna et al. 2019). As a result of these trials, the future of EGFR inhibition combined with radiation remains uncertain, despite FDA approval for cetuximab in HNSCC.

In aggregate, the data are consistent with the notion that EGFR inhibition may only be successful in subsets of patients, thus requiring predictive biomarkers to select patients most like to benefit from combination therapy (Fig. 2.2). In addition, the data point to the need for more thorough preclinical evaluation of combining targeted drugs not only with radiation but also with chemoradiation.

10 Conclusions and Future Directions

Numerous candidate radiosensitizers have been studied and found effective in pre-clinical model systems. Clinical translation and testing of radiosensitizers present unique challenges, including sequencing of agents, establishing biomarkers of efficacy, and integration into the current standard of care. The development of radiosensitizers offers a unique opportunity to reduce toxicity of therapy by selectively sensitizing cancer tissues relative to normal tissue. Recent developments in molecular profiling of tumors may allow selection of sensitizers tailored to the signaling and mutational profile of a tumor, which in turn may increase the likelihood of efficacy. Although few targeted radiosensitizers have effectively been integrated into clinical practice to date, an expanding knowledge of the underlying mechanisms of resistance and recurrence after radiation therapy coupled with the growing capacity to profile the molecular phenotype of tumors provides great hope for future progress in this field.

References

Ang KK, Zhang Q, Rosenthal DI, Nguyen-Tan PF, Sherman EJ, Weber RS, Galvin JM, Bonner JA, Harris J, El-Naggar AK, Gillison ML, Jordan RC, Konski AA, Thorstad WL, Trotti A, Beitler JJ, Garden AS, Spanos WJ, Yom SS, Axelrod RS (2014) Randomized phase III trial of concurrent accelerated radiation plus cisplatin with or without cetuximab for stage III to IV head and neck carcinoma: RTOG 0522. J Clin Oncol 32(27):2940–2950. https://doi.org/10.1200/JCO.2013.53.5633

Basch E (2010) The missing voice of patients in drug-safety reporting. N Engl J Med 362(10):865–869. https://doi.org/10.1056/NEJMp0911494

Basch E, Reeve BB, Mitchell SA, Clauser SB, Minasian LM, Dueck AC, Mendoza TR, Hay J, Atkinson TM, Abernethy AP, Bruner DW, Cleeland CS, Sloan JA, Chilukuri R, Baumgartner P, Denicoff A, St Germain D, O'Mara AM, Chen A, Kelaghan J, Bennett AV, Sit L, Rogak L, Barz A, Paul DB, Schrag D (2014) Development of the National Cancer Institute's patient-reported outcomes version of the common terminology criteria for adverse events (PRO-CTCAE). J Natl Cancer Inst 106(9):dju244. https://doi.org/10.1093/jnci/dju244

Berry SM, Connor JT, Lewis RJ (2015) The platform trial: an efficient strategy for evaluating multiple treatments. JAMA 313(16):1619–1620. https://doi.org/10.1001/jama.2015.2316

Bonner JA, Harari PM, Giralt J, Azarnia N, Shin DM, Cohen RB, Jones CU, Sur R, Raben D, Jassem J, Ove R, Kies MS, Baselga J, Youssoufian H, Amellal N, Rowinsky EK, Ang KK (2006) Radiotherapy plus cetuximab for squamous-cell carcinoma of the head and neck. N Engl J Med 354(6):567–578. https://doi.org/10.1056/NEJMoa053422

Bonner JA, Harari PM, Giralt J, Cohen RB, Jones CU, Sur RK, Raben D, Baselga J, Spencer SA, Zhu J, Youssoufian H, Rowinsky EK, Ang KK (2010) Radiotherapy plus cetuximab for locoregionally advanced head and neck cancer: 5-year survival data from a phase 3 randomised trial, and relation between cetuximab-induced rash and survival. Lancet Oncol 11(1):21–28. https://doi.org/10.1016/S1470-2045(09)70311-0

Bradley JD, Paulus R, Komaki R, Masters G, Blumenschein G, Schild S, Bogart J, Hu C, Forster K, Magliocco A, Kavadi V, Garces YI, Narayan S, Iyengar P, Robinson C, Wynn RB, Koprowski C, Meng J, Beitler J, Gaur R, Curran W Jr, Choy H (2015) Standard-dose versus high-dose conformal radiotherapy with concurrent and consolidation carboplatin plus paclitaxel with or without cetuximab for patients with stage IIIA or IIIB non-small-cell lung cancer (RTOG 0617): a randomised, two-by-two factorial phase 3 study. Lancet Oncol 16(2):187–199. https://doi.org/10.1016/S1470-2045(14)71207-0

Calais G, Alfonsi M, Bardet E, Sire C, Germain T, Bergerot P, Rhein B, Tortochaux J, Oudinot P, Bertrand P (1999) Randomized trial of radiation therapy versus concomitant chemotherapy and radiation therapy for advanced-stage oropharynx carcinoma. J Natl Cancer Inst 91(24):2081–2086

Chinot OL, Wick W, Mason W, Henriksson R, Saran F, Nishikawa R, Carpentier AF, Hoang-Xuan K, Kavan P, Cernea D, Brandes AA, Hilton M, Abrey L, Cloughesy T (2014) Bevacizumab plus radiotherapy-temozolomide for newly diagnosed glioblastoma. N Engl J Med 370(8):709–722. https://doi.org/10.1056/NEJMoa1308345

Cuneo KC, Nyati MK, Ray D, Lawrence TS (2015) EGFR targeted therapies and radiation: optimizing efficacy by appropriate drug scheduling and patient selection. Pharmacol Ther 154:67–77. https://doi.org/10.1016/j.pharmthera.2015.07.002

Curran WJ Jr, Paulus R, Langer CJ, Komaki R, Lee JS, Hauser S, Movsas B, Wasserman T, Rosenthal SA, Gore E, Machtay M, Sause W, Cox JD (2011) Sequential vs. concurrent chemoradiation for stage III non-small cell lung cancer: randomized phase III trial RTOG 9410. J Natl Cancer Inst 103(19):1452–1460. https://doi.org/10.1093/jnci/djr325

Davies AM, Ho C, Lara PN Jr, Mack P, Gumerlock PH, Gandara DR (2006) Pharmacodynamic separation of epidermal growth factor receptor tyrosine kinase inhibitors and chemotherapy in non-small-cell lung cancer. Clin Lung Cancer 7(6):385–388. https://doi.org/10.3816/CLC.2006.n.021

Dueck AC, Mendoza TR, Mitchell SA, Reeve BB, Castro KM, Rogak LJ, Atkinson TM, Bennett AV, Denicoff AM, O'Mara AM, Li Y, Clauser SB, Bryant DM, Bearden JD 3rd, Gillis TA, Harness JK, Siegel RD, Paul DB, Cleeland CS, Schrag D, Sloan JA, Abernethy AP, Bruner DW, Minasian LM, Basch E, National Cancer Institute PROCSG (2015) Validity and reliability of the US National Cancer Institute's Patient-Reported Outcomes Version of the Common Terminology Criteria for Adverse Events (PRO-CTCAE). JAMA Oncol 1(8):1051–1059. https://doi.org/10.1001/jamaoncol.2015.2639

Garg MK, Zhao F, Sparano JA, Palefsky J, Whittington R, Mitchell EP, Mulcahy MF, Armstrong KI, Nabbout NH, Kalnicki S, El-Rayes BF, Onitilo AA, Moriarty DJ, Fitzgerald TJ, Benson AB 3rd (2017) Cetuximab plus chemoradiotherapy in immunocompetent patients with anal carcinoma: a phase II Eastern Cooperative Oncology Group-American College of Radiology Imaging Network Cancer Research Group Trial (E3205). J Clin Oncol 35(7):718–726. https://doi.org/10.1200/JCO.2016.69.1667

Gilbert MR, Dignam JJ, Armstrong TS, Wefel JS, Blumenthal DT, Vogelbaum MA, Colman H, Chakravarti A, Pugh S, Won M, Jeraj R, Brown PD, Jaeckle KA, Schiff D, Stieber VW, Brachman DG, Werner-Wasik M, Tremont-Lukats IW, Sulman EP, Aldape KD, Curran WJ Jr, Mehta MP (2014) A randomized trial of bevacizumab for newly diagnosed glioblastoma. N Engl J Med 370(8):699–708. https://doi.org/10.1056/NEJMoa1308573

Gillison ML, Trotti AM, Harris J, Eisbruch A, Harari PM, Adelstein DJ, Sturgis EM, Burtness B, Ridge JA, Ringash J, Galvin J, Yao M, Koyfman SA, Blakaj DM, Razaq MA, Colevas AD, Beitler JJ, Jones CU, Dunlap NE, Seaward SA, Spencer S, Galloway TJ, Phan J, Dignam JJ, Le QT (2019) Radiotherapy plus cetuximab or cisplatin in human papillomavirus-positive oropharyngeal cancer (NRG oncology RTOG 1016): a randomised, multicentre, non-inferiority trial. Lancet 393(10166):40–50. https://doi.org/10.1016/S0140-6736(18)32779-X

Glynne-Jones R, Harrison M (2017) Cetuximab in the context of current treatment of squamous cell carcinoma of the anus. J Clin Oncol 35(7):699–701. https://doi.org/10.1200/JCO.2016.70.9394

Harrington KJ, Billingham LJ, Brunner TB, Burnet NG, Chan CS, Hoskin P, Mackay RI, Maughan TS, Macdougall J, McKenna WG, Nutting CM, Oliver A, Plummer R, Stratford IJ, Illidge T (2011) Guidelines for preclinical and early phase clinical assessment of novel radiosensitisers. Br J Cancer 105(5):628–639. https://doi.org/10.1038/bjc.2011.240

Herskovic A, Martz K, al-Sarraf M, Leichman L, Brindle J, Vaitkevicius V, Cooper J, Byhardt R, Davis L, Emami B (1992) Combined chemotherapy and radiotherapy compared with radiotherapy alone in patients with cancer of the esophagus. N Engl J Med 326(24):1593–1598. https://doi.org/10.1056/NEJM199206113262403

Keys HM, Bundy BN, Stehman FB, Muderspach LI, Chafe WE, Suggs CL 3rd, Walker JL, Gersell D (1999) Cisplatin, radiation, and adjuvant hysterectomy compared with radiation and adjuvant hysterectomy for bulky stage IB cervical carcinoma. N Engl J Med 340(15):1154–1161. https://doi.org/10.1056/NEJM199904153401503

Kreisl TN, Kim L, Moore K, Duic P, Royce C, Stroud I, Garren N, Mackey M, Butman JA, Camphausen K, Park J, Albert PS, Fine HA (2009) Phase II trial of single-agent bevacizumab followed by bevacizumab plus irinotecan at tumor progression in recurrent glioblastoma. J Clin Oncol 27(5):740–745. https://doi.org/10.1200/JCO.2008.16.3055

Kuban DA, Tucker SL, Dong L, Starkschall G, Huang EH, Cheung MR, Lee AK, Pollack A (2008) Long-term results of the M. D. Anderson randomized dose-escalation trial for prostate cancer. Int J Radiat Oncol Biol Phys 70(1):67–74. https://doi.org/10.1016/j.ijrobp.2007.06.054. S0360-3016(07)01173-X [pii] 23

Lai A, Tran A, Nghiemphu PL, Pope WB, Solis OE, Selch M, Filka E, Yong WH, Mischel PS, Liau LM, Phuphanich S, Black K, Peak S, Green RM, Spier CE, Kolevska T, Polikoff J, Fehrenbacher L, Elashoff R, Cloughesy T (2011) Phase II study of bevacizumab plus temozolomide during and after radiation therapy for patients with newly diagnosed glioblastoma multiforme. J Clin Oncol 29(2):142–148. https://doi.org/10.1200/JCO.2010.30.2729

Machtay M, Moughan J, Trotti A, Garden AS, Weber RS, Cooper JS, Forastiere A, Ang KK (2008) Factors associated with severe late toxicity after concurrent chemoradiation for locally advanced head and neck cancer: an RTOG analysis. J Clin Oncol 26(21):3582–3589. https://doi.org/10.1200/JCO.2007.14.8841

Magrini SM, Buglione M, Corvo R, Pirtoli L, Paiar F, Ponticelli P, Petrucci A, Bacigalupo A, Crociani M, Lastrucci L, Vecchio S, Bonomo P, Pasinetti N, Triggiani L, Cavagnini R, Costa L, Tonoli S, Maddalo M, Grisanti S (2016) Cetuximab and radiotherapy versus cisplatin and radiotherapy for locally advanced head and neck cancer: a randomized phase II trial. J Clin Oncol 34(5):427–435. https://doi.org/10.1200/JCO.2015.63.1671

Marti FEM, Jayson GC, Manoharan P, O'Connor J, Renehan AG, Backen AC, Mistry H, Ortega F, Li K, Simpson KL, Allen J, Connell J, Underhill S, Misra V, Williams KJ, Stratford I, Jackson A, Dive C, Saunders MP (2019) Novel phase I trial design to evaluate the addition of cediranib or selumetinib to preoperative chemoradiotherapy for locally advanced rectal cancer: the DREAMtherapy trial. Eur J Cancer 117:48–59. https://doi.org/10.1016/j.ejca.2019.04.029

Mehanna H, Robinson M, Hartley A, Kong A, Foran B, Fulton-Lieuw T, Dalby M, Mistry P, Sen M, O'Toole L, Al Booz H, Dyker K, Moleron R, Whitaker S, Brennan S, Cook A, Griffin M, Aynsley E, Rolles M, De Winton E, Chan A, Srinivasan D, Nixon I, Grumett J, Leemans CR, Buter J, Henderson J, Harrington K, McConkey C, Gray A, Dunn J, De EHPVTG (2019) Radiotherapy plus cisplatin or cetuximab in low-risk human papillomavirus-positive oropharyngeal cancer (De-ESCALaTE HPV): an open-label randomised controlled phase 3 trial. Lancet 393(10166):51–60. https://doi.org/10.1016/S0140-6736(18)32752-1

Milas L, Fan Z, Andratschke NH, Ang KK (2004) Epidermal growth factor receptor and tumor response to radiation: in vivo preclinical studies. Int J Radiat Oncol Biol Phys 58(3):966–971. https://doi.org/10.1016/j.ijrobp.2003.08.035

Minsky BD, Pajak TF, Ginsberg RJ, Pisansky TM, Martenson J, Komaki R, Okawara G, Rosenthal SA, Kelsen DP (2002) INT 0123 (Radiation Therapy Oncology Group 94-05) phase III trial of combined-modality therapy for esophageal cancer: high-dose versus standard-dose radiation therapy. J Clin Oncol 20(5):1167–1174. https://doi.org/10.1200/JCO.2002.20.5.1167

Morris M, Eifel PJ, Lu J, Grigsby PW, Levenback C, Stevens RE, Rotman M, Gershenson DM, Mutch DG (1999) Pelvic radiation with concurrent chemotherapy compared with pelvic and para-aortic radiation for high-risk cervical cancer. N Engl J Med 340(15):1137–1143. https://doi.org/10.1056/NEJM199904153401501

Movsas B, Vikram B, Hauer-Jensen M, Moulder JE, Basch E, Brown SL, Kachnic LA, Dicker AP, Coleman CN, Okunieff P (2011) Decreasing the adverse effects of cancer therapy: National

Cancer Institute guidance for the clinical development of radiation injury mitigators. Clin Cancer Res 17(2):222–228. https://doi.org/10.1158/1078-0432.CCR-10-1402

Nasu S, Ang KK, Fan Z, Milas L (2001) C225 antiepidermal growth factor receptor antibody enhances tumor radiocurability. Int J Radiat Oncol Biol Phys 51(2):474–477. https://doi.org/10.1016/s0360-3016(01)01671-6

Normolle D, Lawrence T (2006) Designing dose-escalation trials with late-onset toxicities using the time-to-event continual reassessment method. J Clin Oncol 24(27):4426–4433. https://doi.org/10.1200/JCO.2005.04.3844

Pignon JP, Bourhis J, Domenge C, Designe L (2000) Chemotherapy added to locoregional treatment for head and neck squamous-cell carcinoma: three meta-analyses of updated individual data. MACH-NC Collaborative Group. Meta-analysis of chemotherapy on head and neck cancer. Lancet 355(9208):949–955

Pignon JP, le Maitre A, Maillard E, Bourhis J, MACH-NC Collaborative Group (2009) Meta-analysis of chemotherapy in head and neck cancer (MACH-NC): an update on 93 randomised trials and 17,346 patients. Radiother Oncol 92(1):4–14. https://doi.org/10.1016/j.radonc.2009.04.014

Polley MY (2011) Practical modifications to the time-to-event continual reassessment method for phase I cancer trials with fast patient accrual and late-onset toxicities. Stat Med 30(17):2130–2143. https://doi.org/10.1002/sim.4255

Raben D, Helfrich B, Chan DC, Ciardiello F, Zhao L, Franklin W, Baron AE, Zeng C, Johnson TK, Bunn PA Jr (2005) The effects of cetuximab alone and in combination with radiation and/or chemotherapy in lung cancer. Clin Cancer Res 11(2 Pt 1):795–805

Rose PG, Bundy BN, Watkins EB, Thigpen JT, Deppe G, Maiman MA, Clarke-Pearson DL, Insalaco S (1999) Concurrent cisplatin-based radiotherapy and chemotherapy for locally advanced cervical cancer. N Engl J Med 340(15):1144–1153. https://doi.org/10.1056/NEJM199904153401502

Schilsky RL, Doroshow JH, Leblanc M, Conley BA (2012) Development and use of integral assays in clinical trials. Clin Cancer Res 18(6):1540–1546. https://doi.org/10.1158/1078-0432.CCR-11-2202

Schmidt-Ullrich RK, Mikkelsen RB, Dent P, Todd DG, Valerie K, Kavanagh BD, Contessa JN, Rorrer WK, Chen PB (1997) Radiation-induced proliferation of the human A431 squamous carcinoma cells is dependent on EGFR tyrosine phosphorylation. Oncogene 15(10):1191–1197. https://doi.org/10.1038/sj.onc.1201275

Sparano JA, Lee JY, Palefsky J, Henry DH, Wachsman W, Rajdev L, Aboulafia D, Ratner L, Fitzgerald TJ, Kachnic L, Mitsuyasu R (2017) Cetuximab plus chemoradiotherapy for HIV-associated anal carcinoma: a phase II AIDS Malignancy Consortium Trial. J Clin Oncol 35(7):727–733. https://doi.org/10.1200/JCO.2016.69.1642

Stupp R, Dietrich PY, Ostermann Kraljevic S, Pica A, Maillard I, Maeder P, Meuli R, Janzer R, Pizzolato G, Miralbell R, Porchet F, Regli L, de Tribolet N, Mirimanoff RO, Leyvraz S (2002) Promising survival for patients with newly diagnosed glioblastoma multiforme treated with concomitant radiation plus temozolomide followed by adjuvant temozolomide. J Clin Oncol 20(5):1375–1382. https://doi.org/10.1200/JCO.2002.20.5.1375

Stupp R, Mason WP, van den Bent MJ, Weller M, Fisher B, Taphoorn MJ, Belanger K, Brandes AA, Marosi C, Bogdahn U, Curschmann J, Janzer RC, Ludwin SK, Gorlia T, Allgeier A, Lacombe D, Cairncross JG, Eisenhauer E, Mirimanoff RO, European Organisation for Research and Treatment of Cancer Brain Tumor and Radiotherapy Groups; National Cancer Institute of Canada Clinical Trials Group (2005) Radiotherapy plus concomitant and adjuvant temozolomide for glioblastoma. N Engl J Med 352(10):987–996. https://doi.org/10.1056/NEJMoa043330

Wang M, Morsbach F, Sander D, Gheorghiu L, Nanda A, Benes C, Kriegs M, Krause M, Dikomey E, Baumann M, Dahm-Daphi J, Settleman J, Willers H (2011) EGF receptor inhibition radiosensitizes NSCLC cells by inducing senescence in cells sustaining DNA double-strand breaks. Cancer Res 71(19):6261–6269. https://doi.org/10.1158/0008-5472.CAN-11-0213

Chapter 3
Mapping the Radiogenome of Human Cancers

Priyanka Gopal, Jessica A. Castrillon, and Mohamed E. Abazeed

Abstract Precision oncology enables individualized treatment decisions on the basis of patient - and tumor-specific features. Despite growing evidence that inter-patient variation in tumor genomes affects treatment responses after radiation therapy, patients receiving these treatments continue to be treated with the same or similar doses. Herein, we discuss past, contemporary, and potential future forays into the mapping of the radiogenome of humans and their tumors. We contend that the incorporation of genomic information into radiation treatment approaches represents a critical step toward the individualization of radiation dose, which considers both treatment-related toxicity as well as tumor control probability. Specifically, we describe the role of somatic and germline genetic features on radiation tumor sensitivity and normal tissue toxicity. We also discuss potential barriers for the implementation of genomic predictors in clinical practices and strategies to overcome these barriers. The following discourse seeks to inform and guide the future use of genotype-directed radiation dose delivery and targeted radiosensitization.

Keywords Biomarkers · BRAF · EGFR · Genetic testing · Genotype · Germline testing · Inter-tumoral heterogeneity · KRAS · Mutations · Preclinical models · Radiogenome · Radiosensitivity · Therapeutic ratio

Priyanka Gopal and Jessica A. Castrillon contributed equally to this work.

P. Gopal · M. E. Abazeed (✉)
Department of Radiation Oncology, Northwestern Memorial Hospital, Northwestern University, Chicago, IL, USA
e-mail: mabazeed@northwestern.edu

J. A. Castrillon
Department of Translational Hematology Oncology Research, Cleveland Clinic, Cleveland, OH, USA

© Springer Nature Switzerland AG 2020
H. Willers, I. Eke (eds.), *Molecular Targeted Radiosensitizers*, Cancer Drug Discovery and Development, https://doi.org/10.1007/978-3-030-49701-9_3

1   Introduction

In clinical radiation therapy, the ability to maneuver incident beams to conform to the shape of target tumors has reached asymptotic precision. Juxtaposed with this technical precision, however, are widely used generic dose schemas converged upon after decades of population toxicity data and communal consensus of "acceptable" toxicity risk (Marks et al. 2010). In the post-comprehensive genome sequencing era, it is increasingly evident that there exists significant genetic variation across patients and their tumors (Hoadley et al. 2018). Genetic variation, a priori, suggests that doses optimized for populations of patients rather than individuals can lead to significant under- or over-treatment. Similarly, the clinical utility of radiosensitizing targeted agents may be impacted by inter-tumoral genetic differences. Such prescriptive imprecision limits the efficacy of radiation therapy and radiation/drug combinations and could also lead to potentially avoidable normal tissue toxicity. The failure to predict treatment efficacy using genetic variables represents one of the most significant obstacles to the personalization of radiation-based treatment regimens (Dancey Janet et al. 2012; Yard et al. 2015).

The profiling of the genomes of several solid tumors has led to the tailoring of drug treatments on the basis of specific genetic alterations or other biomarkers (De Palma and Hanahan 2012; Tripathy et al. 2014). The identification and cataloguing of genes associated with oncogenesis and tumor phenotypes has led to drug treatments that are guided by individual (e.g., *BRAF* V600E) or categories of mutations (e.g., hypermorphic mutations in *EGFR*) (Demetri et al. 2002; Druker et al. 2001; King et al. 1985). Despite this, the genetic features that determine whether a tumor is more or less likely to be sensitive to radiation therapy remain poorly understood. This is mainly due to a dearth of studies on the functional genomics of radiation sensitivity in cells, animals, and humans.

Prior to embarking on a daunting mission to map the radiogenomes of patients and their tumors, the probability of culling data that can guide clinical predictions is worthy of some discussion. Cancers represent complex systems, comprising a large number of potentially interacting variables (Fig. 3.1). Some of these variables may be encoded in the genome and others may be epi- ("near") or dis- ("apart") genetic (Schwab and Pienta 1996). A salient feature of a complex system is that its behavior cannot be easily implied from its parts. Therefore, it is critical that models that capture the inherent complexity are utilized. This recommends the use of primary human samples or translational systems that approximate those tumors (e.g., patient-derived models like xenografts or organoids) (Williams 2018; Nagle et al. 2018). Alternatively, reductionist approaches that serve as scaffolds for building toward greater complexity have been shown to provide some value (Amundson et al. 2008; Yard et al. 2016).

Typically, the interacting components of a complex system form a network. Networks are useful because they can describe the state of the system as a collection of discrete objects and relationships between them (e.g., gene expression regulatory networks) (Conte et al. 2020). Another common feature of a complex system is its

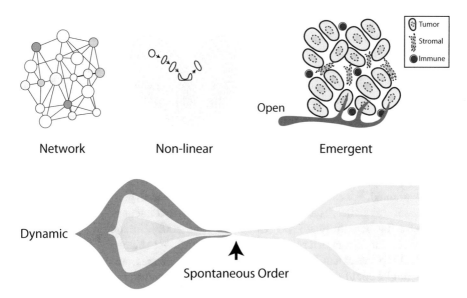

Network   Non-linear   Open   Emergent

Dynamic   Spontaneous Order

Fig. 3.1 Tumors are composed of many components that interact with each other, suggesting that they may abide the behaviors of a complex system. Each feature is described in detail in the main text. The vasculature depicted in the property of emergence suggests that tumors in situ represent "open" versus "closed" complex systems, allowing for exchange of components with another system (i.e. circulation)

emergent properties, which is the appearance of properties (genotypes) and/or behaviors (phenotypes) that are difficult to predict from the original or limited parts of the system (Finzer 2017). Since tumors are inherently genetically unstable, their properties can also be dynamic. This can be manifested by tumor subclones (genetically diverse sub-population of cells) that emerge or collapse on the basis of adaptation to flux in the environment or selective pressure (e.g., therapeutic stress) (McGranahan and Swanton 2017). This has implications for biomarker studies since models that capture patients' tumors at fixed time points (pre-therapy biopsy) are not likely to capture the full extent of the tumor's dynamism and emergent properties. Lastly, and perhaps the most challenging property from the perspective of predicting efficacy, is that complex systems have relationships that are nonlinear. That is, small perturbation in the input variables may cause a large effect on outcomes. Since the survival of a small number of clonogenic cells after radiation therapy can lead to tumor recurrence, this nonlinearity is particularly important when predicting a binary outcome (local failure *v.* control) (Cutanda Henriquez and Vargas Castrillon 2011).

The extent that tumors display each of these features: complexity, network relationships, dynamism, emergence, and non-linearity, can confound our ability to construct useful models and predict behavior. Contributing to this uncertainty is the conditional ability of sparsely ionizing radiation to cause lethal cellular damage due to the orientation of the DNA, its compactness, and the probabilistic trajectories of the ionization tracks (Goodhead 1989, 1994; Howard-Flanders 1958). Nevertheless, it is increasingly evident that there is a genetic basis for the vulnerability of many cancers to radiation therapy (Yard et al. 2016). Furthermore, acquiring comprehensive genomic information (DNA, RNA, protein, metabolites, etc.) on primary and longitudinal models of cancer coupled with the use of facile cellular systems that lend themselves to genetic manipulation represent critical steps toward capturing complexity, accounting for "noise," and predicting system-wide behaviors.

A countervailing perspective to the gene-centric view for predicting the radio-phenotype is that the tumor environment may be substantially more important than the genes encoded by the host or the tumor (Barker et al. 2015). A discussion concerning the relative contribution of genetic features on radiation sensitivity is, therefore, warranted. For example, intra-tumoral dynamic phenotypic states, attributed to epi-genetic "switches," have been shown to impact treatment responses although they have not been fully studied (Creighton et al. 2009). In addition, many other host and tumor factors that represent sources of additional heterogeneity have been identified. To the extent that these variables are dis-genetic, an exclusively gene-centric model could fail to capture their influences. However, there appears to a be a genetic basis for at least some of these variables (e.g., epigenome (Barker et al. 2015), histopathology (Tizhoosh and Pantanowitz 2018), hypoxia (Bhandari et al. 2019), metabolism (Ward et al. 2010; Tang et al. 2014), or image features (Aerts et al. 2014)). Therefore, future predictive models that use genome-guided markers as a surrogate marker of these and other features is still possible and desirable, reducing the debate of the influences of gene versus environment, in part, to pedagogy.

This chapter will discuss past, contemporary, and potential future forays into mapping the radiogenome of humans and their tumors. It contends that the incorporation of genetic information into radiation treatment planning represents a critical step toward the individualization of radiation dose probability. Specifically, we describe the role of germline and somatic genetic features on radiation tumor sensitivity and normal tissue toxicity annotated to date and pending efforts that seek to expand this information capability. We also discuss potential barriers for the implementation of genomic predictors in clinical practices and strategies to overcome these barriers. Together, these considerations form a critical basis for the future use of genotype-directed targeted radiosensitizers.

2   Biomarkers

A biomarker is a measurable biological signal whose presence is indicative of some phenomenon. Biomarkers can be used for early cancer detection, risk stratification, prediction of therapeutic responses, and the monitoring of recurrences (Dienstmann et al. 2013). Accordingly, biomarkers can be diagnostic, prognostic, and/or predictive. Some obstacles in validating and implementing biological biomarkers for therapeutic predictions include sample accessibility (e.g., tumor biopsy, surgery), intra-tumoral heterogeneity (e.g., tumor geographic stratification of the putative biomarker) (Biswas et al. 2019), the stability of the measurement (e.g., labile nature of gene expression networks) (Domany 2014), demonstration of biological plausibility, and confirmation in several external validation cohorts (Domany 2014). Moreover, there are multiple non-genetic determinants that impact radiation sensitivity and resistance (e.g., total treatment dose, fractionation, clinical variables) that must be accounted for when measuring isoeffects.

Despite these limitations, elucidating genomic determinants of radiation sensitivity is vital to developing biologically guided dose optimization strategies for a patient's tumor. These strategies can inform decisions of definitive radiation therapy versus alternative strategies (i.e., surgery or systemic therapies). In addition, since radiation therapy is unique among cancer therapies in that the dose of treatment can be calibrated on the basis of the probability of local tumor failure, such predictive assays could represent a unique opportunity to modulate dose in granular increments of Gray or combinations with tumor-specific radiosensitizers.

Efforts to translate biomarker-guided radiation therapy into clinical practice have had limited success to date (Hall et al. 2018). Optimization is needed for the unbiased selection of candidate radiation biomarkers as well as the design and quality of preclinical studies that seek to validate them. A goal that has been articulated is to accelerate the discovery, translational speed, and success of clinical studies that seek to utilize biomarker-driven stratification to tailor radiation prescriptions and schedules. To effect this goal, an integrated laboratory and clinical effort for radiation biomarker development should have several key features, including: (1) in vitro studies using a large panel of cell lines, (2) validation of the biomarker in an in vivo model, (3) elucidation of mechanistic details that indicate biological relevance, (4) the use of patient-derived models that better reflect tumoral mutational burden, heterogeneity, and transcriptional fidelity, (5) preclinical evaluation of clinically relevant treatment schedules, (6) the use of local tumor control as a clinical end point rather than surrogates (progression-free survival or overall survival), (7) rigorous standards for the reproducibility of biomarker data, (8) integrative omic diagnostics that measure both pathway alterations and activity, accounting for the distinct functional consequence for categories of mutations in genes of interest, and (9) large-scale correlative clinical studies in distinct and large populations of patients. The implementation of these features is poised to improve success rates in biomarker-driven or -stratified clinical trials in radiation oncology (Baumann et al. 2016).

3 Experimental Models and Approaches

There are several model systems with distinct attributes and ranges of facility and relevance to human tumors in situ (Fig. 3.2).

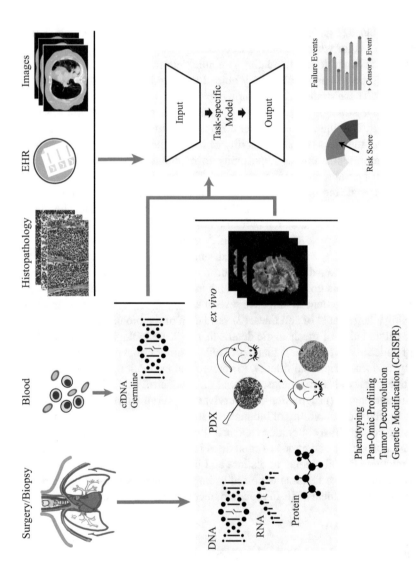

Fig. 3.2 Complementary and possibly tautological variables that span the research continuum including basic, translational, and clinical research are needed to nominate and validate biomarkers that can guide radiation therapy and radiation/drug combinations. The schematic depicts the use of several models and tools that can provide the information necessary to annotate the radiogenome

3.1 2D Cellular Models

Most studies to date that have examined genetic determinants of radiation sensitivity have relied on two-dimensional (2D) culture systems. 2D cellular models have advantages including rapid growth, amenability for high-content profiling, and genetic manipulation potential. As such, cell lines grown in vitro have served as a valuable resource to identify tumor intrinsic determinants of radiation sensitivity (Yard et al. 2016; Amundson et al. 2008). However, cells derived from patients are immortalized and cultured over time, inducing phenotypic changes and inevitable selection of cell subpopulations. Cells are also grown in medium that contain high concentrations of serum and in an abundance of oxygen, which are distinct from the nutrient- and oxygen-challenged microenvironments of a tumor in situ. Moreover, 2D models lack the three-dimensional organization of tumors in vivo (Griffith and Swartz 2006; Hutmacher et al. 2009). Altogether, these differences have direct implications for the identification of genetic features that may be more or less prevalent in patients.

3.2 High-Content Profiling of Cancer Cell Lines

The first large-scale cancer cell line radiation profiling effort measured radiation survival across the NCI-60 panel of cell lines, which represented nine tumor types (breast, central nervous system, colon, leukemia, lung, melanoma, ovarian, prostate, and renal) (Amundson et al. 2008). The study, which focused on basal and induced gene expression patterns across sensitive and resistance cell lines, revealed patterns of induced gene expression that seemed to be unaffected by the genetic variation across the collection of cells.

The largest analysis to date of cancer cell line survival after irradiation comprised the profiling of 533 cancer cell lines from 26 distinct cancer types (Yard et al. 2016). The source of the cell lines used in this study was the Cancer Cell Line Encyclopedia (CCLE), a large panel of comprehensively characterized human cancer models including a compilation of gene expression, copy number, and massively parallel sequencing data (Barretina et al. 2012). The high-content irradiation platform used a 384-well plate format and relied on delayed time to read out of proliferation measures as a surrogate for clonogenicity. The study used new statistical methodology to correlate radiation sensitivity and genomic parameters, identifying single-nucleotide variants (SNVs), copy number alterations, and gene expression changes associated with radiation survival.

3.3 3D Cellular Models

Modeling relevant genotype-phenotype associations can be challenging in 2D culture systems because adherence on a flat surface does not mimic in vivo cell shapes, which can influence biophysical cues (Kenny et al. 2007). In addition, homogeneous access to medium (immediately above the cells in 2D cultures) can result in homogeneous growth. Three dimensional (3D) systems can provide both structure and orientation that mimic in vivo spatial organization. Some of these platforms, also referred to as spheroids (Khaitan et al. 2006) or organoids (Drost et al. 2016), have been shown to be more capable of representing in vivo-like cells fates and cellular phenotypes including cell growth rate, drug response, and differentiation.

3.4 In Vivo Models

A major contributor to the high clinical trial failure rate for biomarkers is the apparent discordance between the promising activities observed in cellular-based preclinical systems and clinical outcomes (Johnson et al. 2001; Kung 2007). This is attributed, in part, to biological differences between cell line-derived models and the original tumors from which they were developed. In contrast, patient-derived xenograft (PDX) models faithfully recapitulate their tumors of origin by histology and transcriptomic, proteomic, and genomic parameters, and in some cases have been shown to have comparable treatment responses to those observed clinically (Bertotti et al. 2011; Daniel et al. 2009; Fichtner et al. 2008; Hidalgo et al. 2014; Hidalgo et al. 2011; Julien et al. 2012; Vargas et al. 2018). These models are poised to serve as powerful tools to enhance prediction and, ultimately, clinical trial success.

The use of NOD-SCID gamma (NSG) mice has facilitated the development of PDX models. Fresh human tissue obtained via biopsy or surgery is processed and injected into the subcutaneous tissue or, in some cases orthotopically, into the animal (Hidalgo et al. 2011). The engrafted tumor can then be harvested and stored for downstream applications. The practice of using PDXs to guide treatment decisions can be limited by implant geographic stratification bias and genetic divergence in the rodent host (usually after serial passages) (Ben-David et al. 2017). Despite this, previous work has suggested that the approach is possible and can potentially correlate with patient responses (Vargas et al. 2018). Due to their genetic diversity, PDX studies should be conducted on a larger scale, hence capturing the inter-tumoral variation of target patient populations (Gao et al. 2015). Although such studies have been completed for anti-cancer drugs, large-scale radiation studies of PDXs have yet to be reported. Such a profiling effort, especially when integrated with orthogonal data including clinical, image, and omic outputs, can provide both tumor intrinsic and microenvironmental variables that regulate radiation sensitivity as well as the response to radiosensitizing drugs.

Genetically engineered mouse model (GEMM) can also inform our ability to predict tumor responses to irradiation (Kersten et al. 2017). GEMMs enable the conditional expression of a genetic variant at the endogenous locus, mainly within the target tissue, and in an immunocompetent host (Huijbers et al. 2011; Sinn et al. 1987; Sutherland et al. 2011). Experiments conducted using these models can have predictive utility if assessing a variant in unary systematic fashion (one variant at a time). However, a major limitation to GEMMs is the lack of genetic complexity frequently observed in human tumors. Moreover, new GEMMs require significant lead-time and can be costly to develop and maintain. Lastly, it is not clear how GEMMs can be used to validate the multitude of putative genetic variants nominated by forward or reverse genetic approaches at scale.

4 The Use of Genetics to Guide Radiation Therapy in the Clinical Setting

Although the challenges of integrating genomic testing into radiation treatment decisions are wide-ranging and complex, there is a scientific and ethical imperative to realize the benefits of personalized cancer medicine given the overwhelming burden of cancer and the unprecedented opportunities for advancements in outcomes for patients. There is a growing appreciation for the influences of germline and tumor genetics on patient outcomes after radiation and chemoradiation, including estimates of the risk of radiation toxicity, radiation-induced secondary malignancies, and tumor response estimates (Bergom et al. 2019). Advances in genomic sequencing have enabled cataloguing of cancer genes into categories of cancer susceptibility genes and passenger mutations. Such advances, however, have outpaced clinical interpretation and utility. Variants identified via genomic testing should provide some information about the functional nature of the variant in question. Clinically, it is vital to distinguish driver variants, which have phenotypic consequences, from functionally neutral alterations. Hence, classification is nuanced and requires information beyond binary annotation. Moreover, actionability is likely to require expert interpretation and recommendations (Leichsenring et al. 2019).

4.1 Germline Testing and Potential Impact on the Therapeutic Ratio

Germline pathogenic variants, either inherited from previous generations or de novo, can increase the susceptibility to develop cancer. These variants are omnipresent (in every cell within an affected individual). Despite this, not every cell manifests the functional loss or gain of a particular pathogenic variant. Mechanisms that result in manifestations of the variant (e.g., development of cancer) include loss of heterozygosity or somatic uniparental disomy. This distinction is critical as it relates directly to haplosufficient variants and the therapeutic ratio: the tumor may manifest the functional alteration but the neighboring normal tissue may not (Bergom et al. 2019).

Several tests exist to assess the germline predisposition to cancer development in many genes. Some well-known genes for germline mutations include: *PTEN* (Cowden), *TP53* (Li-Fraumeni), *CDH1* (Diffuse Gastric Cancer Syndrome), *STK1* (Peutz-Jeghers), and BRCA1/2 (hereditary breast and ovarian cancer) (Liaw et al. 1997; Malkin et al. 1990; Berx et al. 1998; Jenne et al. 1998; Petrucelli et al. 2010). Germline mutations in specific genes resulting in mono- or bi-allelic inactivation can predispose to hereditary forms of cancer, which could impact radiation and radiation/drug sensitivity. These particular alterations affect patients with ataxia telangiectasia (AT), ataxia telangiectasia-like disorder, Nijmegen breakage syndrome (NBS), NBS-like syndrome, RIDDLE syndrome, DNA ligase IV deficiency, Cornelia de Lange syndrome, and Fanconi anemia (FA) (Pollard and Gatti 2009). Correlation of clinical features, prior annotation of a pathogenic variant or a functional assay that measures gene function could help parse the relevance of variant identification. It must be noted that a significant number of variants in these mainly large (in kilobases) genes remain categorized as variants of unknown significance (see below).

4.2   *Somatic Genetic Testing*

There are >19,000 genes in the human genome. Despite the mutation burden in solid human cancers, only some of the altered genes have validated or putative associations with cancer development and/or phenotypes. Accordingly, cancer gene panels have been used to genotype cancers for the purpose of diagnosis [e.g., cancers of unknown origin or cancer subtyping (squamous *v.* adenocarcinoma)] or to guide therapies. In the United States, FDA-approved tests include FoundationOne by Foundation Medicine (Cambridge, MA, USA), Oncomine by ThermoFisher (Waltham, MA, USA), and MSK-IMPACT by Memorial Sloan Kettering Cancer Center (New York, NY, USA) (Zehir et al. 2017; Nagahashi et al. 2019). While these panels could lead to actionable targets, they only capture limited coverage of the genome. Whole genome sequencing (WGS) or whole exome sequencing (WES) represent more comprehensive strategies for the identification of functionally relevant variants that may be missed by panel sequencing. Their benefits extend to the scientific community at large since a cataloguing of less common alterations can better inform large-scale association studies and, ultimately, treatment predictions. Moreover, there are some indications that WGS/WES result in cost saving and shorter time-to-test results compared to gene panel sequencing (Pennell et al. 2019).

5 Genetic Variants that Impact the Radiation Sensitivity Phenotype

The genetic composition of tumors is forged by environmental genotoxins (e.g., tobacco) and/or inherent genetic instability leading to sequence alterations that are pruned by clonal selection. The consequences of these processes result in variants in critical or non-critical (passenger) positions in the genome. Somatic mutations in proto-oncogenes lead to dysregulated cell growth and proliferation (Dixon and Kopras 2004). Frequent alterations in genes that encode for growth factors (e.g., *EGFR*), signal transduction pathways (e.g., *NRAS*), or nuclear transcription factors (e.g., *NFE2L2*) often represent recurrent and frequent alterations resulting in mutational "hot spots." The net effect of activation of these proto-oncogenes is the stimulation of cell proliferation, leading to the expansion of the transformed cell population and augmenting the effects of loss of tumor suppressor function. The latter represents another hallmark of cancer, the evasion of growth suppressors (Hanahan and Weinberg 2011). Cancer cells must also inactivate well-conserved programs that are designed to limit tumor growth and proliferation. Prototypical tumor suppressor genes like *TP53* and *RB1* are frequently inactivated via copy loss and/or functionally disruptive variants. Annotating functional variants of unknown significance in tumor suppressor genes is more challenging since they have a lower propensity for amino acid hot spots. This is especially true for larger genes that can accumulate sequence alterations over time (Lawrence et al. 2014).

5.1 Categories of Mutations

Since oncogenesis requires the activation of some genes and the inactivation of others, a cataloguing of functional variants into categories can be instructive. Mutations, or pathogenic variants, are classified by their phenotypic consequence compared to the wild-type allele as follows:

Loss of function: The mutant allele has less or no function compared to wild-type.

Gain of function: The mutant allele has increased levels of activity compared to wild-type.

Amorphic (dominant negative): These mutations result in a transformed gene product that acts antagonistically to the wild-type allele as a result of altered molecular function.

Neomorphic: These mutations result in a changed activity in the gene product compared the wild-type gene product as a result of altered molecular function (e.g., IDH1/2 mutations).

Variant of unknown significance: These variants result in a transformed gene product but it is unclear whether it affects gene function.

Functionally silent: These variants result in a transformed gene product that does not alter gene function. This category is distinguished from genetically silent mutations, which do not result in a subsequent change in the amino acid of the overall protein.

5.2 Variant Allele Frequency and Clonal Architecture

The prevalence of a gene variant in a tumor can be estimated by the variant allele frequency (VAF). The VAF is calculated by dividing the number of reads (contiguous sequence output from next-generation sequencing data) with the variant allele divided by the total number of reads generated. If the sample is purely tumoral (no contaminating stromal or immune cells) and the ploidy is *2n*, then the VAF of a heterozygous variant present in all tumor cells is 0.50. If the VAF is <0.50 under the same criteria (purity and ploidy), then the variant or the cluster of variants with that VAFs are considered subclonal and a subclone, respectively. This approach allows the identification of genetic spatial heterogeneity in a tumor. Several algorithms have been used to calculate VAFs corrected for purity and ploidy (Deshwar et al. 2015; Roth et al. 2014; Carter et al. 2012). These, coupled with other computational approaches to deconvolute the clonal architecture of tumors from bulk sequencing data have provided significant insight into the extent and content of intra-tumoral genetic heterogeneity. Despite these advances, there has been little work describing the clonal evolution of tumors under ionizing radiation stress (Kamran et al. 2019; Gopal et al. 2019). Therefore, it remains unclear to what extent subclonal frequencies, which can encode emergent properties (genotypes and phenotypes), rise and fall during irradiation.

5.3 Cell Cycle and DNA Repair

Ionizing radiation generates distinct types of DNA alterations, with double-strand breaks (DSBs) representing the principal lethal lesions (Vignard et al. 2013; Jackson and Bartek 2009). DSBs initiate a cascade of events that include cell cycle arrest, DNA repair or abrogation of repair, and induction of cellular death (Ciccia and Elledge 2010). Somatic alterations in cell cycle and DNA repair pathways are frequently found in several cancer types. This is likely attributed to etiology since challenges to genomic integrity via loss of DNA repair capacity increases the probability that cells acquire the requisite complement of alterations that drive uncontrollable growth. Bi-allelic germline or somatic loss of *ATM, ATR, TP53, TP53BP1, RAD51,* and other genes have been shown to confer radiation sensitivity in tumor cells with those alterations. Despite this, the extent that individual variants in these critical genes regulate radiation sensitivity remains unclear.

TP53 encodes a nucleophosphoprotein that acts as a transcriptional regulator of cell division, proliferation, and many other cellular functions. Upon irradiation or other exposures resulting in DNA damage, p53 is induced resulting in the transcriptional activation of a program of genes that regulate cell cycle arrest and DNA repair. *TP53* can undergo inactivation via single base substitution, loss of heterozygosity, or viral inactivation (Tommasino et al. 2003). Somatic alterations of *TP53* are commonly seen in many cancers including those of the upper aerodigestive tract and were nominated as possible biomarkers for local regional recurrence following radiation therapy for head and neck cancers (Alsner et al. 2001; Koch et al. 1996). Loss of p53 function generally does not affect cellular radiation sensitivity (Dahm-Daphi et al. 2005) but some studies have shown that individual *TP53* mutations can confer distinct sensitivities to radiation (Okaichi et al. 2011; Cuddihy and Bristow 2004). Hence, the role of individual *TP53* alterations in radiation sensitivity is far from clear.

5.4   Pathway Modulators

Distinct signaling pathways can alter the sensitivity of tumors to radiation treatments. Active signaling pathways, based on gene set enrichment analyses, suggest that several cellular receptors including RAS/RAF, EGFR, c-MYC, transforming growth factor-β (TGF-β), NFκB, AKT, FGFR, HER2, MEK, and Wnt/β-catenin can confer resistance to radiation (Yard et al. 2016). Although some work on select variants and genes demonstrate that hypermorphic mutations confer resistance to radiation, it remains unclear whether the vast majority of individual alterations in these genes (or others) regulate radiation sensitivity.

5.4.1   KRAS

The Ras family of GTPases comprises three members: *KRAS, HRAS,* and *NRAS* (Simanshu et al. 2017). Activation of the Ras GTPases result in the activation of a cascade of downstream molecules that play essential role in cellular proliferation and differentiation. *KRAS* is the most commonly mutated oncogene among the RAS family with high incidences in colorectal, pancreatic, and lung cancers (Cox and Der 2010). Mutations in *KRAS* constitutively activate the GTPase, independent of ligand binding, resulting in the activation of downstream signals. Alterations in *KRAS* often lead to poor prognosis, in part attributed to treatment resistance (Edkins et al. 2006; Bournet et al. 2016; Cserepes et al. 2014; Izar et al. 2014; Eberhard et al. 2005). Recent data in non-small cell lung carcinoma (NSCLC) has shown that cells with *KRAS* mutations can have stem-like tumor initiating properties, consisting of a subpopulation within *KRAS*-mutated tumors that are enriched with co-occurring mutations in *TP53* and *CDKN2A* (Wang et al. 2017). Moreover, specific mutations in *KRAS*, namely $KRAS^{G12V}$ and $KRAS^{G12C}$, appear to be associated with both poor response rate in NSCLC patients with brain metastasis (Renaud et al. 2016).

5.4.2 *BRAF*

BRAF encodes for a serine/threonine protein kinase that controls cell survival and is a key effector in the MAPK pathway (Xue et al. 2017). Mutations in *BRAF* leads to constitutive activation of the kinase, resulting in increased cell survival and proliferation. *BRAF* mutations occur at a frequency of 8% across all tumors, including melanoma, papillary thyroid cancer, colorectal cancer, and NSCLC (Cancer Genome Atlas Research Network 2014b; Davies et al. 2002; Cancer Genome Atlas Network 2012; The Cancer Genome Atlas Network 2015).

BRAF^{V600E} is the most commonly occurring mutation with a highest incidence in melanomas and thyroid cancers (Shain et al. 2015; Robb et al. 2019). However, other mutations have a higher incidence in other cancers (e.g., *BRAF*^{D594H} in colorectal cancer and *BRAF*^{G466V} in lung adenocarcinomas). *BRAF*-driven cancers can be effectively treated using BRAF and/or MEK inhibitors although in many cases resistance to treatment ultimately develops. Recent studies in lung adenocarcinoma have identified non-canonical *BRAF*-driven cancers with mutations in the highly conserved kinase domain as strongly associated with resistance to radiation (Gopal et al. 2019). Relatedly, *BRAF* mutant PDX models demonstrated *BRAF* mutant subclonal enrichment after radiation therapy, suggesting a putative mechanism of subclonal emergence resulting in treatment failures. In addition to these findings, *BRAF*^{V600E}-driven thyroid cancer cell lines were associated with resistance to radiation, and BRAF inhibition selectively radiosensitized these cells by modulating DNA repair (Robb et al. 2019). Studies to assess different classes of *BRAF* mutations and the efficacy of sequencing treatments using targeted therapies and radiation are poised to add greater clarity to the interaction between targeted agents and radiation in a genotype-specific manner.

5.4.3 *PIK3CA*

Structural and substrate specificity distinguishes the PI3Ks into three classes (Yu et al. 2015). *PIK3CA* belongs to class I PI3Ks and plays an important role in oncogenesis with links to receptor tyrosine kinases (RTKs), G protein-coupled receptors and other oncogenes including RAS (Vanhaesebroeck et al. 2012). *PIK3CA* signaling has been associated with mediating important biological functions such as cell survival, differentiation, and proliferation. Mutations in *PIK3CA* commonly occur across several cancer lineages including breast, colorectal, and pancreatic (Sanchez-Vega et al. 2018). PIK3CA mutations have been known to be associated with radiation resistance (Krasilnikov et al. 1999; Zhang et al. 2010). Specifically, in glioblastomas *PIK3CA* activating mutations with amino acid change at amino acid positions 88, 542–546, and 1047 have been associated with resistance to radiation.

5.4.4   *EGFR*

The epidermal growth factor receptor (EGFR) is a transmembrane protein that belong to the *ERB* family of genes that when active promotes cell survival, migration, and proliferation. Gene amplification and overexpression of EGFR have been observed in glioblastomas (Brennan et al. 2013), NSCLC (Cancer Genome Atlas Research Network 2014b), head and neck cancers (Cancer Genome Atlas Network 2015), bladder cancers (Cancer Genome Atlas Research Network 2014a), and colorectal cancers. *EGFR* mutational status correlates with radiation sensitivity in NSCLC cell lines (Das et al. 2006) Mechanistically, *EGFR* mutations may promote NSCLC apoptosis in response to irradiation through the upregulation of proapoptotic proteins and the DNA-dependent protein kinase catalytic subunit. In addition, phosphorylated histone (γ-H2AX) foci assay showed that *EGFR* mutations sustained irradiation-induced DNA damage (Xie et al. 2018). In a clinical study of head and neck cancer, *EGFR* overexpression was associated with higher failure rates after conventional radiation therapy (Chang et al. 2002). It remains unclear whether this correlative study represent mere association without causation or in fact there exists a functional role for EGFR in modulating radiation sensitivity in cells and tumors.

The above list is not intended to be exhaustive. There are additional variants that alter radiation sensitivity (Abazeed et al. 2013; Jeong et al. 2017). However, the vast majority of currently established associations are derived from hypothesis-directed research. A comprehensive and unbiased profiling of cancer-relevant genes for radiation sensitivity in several cellular contexts has yet to be conducted.

6   The Therapeutic Index and Radiation-Related Toxicities

The relation between the probability of tumor control (TCP) and the normal tissue complication probability (NTCP) provides estimates of the therapeutic ratio and guides radiotherapeutic interventions (Baumann and Petersen 2005). The oncologist seeks to deliver a dose that maximizes the TCP and minimizes NTCP, the investigator seeks to discover interventions that result in optimal separation of the two probabilities, and the annotation of the radiogenome of patients and their tumors seeks to delimit the dose relationship for individual patients in order to better calibrate dose. Late effects of tissue toxicity, for example, due to release of reactive oxygen species and pro-inflammatory cytokines, impair tissue remodeling by stromal cells that have been damaged (Kim et al. 2014), ultimately leading to fibrosis. Examples of late onset radiation effects include damage to blood vessels, central nervous system, heart (valvular defect and atherosclerosis), and lung (De Ruysscher et al. 2019). However, measurements of toxicity do not merely reflect the biological variation in the irradiated population, but can also depend on the type, form, and means by which radiation therapy is delivered.

The genetic basis for toxic effects during and after radiation treatments remains poorly defined. The rate of late effects of radiation in peritumoral organs increases as a function of time. However, these rates can be confounded by several variables including a competing risk of death, tumor recurrence, other treatments (i.e., chemotherapy), somatic acquisition of genetic variations, iatrogenic risks (i.e., procedures), and other epidemiological risks (i.e., tobacco consumption). Moreover, additional factors related to treatment administration (e.g., dosimetric accuracy, organ motion, poor treatment localization, and poor radiation quality assurance) can impact the probability of late toxicity. Notwithstanding these mainly dis-genetic variables, some germline genetic variants (or single nucleotide polymorphisms due to their prevalence in the population) have been shown to be associated with toxicities.

Genome-wide association studies (GWAS) analysis allows for the identification of common polymorphisms enriched in cases of late onset radiation toxicity. In order to confidently identify loci and ameliorate spurious associations, however, a significant number of samples are required. The REQUITE international prospective toxicity profiling effort, initiated by The Radiogenomics Consortium, comprises the largest study to date aimed at identifying common single nucleotide polymorphisms (SNPs) associated with clinical radiation toxicity (West et al. 2014; Kerns et al. 2020). Importantly, this effort has led to the creation of a centralized database which includes clinical information including treatment, dosimetry, toxicity, and genome-wide SNP genotyping data.

The first study using genome-wide association evaluated toxicity in patients with prostate cancer. SNPs *TANC1* locus 2q24.1, *KDM3B* 5q31.2, and *DNAH5* 5p15.2 were found to be associated with the development of erectile dysfunction, urinary symptoms, and proctitis, respectively (Kerns et al. 2013; Kerns et al. 2010). Additionally, a meta-analysis comprising six separate cohorts assessed radiation-related late complications in prostate cancer and identified common SNVs associated with rectal bleeding, decreased urinary stream, and hematuria (Kerns et al. 2020). The same study further validated the *KDM3B, ATM*, and *TANC1* loci and the association with respective toxicities.

These represent initial forays into the annotation of human variation and its role in radiation-related toxicities. In some aspects, the study of toxicity is substantially more challenging than the study of the tumor-associated genetic determinants. In addition to challenges in the clinical annotation of toxicities, other challenges include the relatively low genetic variation between patients compared to the variation between their tumors, the relatively low number of events (low late toxicity rates), and the lack of clinical follow-up compared to tumor recurrence (clinical follow-up and the use of medical images is the highest peri-diagnosis and after treatment completion, tapering significantly overtime).

7 Conclusions

Patient and tumor phenotypes are encoded by germline and somatic genomes, respectively. Analogously, therapies, including radiation therapy and radiation/drug combinations, are likely to vary based on the identity and interaction of these genetic determinants. Population-based estimates of treatment-related effects increasingly cannot be justified considering the extensive and detailed annotations of the genetic landscapes of humans and their cancers. Although additional variables beyond the genome may influence estimates of the probabilities of treatment successes, the lack of incorporation of genetic variables in radiation treatment deliveries represents a significant unmet clinical need. Current and future efforts, using varied methodologies and reviewed herein, are poised to chart the patient and tumor radiogenomes. These ambitious efforts are poised to reveal actionable information that can guide radiation treatments and the use of targeted radiosensitizers.

References

Abazeed ME, Adams DJ, Hurov KE, Tamayo P, Creighton CJ, Sonkin D, Giacomelli AO, Du C, Fries DF, Wong KK, Mesirov JP, Loeffler JS, Schreiber SL, Hammerman PS, Meyerson M (2013) Integrative radiogenomic profiling of squamous cell lung cancer. Cancer Res 73(20):6289–6298

Aerts HJWL, Velazquez ER, Leijenaar RTH, Parmar C, Grossmann P, Carvalho S, Bussink J, Monshouwer R, Haibe-Kains B, Rietveld D, Hoebers F, Rietbergen MM, Leemans CR, Dekker A, Quackenbush J, Gillies RJ, Lambin P (2014) Decoding tumour phenotype by non-invasive imaging using a quantitative radiomics approach. Nat Commun 5:4006. https://doi.org/10.1038/ncomms5644

Alsner J, Sørensen SB, Overgaard J (2001) TP53 mutation is related to poor prognosis after radiotherapy, but not surgery, in squamous cell carcinoma of the head and neck. Radiother Oncol 59(2):179–185. https://doi.org/10.1016/S0167-8140(01)00301-2

Amundson SA, Do KT, Vinikoor LC, Lee RA, Koch-Paiz CA, Ahn J, Reimers M, Chen Y, Scudiero DA, Weinstein JN, Trent JM, Bittner ML, Meltzer PS, Fornace AJ Jr (2008) Integrating global gene expression and radiation survival parameters across the 60 cell lines of the National Cancer Institute Anticancer Drug Screen. Cancer Res 68(2):415–424. https://doi.org/10.1158/0008-5472.CAN-07-2120

Barker HE, Paget JT, Khan AA, Harrington KJ (2015) The tumour microenvironment after radiotherapy: mechanisms of resistance and recurrence. Nat Rev Cancer 15(7):409–425. https://doi.org/10.1038/nrc3958

Barretina J, Caponigro G, Stransky N, Venkatesan K, Margolin AA, Kim S, Wilson CJ, Lehar J, Kryukov GV, Sonkin D, Reddy A, Liu M, Murray L, Berger MF, Monahan JE, Morais P, Meltzer J, Korejwa A, Jane-Valbuena J, Mapa FA, Thibault J, Bric-Furlong E, Raman P, Shipway A, Engels IH, Cheng J, Yu GK, Yu J, Aspesi P Jr, de Silva M, Jagtap K, Jones MD, Wang L, Hatton C, Palescandolo E, Gupta S, Mahan S, Sougnez C, Onofrio RC, Liefeld T, MacConaill L, Winckler W, Reich M, Li N, Mesirov JP, Gabriel SB, Getz G, Ardlie K, Chan V, Myer VE, Weber BL, Porter J, Warmuth M, Finan P, Harris JL, Meyerson M, Golub TR, Morrissey MP, Sellers WR, Schlegel R, Garraway LA (2012) The cancer cell line encyclopedia enables predictive modelling of anticancer drug sensitivity. Nature 483(7391):603–607

Baumann M, Petersen C (2005) TCP and NTCP: a basic introduction. Rays 30(2):99–104

Baumann M, Krause M, Overgaard J, Debus J, Bentzen SM, Daartz J, Richter C, Zips D, Bortfeld T (2016) Radiation oncology in the era of precision medicine. Nat Rev Cancer 16(4):234–249. https://doi.org/10.1038/nrc.2016.18

Ben-David U, Ha G, Tseng YY, Greenwald NF, Oh C, Shih J, McFarland JM, Wong B, Boehm JS, Beroukhim R, Golub TR (2017) Patient-derived xenografts undergo mouse-specific tumor evolution. Nat Genet 49(11):1567–1575. https://doi.org/10.1038/ng.3967

Bergom C, West CM, Higginson DS, Abazeed ME, Arun B, Bentzen SM, Bernstein JL, Evans JD, Gerber NK, Kerns SL, Keen J, Litton JK, Reiner AS, Riaz N, Rosenstein BS, Sawakuchi GO, Shaitelman SF, Powell SN, Woodward WA (2019) The implications of genetic testing on radiation therapy decisions: a guide for radiation oncologists. Int J Radiat Oncol Biol Phys 105(4):698–712. https://doi.org/10.1016/j.ijrobp.2019.07.026

Bertotti A, Migliardi G, Galimi F, Sassi F, Torti D, Isella C, Cora D, Di Nicolantonio F, Buscarino M, Petti C, Ribero D, Russolillo N, Muratore A, Massucco P, Pisacane A, Molinaro L, Valtorta E, Sartore-Bianchi A, Risio M, Capussotti L, Gambacorta M, Siena S, Medico E, Sapino A, Marsoni S, Comoglio PM, Bardelli A, Trusolino L (2011) A molecularly annotated platform of patient-derived xenografts ("xenopatients") identifies HER2 as an effective therapeutic target in cetuximab-resistant colorectal cancer. Cancer Discov 1(6):508–523. https://doi.org/10.1158/2159-8290.CD-11-0109

Berx G, Becker KF, Hofler H, van Roy F (1998) Mutations of the human E-cadherin (CDH1) gene. Hum Mutat 12(4):226–237. https://doi.org/10.1002/(SICI)1098-1004(1998)12:4<226::AID-HUMU2>3.0.CO;2-D

Bhandari V, Hoey C, Liu LY, Lalonde E, Ray J, Livingstone J, Lesurf R, Shiah YJ, Vujcic T, Huang X, Espiritu SMG, Heisler LE, Yousif F, Huang V, Yamaguchi TN, Yao CQ, Sabelnykova VY, Fraser M, Chua MLK, van der Kwast T, Liu SK, Boutros PC, Bristow RG (2019) Molecular landmarks of tumor hypoxia across cancer types. Nat Genet 51(2):308–318. https://doi.org/10.1038/s41588-018-0318-2

Biswas D, Birkbak NJ, Rosenthal R, Hiley CT, Lim EL, Papp K, Boeing S, Krzystanek M, Djureinovic D, La Fleur L, Greco M, Dome B, Fillinger J, Brunnstrom H, Wu Y, Moore DA, Skrzypski M, Abbosh C, Litchfield K, Al Bakir M, Watkins TBK, Veeriah S, Wilson GA, Jamal-Hanjani M, Moldvay J, Botling J, Chinnaiyan AM, Micke P, Hackshaw A, Bartek J, Csabai I, Szallasi Z, Herrero J, McGranahan N, Swanton C, Consortium TR (2019) A clonal expression biomarker associates with lung cancer mortality. Nat Med 25(10):1540–1548. https://doi.org/10.1038/s41591-019-0595-z

Bournet B, Muscari F, Buscail C, Assenat E, Barthet M, Hammel P, Selves J, Guimbaud R, Cordelier P, Buscail L (2016) KRAS G12D mutation subtype is a prognostic factor for advanced pancreatic adenocarcinoma. Clin Transl Gastroenterol 7:e157. https://doi.org/10.1038/ctg.2016.18

Brennan CW, Verhaak RG, McKenna A, Campos B, Noushmehr H, Salama SR, Zheng S, Chakravarty D, Sanborn JZ, Berman SH, Beroukhim R, Bernard B, Wu CJ, Genovese G, Shmulevich I, Barnholtz-Sloan J, Zou L, Vegesna R, Shukla SA, Ciriello G, Yung WK, Zhang W, Sougnez C, Mikkelsen T, Aldape K, Bigner DD, Van Meir EG, Prados M, Sloan A, Black KL, Eschbacher J, Finocchiaro G, Friedman W, Andrews DW, Guha A, Iacocca M, O'Neill BP, Foltz G, Myers J, Weisenberger DJ, Penny R, Kucherlapati R, Perou CM, Hayes DN, Gibbs R, Marra M, Mills GB, Lander E, Spellman P, Wilson R, Sander C, Weinstein J, Meyerson M, Gabriel S, Laird PW, Haussler D, Getz G, Chin L, Network TR (2013) The somatic genomic landscape of glioblastoma. Cell 155(2):462–477. https://doi.org/10.1016/j.cell.2013.09.034

Cancer Genome Atlas Network (2012) Comprehensive molecular characterization of human colon and rectal cancer. Nature 487(7407):330–337. https://doi.org/10.1038/nature11252

Cancer Genome Atlas Network (2015) Comprehensive genomic characterization of head and neck squamous cell carcinomas. Nature 517(7536):576–582. https://doi.org/10.1038/nature14129

Cancer Genome Atlas Research Network (2014a) Comprehensive molecular characterization of urothelial bladder carcinoma. Nature 507(7492):315–322. https://doi.org/10.1038/nature12965

Cancer Genome Atlas Research Network (2014b) Comprehensive molecular profiling of lung adenocarcinoma. Nature 511(7511):543–550. https://doi.org/10.1038/nature13385

Carter SL, Cibulskis K, Helman E, McKenna A, Shen H, Zack T, Laird PW, Onofrio RC, Winckler W, Weir BA, Beroukhim R, Pellman D, Levine DA, Lander ES, Meyerson M, Getz G (2012) Absolute quantification of somatic DNA alterations in human cancer. Nat Biotechnol 30(5):413–421. https://doi.org/10.1038/nbt.2203

Chang BD, Swift ME, Shen M, Fang J, Broude EV, Roninson IB (2002) Molecular determinants of terminal growth arrest induced in tumor cells by a chemotherapeutic agent. Proc Natl Acad Sci U S A 99(1):389–394

Ciccia A, Elledge SJ (2010) The DNA damage response: making it safe to play with knives. Mol Cell 40(2):179–204

Conte F, Fiscon G, Licursi V, Bizzarri D, D'Anto T, Farina L, Paci P (2020) A paradigm shift in medicine: a comprehensive review of network-based approaches. Biochim Biophys Acta Gene Regul Mech 1863:194416. https://doi.org/10.1016/j.bbagrm.2019.194416

Cox AD, Der CJ (2010) Ras history: the saga continues. Small GTPases 1(1):2–27. https://doi.org/10.4161/sgtp.1.1.12178

Creighton CJ, Li X, Landis M, Dixon JM, Neumeister VM, Sjolund A, Rimm DL, Wong H, Rodriguez A, Herschkowitz JI, Fan C, Zhang X, He X, Pavlick A, Gutierrez MC, Renshaw L, Larionov AA, Faratian D, Hilsenbeck SG, Perou CM, Lewis MT, Rosen JM, Chang JC (2009) Residual breast cancers after conventional therapy display mesenchymal as well as tumor-initiating features. Proc Natl Acad Sci U S A 106(33):13820–13825. https://doi.org/10.1073/pnas.0905718106

Cserepes M, Ostoros G, Lohinai Z, Raso E, Barbai T, Timar J, Rozsas A, Moldvay J, Kovalszky I, Fabian K, Gyulai M, Ghanim B, Laszlo V, Klikovits T, Hoda MA, Grusch M, Berger W, Klepetko W, Hegedus B, Dome B (2014) Subtype-specific KRAS mutations in advanced lung adenocarcinoma: a retrospective study of patients treated with platinum-based chemotherapy. Eur J Cancer 50(10):1819–1828. https://doi.org/10.1016/j.ejca.2014.04.001

Cuddihy AR, Bristow RG (2004) The p53 protein family and radiation sensitivity: yes or no? Cancer Metastasis Rev 23(3):237–257. https://doi.org/10.1023/B:CANC.0000031764.81141.e4

Cutanda Henriquez F, Vargas Castrillon S (2011) The use of a mixed Poisson model for tumour control probability computation in non homogeneous irradiations. Australas Phys Eng Sci Med 34(2):267–272. https://doi.org/10.1007/s13246-011-0074-4

Dahm-Daphi J, Hubbe P, Horvath F, El-Awady RA, Bouffard KE, Powell SN, Willers H (2005) Nonhomologous end-joining of site-specific but not of radiation-induced DNA double-strand breaks is reduced in the presence of wild-type p53. Oncogene 24(10):1663–1672

Dancey Janet E, Bedard Philippe L, Onetto N, Hudson Thomas J (2012) The genetic basis for cancer treatment decisions. Cell 148(3):409–420. https://doi.org/10.1016/j.cell.2012.01.014

Daniel VC, Marchionni L, Hierman JS, Rhodes JT, Devereux WL, Rudin CM, Yung R, Parmigiani G, Dorsch M, Peacock CD, Watkins DN (2009) A primary xenograft model of small-cell lung cancer reveals irreversible changes in gene expression imposed by culture in vitro. Cancer Res 69(8):3364–3373. https://doi.org/10.1158/0008-5472.CAN-08-4210

Das AK, Sato M, Story MD, Peyton M, Graves R, Redpath S, Girard L, Gazdar AF, Shay JW, Minna JD, Nirodi CS (2006) Non-small-cell lung cancers with kinase domain mutations in the epidermal growth factor receptor are sensitive to ionizing radiation. Cancer Res 66(19):9601–9608. https://doi.org/10.1158/0008-5472.CAN-06-2627

Davies H, Bignell GR, Cox C, Stephens P, Edkins S, Clegg S, Teague J, Woffendin H, Garnett MJ, Bottomley W, Davis N, Dicks E, Ewing R, Floyd Y, Gray K, Hall S, Hawes R, Hughes J, Kosmidou V, Menzies A, Mould C, Parker A, Stevens C, Watt S, Hooper S, Wilson R, Jayatilake H, Gusterson BA, Cooper C, Shipley J, Hargrave D, Pritchard-Jones K, Maitland N, Chenevix-Trench G, Riggins GJ, Bigner DD, Palmieri G, Cossu A, Flanagan A, Nicholson A, Ho JW, Leung SY, Yuen ST, Weber BL, Seigler HF, Darrow TL, Paterson H, Marais R, Marshall CJ, Wooster R, Stratton MR, Futreal PA (2002) Mutations of the BRAF gene in human cancer. Nature 417(6892):949–954. https://doi.org/10.1038/nature00766

De Palma M, Hanahan D (2012) The biology of personalized cancer medicine: facing individual complexities underlying hallmark capabilities. Mol Oncol 6(2):111–127. https://doi.org/10.1016/j.molonc.2012.01.011

De Ruysscher D, Niedermann G, Burnet NG, Siva S, Lee AWM, Hegi-Johnson F (2019) Radiotherapy toxicity. Nat Rev Dis Primers 5(1):13. https://doi.org/10.1038/s41572-019-0064-5

Demetri GD, von Mehren M, Blanke CD, Van den Abbeele AD, Eisenberg B, Roberts PJ, Heinrich MC, Tuveson DA, Singer S, Janicek M, Fletcher JA, Silverman SG, Silberman SL, Capdeville R, Kiese B, Peng B, Dimitrijevic S, Druker BJ, Corless C, Fletcher CD, Joensuu H (2002) Efficacy and safety of imatinib mesylate in advanced gastrointestinal stromal tumors. N Engl J Med 347(7):472–480. https://doi.org/10.1056/NEJMoa020461

Deshwar AG, Vembu S, Yung CK, Jang GH, Stein L, Morris Q (2015) PhyloWGS: reconstructing subclonal composition and evolution from whole-genome sequencing of tumors. Genome Biol 16:35. https://doi.org/10.1186/s13059-015-0602-8

Dienstmann RRJ, Barretina J, Tabernero J (2013) Genomic medicine frontier in human solid tumors: prospects and challenges. J Clin Oncol 31:1874–1884

Dixon K, Kopras E (2004) Genetic alterations and DNA repair in human carcinogenesis. Semin Cancer Biol 14(6):441–448. https://doi.org/10.1016/j.semcancer.2004.06.007

Domany E (2014) Using high-throughput transcriptomic data for prognosis: a critical overview and perspectives. Cancer Res 74(17):4612–4621. https://doi.org/10.1158/0008-5472.CAN-13-3338

Drost J, Karthaus WR, Gao D, Driehuis E, Sawyers CL, Chen Y, Clevers H (2016) Organoid culture systems for prostate epithelial and cancer tissue. Nat Protoc 11:347. https://doi.org/10.1038/nprot.2016.006

Druker BJ, Talpaz M, Resta DJ, Peng B, Buchdunger E, Ford JM, Lydon NB, Kantarjian H, Capdeville R, Ohno-Jones S, Sawyers CL (2001) Efficacy and safety of a specific inhibitor of the BCR-ABL tyrosine kinase in chronic myeloid leukemia. N Engl J Med 344(14):1031–1037. https://doi.org/10.1056/NEJM200104053441401

Eberhard DA, Johnson BE, Amler LC, Goddard AD, Heldens SL, Herbst RS, Ince WL, Jänne PA, Januario T, Johnson DH, Klein P, Miller VA, Ostland MA, Ramies DA, Sebisanovic D, Stinson JA, Zhang YR, Seshagiri S, Hillan KJ (2005) Mutations in the epidermal growth factor receptor and in KRAS are predictive and prognostic indicators in patients with non–small-cell lung cancer treated with chemotherapy alone and in combination with Erlotinib. J Clin Oncol 23(25):5900–5909. https://doi.org/10.1200/jco.2005.02.857

Edkins S, O'Meara S, Parker A, Stevens C, Reis M, Jones S, Greenman C, Davies H, Dalgliesh G, Forbes S, Hunter C, Smith R, Stephens P, Goldstraw P, Nicholson A, Chan TL, Velculescu VE, Yuen ST, Leung SY, Stratton MR, Futreal PA (2006) Recurrent KRAS codon 146 mutations in human colorectal cancer. Cancer Biol Ther 5(8):928–932. https://doi.org/10.4161/cbt.5.8.3251

Fichtner I, Rolff J, Soong R, Hoffmann J, Hammer S, Sommer A, Becker M, Merk J (2008) Establishment of patient-derived non-small cell lung cancer xenografts as models for the identification of predictive biomarkers. Clin Cancer Res 14(20):6456–6468. https://doi.org/10.1158/1078-0432.CCR-08-0138

Finzer P (2017) How we become ill: investigating emergent properties of biological systems could help to better understand the pathology of diseases. EMBO Rep 18(4):515–518. https://doi.org/10.15252/embr.201743948

Gao H, Korn JM, Ferretti S, Monahan JE, Wang Y, Singh M, Zhang C, Schnell C, Yang G, Zhang Y, Balbin OA, Barbe S, Cai H, Casey F, Chatterjee S, Chiang DY, Chuai S, Cogan SM, Collins SD, Dammassa E, Ebel N, Embry M, Green J, Kauffmann A, Kowal C, Leary RJ, Lehar J, Liang Y, Loo A, Lorenzana E, Robert McDonald E 3rd, McLaughlin ME, Merkin J, Meyer R, Naylor TL, Patawaran M, Reddy A, Roelli C, Ruddy DA, Salangsang F, Santacroce F, Singh AP, Tang Y, Tinetto W, Tobler S, Velazquez R, Venkatesan K, Von Arx F, Wang HQ, Wang Z, Wiesmann M, Wyss D, Xu F, Bitter H, Atadja P, Lees E, Hofmann F, Li E, Keen N, Cozens R, Jensen MR, Pryer NK, Williams JA, Sellers WR (2015) High-throughput screening using patient-derived tumor xenografts to predict clinical trial drug response. Nat Med 21(11):1318–1325. https://doi.org/10.1038/nm.3954

Goodhead DT (1989) The initial physical damage produced by ionizing radiations. Int J Radiat Biol 56(5):623–634

Goodhead DT (1994) Initial events in the cellular effects of ionizing radiations: clustered damage in DNA. Int J Radiat Biol 65(1):7–17

Gopal P, Sarihan EI, Chie EK, Kuzmishin G, Doken S, Pennell NA, Raymond DP, Murthy SC, Ahmad U, Raja S, Almeida F, Sethi S, Gildea TR, Peacock CD, Adams DJ, Abazeed ME (2019) Clonal selection confers distinct evolutionary trajectories in BRAF-driven cancers. Nat Commun 10(1):5143. https://doi.org/10.1038/s41467-019-13161-x

Griffith LG, Swartz MA (2006) Capturing complex 3D tissue physiology in vitro. Nat Rev Mol Cell Biol 7(3):211–224. https://doi.org/10.1038/nrm1858

Hall WA, Bergom C, Thompson RF, Baschnagel AM, Vijayakumar S, Willers H, Li XA, Schultz CJ, Wilson GD, West CML, Capala J, Coleman CN, Torres-Roca JF, Weidhaas J, Feng FY (2018) Precision oncology and Genomically guided radiation therapy: a report from the American Society for Radiation Oncology/American Association of Physicists in Medicine/National Cancer Institute Precision Medicine Conference. Int J Radiat Oncol Biol Phys 101(2):274–284. https://doi.org/10.1016/j.ijrobp.2017.05.044

Hanahan D, Weinberg RA (2011) Hallmarks of cancer: the next generation. Cell 144(5):646–674. https://doi.org/10.1016/j.cell.2011.02.013

Hidalgo M, Bruckheimer E, Rajeshkumar NV, Garrido-Laguna I, De Oliveira E, Rubio-Viqueira B, Strawn S, Wick MJ, Martell J, Sidransky D (2011) A pilot clinical study of treatment guided by personalized tumorgrafts in patients with advanced cancer. Mol Cancer Ther 10(8):1311–1316. https://doi.org/10.1158/1535-7163.MCT-11-0233

Hidalgo M, Amant F, Biankin AV, Budinska E, Byrne AT, Caldas C, Clarke RB, de Jong S, Jonkers J, Maelandsmo GM, Roman-Roman S, Seoane J, Trusolino L, Villanueva A (2014) Patient-derived xenograft models: an emerging platform for translational cancer research. Cancer Discov 4(9):998–1013. https://doi.org/10.1158/2159-8290.CD-14-0001

Hoadley KA, Yau C, Hinoue T, Wolf DM, Lazar AJ, Drill E, Shen R, Taylor AM, Cherniack AD, Thorsson V, Akbani R, Bowlby R, Wong CK, Wiznerowicz M, Sanchez-Vega F, Robertson AG, Schneider BG, Lawrence MS, Noushmehr H, Malta TM, Cancer Genome Atlas N, Stuart JM, Benz CC, Laird PW (2018) Cell-of-origin patterns dominate the molecular classification of 10,000 tumors from 33 types of cancer. Cell 173(2):291–304.e296. https://doi.org/10.1016/j.cell.2018.03.022

Howard-Flanders P (1958) Physical and chemical mechanisms in the injury of cells of ionizing radiations. Adv Biol Med Phys 6:553–603

Huijbers IJ, Krimpenfort P, Berns A, Jonkers J (2011) Rapid validation of cancer genes in chimeras derived from established genetically engineered mouse models. Bioessays 33(9):701–710. https://doi.org/10.1002/bies.201100018

Hutmacher DW, Horch RE, Loessner D, Rizzi S, Sieh S, Reichert JC, Clements JA, Beier JP, Arkudas A, Bleiziffer O, Kneser U (2009) Translating tissue engineering technology platforms into cancer research. J Cell Mol Med 13(8A):1417–1427. https://doi.org/10.1111/j.1582-4934.2009.00853.x

Izar B, Zhou H, Heist RS, Azzoli CG, Muzikansky A, Scribner EE, Bernardo LA, Dias-Santagata D, Iafrate AJ, Lanuti M (2014) The prognostic impact of KRAS, its codon and amino acid specific mutations, on survival in resected stage I lung adenocarcinoma. J Thorac Oncol 9(9):1363–1369. https://doi.org/10.1097/jto.0000000000000266

Jackson SP, Bartek J (2009) The DNA-damage response in human biology and disease. Nature 461(7267):1071–1078. https://doi.org/10.1038/nature08467

Jenne DE, Reimann H, Nezu J, Friedel W, Loff S, Jeschke R, Muller O, Back W, Zimmer M (1998) Peutz-Jeghers syndrome is caused by mutations in a novel serine threonine kinase. Nat Genet 18(1):38–43. https://doi.org/10.1038/ng0198-38

Jeong Y, Hoang NT, Lovejoy A, Stehr H, Newman AM, Gentles AJ, Kong W, Truong D, Martin S, Chaudhuri A, Heiser D, Zhou L, Say C, Carter JN, Hiniker SM, Loo BW Jr, West RB, Beachy P, Alizadeh AA, Diehn M (2017) Role of KEAP1/NRF2 and TP53 mutations in lung squamous cell carcinoma development and radiation resistance. Cancer Discov 7(1):86–101. https://doi.org/10.1158/2159-8290.Cd-16-0127

Johnson JI, Decker S, Zaharevitz D, Rubinstein LV, Venditti JM, Schepartz S, Kalyandrug S, Christian M, Arbuck S, Hollingshead M, Sausville EA (2001) Relationships between drug activity in NCI preclinical in vitro and in vivo models and early clinical trials. Br J Cancer 84(10):1424–1431. https://doi.org/10.1054/bjoc.2001.1796

Julien S, Merino-Trigo A, Lacroix L, Pocard M, Goere D, Mariani P, Landron S, Bigot L, Nemati F, Dartigues P, Weiswald LB, Lantuas D, Morgand L, Pham E, Gonin P, Dangles-Marie V, Job B, Dessen P, Bruno A, Pierre A, De The H, Soliman H, Nunes M, Lardier G, Calvet L, Demers B, Prevost G, Vrignaud P, Roman-Roman S, Duchamp O, Berthet C (2012) Characterization of a large panel of patient-derived tumor xenografts representing the clinical heterogeneity of human colorectal cancer. Clin Cancer Res 18(19):5314–5328. https://doi.org/10.1158/1078-0432.CCR-12-0372

Kamran SC, Lennerz JK, Margolis CA, Liu D, Reardon B, Wankowicz SA, Van Seventer EE, Tracy A, Wo JY, Carter SL, Willers H, Corcoran RB, Hong TS, Van Allen EM (2019) Integrative molecular characterization of resistance to neoadjuvant chemoradiation in rectal cancer. Clin Cancer Res 25(18):5561–5571. https://doi.org/10.1158/1078-0432.CCR-19-0908

Kenny PA, Lee GY, Myers CA, Neve RM, Semeiks JR, Spellman PT, Lorenz K, Lee EH, Barcellos-Hoff MH, Petersen OW, Gray JW, Bissell MJ (2007) The morphologies of breast cancer cell lines in three-dimensional assays correlate with their profiles of gene expression. Mol Oncol 1(1):84–96. https://doi.org/10.1016/j.molonc.2007.02.004

Kerns SL, Ostrer H, Stock R, Li W, Moore J, Pearlman A, Campbell C, Shao Y, Stone N, Kusnetz L, Rosenstein BS (2010) Genome-wide association study to identify single nucleotide polymorphisms (SNPs) associated with the development of erectile dysfunction in African-American men after radiotherapy for prostate cancer. Int J Radiat Oncol Biol Phys 78(5):1292–1300. https://doi.org/10.1016/j.ijrobp.2010.07.036

Kerns SL, Stone NN, Stock RG, Rath L, Ostrer H, Rosenstein BS (2013) A 2-stage genome-wide association study to identify single nucleotide polymorphisms associated with development of urinary symptoms after radiotherapy for prostate cancer. J Urol 190(1):102–108. https://doi.org/10.1016/j.juro.2013.01.096

Kerns SL, Fachal L, Dorling L, Barnett GC, Baran A, Peterson DR, Hollenberg M, Hao K, Narzo AD, Ahsen ME, Pandey G, Bentzen SM, Janelsins M, Elliott RM, Pharoah PDP, Burnet NG, Dearnaley DP, Gulliford SL, Hall E, Sydes MR, Aguado-Barrera ME, Gomez-Caamano A, Carballo AM, Peleteiro P, Lobato-Busto R, Stock R, Stone NN, Ostrer H, Usmani N, Singhal S, Tsuji H, Imai T, Saito S, Eeles R, DeRuyck K, Parliament M, Dunning AM, Vega A, Rosenstein BS, West CML (2020) Radiogenomics consortium genome-wide association study meta-analysis of late toxicity after prostate cancer radiotherapy. J Natl Cancer Inst 112(2):179–190. https://doi.org/10.1093/jnci/djz075

Kersten K, de Visser KE, van Miltenburg MH, Jonkers J (2017) Genetically engineered mouse models in oncology research and cancer medicine. EMBO Mol Med 9(2):137–153. https://doi.org/10.15252/emmm.201606857

Khaitan D, Chandna S, Arya MB, Dwarakanath BS (2006) Establishment and characterization of multicellular spheroids from a human glioma cell line; implications for tumor therapy. J Transl Med 4:12. https://doi.org/10.1186/1479-5876-4-12

Kim JH, Jenrow KA, Brown SL (2014) Mechanisms of radiation-induced normal tissue toxicity and implications for future clinical trials. Radiat Oncol J 32(3):103–115. https://doi.org/10.3857/roj.2014.32.3.103

King CR, Kraus MH, Aaronson SA (1985) Amplification of a novel v-erbB-related gene in a human mammary carcinoma. Science 229(4717):974–976

Koch WM, Brennan JA, Zahurak M, Goodman SN, Westra WH, Schwab D, Yoo GH, Lee DJ, Forastiere AA, Sidransky D (1996) p53 mutation and locoregional treatment failure in head and neck squamous cell carcinoma. JNCI J Natl Cancer Inst 88(21):1580–1586. https://doi.org/10.1093/jnci/88.21.1580

Krasilnikov M, Adler V, Fuchs SY, Dong Z, Haimovitz-Friedman A, Herlyn M, Ronai Z (1999) Contribution of phosphatidylinositol 3-kinase to radiation resistance in human melanoma cells. Mol Carcinog 24(1):64–69

Kung AL (2007) Practices and pitfalls of mouse cancer models in drug discovery. Adv Cancer Res 96:191–212. https://doi.org/10.1016/S0065-230X(06)96007-2

Lawrence MS, Stojanov P, Mermel CH, Robinson JT, Garraway LA, Golub TR, Meyerson M, Gabriel SB, Lander ES, Getz G (2014) Discovery and saturation analysis of cancer genes across 21 tumour types. Nature 505(7484):495–501. https://doi.org/10.1038/nature12912

Leichsenring J, Horak P, Kreutzfeldt S, Heining C, Christopoulos P, Volckmar AL, Neumann O, Kirchner M, Ploeger C, Budczies J, Heilig CE, Hutter B, Frohlich M, Uhrig S, Kazdal D, Allgauer M, Harms A, Rempel E, Lehmann U, Thomas M, Pfarr N, Azoitei N, Bonzheim I, Marienfeld R, Moller P, Werner M, Fend F, Boerries M, von Bubnoff N, Lassmann S, Longerich T, Bitzer M, Seufferlein T, Malek N, Weichert W, Schirmacher P, Penzel R, Endris V, Brors B, Klauschen F, Glimm H, Frohling S, Stenzinger A (2019) Variant classification in precision oncology. Int J Cancer 145(11):2996–3010. https://doi.org/10.1002/ijc.32358

Liaw D, Marsh DJ, Li J, Dahia PL, Wang SI, Zheng Z, Bose S, Call KM, Tsou HC, Peacocke M, Eng C, Parsons R (1997) Germline mutations of the PTEN gene in Cowden disease, an inherited breast and thyroid cancer syndrome. Nat Genet 16(1):64–67. https://doi.org/10.1038/ng0597-64

Malkin D, Li FP, Strong LC, Fraumeni JF Jr, Nelson CE, Kim DH, Kassel J, Gryka MA, Bischoff FZ, Tainsky MA et al (1990) Germ line p53 mutations in a familial syndrome of breast cancer, sarcomas, and other neoplasms. Science 250(4985):1233–1238. https://doi.org/10.1126/science.1978757

Marks LB, Yorke ED, Jackson A, Ten Haken RK, Constine LS, Eisbruch A, Bentzen SM, Nam J, Deasy JO (2010) Use of normal tissue complication probability models in the clinic. Int J Radiat Oncol Biol Phys 76(3 Suppl):S10–S19. https://doi.org/10.1016/j.ijrobp.2009.07.1754

McGranahan N, Swanton C (2017) Clonal heterogeneity and tumor evolution: past, present, and the future. Cell 168(4):613–628. https://doi.org/10.1016/j.cell.2017.01.018

Nagahashi M, Shimada Y, Ichikawa H, Kameyama H, Takabe K, Okuda S, Wakai T (2019) Next generation sequencing-based gene panel tests for the management of solid tumors. Cancer Sci 110(1):6–15. https://doi.org/10.1111/cas.13837

Nagle PW, Plukker JTM, Muijs CT, van Luijk P, Coppes RP (2018) Patient-derived tumor organoids for prediction of cancer treatment response. Semin Cancer Biol 53:258–264. https://doi.org/10.1016/j.semcancer.2018.06.005

Okaichi K, Nose K, Kotake T, Izumi N, Kudo T (2011) Phosphorylation of p53 modifies sensitivity to ionizing radiation. Anticancer Res 31(6):2255–2258

Pennell NA, Mutebi A, Zhou Z-Y, Ricculli ML, Tang W, Wang H, Guerin A, Arnhart T, Dalal A, Sasane M, Wu KY, Culver KW, Otterson GA (2019) Economic impact of next-generation sequencing versus single-gene testing to detect genomic alterations in metastatic non–small-cell lung cancer using a decision analytic model. JCO Precis Oncol 3:1–9. https://doi.org/10.1200/PO.18.00356

Petrucelli N, Daly MB, Feldman GL (2010) Hereditary breast and ovarian cancer due to mutations in BRCA1 and BRCA2. Genet Med 12(5):245–259. https://doi.org/10.1097/GIM.0b013e3181d38f2f

Pollard JM, Gatti RA (2009) Clinical radiation sensitivity with DNA repair disorders: an overview. Int J Radiat Oncol Biol Phys 74(5):1323–1331. https://doi.org/10.1016/j.ijrobp.2009.02.057

Renaud S, Schaeffer M, Voegeli A-C, Legrain M, Guérin E, Meyer N, Mennecier B, Quoix E, Falcoz P-E, Guénot D, Massard G, Noël G, Beau-Faller M (2016) Impact of EGFR mutations and KRAS amino acid substitution on the response to radiotherapy for brain metastasis of non-small-cell lung cancer. Future Oncol 12(1):59–70. https://doi.org/10.2217/fon.15.273

Robb R, Yang L, Shen C, Wolfe A, Webb A, Zhang X, Vedaie M, Saji M, Jhiang SM, Ringel MD,
    Williams TM (2019) Inhibiting BRAF oncogene-mediated radioresistance effectively radio-
    sensitizes BRAF^{V600E}mutant thyroid cancer cells by constraining DNA double-
    strand break repair. Clin Cancer Res 25(15):4749–4760. https://doi.org/10.1158/1078-0432.
    Ccr-18-3625
Roth A, Khattra J, Yap D, Wan A, Laks E, Biele J, Ha G, Aparicio S, Bouchard-Cote A, Shah SP
    (2014) PyClone: statistical inference of clonal population structure in cancer. Nat Methods
    11(4):396–398. https://doi.org/10.1038/nmeth.2883
Sanchez-Vega F, Mina M, Armenia J, Chatila WK, Luna A, La KC, Dimitriadoy S, Liu DL,
    Kantheti HS, Saghafinia S, Chakravarty D, Daian F, Gao Q, Bailey MH, Liang W-W, Foltz SM,
    Shmulevich I, Ding L, Heins Z, Ochoa A, Gross B, Gao J, Zhang H, Kundra R, Kandoth C,
    Bahceci I, Dervishi L, Dogrusoz U, Zhou W, Shen H, Laird PW, Way GP, Greene CS, Liang H,
    Xiao Y, Wang C, Iavarone A, Berger AH, Bivona TG, Lazar AJ, Hammer GD, Giordano T,
    Kwong LN, McArthur G, Huang C, Tward AD, Frederick MJ, McCormick F, Meyerson M,
    Caesar-Johnson SJ, Demchok JA, Felau I, Kasapi M, Ferguson ML, Hutter CM, Sofia HJ,
    Tarnuzzer R, Wang Z, Yang L, Zenklusen JC, Zhang J, Chudamani S, Liu J, Lolla L, Naresh R,
    Pihl T, Sun Q, Wan Y, Wu Y, Cho J, DeFreitas T, Frazer S, Gehlenborg N, Getz G, Heiman DI,
    Kim J, Lawrence MS, Lin P, Meier S, Noble MS, Saksena G, Voet D, Zhang H, Bernard B,
    Chambwe N, Dhankani V, Knijnenburg T, Kramer R, Leinonen K, Liu Y, Miller M, Reynolds
    S, Shmulevich I, Thorsson V, Zhang W, Akbani R, Broom BM, Hegde AM, Ju Z, Kanchi RS,
    Korkut A, Li J, Liang H, Ling S, Liu W, Lu Y, Mills GB, Ng K-S, Rao A, Ryan M, Wang J,
    Weinstein JN, Zhang J, Abeshouse A, Armenia J, Chakravarty D, Chatila WK, de Bruijn I, Gao
    J, Gross BE, Heins ZJ, Kundra R, La K, Ladanyi M, Luna A, Nissan MG, Ochoa A, Phillips
    SM, Reznik E, Sanchez-Vega F, Sander C, Schultz N, Sheridan R, Sumer SO, Sun Y, Taylor BS,
    Wang J, Zhang H, Anur P, Peto M, Spellman P, Benz C, Stuart JM, Wong CK, Yau C, Hayes
    DN, Parker JS, Wilkerson MD, Ally A, Balasundaram M, Bowlby R, Brooks D, Carlsen R,
    Chuah E, Dhalla N, Holt R, Jones SJM, Kasaian K, Lee D, Ma Y, Marra MA, Mayo M, Moore
    RA, Mungall AJ, Mungall K, Robertson AG, Sadeghi S, Schein JE, Sipahimalani P, Tam A,
    Thiessen N, Tse K, Wong T, Berger AC, Beroukhim R, Cherniack AD, Cibulskis C, Gabriel SB,
    Gao GF, Ha G, Meyerson M, Schumacher SE, Shih J, Kucherlapati MH, Kucherlapati RS,
    Baylin S, Cope L, Danilova L, Bootwalla MS, Lai PH, Maglinte DT, Van Den Berg DJ,
    Weisenberger DJ, Auman JT, Balu S, Bodenheimer T, Fan C, Hoadley KA, Hoyle AP, Jefferys
    SR, Jones CD, Meng S, Mieczkowski PA, Mose LE, Perou AH, Perou CM, Roach J, Shi Y,
    Simons JV, Skelly T, Soloway MG, Tan D, Veluvolu U, Fan H, Hinoue T, Laird PW, Shen H,
    Zhou W, Bellair M, Chang K, Covington K, Creighton CJ, Dinh H, Doddapaneni H, Donehower
    LA, Drummond J, Gibbs RA, Glenn R, Hale W, Han Y, Hu J, Korchina V, Lee S, Lewis L, Li
    W, Liu X, Morgan M, Morton D, Muzny D, Santibanez J, Sheth M, Shinbrot E, Wang L, Wang
    M, Wheeler DA, Xi L, Zhao F, Hess J, Appelbaum EL, Bailey M, Cordes MG, Ding L, Fronick
    CC, Fulton LA, Fulton RS, Kandoth C, Mardis ER, McLellan MD, Miller CA, Schmidt HK,
    Wilson RK, Crain D, Curley E, Gardner J, Lau K, Mallery D, Morris S, Paulauskis J, Penny R,
    Shelton C, Shelton T, Sherman M, Thompson E, Yena P, Bowen J, Gastier-Foster JM, Gerken
    M, Leraas KM, Lichtenberg TM, Ramirez NC, Wise L, Zmuda E, Corcoran N, Costello T,
    Hovens C, Carvalho AL, de Carvalho AC, Fregnani JH, Longatto-Filho A, Reis RM,
    Scapulatempo-Neto C, Silveira HCS, Vidal DO, Burnette A, Eschbacher J, Hermes B, Noss A,
    Singh R, Anderson ML, Castro PD, Ittmann M, Huntsman D, Kohl B, Le X, Thorp R, Andry
    C, Duffy ER, Lyadov V, Paklina O, Setdikova G, Shabunin A, Tavobilov M, McPherson C,
    Warnick R, Berkowitz R, Cramer D, Feltmate C, Horowitz N, Kibel A, Muto M, Raut CP,
    Malykh A, Barnholtz-Sloan JS, Barrett W, Devine K, Fulop J, Ostrom QT, Shimmel K,
    Wolinsky Y, Sloan AE, De Rose A, Giuliante F, Goodman M, Karlan BY, Hagedorn CH,
    Eckman J, Harr J, Myers J, Tucker K, Zach LA, Deyarmin B, Hu H, Kvecher L, Larson C,
    Mural RJ, Somiari S, Vicha A, Zelinka T, Bennett J, Iacocca M, Rabeno B, Swanson P, Latour
    M, Lacombe L, Têtu B, Bergeron A, McGraw M, Staugaitis SM, Chabot J, Hibshoosh H,
    Sepulveda A, Su T, Wang T, Potapova O, Voronina O, Desjardins L, Mariani O, Roman-Roman

S, Sastre X, Stern M-H, Cheng F, Signoretti S, Berchuck A, Bigner D, Lipp E, Marks J, McCall S, McLendon R, Secord A, Sharp A, Behera M, Brat DJ, Chen A, Delman K, Force S, Khuri F, Magliocca K, Maithel S, Olson JJ, Owonikoko T, Pickens A, Ramalingam S, Shin DM, Sica G, Van Meir EG, Zhang H, Eijckenboom W, Gillis A, Korpershoek E, Looijenga L, Oosterhuis W, Stoop H, van Kessel KE, Zwarthoff EC, Calatozzolo C, Cuppini L, Cuzzubbo S, DiMeco F, Finocchiaro G, Mattei L, Perin A, Pollo B, Chen C, Houck J, Lohavanichbutr P, Hartmann A, Stoehr C, Stoehr R, Taubert H, Wach S, Wullich B, Kycler W, Murawa D, Wiznerowicz M, Chung K, Edenfield WJ, Martin J, Baudin E, Bubley G, Bueno R, De Rienzo A, Richards WG, Kalkanis S, Mikkelsen T, Noushmehr H, Scarpace L, Girard N, Aymerich M, Campo E, Giné E, Guillermo AL, Van Bang N, Hanh PT, Phu BD, Tang Y, Colman H, Evason K, Dottino PR, Martignetti JA, Gabra H, Juhl H, Akeredolu T, Stepa S, Hoon D, Ahn K, Kang KJ, Beuschlein F, Breggia A, Birrer M, Bell D, Borad M, Bryce AH, Castle E, Chandan V, Cheville J, Copland JA, Farnell M, Flotte T, Giama N, Ho T, Kendrick M, Kocher J-P, Kopp K, Moser C, Nagorney D, O'Brien D, O'Neill BP, Patel T, Petersen G, Que F, Rivera M, Roberts L, Smallridge R, Smyrk T, Stanton M, Thompson RH, Torbenson M, Yang JD, Zhang L, Brimo F, Ajani JA, Gonzalez AMA, Behrens C, Bondaruk J, Broaddus R, Czerniak B, Esmaeli B, Fujimoto J, Gershenwald J, Guo C, Lazar AJ, Logothetis C, Meric-Bernstam F, Moran C, Ramondetta L, Rice D, Sood A, Tamboli P, Thompson T, Troncoso P, Tsao A, Wistuba I, Carter C, Haydu L, Hersey P, Jakrot V, Kakavand H, Kefford R, Lee K, Long G, Mann G, Quinn M, Saw R, Scolyer R, Shannon K, Spillane A, Stretch J, Synott M, Thompson J, Wilmott J, Al-Ahmadie H, Chan TA, Ghossein R, Gopalan A, Levine DA, Reuter V, Singer S, Singh B, Tien NV, Broudy T, Mirsaidi C, Nair P, Drwiega P, Miller J, Smith J, Zaren H, Park J-W, Hung NP, Kebebew E, Linehan WM, Metwalli AR, Pacak K, Pinto PA, Schiffman M, Schmidt LS, Vocke CD, Wentzensen N, Worrell R, Yang H, Moncrieff M, Goparaju C, Melamed J, Pass H, Botnariuc N, Caraman I, Cernat M, Chemencedji I, Clipca A, Doruc S, Gorincioi G, Mura S, Pirtac M, Stancul I, Tcaciuc D, Albert M, Alexopoulou I, Arnaout A, Bartlett J, Engel J, Gilbert S, Parfitt J, Sekhon H, Thomas G, Rassl DM, Rintoul RC, Bifulco C, Tamakawa R, Urba W, Hayward N, Timmers H, Antenucci A, Facciolo F, Grazi G, Marino M, Merola R, de Krijger R, Gimenez-Roqueplo A-P, Piché A, Chevalier S, McKercher G, Birsoy K, Barnett G, Brewer C, Farver C, Naska T, Pennell NA, Raymond D, Schilero C, Smolenski K, Williams F, Morrison C, Borgia JA, Liptay MJ, Pool M, Seder CW, Junker K, Omberg L, Dinkin M, Manikhas G, Alvaro D, Bragazzi MC, Cardinale V, Carpino G, Gaudio E, Chesla D, Cottingham S, Dubina M, Moiseenko F, Dhanasekaran R, Becker K-F, Janssen K-P, Slotta-Huspenina J, Abdel-Rahman MH, Aziz D, Bell S, Cebulla CM, Davis A, Duell R, Elder JB, Hilty J, Kumar B, Lang J, Lehman NL, Mandt R, Nguyen P, Pilarski R, Rai K, Schoenfield L, Senecal K, Wakely P, Hansen P, Lechan R, Powers J, Tischler A, Grizzle WE, Sexton KC, Kastl A, Henderson J, Porten S, Waldmann J, Fassnacht M, Asa SL, Schadendorf D, Couce M, Graefen M, Huland H, Sauter G, Schlomm T, Simon R, Tennstedt P, Olabode O, Nelson M, Bathe O, Carroll PR, Chan JM, Disaia P, Glenn P, Kelley RK, Landen CN, Phillips J, Prados M, Simko J, Smith-McCune K, VandenBerg S, Roggin K, Fehrenbach A, Kendler A, Sifri S, Steele R, Jimeno A, Carey F, Forgie I, Mannelli M, Carney M, Hernandez B, Campos B, Herold-Mende C, Jungk C, Unterberg A, von Deimling A, Bossler A, Galbraith J, Jacobus L, Knudson M, Knutson T, Ma D, Milhem M, Sigmund R, Godwin AK, Madan R, Rosenthal HG, Adebamowo C, Adebamowo SN, Boussioutas A, Beer D, Giordano T, Mes-Masson A-M, Saad F, Bocklage T, Landrum L, Mannel R, Moore K, Moxley K, Postier R, Walker J, Zuna R, Feldman M, Valdivieso F, Dhir R, Luketich J, Pinero EMM, Quintero-Aguilo M, Carlotti CG, Dos Santos JS, Kemp R, Sankarankuty A, Tirapelli D, Catto J, Agnew K, Swisher E, Creaney J, Robinson B, Shelley CS, Godwin EM, Kendall S, Shipman C, Bradford C, Carey T, Haddad A, Moyer J, Peterson L, Prince M, Rozek L, Wolf G, Bowman R, Fong KM, Yang I, Korst R, Rathmell WK, Fantacone-Campbell JL, Hooke JA, Kovatich AJ, Shriver CD, DiPersio J, Drake B, Govindan R, Heath S, Ley T, Van Tine B, Westervelt P, Rubin MA, Lee JI, Aredes ND, Mariamidze A, Van Allen EM, Cherniack AD, Ciriello G, Sander C, Schultz N (2018) Oncogenic signaling pathways in The Cancer Genome Atlas. Cell 173(2):321–337.e310. https://doi.org/10.1016/j.cell.2018.03.035

Schwab ED, Pienta KJ (1996) Cancer as a complex adaptive system. Med Hypotheses 47(3):235–241. https://doi.org/10.1016/s0306-9877(96)90086-9

Shain AH, Yeh I, Kovalyshyn I, Sriharan A, Talevich E, Gagnon A, Dummer R, North J, Pincus L, Ruben B, Rickaby W, D'Arrigo C, Robson A, Bastian BC (2015) The genetic evolution of melanoma from precursor lesions. N Engl J Med 373(20):1926–1936. https://doi.org/10.1056/NEJMoa1502583

Simanshu DK, Nissley DV, McCormick F (2017) RAS proteins and their regulators in human disease. Cell 170(1):17–33. https://doi.org/10.1016/j.cell.2017.06.009

Sinn E, Muller W, Pattengale P, Tepler I, Wallace R, Leder P (1987) Coexpression of MMTV/v--Ha-ras and MMTV/c-myc genes in transgenic mice: synergistic action of oncogenes in vivo. Cell 49(4):465–475. https://doi.org/10.1016/0092-8674(87)90449-1

Sutherland KD, Proost N, Brouns I, Adriaensen D, Song JY, Berns A (2011) Cell of origin of small cell lung cancer: inactivation of Trp53 and Rb1 in distinct cell types of adult mouse lung. Cancer Cell 19(6):754–764. https://doi.org/10.1016/j.ccr.2011.04.019

Tang X, Lin CC, Spasojevic I, Iversen ES, Chi JT, Marks JR (2014) A joint analysis of metabolomics and genetics of breast cancer. Breast Cancer Res 16(4):415. https://doi.org/10.1186/s13058-014-0415-9

The Cancer Genome Atlas Network (2015) Genomic classification of cutaneous melanoma. Cell 161(7):1681–1696. https://doi.org/10.1016/j.cell.2015.05.044

Tizhoosh HR, Pantanowitz L (2018) Artificial intelligence and digital pathology: challenges and opportunities. J Pathol Inform 9:38. https://doi.org/10.4103/jpi.jpi_53_18

Tommasino M, Accardi R, Caldeira S, Dong W, Malanchi I, Smet A, Zehbe I (2003) The role of TP53 in cervical carcinogenesis. Hum Mutat 21(3):307–312. https://doi.org/10.1002/humu.10178

Tripathy D, Harnden K, Blackwell K, Robson M (2014) Next generation sequencing and tumor mutation profiling: are we ready for routine use in the oncology clinic? BMC Med 12(1):140. https://doi.org/10.1186/s12916-014-0140-3

Vanhaesebroeck B, Stephens L, Hawkins P (2012) PI3K signalling: the path to discovery and understanding. Nat Rev Mol Cell Biol 13:195. https://doi.org/10.1038/nrm3290

Vargas R, Gopal P, Kuzmishin GB, DeBernardo R, Koyfman SA, Jha BK, Mian OY, Scott J, Adams DJ, Peacock CD, Abazeed ME (2018) Case study: patient-derived clear cell adenocarcinoma xenograft model longitudinally predicts treatment response. NPJ Prec Oncol 2(1):14. https://doi.org/10.1038/s41698-018-0060-3

Vignard J, Mirey G, Salles B (2013) Ionizing-radiation induced DNA double-strand breaks: a direct and indirect lighting up. Radiother Oncol 108(3):362–369

Wang M, Han J, Marcar L, Black J, Liu Q, Li X, Nagulapalli K, Sequist LV, Mak RH, Benes CH, Hong TS, Gurtner K, Krause M, Baumann M, Kang JX, Whetstine J, Willers H (2017) Radiation resistance in KRAS-mutated lung cancer is enabled by stem-like properties mediated by an osteopontin-EGFR pathway. Clin Cancer Res 77(8):2018–2028. https://doi.org/10.1158/0008-5472.CAN-16-0808

Ward PS, Patel J, Wise DR, Abdel-Wahab O, Bennett BD, Coller HA, Cross JR, Fantin VR, Hedvat CV, Perl AE, Rabinowitz JD, Carroll M, Su SM, Sharp KA, Levine RL, Thompson CB (2010) The common feature of leukemia-associated IDH1 and IDH2 mutations is a neomorphic enzyme activity converting alpha-ketoglutarate to 2-hydroxyglutarate. Cancer Cell 17(3):225–234. https://doi.org/10.1016/j.ccr.2010.01.020

West C, Azria D, Chang-Claude J, Davidson S, Lambin P, Rosenstein B, De Ruysscher D, Talbot C, Thierens H, Valdagni R, Vega A, Yuille M (2014) The REQUITE project: validating predictive models and biomarkers of radiotherapy toxicity to reduce side-effects and improve quality of life in cancer survivors. Clin Oncol (R Coll Radiol) 26(12):739–742. https://doi.org/10.1016/j.clon.2014.09.008

Williams JA (2018) Using PDX for preclinical cancer drug discovery: the evolving field. J Clin Med 7(3). https://doi.org/10.3390/jcm7030041

Xie B, Sun L, Cheng Y, Zhou J, Zheng J, Zhang W (2018) Epidermal growth factor receptor gene mutations in non-small-cell lung cancer cells are associated with increased radiosensitivity in vitro. Cancer Manag Res 10:3551–3560. https://doi.org/10.2147/CMAR.S165831

Xue Y, Martelotto L, Baslan T, Vides A, Solomon M, Mai TT, Chaudhary N, Riely GJ, Li BT, Scott K, Cechhi F, Stierner U, Chadalavada K, de Stanchina E, Schwartz S, Hembrough T, Nanjangud G, Berger MF, Nilsson J, Lowe SW, Reis-Filho JS, Rosen N, Lito P (2017) An approach to suppress the evolution of resistance in BRAF(V600E)-mutant cancer. Nat Med 23(8):929–937. https://doi.org/10.1038/nm.4369

Yard B, Chie EK, Adams DJ, Peacock C, Abazeed ME (2015) Radiotherapy in the era of precision medicine. Semin Radiat Oncol 25(4):227–236. https://doi.org/10.1016/j.semradonc.2015.05.003

Yard BD, Adams DJ, Chie EK, Tamayo P, Battaglia JS, Gopal P, Rogacki K, Pearson BE, Phillips J, Raymond DP, Pennell NA, Almeida F, Cheah JH, Clemons PA, Shamji A, Peacock CD, Schreiber SL, Hammerman PS, Abazeed ME (2016) A genetic basis for the variation in the vulnerability of cancer to DNA damage. Nat Commun 7:11428. https://doi.org/10.1038/ncomms11428

Yu X, Long YC, Shen H-M (2015) Differential regulatory functions of three classes of phosphatidylinositol and phosphoinositide 3-kinases in autophagy. Autophagy 11(10):1711–1728. https://doi.org/10.1080/15548627.2015.1043076

Zehir A, Benayed R, Shah RH, Syed A, Middha S, Kim HR, Srinivasan P, Gao J, Chakravarty D, Devlin SM, Hellmann MD, Barron DA, Schram AM, Hameed M, Dogan S, Ross DS, Hechtman JF, DeLair DF, Yao J, Mandelker DL, Cheng DT, Chandramohan R, Mohanty AS, Ptashkin RN, Jayakumaran G, Prasad M, Syed MH, Rema AB, Liu ZY, Nafa K, Borsu L, Sadowska J, Casanova J, Bacares R, Kiecka IJ, Razumova A, Son JB, Stewart L, Baldi T, Mullaney KA, Al-Ahmadie H, Vakiani E, Abeshouse AA, Penson AV, Jonsson P, Camacho N, Chang MT, Won HH, Gross BE, Kundra R, Heins ZJ, Chen HW, Phillips S, Zhang H, Wang J, Ochoa A, Wills J, Eubank M, Thomas SB, Gardos SM, Reales DN, Galle J, Durany R, Cambria R, Abida W, Cercek A, Feldman DR, Gounder MM, Hakimi AA, Harding JJ, Iyer G, Janjigian YY, Jordan EJ, Kelly CM, Lowery MA, Morris LGT, Omuro AM, Raj N, Razavi P, Shoushtari AN, Shukla N, Soumerai TE, Varghese AM, Yaeger R, Coleman J, Bochner B, Riely GJ, Saltz LB, Scher HI, Sabbatini PJ, Robson ME, Klimstra DS, Taylor BS, Baselga J, Schultz N, Hyman DM, Arcila ME, Solit DB, Ladanyi M, Berger MF (2017) Mutational landscape of metastatic cancer revealed from prospective clinical sequencing of 10,000 patients. Nat Med 23(6):703–713. https://doi.org/10.1038/nm.4333

Zhang T, Cui GB, Zhang J, Zhang F, Zhou YA, Jiang T, Li XF (2010) Inhibition of PI3 kinases enhances the sensitivity of non-small cell lung cancer cells to ionizing radiation. Oncol Rep 24(6):1683–1689

Chapter 4
Mechanisms and Markers of Clinical Radioresistance

Michael S. Binkley, Maximilian Diehn, Iris Eke, and Henning Willers

Abstract Predictive biomarkers that allow rational selection of treatments for individual patients have played a central role in precision oncology. While such biomarkers have transformed approaches for systemic drug-based therapies, few markers are currently available clinically for aiding therapeutic decisions involving radiation therapy and radiation/drug combination. Given the considerable heterogeneity of tumor responses to radiation and chemoradiation in the clinic, there exists a critical need to establish biomarkers for stratifying tumors according to their relative treatment sensitivity/resistance. This will aid the development of radiation/drug combinations which to date have largely followed the historical "one-size-fits-all" approach. The use of targeted radiosensitizers may be especially beneficial for radioresistant cancers where pure radiation dose escalation may be limited by the radiation tolerance of the normal tissues surrounding a tumor. In particular, the therapeutic index could be widened if radiosensitizers take aim at molecular targets that are present or overexpressed in the tumor but not normal tissues. Here, we review not only established radiobiological parameters that impact clinical radioresistance but also genomic tumor alterations such as mutations in *KEAP1/NFE2L2* or *KRAS* that are emerging as clinically useful biomarkers in this regard. There exists tremendous opportunity to realize the precision radiation medicine concept in the clinic through the rational development of radiation/drug or chemoradiation/drug combinations that are guided by these biomarkers.

Keywords Accelerated repopulation · Biomarkers · Cancer stem cells · Clonogenicity · DNA repair · Genotype · Intrinsic radioresistance · KEAP1 · Kinase inhibitors · KRAS · NFE2L2 · TP53 · Radioresistance · Radiosensitivity index (RSI) · Tumor control probability · Tumor heterogeneity · Tumor spheres

M. S. Binkley · M. Diehn · I. Eke
Department of Radiation Oncology, Stanford University School of Medicine, Stanford, CA, USA
e-mail: msb996@stanford.edu; diehn@stanford.edu; iris.eke@stanford.edu

H. Willers (✉)
Department of Radiation Oncology, Massachusetts General Hospital, Harvard Medical School, Boston, MA, USA
e-mail: hwillers@mgh.harvard.edu

© Springer Nature Switzerland AG 2020
H. Willers, I. Eke (eds.), *Molecular Targeted Radiosensitizers*, Cancer Drug Discovery and Development, https://doi.org/10.1007/978-3-030-49701-9_4

1 Introduction

In radiation oncology, clonogenic tumor cells have been historically defined as cells that have the capacity to produce an expanding family of daughter cells and form colonies following irradiation in an in vitro assay or give rise to a locally recurrent tumor in in vivo models (Willers et al. 2019). To what extent clonogenic cells resemble cancer stem cells (CSC) or CSC-like cells is poorly understood but the terms have been used interchangeably (Baumann et al. 2016; Krause et al. 2011, 2017; Willers et al. 2013). To eradicate or locally control a tumor, all CSCs have to be inactivated. Treatment may fail if only one CSC survives because that cell can regenerate the tumor. The success rate of radiation therapy is determined by the fraction of tumors that are without any surviving CSCs after the final radiation dose is delivered. At first approximation, CSC inactivation by radiation is both random and logarithmic (Willers and Held 2006). Logarithmic cell inactivation translates into a sigmoid dose-response curve, i.e., a curve of tumor control probability (TCP) (Fig. 4.1a). It follows that increasing the radiation dose—for a given number of CSCs—will increase the probability that a CSC is lethally injured, thereby decreasing the number of surviving CSCs. This dose-response relationship suggests that absolute radioresistance does not exist. Any number of tumor cells can be eradicated as long as the total dose of radiation is high enough. However, the radiation tolerance of normal organs and tissues surrounding a tumor restricts the maximum amount of radiation that can be safely administered to a patient (Willers et al. 2013).

Based on experimental evidence and clinical observations, it can be assumed that in a population of cancer patients, a spectrum of dose-response curves exists (Krause et al. 2017). Figures 4.1b and c depict hypothetical individual TCP curves to illustrate this concept. In clinical practice, the TCP curve for a patient population is flatter than in individual patients because of underlying inter-patient and inter-tumoral heterogeneity (Fig. 4.1c). Thus, the more heterogeneous a patient population is, the flatter the average TCP curve becomes and the more difficult it is to detect an improvement in treatment outcome with increasing radiation dose. Therefore, it is difficult to apply the dose-response findings observed in a population accurately to a given individual patient whose individual tumor dose-response curve is unknown. Here, predictive biomarkers would be extremely useful, if not to identify individual patient curves but at least to stratify tumors into radiosensitive, radioresistant, and intermediate bins (Krause et al. 2017). Within most cancer types tumors exist that are (relatively) resistant to radiation or concurrent chemoradiation therapy. For these tumors, approaches other than pure radiation dose escalation may be needed to increase the TCP, for instance, through the addition of molecular targeted radiosensitizers.

Historically, the framework of the so-called five "R's" of Radiation Therapy has been used to try to explain the sensitivity of tumors and normal tissues to fractionated radiation treatment: Recovery, Repopulation, Reoxygenation, Redistribution, and Radiosensitivity (reviewed in (Willers and Held 2006; Willers et al. 2019)). However, these factors have only partial clinical relevance, especially with regard to

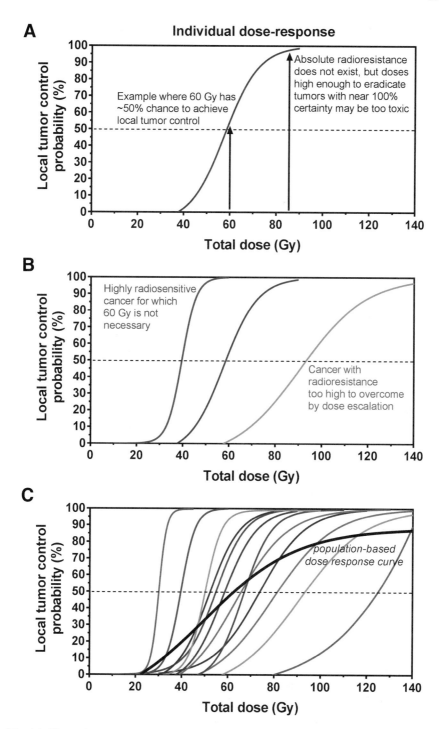

Fig. 4.1 Illustration of tumor control probability curves assumed to exist in humans of (**a**) an individual tumor, (**b**) several individual tumors with varying radiosensitivity, and (**c**) of a population-based dose response curve

the characterization of radioresistant tumors. In this chapter, we review mechanisms and biomarkers of tumor radioresistance that are of clinical significance. Readers are also referred to excellent recent reviews on this topic (Baumann et al. 2016; Kirsch et al. 2018). We will expand on emerging genomic biomarkers such as mutations in *KEAP1*, *NFE2L2*, and *KRAS*, which may be able to impact clinical practice in the not too distant future. For a discussion of hypoxia, tumor microenvironment, and immune response, and their relationship to tumor radioresistance, readers are referred to Chaps. 11–13.

2 Intrinsic or Cellular Radioresistance

Despite advances in radiation therapy leading to more efficient eradication of cancer and improved patient outcomes, a significant percentage of tumors are still able to withstand treatment which eventually leads to recurrent disease. In addition to extrinsic or microenvironmental factors such as hypoxia (reviewed in Chap. 11), tissue stiffness or the composition of the extracellular matrix, intrinsic, or cellular characteristics, such as DNA repair capacity or pro-survival signaling, constitute an important determinant of a tumor's ability to survive irradiation (Kirsch et al. 2018).

Analyzing in vitro survival curves, Fertil and Malaise found that cell lines derived from human cancer patients vary in their radiosensitivity, in particular in the low dose range which could not be explained by external or technical parameters (Fertil and Malaise 1981). Comparison between the surviving fraction after 2 Gy (SF2) and clinical data of different cancer types revealed a significant association between high in vitro radiosensitivity and a low radiation dose necessary to obtain a 95% tumor control probability (TCD 95%). These results were confirmed by Deacon and colleagues who showed that the initial slope of the survival curve correlates with clinical radiosensitivity but not clonogenic survival at higher doses (Deacon et al. 1984). Although attempts to use the SF2 as well as the colony-forming efficiency of tumors to predict local control and patient survival after radiation therapy showed encouraging prognostic value (Björk-Eriksson et al. 2000; Buffa et al. 2001), these parameters have not been implemented into standard clinical care. Reasons for this included the challenges to establish an easy-to-perform, automated, and observer-independent assay to measure clonogenic survival as well as the long time which is required to allow the colonies to grow, making this approach impracticable for clinical routine.

An alternative, genomics-based method has been pursued by Torres-Roca and others (Eschrich et al. 2009; Torres-Roca 2012; Hall et al. 2018). These investigators determined clonogenic SF2 values in a panel of 48 annotated human cancer cell lines. A gene expression signature consisting of 10 genes was identified and used to build a rank-based linear regression algorithm to predict a radiosensitivity index (RSI) where high index signals are relative to radioresistance. Eschrich et al. showed in a retrospective analysis that RSI correlates with 5-year disease-free survival of breast cancer patients treated with radiation therapy but has no association with survival of patients treated without irradiation (Eschrich et al. 2012). Further, RSI was found to be an independent predictor for the clinical outcome of radiation treated-patients suffering from a number of different cancer types including radio-resistant glioblastoma, pancreatic adenocarcinoma, triple-negative breast cancer, and metastatic colon cancer (Ahmed et al. 2015a, b, 2019; Strom et al. 2015). Recently, a genomic-adjusted radiation dose (GARD) was derived from the RSI and linear quadratic model. A patient-specific GARD served as a marker for the expected individual tumor sensitivity to radiation and was found to be associated with sur-vival and local control endpoints (Ahmed et al. 2019; Scott et al. 2017). This data strongly suggests that a one-size-fits-all radiation dose prescription is suboptimal for at least some patients given the genomic heterogeneity in intrinsic radiosensitiv-ity observed.

Thus, there exists accumulating evidence that assessing the intrinsic radiosensi-tivity of tumors may be useful to identify radioresistant tumors and select those patients for intensified multimodal cancer therapy including treatment with targeted radiosensitizers. Nevertheless, prospective studies are warranted to confirm that use of these methods for treatment planning results in a significant benefit in clinical outcome.

3 Cancer Stem Cells and Radioresistance

In recent years, the significance of CSCs, or CSC-like cells, for radiation and che-motherapy resistance resulting in treatment failure and disease relapse has emerged. Because CSCs have a capability for unlimited cell division and are able to differen-tiate into heterogeneous cancer cell types, one surviving CSC can potentially rebuild a complete tumor (Fig. 4.2) (Clarke et al. 2006). Therefore, as the goal for success-ful curative therapy is to eradicate all CSCs, a lot of effort has been made to develop novel treatment strategies that specifically target CSCs. A preferred method to iden-tify and isolate CSCs in tumors for studying their unique molecular characteristics is using the expression of cell surface markers and proteins. For example, the cluster of differentiation (CD)133 has been linked to CSC-like behavior of glioblastoma and colon cancer cells (Singh et al. 2004; O'Brien et al. 2007), while tumorigenic breast cancer cells exhibit a combination of high CD44 and low CD24 levels (Al-Hajj et al. 2003). Moreover, it has been shown that CSCs of several cancer types have an enhanced activity of aldehyde dehydrogenase 1 (ALDH1) which is why measuring the enzymatic activity of ALDH1 can be exploited to identify CSC-like cells (Huang et al. 2009).

A variety of different mechanisms have been reported to promote the radioresis-tance of CSCs. For instance, CSCs of breast cancers have lower concentrations of reactive oxygen species (ROS) than non-tumorigenic cells by overexpression of free radical scavenging systems (Diehn et al. 2009). Since ROS are crucial for the effi-cacy of ionizing radiation, CSCs exhibited less radiation-induced DNA damage, while inhibition of ROS scavengers resulted in radiosensitization of CSCs. Similarly,

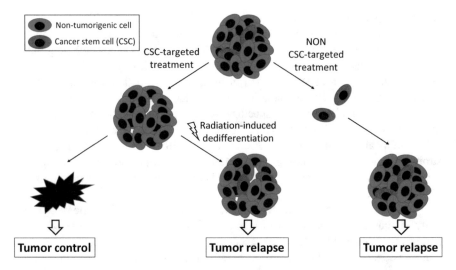

Fig. 4.2 Illustration of the response of cancer stem cells (CSC) to radiation treatment

Chang and colleagues found that squamous cell carcinoma cells of the head and neck with low ROS levels frequently expressed CSC markers and had high tumorigenicity (Chang et al. 2014). Further, there have been studies showing increased DNA repair in CSCs which may also contribute to the observed radioresistance (Bao et al. 2006; Yin and Glass 2011). In glioma, CD133-positive tumor cells are enriched after radiation treatment indicating that these cells may survive irradiation to a greater extent (Bao et al. 2006). Additionally, CD133-expressing glioma cells showed a significantly increased radiation-induced phosphorylation of ataxia-telangiectasia-mutated (ATM), CHK1, and CHK2 and a more efficient repair of DNA breaks than CD133-negative cells. In line with these results, ATM signaling is also enhanced in CSC-like CD44⁺/CD24⁻ breast cancer cells resulting in higher radiation resistance, whereas ATM inhibition reverses this effect (Yin and Glass 2011).

Although increased DNA repair capacity and reduced DNA damage induction can explain the enrichment of CSCs after radiation therapy, there is also evidence that cancer cell plasticity may play a role for this finding (Fig. 4.2) (Vlashi and Pajonk 2015). Interestingly in breast cancer, radiation has been shown to upregulate CSC markers and enable differentiated cancer cells to re-acquire stem-like characteristics (Lagadec et al. 2012). Similar results were obtained in hepatocellular carcinoma cells (Ghisolfi et al. 2012). One mechanism how irradiation might trigger non-tumorigenic cells to dedifferentiate and turn into CSCs or CSC-like cells is the induction of epithelial–mesenchymal transition (EMT). Mani and colleagues showed that forced EMT of immortalized human mammary epithelial cells not only enhanced the ability to form mammospheres but also resulted in expression of various CSC markers (Mani et al. 2008). Additionally, stem-like normal and cancer cells obtained from mammary gland tissue or mamma carcinoma expressed EMT markers indicating an association between EMT and stem cell properties. In line with these results, radiation therapy has been shown to induce EMT in endometrial carcinoma, breast cancer, and lung carcinoma, and impacts tumor radioresistance (Chiba et al. 2012; Jung et al. 2007; Theys et al. 2011; Tsukamoto et al. 2007; Zhang et al. 2011).

4 Cancer Stem Cells: Tumor Volume and Repopulation

Human tumors are thought to contain variable fractions of CSCs (Baumann et al. 2016; Krause et al. 2017). Therefore, radioresistance increases with enlarging tumor volume, i.e., an increasing number of CSCs, which has been consistently shown in experimental (immunodeficient) mouse models and in clinical cohorts, particularly non-small lung carcinoma (NSCLC) (Yaromina et al. 2007; Baumann et al. 1990; Alexander et al. 2011; Dubben et al. 1998; Johnson et al. 1995; Soliman et al. 2013; Werner-Wasik et al. 2008). At the same time, for tumors of equal volume, a higher density of CSCs will negatively impact local control after radiation therapy. It follows that larger tumors, with a higher fraction of CSCs, will require a higher dose of radiation (or/and a radiosensitizing drug) to maintain adequate levels of local tumor control compared to smaller tumors (Willers et al. 2013).

The time over which the total dose of radiation is delivered becomes important if there is repopulation of CSCs within the irradiated tumor during a several-week course of radiation therapy (Willers et al. 2013; Willers and Held 2006). CSC repopulation is likely an adaptive response to the cytotoxic effects of radiation and may be due to several factors including cellular plasticity where radiation transforms bulk tumor cells into CSCs and a reduction of the fraction of cells lost from the tumor. Because repopulation compensates for radiation-induced cell death during fractionated treatment, it leads to an increased likelihood of CSCs and local relapse. Repopulation is accelerated when the doubling time of the proliferative cell pool is shorter than the doubling time before the start of radiation therapy. During treatment, the doubling time of the CSC fraction may be as short as 4–5 days (so-called T_{pot}) compared with an average doubling time of many months or even longer prior to treatment. As a result, repopulation can compensate for ~0.6–1 Gy per day in some tumor types such as head and neck squamous cell cancers (HNSCC) (Withers et al. 1988). This kind of dose compensation may reduce the TCP by ~1% per day. Clinical and experimental data suggest that accelerated CSC repopulation may commence after a lag period of 3–4 weeks (Withers et al. 1988; Baumann et al. 1994, 2003), but whether some tumors have the ability to repopulate earlier than that remains unknown. Thus, prolonging the overall treatment time will be associated with radioresistance. The role of overall treatment time and the importance of accelerated repopulation are complicated by the administration of chemotherapy in many tumor types. There are data that suggest that overall treatment time is less important when concurrent chemotherapy is administered though this is not universally the case (Nguyen-Tan et al. 2014; Bourhis et al. 2012; Meade et al. 2013; Machtay et al. 2005; Turrisi 3rd et al. 1999).

The tissue, cellular, and molecular mechanisms of accelerated repopulation are poorly studied (Krause et al. 2011; Huang et al. 2011). Interestingly, in head and neck squamous cell carcinoma, shortening the overall treatment time was shown to only benefits patients whose tumors have high expression of epiderma growth factor receptor (EGFR), whereas experimental data suggest that EGFR blockade may reduce tumor cell repopulation (Krause et al. 2005; Bentzen et al. 2005). There are currently no targeted agents in use with radiation to prevent or overcome accelerated repopulation.

5 The KEAP1/NFE2L2 Pathway and its Role in Clinical Radioresistance

5.1 Overview of the KEAP1/NFE2L2 Pathway and Proteins

One radioresistance pathway that is becoming increasingly recognized as clinically significant in oncology is the Kelch-like ECH-associated protein 1/nuclear factor erythroid 2-related factor 2 (*KEAP1/NFE2L2*) pathway, which plays a crucial role in both normal cell and tumor cell oxygen and free radical homeostasis (Itoh et al. 1997). The transcription factor NFE2L2 (also known as NRF2) is responsible for initiating transcription of hundreds of genes involved in cellular stress responses. The far-reaching effects of NFE2L2 activation include free radical detoxification and changes in cellular metabolism with a shift towards non-oxidative metabolism (Best and Sutherland 2018). For example, Blake et al. have shown that cellular stress following exposure to cigarette smoke leads to an increase in NFE2L2 downstream target genes in respiratory epithelial cells due to an increase in free radical formation (Blake et al. 2010). Thus, the KEAP1/NFE2L2 pathway is a critical component of cellular stress responses.

The NFE2L2 protein is 605 amino acids in length and contains seven conserved regions known as NRF2-ECH homology domains (Neh). The C-terminal Neh1 domain contains a basic leucine zipper (bZip) and mediates hetero-dimerization with Maf proteins. This heterodimer binds antioxidant response elements (AREs) in promoters and leads to the transcription of downstream targets (Canning et al. 2015). In the absence of oxidative stress, NFE2L2 proteins are bound by KEAP1 homodimers that contact NFE2L2 at the N-terminal Neh2 domain (Fig. 4.3) (Eggler et al. 2005; Itoh et al. 1999). The Neh2 domain contains two motifs responsible for KEAP1 binding. The first is the ETGE motif, which extends from residues Asp77 to Glu82 (with conserved Glu79 and Glu82) and mediates strong binding via hydrogen bonds to the one member of the KEAP1 homodimer (Canning et al. 2015; Fukutomi et al. 2014). The second is the DLG motif, which extends from Trp24 to Arg34 and binds the second KEAP1 protein more weakly.

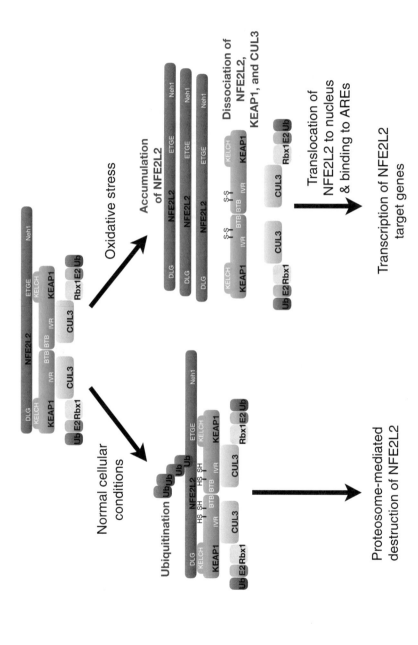

Fig. 4.3 Schematic of the KEAP1 and NFE2L2 pathway under normal homeostasis (left pathway) and during oxidative stress (right pathway)

KEAP1 is a member of the BTB-Kelch family of proteins and is 624 amino acids in length. KEAP1 serves as an adapter protein to recruit substrates for the Cullin3 (CUL3)-based E3 ubiquitin ligase, resulting in ubiquitination and subsequent proteasomal destruction of targets such as NFE2L2 (Kobayashi et al. 2004). KEAP1 contains highly conserved cysteine residues in its BTB domain that mediate homodimerization and binding to CUL3 under normal cellular conditions (Fig. 4.3). It binds NFE2L2 via 6 Kelch repeats that form a 6-bladed *beta*-propeller structure (Canning et al. 2015). However, when exposed to oxidative stress, key cysteine residues in KEAP1 become oxidized resulting in a conformational change that disrupts binding of KEAP1 and CUL3 (Eggler et al. 2005; Eggler et al. 2009). This results in accumulation of NFE2L2 proteins, facilitating translocation from the cytoplasm, binding to AREs, and transcription of *NFE2L2* target genes (Best and Sutherland 2018; Kobayashi et al. 2004).

5.2 Mutations in the KEAP1/NFE2L2 Pathway and Their Role in Cancer

Mutations in *KEAP1* or *NFE2L2* occur most commonly in NSCLC but are also seen recurrently in a number of other tumor types (Fig. 4.4) (Hoadley et al. 2018). In NSCLC, mutations in *KEAP1* and *NFE2L2* are mutually exclusive, and *KEAP1* mutations occur more frequently in adenocarcinoma while mutations in *NFE2L2* are more frequently observed in squamous cell carcinoma (Campbell et al. 2016; Hoadley et al. 2018). The exact role of these mutations in cancer development remains to be elucidated as activation of the KEAP1/NFE2L2 pathway is by itself insufficient for tumorigenesis. However, several mouse studies have shown that deletion of *Keap1* synergizes with mutations in other pathways such as *Trp53* or *Pik3ca* (Best et al. 2018; Jeong et al. 2017).

Mutations in *KEAP1* or *NFE2L2* are typically loss of function and gain of function, respectively (Shibata et al. 2008). However, the resultant phenotype is similar, leading to upregulation of *NFE2L2* target genes. The mutational pattern in *NFE2L2* is akin to an oncogene, with hotspots occurring in the ETGE and the DGR motifs (located within the Neh2 domain, Fig. 4.5a). These mutations disrupt binding between NFE2L2 and KEAP1, interfere with the ubiquitination of NFE2L2, and lead to its constitutive activation. In contrast, *KEAP1* mutations occur throughout the protein and have a pattern akin to a tumor suppressor, including gain of stop codon mutations. This is consistent with KEAP1's role as a suppressor of NFE2L2 function (Fig. 4.5b) (Eggler et al. 2005, 2009; Best and Sutherland 2018; Canning et al. 2015). Interestingly, three categories of pathogenic *KEAP1* mutations have been described: (1) dominant-negative, (2) loss of function, (3) hypomorph (Berger et al. 2016; Cloer et al. 2018; Hast et al. 2014). Thus, there is a spectrum of pathologic phenotypes of *KEAP1* mutations and their effect on clinical phenotypes has not been well studied.

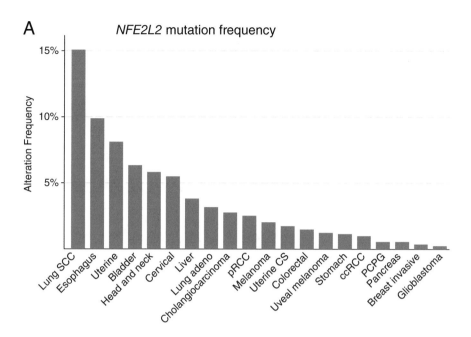

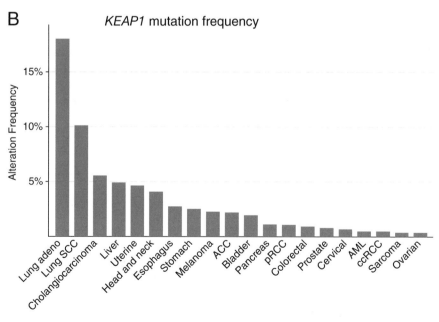

Fig. 4.4 Frequency of point mutations and insertion/deletions for the 20 cancer types most frequently harboring *KEAP1/NFE2L2* somatic tumor mutations reported by The Cancer Genome Atlas PanCancer Atlas (figure generated via cbioportal.org) (Hoadley et al. 2018). *adeno* adenocarcinoma, *SCC* squamous cell carcinoma, *Uterine CC* uterine clear cell, *PCPG* Pheochromocytoma and Paraganglioma, *ACC* adrenocortical carcinoma, *pRCC* renal papillary cell carcinoma, *ccRCC* clear cell renal cell carcinoma

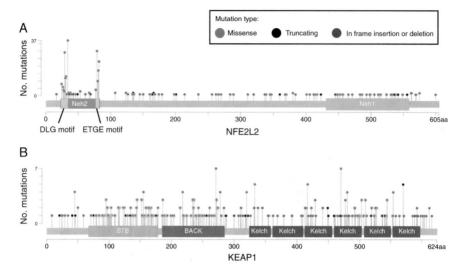

Fig. 4.5 Distribution of *KEAP1* (panel **a**) and *NFE2L2* (panel **b**) and mutations reported by The Cancer Genome Atlas PanCancer Atlas (Modified figure generated via cbioportal.org) (Hoadley et al. 2018)

Ultimately, loss-of-function mutations in *KEAP1* or gain-of-function mutations in *NFE2L2* result in similar gene expression phenotypes (Namani et al. 2018). Of note, some studies have found associations between *NFE2L2* pathway gene expression and prognosis in cancers where *KEAP1/NFE2L2* mutations are not common, suggesting that there may be mutation-independent mechanisms of NFE2L2 activation that could be of clinical relevance (O'Cathail et al. 2019; Yang et al. 2011; Zhang et al. 2018).

5.3 Clinical Evidence of KEAP1/NFE2L2 Mutant Resistance to Therapy

Cancer therapy including some cytotoxic chemotherapies and radiation therapy generate free radicals that result in tumor cell killing. Thus, a tumor cell with upregulation of the NFE2L2 pathway would be expected to have inherent resistance to therapies that rely on free radical induced DNA damage. Focusing on resistance to radiation, several in vitro studies using human lung cancer cell lines have suggested that these mutations promote a cancer cell-intrinsic radioresistant phenotype that is dependent on NFE2L2-mediated transcription (Singh et al. 2010; Abazeed et al. 2013). More recently, data supporting a role of *KEAP1* loss-of-function mutations in radioresistance also come from a genetically engineered mouse model of lung squamous cell carcinoma based on deletion of *Keap1* and *Trp53* (Jeong et al. 2017). In these tumors, *Keap1* deletion results in upregulation of NFE2L2-mediated transcription, decrease in baseline ROS levels, and radioresistance both in clonogenic assays and in vivo.

While mounting preclinical data suggest a role for *KEAP1/NFE2L2* mutations in radioresistance, until recently clinical data supporting this hypothesis were lacking. The clinical outcome that should most specifically reflect radioresistance is local recurrence within an irradiated volume. Distant recurrence outside of the high dose treatment volume can be due to micrometastases that were present prior to radiation therapy and therefore does not clearly reflect radioresistance of tumor cells. Along these lines, in 2017 Jeong et al. reported on a cohort of 42 localized NSCLC patients whose tumors were genotyped for *KEAP1* and *NFE2L2* mutations and who were treated with radiation therapy (Jeong et al. 2017). Strikingly, patients with *KEAP1/NFE2L2* mutant tumors had extremely high rates of in-field local recurrence (~60%) compared to patients with wild-type tumors (~20%). Similar results were observed in an independent cohort of 20 patients genotyped using circulating tumor DNA, providing initial evidence of validation of this finding. Both cohorts included patients treated with conventionally fractionated radiation therapy or stereotactic body radiation therapy (SBRT) but were not powered to determine a difference between these two types of approaches. Similar evidence for increased local recurrence of *KEAP1/NFE2L2* mutant tumors following radiation therapy in other tumor types remain limited to date although two studies only published in abstract form, one in head and neck cancer and another in metastatic NSCLC, suggest similar results (Farquhar et al. 2018; Anderson et al. 2018). Furthermore, although there have been several reports suggesting gene expression of *NFE2L2* target genes may identify patients with poorer prognoses after radiation therapy, none of these studies have specifically examined local tumor control, and therefore it remains unclear if *NFE2L2* gene expression in the absence of *KEAP1/NFE2L2* mutations is associated with increased local recurrence (Anderson et al. 2018; Namani et al. 2018; O'Cathail et al. 2019; Singh et al. 2010; Zhang et al. 2018). Finally, regarding resistance to systemic therapy, there have been multiple reports of worse response to chemotherapy or EGFR tyrosine kinase inhibitor in *KEAP1/NFE2L2* mutant metastatic NSCLC (Bollong et al. 2015; Goeman et al. 2019; Jeong et al. 2020).

5.4 Strategies to Overcome KEAP1/NFE2L2 Resistance to Therapy

Given the radioresistant phenotype of tumors with *KEAP1/NFE2L2* mutations, approaches for overcoming the high local failure rates observed clinically are urgently needed. One potential strategy is dose escalation although it remains to be seen if more intense dose regimens such as SBRT can overcome *KEAP1/NFE2L2*-mediated radioresistance. A second potential strategy involves radiosensitization using pharmacologic agents and a variety of strategies for inhibiting the KEAP1/NFE2L2 pathway have been explored preclinically. For example, depletion of

NFE2L2 using siRNA or shRNA can radiosensitize cells with *KEAP1* or *NFE2L2* alterations (Abazeed et al. 2013; Singh et al. 2010; Jeong et al. 2017). However, clinical translation of such approaches remains challenging. Potentially more readily translatable, several small molecule inhibitors have been identified that can inhibit cells with NFE2L2 activation (Abazeed et al. 2013; Bollong et al. 2015; Lee et al. 2012; Moore et al. 2018; Singh et al. 2016; Sun et al. 2016). Currently, none of these approaches are being tested clinically in the context of radiation therapy. However, two drugs are being tested as monotherapy in patients with metastatic NSCLC. The first is based on the observation that *KEAP1* mutant tumor cells exhibit increased dependence on glutaminolysis that can be targeted using pharmacologic inhibitors of glutaminase (Romero et al. 2017; Shibata et al. 2010). A phase 2 basket trial testing the glutaminase inhibitor CB-839 in patients with advanced *KEAP1* mutant tumors is currently underway (NCT03872427). Separately, preclinical data suggest that *KEAP1/NFE2L2* mutations lead to mTOR pathway activation and induce sensitivity to mTOR inhibitors (Shibata et al. 2010). This work has motivated a phase 2 trial testing the activity of the mTOR inhibitor sapanisertib in patients with metastatic NSCLC harboring *KEAP1/NFE2L2* mutations (NCT02417701).

5.5 Conclusions

Preclinical and emerging clinical evidence suggests that tumors harboring *KEAP1/ NFE2L2* mutations are resistant to radiation therapy and other treatments that involve production of free radicals. Currently, the strongest evidence for the association of *KEAP1/NFE2L2* mutations with clinical radioresistance is in NSCLC, but it is likely these mutations have similar effects in other tumor types in which they are recurrently mutated. In addition to further validation of these observations, approaches for overcoming *KEAP1/NFE2L2* mutation-mediated radioresistance are urgently needed.

6 *KRAS* Mutations and Their Role in Clinical Radioresistance

6.1 The KRAS Oncogene and Cellular Radioresistance

Another radioresistance pathway with emerging clinical significance is defined by the *KRAS* gene, which encodes a GTPase involved in relaying signals from the cell membrane to the nucleus (Stephen et al. 2014; Simanshu et al. 2017). Upon the introduction of point mutations, most commonly at codons 12 and 13, the KRAS protein becomes constitutively active and acquires oncogenic properties. *KRAS* is commonly mutated in many malignancies, including approximately 30% of NSCLC, 40% of colorectal cancers, and 95% of pancreatic cancers (Stephen et al. 2014). *KRAS* mutant cancers often exhibit poor drug responses and prognosis (Blons et al. 2014; Eberhard et al. 2005; Han et al. 2006; Richman et al. 2009; Tao et al. 2007; Winton et al. 2005).

For more than two decades, it has been known that *KRAS* mutation also promotes cellular resistance to ionizing radiation (Bernhard et al. 2000; Cengel et al. 2007; Kim et al. 2005). A variety of underlying mechanisms have been proposed to explain KRAS-mediated radioresistance (Grana et al. 2002; Kim et al. 2005; Kleiman et al. 2013; Minjgee et al. 2011; Toulany et al. 2005; Williams et al. 2012; Xu et al. 2011). Some groups have suggested a role of PI3K-AKT and FAK pathways in mediating DNA double-strand break (DSB) repair and radioresistance downstream of KRAS (Minjgee et al. 2011; Tang et al. 2016; Toulany et al. 2005). However, the potentially complex roles of AKT in DSB repair remain far from being understood, and how FAK connects to DSB repair is poorly defined as well (Fraser et al. 2011; Plo et al. 2008; Toulany et al. 2008, 2012; Xiang et al. 2008). Another mechanism was proposed by Wang et al. who reported that *KRAS* mutation was associated with a suppression of the induction of DSBs rather than an enhancement of DSB repair in NSCLC models (Wang et al. 2014). In that study, the suppression of DSB induction was dependent on EGFR and PKCα signaling in KRAS mutant cells and potentially related to chromatin condensation that shielded genomic DNA from ionizing radiation. In a follow-up study, Wang et al. tied KRAS mutant-dependent radioresistance to an osteopontin- and EGFR-mediated CSC-like phenotype (Wang et al. 2017). This data is consistent with accumulating observations that link KRAS to CSC-like properties (Ali et al. 2016; Barcelo et al. 2013; Moon et al. 2014; Seguin et al. 2014; Stephen et al. 2014; Wang et al. 2015). In contrast, in a large screen of more than 500 cancer cell lines, *KRAS* mutation was unexpectedly not found to be associated with radioresistance (Yard et al. 2016). Taken together, these conflicting observations may be related to the complexity of KRAS function and heterogeneity across KRAS mutant tumors, which are only recently being more appreciated.

6.2 In Vivo and Clinical Radioresistance Associated with KRAS Mutation

Despite extensive preclinical work on the link between *KRAS* mutation and radioresistance over the past two decades, evidence that *KRAS* status can indeed impact local tumor control has been lacking until recently. Table 4.1 summarizes clinical data mostly in lung and rectal cancers that demonstrate a link between mutant *KRAS* and either pathological tumor response or local control at 1–2 years after radiation treatment (Hong et al. 2017; Mak et al. 2015; Kamran et al. 2019; Russo et al. 2014; Chow et al. 2016; Cassidy et al. 2017; Jethwa et al. 2020). For example, in a prospective phase II trial of SBRT for liver metastases from different tumor types

Table 4.1 Accumulating clinical evidence for the predictive value of *KRAS/TP53* (KP) mutation in cancer patients undergoing radiation therapy

Reference	Institution	Geno-typed pts (*n*)	Cancer type	Radiation	Dose (Gy)	Endpoint	*KRAS* mut vs. wt (%)	KP vs. others (%)
Russo et al., *J Gastrointest Cancer* (2014)	MGH	47	Rectal cancer	Preop RT + 5FU	50.4	pCR	5 vs. 15	N/A
Mak et al., *Clin Lung Cancer* (2015)	DFCI	9	NSCLC	SBRT	Median 54	1-year LC	57 vs. 74	N/A
Chow et al., *Ann Surg Oncol* (2016)	Multicenter	229	Rectal cancer	Preop RT + 5FU	N/A	pCR	15 vs. 34	6 vs. 53
Cassidy et al., *Cancer* (2017)	Emory	45	NSCLC	SBRT	Median 50	2-year LC	44 vs. 74	N/A
Hong et al., *JNCI* (2017)	MGH Phase II Trial	57	Liver metastases	SBRT protons	Median 50	1-year LC	43 vs. 72	20 vs. 69
Kamran et al., *Clin Cancer Res* (2019)	MGH/ Broad	17	Rectal cancer	Preop RT + 5FU	50.4	Path response	30 vs. 71	14 vs. 64
Jethwa et al., *Radiother Oncol* (2020)	Mayo	85	Colorectal metastases	SBRT	Median 50	2-year LC	NS	56 vs. 89

Pts patients, *NSCLC* non-small cell lung carcinoma, *Preop* preoperative, *RT* radiation therapy, *5FU* 5-fluorouracil, *SBRT* stereotactic body radiation therapy, *pCR* pathologically complete response, *LC* local control, *mut* mutant, *wt* wild-type, *N/A* not applicable, *NS* no statistically significant

including NSCLC, colorectal cancers, and pancreatic cancer, Hong and colleagues were able to obtain *KRAS* mutation status for 57 out of a total of 89 tumors using a next-generation sequencing-based clinical assay (Hong et al. 2017). The presence of a *KRAS* mutation in codon 12, 13, or 61 was the strongest predictor of inferior local treatment outcome, with a 1-year local control rate of 43% vs. 72% for tumors without detected mutation ($p = 0.02$). In support of the patient data, Gurtner et al. conducted a co-clinical trial using a clinical radiation regimen with a range of total doses delivered in 30 fractions over 6 weeks to nude mice harboring NSCLC xenografts (Gurtner et al. 2020) (Fig. 4.6). To locally control 50% of KRAS wild-type xenografts, a dose of 43.1 Gy (TCD_{50}) was required while KRAS mutant tumors needed a 1.9-fold higher TCD_{50} of 81.4 Gy.

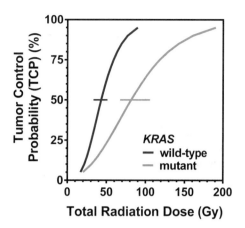

Fig. 4.6 Tumor control probability curves in a heterotopic lung cancer xenograft model treated with 30 fractions of radiation. Tumors were either *KRAS* mutant or wild-type in a *TP53* mutant background. (Redrawn from Gurtner et al. (2020))

6.3   Inter-tumoral heterogeneity and the Role of KRAS/TP53 (KP) Co-Mutation

KRAS mutant tumors are heterogenous with regard to their treatment sensitivity which may depend on histology, specific allelic mutation, and co-mutations in other cancer genes (Stephen et al. 2014; Haigis 2017; Skoulidis and Heymach 2019). In NSCLC, there exists growing evidence for distinct KRAS subgroups depending on co-mutation of either the *TP53* or *LKB1* (*STK-11*) tumor suppressor gene (Skoulidis et al. 2015, 2018). In addition, *KEAP1* co-mutation or increased MYC activity may impact the immune environment of these cancers (Skoulidis and Heymach 2019). Loss of *TP53* is associated with an inflamed tumor microenvironment and increased PD-L1 expression in tumor cells. As a result, these tumors show high response rates to immune checkpoint inhibition (Skoulidis et al. 2018).

At the same time, co-occurrence of *TP53* mutation has been linked with increased resistance to radiation compared to wild-type *TP53* in lung and rectal cancers (Chow et al. 2016; Jethwa et al. 2020; Kamran et al. 2018; Wang et al. 2017; Hong et al. 2017) (Table 4.1). In a preclinical study of 17 NSCLC cell lines, KP mutant status was associated with the highest clonogenic survival fraction (Gurtner et al. 2020). In two retrospective clinical analyses, poor pathological response following neoadjuvant concurrent chemotherapy and radiation was more common in rectal cancer patients with KP mutant tumors (Chow et al. 2016; Kamran et al. 2019). In one of these, Kamran et al. performed integrated genomic profiling of tumors before and after chemoradiation (Kamran et al. 2019). Interestingly, one *KRAS*-mutated tumor with a non-response harbored a *TP53* mutation post-chemoradiation that was not detected in the pre-treatment tumor despite sufficient power to detect a mutation, suggesting the emergence of a radioresistant subclone. The analysis also suggested that local immune escape during or after chemoradiation in KP mutant tumors may contribute to distant disease progression. Two additional clinical cohorts have shown reduced local tumor control after irradiation of metastases. In the prospective trial by Hong et al., patients with KP mutant tumors experienced a 1-year local control rate of 20% after SBRT compared to 69% for all other genotypes ($p = 0.001$) (Hong et al. 2017). In a retrospective cohort of colorectal metastases treated with SBRT, 1-year local control was 56% and 89% for KP mutants versus all other tumors, respectively ($p = 0.04$) (Jethwa et al. 2020). In this context, the radioresistance of pancreatic adenocarcinomas, which are characterized by a very high prevalence of KP mutations, is noteworthy (Seshacharyulu et al. 2017). It remains to be elucidated whether *TP53* mutation is merely a marker for radioresistance or directly modulates radiation response in *KRAS* mutant tumors. While DNA repair functions have been ascribed to TP53, it is unclear if *TP53* status in of itself can affect radioresistance (Dahm-Daphi et al. 2005; DiBiase et al. 1999).

There currently exist no good data to define the radioresistance of *KRAS/LKB1* (KL) mutant NSCLCs. These tumors are distinct from KP tumors by virtue of resistance to anti-PD-1 and anti-PD-L1 therapies (Skoulidis et al. 2018). They exhibit impaired innate immunity (Kitajima et al. 2019), and this could conceivably affect clinical radiation responsiveness. In addition, somatic mutations in *LKB1* and *KEAP1* commonly co-occur in *KRAS* mutant NSCLC which is expected to impact radioresistance (Skoulidis and Heymach 2019). In a genetically engineered mouse model of NSCLCs with different genotypes, Wong and others observed rapid regrowth of KL tumors >6 weeks following 17 Gy in two fractions which was not seen in KP tumors or *KRAS* mutant tumors that were otherwise wild-type (Herter-Sprie et al. 2014). Experimental local tumor control data for KL mutants are not available to the best of the authors' knowledge.

6.4 Targeting of KRAS Mutant Cancers

There has been a longstanding interest in using molecular targeted agents to overcome the radioresistance of KRAS mutant tumors and cells (Minjgee et al. 2011; Tang et al. 2016; Toulany et al. 2005, 2006; Cengel et al. 2007); however, no treatment combination has yet been clinically successful. Here, we highlight four potential approaches based on more recent preclinical data:

6.4.1 MEK Inhibitor Trametinib

In a high-content clonogenic radiation/drug screen, Lin and colleagues identified several MEK inhibitors as radiosensitizers in KRAS mutant NSCLC cells (Lin et al. 2014). One of these, trametinib, sensitized KRAS mutant NSCLC to radiation both in vitro and in vivo (Lin et al. 2014; Wang et al. 2018). Importantly, trametinib also sensitized xenografts to chemoradiation which is the standard-of-care treatment for locally advanced NSCLC. Furthermore, on the basis of 8 KP and KL models trametinib appeared to preferentially sensitize tumors with an *LKB1* co-mutation (Wang et al. 2018). Mechanistically, MEK inhibition and radiation caused premature senescence, from which cells could be rescued through an AMPK autophagy pathway in *LKB1* wild-type but not in KL mutant tumors. Trametinib is currently in a phase I clinical trial in combination with chemoradiation for locally advanced NSCLC (NCT01912625).

6.4.2 Multikinase Inhibitor Midostaurin

In an in vitro screen of 12 NSCLC cell lines, Liu et al. identified the multikinase inhibitor midostaurin, FDA approved for the treatment of FLT3-positive acute myeloid leukemia, as a preferential radiosensitizer of cells harboring *KRAS* codon 12/13 mutations (Liu et al. 2015). This was confirmed in isogenic cell pairs and a clonogenic suvival assay. Midostaurin also increased the number of residual radiation-induced DNA double-strand breaks (DSB) and caused apoptosis or senescence in irradiated *KRAS* mutant cells. Further study suggested that PKCα is the relevant radiosensitization target of midostaurin (Liu et al. 2015; Wang et al. 2014). Even though the radiosensitizing effect of midostaurin was not validated in vivo, a clinical phase Ib trial of this compound in conjunction with neoadjuvant chemoradiation was completed in 19 rectal cancer patients (NCT01282502) (Hong et al. 2018). Treatment was well tolerated, and all patients underwent surgical resection. Correlation of pathological response with tumor genotype suggests that midostaurin has efficacy in *KRAS* mutant cancers (Kamran et al., unpublished).

6.4.3 EGFR Inhibitor Erlotinib

Wang et al. screened 40 NSCLC cell lines to assess the radiosensitizing properties of the EGFR tyrosine kinase inhibitor erlotinib and the anti-EGFR monoclonal antibody cetuximab (Wang et al. 2014). Unexpectedly, radiosensitization by these agents was correlated with *KRAS* mutation, which was confirmed in several isogenic cell pairs and additional assays. The radiosensitizing effect of erlotinib was validated by Gurtner et al. who treated nude mice bearing isogenic NSCLC xenografts with or without mutant *KRAS* (in a *TP53* mutant background) (Gurtner et al. 2020). Erlotinib reduced the TCD_{50} by 1.4-fold, a degree of magnitude that was similar to that observed in vitro. Cetuximab unexpectedly did not have any radiosensitizing effect, consistent with prior xenograft and clinical data (Kriegs et al. 2015; Bradley et al. 2020). In a subset analysis of the CALGB 30106 phase II clinical trial, patients with locally advanced NSCLC were treated with chemoradiation and the EGFR inhibitor gefitinib (Ready et al. 2010). Only 45 patients had *KRAS* status available with a mutation present in just 7 patients. There was no difference in overall and progress-free survival between *KRAS* wild-type and mutant tumors but the sample size was too small to derive any meaningful conclusions. The sensitivity of *KRAS* mutant cancer cells to radiation/erlotinib seen preclinically stands in contrast to the known resistance of KRAS mutant cancers to EGFR inhibitors in monotherapy (Aviel-Ronen et al. 2006). Cancer cells with activating mutations in *KRAS* become independent of upstream EGFR signaling for growth and survival and thus resistant to EGFR inhibitors alone. However, it appears that in some settings EGFR maintains survival promoting functions that are independent of canonical PI3K-AKT and MEK-ERK signaling downstream of mutant KRAS. Wang and colleagues proposed a pathway in which EGFR and PKCα signaling protected KRAS mutant cells from the induction of potentially lethal DSB by ionizing radiation (Wang et al. 2014).

6.4.4 DNA Damage Response (DDR) Inhibitors

There has been renewed interest in the clinical testing of DDR inhibitors. While their efficacy and safety in conjunction with chemoradiation remains to be established, potentially increased toxicity may be justified in the treatment of radioresistant tumors such as those with *KRAS* mutations. Alternatively, *KRAS* mutant tumors conceivably could harbor altered DDR responses that can be therapeutically exploited. For example, *ATM* mutations are found in these tumors which may provide an opportunity for ATR or PARP inhibitors (Skoulidis and Heymach 2019). There has also been a growing notion that *KRAS* mutant tumors exhibit increased DNA replication stress which affects radioresistance and could make them vulnerable to inhibitors of kinases involved in replication (Grabocka et al. 2015; Carruthers et al. 2018; Wurster et al. 2016). Potentially related to this notion, preclinical in vitro data suggest that inhibitors of CHK1 kinase may be effective radiosensitizers in these tumors (Dinkelborg et al. 2019; Kleiman et al. 2013).

6.5 Conclusions

More than 20 years since the realization that *KRAS* mutation confers cellular radioresistance, there is now emerging clinical evidence that this relationship holds in patients. Owing to routine clinical testing for *KRAS* in metastatic cancer patients there exists considerable opportunity to leverage this genomic data for informing radiation therapy decisions. This is best done in a prospective fashion. Furthermore, KRAS-like signaling alterations and associated radioresistance may exist in tumor types that do not harbor mutations in *KRAS*, such as *BRAF* mutant cancers or triple-negative breast cancer (Dinkelborg et al. 2019; Robb et al. 2019). This is likely a rewarding space for future studies into molecular markers of clinical radioresistance.

7 Outlook

A number of predictive biomarkers already exist or are emerging for clinical use in radiation oncology (Baumann et al. 2016; Kirsch et al. 2018; Krause et al. 2017; Hall et al. 2018). While it may ultimately not be possible to predict dose-tumor response curves in individual patients, stratifying patients into subsets of high, intermediate, and low tumor radiosensitivity would be extremely helpful to guide decision-making. Biomarker combinations to define these patient strata would include tumor volume, hypoxia markers, genomic markers such as *KEAP1*, *KRAS*, and others, as well as measures of intrinsic radiosensitivity such as RSI. For certain tumor types, such as head and neck cancer squamous cell cancers, HPV status will also impact radiation approaches. Targeted radiosensitizers will have particular utility in patient subsets with radioresistant tumors. For some of these, it may be possible to develop radiosensitizer treatments with tumor specificity, for example, through targeting *KRAS* or *KEAP1* mutation-specific signaling pathways which are not or less active in normal tissues, thereby achieving therapeutic gain. Ultimately, prospective intervention studies will be needed to test the predictive value of these biomarkers.

References

Abazeed ME, Adams DJ, Hurov KE, Tamayo P, Creighton CJ, Sonkin D, Giacomelli AO, Du C, Fries DF, Wong KK, Mesirov JP, Loeffler JS, Schreiber SL, Hammerman PS, Meyerson M (2013) Integrative radiogenomic profiling of squamous cell lung cancer. Cancer Res 73(20):6289–6298. https://doi.org/10.1158/0008-5472.CAN-13-1616

Ahmed KA, Chinnaiyan P, Fulp WJ, Eschrich S, Torres-Roca JF, Caudell JJ, Ahmed KA, Chinnaiyan P, Fulp WJ, Eschrich S, Torres-Roca JF, Caudell JJ (2015a) The radiosensitivity index predicts for overall survival in glioblastoma. Oncotarget 6:34414–34422. https://doi.org/10.18632/oncotarget.5437

Ahmed KA, Fulp WJ, Berglund AE, Hoffe SE, Dilling TJ, Eschrich SA, Shridhar R, Torres-Roca JF (2015b) Differences between colon cancer primaries and metastases using a molecular assay for tumor radiation sensitivity suggest implications for potential oligometastatic SBRT patient selection. Int J Radiat Oncol Biol Phys 92:837–842. https://doi.org/10.1016/j.ijrobp.2015.01.036

Ahmed KA, Liveringhouse CL, Mills MN, Figura NB, Grass GD, Washington IR, Harris EE, Czerniecki BJ, Blumencranz PW, Eschrich SA, Scott JG, Diaz R, Torres-Roca JF (2019) Utilizing the genomically adjusted radiation dose (GARD) to personalize adjuvant radiotherapy in triple negative breast cancer management. EBioMedicine 47:163–169. https://doi.org/10.1016/j.ebiom.2019.08.019

Alexander BM, Othus M, Caglar HB, Allen AM (2011) Tumor volume is a prognostic factor in non-small-cell lung cancer treated with chemoradiotherapy. Int J Radiat Oncol Biol Phys 79(5):1381–1387. https://doi.org/10.1016/j.ijrobp.2009.12.060

Al-Hajj M, Wicha MS, Benito-Hernandez A, Morrison SJ, Clarke MF (2003) Prospective identification of tumorigenic breast cancer cells. Proc Natl Acad Sci U S A 100:3983–3988. https://doi.org/10.1073/PNAS.0530291100

Ali SA, Justilien V, Jamieson L, Murray NR, Fields AP (2016) Protein kinase Ciota drives a NOTCH3-dependent stem-like phenotype in mutant KRAS lung adenocarcinoma. Cancer Cell 29(3):367–378. https://doi.org/10.1016/j.ccell.2016.02.012

Anderson ES, Lockney NA, Lockney DT, Samstein R, Higginson DS, Bilsky M, Laufer I, Yamada Y, Schmitt A (2018) KEAP1 mutation is correlated to increased rates of local failure after radiation therapy for spine metastases from non-small cell lung cancer. Int J Radiat Oncol Biol Phys 102(3):S187. https://doi.org/10.1016/j.ijrobp.2018.07.072

Aviel-Ronen S, Blackhall FH, Shepherd FA, Tsao MS (2006) K-ras mutations in non-small-cell lung carcinoma: a review. Clin Lung Cancer 8(1):30–38

Bao S, Wu Q, McLendon RE, Hao Y, Shi Q, Hjelmeland AB, Dewhirst MW, Bigner DD, Rich JN (2006) Glioma stem cells promote radioresistance by preferential activation of the DNA damage response. Nature 444:756–760. https://doi.org/10.1038/nature05236

Barcelo C, Paco N, Morell M, Alvarez-Moya B, Bota-Rabassedas N, Jaumot M, Vilardell F, Capella G, Agell N (2013) Phosphorylation at Ser-181 of oncogenic KRAS is required for tumor growth. Cancer Res 74(4):1190–1199

Baumann M, Dubois W, Suit HD (1990) Response of human squamous cell carcinoma xenografts of different sizes to irradiation: relationship of clonogenic cells, cellular radiation sensitivity in vivo, and tumor rescuing units. Radiat Res 123(3):325–330

Baumann M, Liertz C, Baisch H, Wiegel T, Lorenzen J, Arps H (1994) Impact of overall treatment time of fractionated irradiation on local control of human FaDu squamous cell carcinoma in nude mice. Radiother Oncol 32(2):137–143

Baumann M, Dorr W, Petersen C, Krause M (2003) Repopulation during fractionated radiotherapy: much has been learned, even more is open. Int J Radiat Biol 79(7):465–467. https://doi.org/10.1080/0955300031000160259

Baumann M, Krause M, Overgaard J, Debus J, Bentzen SM, Daartz J, Richter C, Zips D, Bortfeld T (2016) Radiation oncology in the era of precision medicine. Nat Rev Cancer 16(4):234–249. https://doi.org/10.1038/nrc.2016.18

Bentzen SM, Atasoy BM, Daley FM, Dische S, Richman PI, Saunders MI, Trott KR, Wilson GD (2005) Epidermal growth factor receptor expression in pretreatment biopsies from head and neck squamous cell carcinoma as a predictive factor for a benefit from accelerated radiation therapy in a randomized controlled trial. J Clin Oncol 23(24):5560–5567. https://doi.org/10.1200/JCO.2005.06.411

Berger AH, Brooks AN, Wu X, Shrestha Y, Chouinard C, Piccioni F, Bagul M, Kamburov A, Imielinski M, Hogstrom L, Zhu C, Yang X, Pantel S, Sakai R, Watson J, Kaplan N, Campbell JD, Singh S, Root DE, Narayan R, Natoli T, Lahr DL, Tirosh I, Tamayo P, Getz G, Wong B, Doench J, Subramanian A, Golub TR, Meyerson M, Boehm JS (2016) High-throughput phenotyping of lung cancer somatic mutations. Cancer Cell 30(2):214–228. https://doi.org/10.1016/j.ccell.2016.06.022

Bernhard EJ, Stanbridge EJ, Gupta S, Gupta AK, Soto D, Bakanauskas VJ, Cerniglia GJ, Muschel RJ, McKenna WG (2000) Direct evidence for the contribution of activated N-ras and K-ras oncogenes to increased intrinsic radiation resistance in human tumor cell lines. Cancer Res 60(23):6597–6600

Best SA, Sutherland KD (2018) "Keaping" a lid on lung cancer: the Keap1-Nrf2 pathway. Cell Cycle 17(14):1696–1707. https://doi.org/10.1080/15384101.2018.1496756

Best SA, De Souza DP, Kersbergen A, Policheni AN, Dayalan S, Tull D, Rathi V, Gray DH, Ritchie ME, McConville MJ, Sutherland KD (2018) Synergy between the KEAP1/NRF2 and PI3K pathways drives non-small-cell lung cancer with an altered immune microenvironment. Cell Metab 27(4):935–943.e934. https://doi.org/10.1016/j.cmet.2018.02.006

Björk-Eriksson T, West C, Karlsson E, Mercke C (2000) Tumor radiosensitivity (SF2) is a prognostic factor for local control in head and neck cancers. Int J Radiat Oncol Biol Phys 46:13–19. https://doi.org/10.1016/s0360-3016(99)00373-9

Blake DJ, Singh A, Kombairaju P, Malhotra D, Mariani TJ, Tuder RM, Gabrielson E, Biswal S (2010) Deletion of Keap1 in the lung attenuates acute cigarette smoke–induced oxidative stress and inflammation. Am J Respir Cell Mol Biol 42(5):524–536. https://doi.org/10.1165/rcmb.2009-0054OC

Blons H, Emile JF, Le Malicot K, Julie C, Zaanan A, Tabernero J, Mini E, Folprecht G, Van Laethem JL, Thaler J, Bridgewater J, Norgard-Petersen L, Van Cutsem E, Lepage C, Zawadi MA, Salazar R, Laurent-Puig P, Taieb J (2014) Prognostic value of KRAS mutations in stage III colon cancer: post hoc analysis of the PETACC8 phase III trial dataset. Ann Oncol 25(12):2378–2385. https://doi.org/10.1093/annonc/mdu464

Bollong MJ, Yun H, Sherwood L, Woods AK, Lairson LL, Schultz PG (2015) A small molecule inhibits deregulated NRF2 transcriptional activity in cancer. ACS Chem Biol 10(10):2193–2198. https://doi.org/10.1021/acschembio.5b00448

Bourhis J, Sire C, Graff P, Gregoire V, Maingon P, Calais G, Gery B, Martin L, Alfonsi M, Desprez P, Pignon T, Bardet E, Rives M, Geoffrois L, Daly-Schveitzer N, Sen S, Tuchais C, Dupuis O, Guerif S, Lapeyre M, Favrel V, Hamoir M, Lusinchi A, Temam S, Pinna A, Tao YG, Blanchard P, Auperin A (2012) Concomitant chemoradiotherapy versus acceleration of radiotherapy with or without concomitant chemotherapy in locally advanced head and neck carcinoma (GORTEC 99-02): an open-label phase 3 randomised trial. Lancet Oncol 13(2):145–153. https://doi.org/10.1016/S1470-2045(11)70346-1

Bradley JD, Hu C, Komaki RR, Masters GA, Blumenschein GR, Schild SE, Bogart JA, Forster KM, Magliocco AM, Kavadi VS, Narayan S, Iyengar P, Robinson CG, Wynn RB, Koprowski CD, Olson MR, Meng J, Paulus R, Curran WJ Jr, Choy H (2020) Long-term results of NRG oncology RTOG 0617: standard- versus high-dose chemoradiotherapy with or without Cetuximab for unresectable stage III non-small-cell lung cancer. J Clin Oncol 38(7):706–714. https://doi.org/10.1200/JCO.19.01162

Buffa FM, Davidson SE, Hunter RD, Nahum AE, West CM (2001) Incorporating biologic measurements (SF(2), CFE) into a tumor control probability model increases their prognostic significance: a study in cervical carcinoma treated with radiation therapy. Int J Radiat Oncol Biol Phys 50:1113–1122. https://doi.org/10.1016/s0360-3016(01)01584-x

Campbell JD, Alexandrov A, Kim J, Wala J, Berger AH, Pedamallu CS, Shukla SA, Guo G, Brooks AN, Murray BA, Imielinski M, Hu X, Ling S, Akbani R, Rosenberg M, Cibulskis C, Ramachandran A, Collisson EA, Kwiatkowski DJ, Lawrence MS, Weinstein JN, Verhaak RGW, Wu CJ, Hammerman PS, Cherniack AD, Getz G, Cancer Genome Atlas Research Network, Artyomov MN, Schreiber R, Govindan R, Meyerson M (2016) Distinct patterns of somatic genome alterations in lung adenocarcinomas and squamous cell carcinomas. Nat Genet 48(6):607–616. https://doi.org/10.1038/ng.3564

Canning P, Sorrell FJ, Bullock AN (2015) Structural basis of Keap1 interactions with Nrf2. Free Radic Biol Med 88:101–107. https://doi.org/10.1016/j.freeradbiomed.2015.05.034

Carruthers RD, Ahmed SU, Ramachandran S, Strathdee K, Kurian KM, Hedley A, Gomez-Roman N, Kalna G, Neilson M, Gilmour L, Stevenson KH, Hammond EM, Chalmers AJ (2018) Replication stress drives constitutive activation of the DNA damage response and radioresistance in glioblastoma stem-like cells. Cancer Res 78(17):5060–5071. https://doi.org/10.1158/0008-5472.CAN-18-0569

Cassidy RJ, Zhang X, Patel PR, Shelton JW, Escott CE, Sica GL, Rossi MR, Hill CE, Steuer CE, Pillai RN, Ramalingam SS, Owonikoko TK, Behera M, Force SD, Fernandez FG, Curran WJ, Higgins KA (2017) Next-generation sequencing and clinical outcomes of patients with lung adenocarcinoma treated with stereotactic body radiotherapy. Cancer 123(19):3681–3690. https://doi.org/10.1002/cncr.30794

Cengel KA, Voong KR, Chandrasekaran S, Maggiorella L, Brunner TB, Stanbridge E, Kao GD, McKenna WG, Bernhard EJ (2007) Oncogenic K-Ras signals through epidermal growth factor receptor and wild-type H-Ras to promote radiation survival in pancreatic and colorectal carcinoma cells. Neoplasia 9(4):341–348

Chang C-W, Chen Y-S, Chou S-H, Han C-L, Chen Y-J, Yang C-C, Huang C-Y, Lo J-F (2014) Distinct subpopulations of head and neck cancer cells with different levels of intracellular reactive oxygen species exhibit diverse stemness, proliferation, and chemosensitivity. Cancer Res 74:6291–6305. https://doi.org/10.1158/0008-5472.CAN-14-0626

Chiba N, Comaills V, Shiotani B, Takahashi F, Shimada T, Tajima K, Winokur D, Hayashida T, Willers H, Brachtel E, Vivanco MD, Haber DA, Zou L, Maheswaran S (2012) Homeobox B9 induces epithelial-to-mesenchymal transition-associated radioresistance by accelerating DNA damage responses. Proc Natl Acad Sci U S A 109(8):2760–2765. https://doi.org/10.1073/pnas.1018867108

Chow OS, Kuk D, Keskin M, Smith JJ, Camacho N, Pelossof R, Chen CT, Chen Z, Avila K, Weiser MR, Berger MF, Patil S, Bergsland E, Garcia-Aguilar J (2016) KRAS and combined KRAS/TP53 mutations in locally advanced rectal cancer are independently associated with decreased response to Neoadjuvant therapy. Ann Surg Oncol 23(8):2548–2555. https://doi.org/10.1245/s10434-016-5205-4

Clarke MF, Dick JE, Dirks PB, Eaves CJ, Jamieson CHM, Jones DL, Visvader J, Weissman IL, Wahl GM (2006) Cancer stem cells—perspectives on current status and future directions: AACR workshop on cancer stem cells. Cancer Res 66:9339–9344. https://doi.org/10.1158/0008-5472.CAN-06-3126

Cloer EW, Siesser PF, Cousins EM, Goldfarb D, Mowrey DD, Harrison JS, Weir SJ, Dokholyan NV, Major MB (2018) p62-dependent phase separation of patient-derived KEAP1 mutations and NRF2. Mol Cell Biol 38(22). https://doi.org/10.1128/MCB.00644-17

Dahm-Daphi J, Hubbe P, Horvath F, El-Awady RA, Bouffard KE, Powell SN, Willers H (2005) Nonhomologous end-joining of site-specific but not of radiation-induced DNA double-strand breaks is reduced in the presence of wild-type p53. Oncogene 24(10):1663–1672

Deacon J, Peckham MJ, Steel GG (1984) The radioresponsiveness of human tumours and the initial slope of the cell survival curve. Radiother Oncol 2:317–323. https://doi.org/10.1016/s0167-8140(84)80074-2

DiBiase SJ, Guan J, Curran WJ Jr, Iliakis G (1999) Repair of DNA double-strand breaks and radiosensitivity to killing in an isogenic group of p53 mutant cell lines. Int J Radiat Oncol Biol Phys 45(3):743–751. https://doi.org/10.1016/s0360-3016(99)00229-1

Diehn M, Cho RW, Lobo NA, Kalisky T, Dorie MJ, Kulp AN, Qian D, Lam JS, Ailles LE, Wong M, Joshua B, Kaplan MJ, Wapnir I, Dirbas FM, Somlo G, Garberoglio C, Paz B, Shen J, Lau SK, Quake SR, Brown JM, Weissman IL, Clarke MF (2009) Association of reactive oxygen species levels and radioresistance in cancer stem cells. Nature 458:780–783. https://doi.org/10.1038/nature07733

Dinkelborg PH, Wang M, Gheorghiu L, Gurski JM, Hong TS, Benes CH, Juric D, Jimenez RB, Borgmann K, Willers H (2019) A common Chk1-dependent phenotype of DNA double-strand break suppression in two distinct radioresistant cancer types. Breast Cancer Res Treat 174(3):605–613. https://doi.org/10.1007/s10549-018-05079-7

Dubben HH, Thames HD, Beck-Bornholdt HP (1998) Tumor volume: a basic and specific response predictor in radiotherapy. Radiother Oncol 47(2):167–174. https://doi.org/10.1016/s0167-8140(97)00215-6

Eberhard DA, Johnson BE, Amler LC, Goddard AD, Heldens SL, Herbst RS, Ince WL, Janne PA, Januario T, Johnson DH, Klein P, Miller VA, Ostland MA, Ramies DA, Sebisanovic D, Stinson JA, Zhang YR, Seshagiri S, Hillan KJ (2005) Mutations in the epidermal growth factor receptor and in KRAS are predictive and prognostic indicators in patients with non-small-cell lung cancer treated with chemotherapy alone and in combination with erlotinib. J Clin Oncol 23(25):5900–5909

Eggler AL, Liu G, Pezzuto JM, van Breemen RB, Mesecar AD (2005) Modifying specific cysteines of the electrophile-sensing human Keap1 protein is insufficient to disrupt binding to the Nrf2 domain Neh2. Proc Natl Acad Sci U S A 102(29):10070–10075. https://doi.org/10.1073/pnas.0502402102

Eggler AL, Small E, Hannink M, Mesecar AD (2009) Cul3-mediated Nrf2 ubiquitination and ARE activation are dependent on the partial molar volume at position 151 of Keap1. Biochem J 422(1):171–180. https://doi.org/10.1042/BJ20090471

Eschrich SA, Pramana J, Zhang H, Zhao H, Boulware D, Lee JH, Bloom G, Rocha-Lima C, Kelley S, Calvin DP, Yeatman TJ, Begg AC, Torres-Roca JF (2009) A gene expression model of intrinsic tumor radiosensitivity: prediction of response and prognosis after chemoradiation. Int J Radiat Oncol Biol Phys 75(2):489–496. https://doi.org/10.1016/j.ijrobp.2009.06.014

Eschrich SA, Fulp WJ, Pawitan Y, Foekens JA, Smid M, Martens JWM, Echevarria M, Kamath V, Lee J-H, Harris EE, Bergh J, Torres-Roca JF (2012) Validation of a radiosensitivity molecular signature in breast cancer. Clin Cancer Res 18:5134–5143. https://doi.org/10.1158/1078-0432.CCR-12-0891

Farquhar D, Sheth S, Mazul A, Little P, Hayes DN, Zevallos JP (2018) Genetic mutations in KEAP/NFE2L2 associated with radiation resistance in early-stage laryngeal squamous cell carcinoma: a case series. Int J Radiat Oncol Biol Phys 100(5):1375–1376. https://doi.org/10.1016/j.ijrobp.2017.12.176

Fertil B, Malaise EP (1981) Inherent cellular radiosensitivity as a basic concept for human tumor radiotherapy. Int J Radiat Oncol Biol Phys 7:621–629. https://doi.org/10.1016/0360-3016(81)90377-1

Fraser M, Harding SM, Zhao H, Coackley C, Durocher D, Bristow RG (2011) MRE11 promotes AKT phosphorylation in direct response to DNA double-strand breaks. Cell Cycle 10(13):2218–2232

Fukutomi T, Takagi K, Mizushima T, Ohuchi N, Yamamoto M (2014) Kinetic, thermodynamic, and structural characterizations of the association between Nrf2-DLGex Degron and Keap1. Mol Cell Biol 34(5):832. https://doi.org/10.1128/MCB.01191-13

Ghisolfi L, Keates AC, Hu X, Lee D-k, Li CJ (2012) Ionizing radiation induces stemness in cancer cells. PLoS One 7:e43628. https://doi.org/10.1371/journal.pone.0043628

Goeman F, Nicola FD, Scalera S, Sperati F, Gallo E, Ciuffreda L, Pallocca M, Pizzuti L, Krasniqi E, Barchiesi G, Vici P, Barba M, Buglioni S, Casini B, Visca P, Pescarmona E, Mazzotta M, Maria RD, Fanciulli M, Ciliberto G, Maugeri-Saccà M (2019) Mutations in the KEAP1-NFE2L2 pathway define a molecular subset of rapidly progressing lung adenocarcinoma. J Thorac Oncol 14(11):1924–1934. https://doi.org/10.1016/j.jtho.2019.07.003

Grabocka E, Commisso C, Bar-Sagi D (2015) Molecular pathways: targeting the dependence of mutant RAS cancers on the DNA damage response. Clin Cancer Res 21(6):1243–1247. https://doi.org/10.1158/1078-0432.CCR-14-0650

Grana TM, Rusyn EV, Zhou H, Sartor CI, Cox AD (2002) Ras mediates radioresistance through both phosphatidylinositol 3-kinase-dependent and Raf-dependent but mitogen-activated protein kinase/extracellular signal-regulated kinase kinase-independent signaling pathways. Cancer Res 62(14):4142–4150

Gurtner K, Mikołajczak Z, Koi L, Wang M, Benes CH, Hering S, Willers H, Baumann M, Krause M (2020) Radioresistance of KRAS/TP53-mutated lung cancer can be overcome by radiation dose escalation or EGFR tyrosine kinase inhibition in vivo. Int J Cancer 147(2):472–477

Haigis KM (2017) KRAS alleles: the devil is in the detail. Trends Cancer 3(10):686–697. https://doi.org/10.1016/j.trecan.2017.08.006

Hall WA, Bergom C, Thompson RF, Baschnagel AM, Vijayakumar S, Willers H, Li A, Schultz CJ, Wilson GD, West CML, Capala J, Coleman CN, Torres-Roca JF, Weidhaas J, Feng FY (2018) Precision oncology and genomically guided radiation therapy, a report from the ASTRO/AAPM/NCI precision medicine conference. Int J Radiat Oncol Biol Phys 101(2):274–284

Han SW, Kim TY, Jeon YK, Hwang PG, Im SA, Lee KH, Kim JH, Kim DW, Heo DS, Kim NK, Chung DH, Bang YJ (2006) Optimization of patient selection for gefitinib in non-small cell lung cancer by combined analysis of epidermal growth factor receptor mutation, K-ras mutation, and Akt phosphorylation. Clin Cancer Res 12(8):2538–2544

Hast BE, Cloer EW, Goldfarb D, Li H, Siesser PF, Yan F, Walter V, Zheng N, Hayes DN, Major MB (2014) Cancer-derived mutations in KEAP1 impair NRF2 degradation but not ubiquitination. Cancer Res 74(3):808–817. https://doi.org/10.1158/0008-5472.CAN-13-1655

Herter-Sprie GS, Korideck H, Christensen CL, Herter JM, Rhee K, Berbeco RI, Bennett DG, Akbay EA, Kozono D, Mak RH, Mike Makrigiorgos G, Kimmelman AC, Wong KK (2014)

Image-guided radiotherapy platform using single nodule conditional lung cancer mouse models. Nat Commun 5:5870

Hoadley KA, Yau C, Hinoue T, Wolf DM, Lazar AJ, Drill E, Shen R, Taylor AM, Cherniack AD, Thorsson V, Akbani R, Bowlby R, Wong CK, Wiznerowicz M, Sanchez-Vega F, Robertson AG, Schneider BG, Lawrence MS, Noushmehr H, Malta TM, Caesar-Johnson SJ, Demchok JA, Felau I, Kasapi M, Ferguson ML, Hutter CM, Sofia HJ, Tarnuzzer R, Wang Z, Yang L, Zenklusen JC, Zhang JJ, Chudamani S, Liu J, Lolla L, Naresh R, Pihl T, Sun Q, Wan Y, Wu Y, Cho J, DeFreitas T, Frazer S, Gehlenborg N, Getz G, Heiman DI, Kim J, Lawrence MS, Lin P, Meier S, Noble MS, Saksena G, Voet D, Zhang H, Bernard B, Chambwe N, Dhankani V, Knijnenburg T, Kramer R, Leinonen K, Liu Y, Miller M, Reynolds S, Shmulevich I, Thorsson V, Zhang W, Akbani R, Broom BM, Hegde AM, Ju Z, Kanchi RS, Korkut A, Li J, Liang H, Ling S, Liu W, Lu Y, Mills GB, Ng K-S, Rao A, Ryan M, Wang J, Weinstein JN, Zhang J, Abeshouse A, Armenia J, Chakravarty D, Chatila WK, Id B, Gao J, Gross BE, Heins ZJ, Kundra R, La K, Ladanyi M, Luna A, Nissan MG, Ochoa A, Phillips SM, Reznik E, Sanchez-Vega F, Sander C, Schultz N, Sheridan R, Sumer SO, Sun Y, Taylor BS, Wang J, Zhang H, Anur P, Peto M, Spellman P, Benz C, Stuart JM, Wong CK, Yau C, Hayes DN, Parker JS, Wilkerson MD, Ally A, Balasundaram M, Bowlby R, Brooks D, Carlsen R, Chuah E, Dhalla N, Holt R, Jones SJM, Kasaian K, Lee D, Ma Y, Marra MA, Mayo M, Moore RA, Mungall AJ, Mungall K, Robertson AG, Sadeghi S, Schein JE, Sipahimalani P, Tam A, Thiessen N, Tse K, Wong T, Berger AC, Beroukhim R, Cherniack AD, Cibulskis C, Gabriel SB, Gao GF, Ha G, Meyerson M, Schumacher SE, Shih J, Kucherlapati MH, Kucherlapati RS, Baylin S, Cope L, Danilova L, Bootwalla MS, Lai PH, Maglinte DT, Berg DJVD, Weisenberger DJ, Auman JT, Balu S, Bodenheimer T, Fan C, Hoadley KA, Hoyle AP, Jefferys SR, Jones CD, Meng S, Mieczkowski PA, Mose LE, Perou AH, Perou CM, Roach J, Shi Y, Simons JV, Skelly T, Soloway MG, Tan D, Veluvolu U, Fan H, Hinoue T, Laird PW, Shen H, Zhou W, Bellair M, Chang K, Covington K, Creighton CJ, Dinh H, Doddapaneni H, Donehower LA, Drummond J, Gibbs RA, Glenn R, Hale W, Han Y, Hu J, Korchina V, Lee S, Lewis L, Li W, Liu X, Morgan M, Morton D, Muzny D, Santibanez J, Sheth M, Shinbrot E, Wang L, Wang M, Wheeler DA, Xi L, Zhao F, Hess J, Appelbaum EL, Bailey M, Cordes MG, Ding L, Fronick CC, Fulton LA, Fulton RS, Kandoth C, Mardis ER, McLellan MD, Miller CA, Schmidt HK, Wilson RK, Crain D, Curley E, Gardner J, Lau K, Mallery D, Morris S, Paulauskis J, Penny R, Shelton C, Shelton T, Sherman M, Thompson E, Yena P, Bowen J, Gastier-Foster JM, Gerken M, Leraas KM, Lichtenberg TM, Ramirez NC, Wise L, Zmuda E, Corcoran N, Costello T, Hovens C, Carvalho AL, Carvalho ACD, Fregnani JH, Longatto-Filho A, Reis RM, Scapulatempo-Neto C, HCS S, Vidal DO, Burnette A, Eschbacher J, Hermes B, Noss A, Singh R, Anderson ML, Castro PD, Ittmann M, Huntsman D, Kohl B, Le X, Thorp R, Andry C, Duffy ER, Lyadov V, Paklina O, Setdikova G, Shabunin A, Tavobilov M, McPherson C, Warnick R, Berkowitz R, Cramer D, Feltmate C, Horowitz N, Kibel A, Muto M, Raut CP, Malykh A, Barnholtz-Sloan JS, Barrett W, Devine K, Fulop J, Ostrom QT, Shimmel K, Wolinsky Y, Sloan AE, Rose AD, Giuliante F, Goodman M, Karlan BY, Hagedorn CH, Eckman J, Harr J, Myers J, Tucker K, Zach LA, Deyarmin B, Hu H, Kvecher L, Larson C, Mural RJ, Somiari S, Vicha A, Zelinka T, Bennett J, Iacocca M, Rabeno B, Swanson P, Latour M, Lacombe L, Têtu B, Bergeron A, McGraw M, Staugaitis SM, Chabot J, Hibshoosh H, Sepulveda A, Su T, Wang T, Potapova O, Voronina O, Desjardins L, Mariani O, Roman-Roman S, Sastre X, Stern M-H, Cheng F, Signoretti S, Berchuck A, Bigner D, Lipp E, Marks J, McCall S, McLendon R, Secord A, Sharp A, Behera M, Brat DJ, Chen A, Delman K, Force S, Khuri F, Magliocca K, Maithel S, Olson JJ, Owonikoko T, Pickens A, Ramalingam S, Shin DM, Sica G, Meir EVG, Zhang H, Eijckenboom W, Gillis A, Korpershoek E, Looijenga L, Oosterhuis W, Stoop H, Kessel KEV, Zwarthoff EC, Calatozzolo C, Cuppini L, Cuzzubbo S, DiMeco F, Finocchiaro G, Mattei L, Perin A, Pollo B, Chen C, Houck J, Lohavanichbutr P, Hartmann A, Stoehr C, Stoehr R, Taubert H, Wach S, Wullich B, Kycler W, Murawa D, Wiznerowicz M, Chung K, Edenfield WJ, Martin J, Baudin E, Bubley G, Bueno R, Rienzo AD, Richards WG, Kalkanis S, Mikkelsen T, Noushmehr H, Scarpace L, Girard N, Aymerich M, Campo E, Giné E, Guillermo AL, Bang NV, Hanh PT, Phu BD, Tang Y, Colman H, Evason K,

Dottino PR, Martignetti JA, Gabra H, Juhl H, Akeredolu T, Stepa S, Hoon D, Ahn K, Kang KJ, Beuschlein F, Breggia A, Birrer M, Bell D, Borad M, Bryce AH, Castle E, Chandan V, Cheville J, Copland JA, Farnell M, Flotte T, Giama N, Ho T, Kendrick M, Kocher J-P, Kopp K, Moser C, Nagorney D, O'Brien D, O'Neill BP, Patel T, Petersen G, Que F, Rivera M, Roberts L, Smallridge R, Smyrk T, Stanton M, Thompson RH, Torbenson M, Yang JD, Zhang L, Brimo F, Ajani JA, AMA G, Behrens C, Bondaruk O, Broaddus R, Czerniak B, Esmaeli B, Fujimoto J, Gershenwald J, Guo C, Lazar AJ, Logothetis C, Meric-Bernstam F, Moran C, Ramondetta L, Rice D, Sood A, Tamboli P, Thompson T, Troncoso P, Tsao A, Wistuba I, Carter C, Haydu L, Hersey P, Jakrot V, Kakavand H, Kefford R, Lee K, Long G, Mann G, Quinn M, Saw R, Scolyer R, Shannon K, Spillane A, Stretch J, Synott M, Thompson J, Wilmott J, Al-Ahmadie H, Chan TA, Ghossein R, Gopalan A, Levine DA, Reuter V, Singer S, Singh B, Tien NV, Broudy T, Mirsaidi C, Nair P, Drwiega P, Miller J, Smith J, Zaren H, Park J-W, Hung NP, Kebebew E, Linehan WM, Metwalli AR, Pacak K, Pinto PA, Schiffman M, Schmidt LS, Vocke CD, Wentzensen N, Worrell R, Yang H, Moncrieff M, Goparaju C, Melamed J, Pass H, Botnariuc N, Caraman I, Cernat M, Chemencedji I, Clipca A, Doruc S, Gorincioi G, Mura S, Pirtac M, Stancul I, Tcaciuc D, Albert M, Alexopoulou I, Arnaout A, Bartlett J, Engel J, Gilbert S, Parfitt J, Sekhon H, Thomas G, Rassl DM, Rintoul RC, Bifulco C, Tamakawa R, Urba W, Hayward N, Timmers H, Antenucci A, Facciolo F, Grazi G, Marino M, Merola R, Rd K, Gimenez-Roqueplo A-P, Piché A, Chevalier S, McKercher G, Birsoy K, Barnett G, Brewer C, Farver C, Naska T, Pennell NA, Raymond D, Schilero C, Smolenski K, Williams F, Morrison C, Borgia JA, Liptay MJ, Pool M, Seder CW, Junker K, Omberg L, Dinkin M, Manikhas G, Alvaro D, Bragazzi MC, Cardinale V, Carpino G, Gaudio E, Chesla D, Cottingham S, Dubina M, Moiseenko F, Dhanasekaran R, Becker K-F, Janssen K-P, Slotta-Huspenina J, Abdel-Rahman MH, Aziz D, Bell S, Cebulla CM, Davis A, Duell R, Elder JB, Hilty J, Kumar B, Lang J, Lehman NL, Mandt R, Nguyen P, Pilarski R, Rai K, Schoenfield L, Senecal K, Wakely P, Hansen P, Lechan R, Powers J, Tischler A, Grizzle WE, Sexton KC, Kastl A, Henderson J, Porten S, Waldmann J, Fassnacht M, Asa SL, Schadendorf D, Couce M, Graefen M, Huland H, Sauter G, Schlomm T, Simon R, Tennstedt P, Olabode O, Nelson M, Bathe O, Carroll PR, Chan JM, Disaia P, Glenn P, Kelley RK, Landen CN, Phillips J, Prados M, Simko J, Smith-McCune K, VandenBerg S, Roggin K, Fehrenbach A, Kendler A, Sifri S, Steele R, Jimeno A, Carey F, Forgie I, Mannelli M, Carney M, Hernandez B, Campos B, Herold-Mende C, Jungk C, Unterberg A, Deimling AV, Bossler A, Galbraith J, Jacobus L, Knudson M, Knutson T, Ma D, Milhem M, Sigmund R, Godwin AK, Madan R, Rosenthal HG, Adebamowo C, Adebamowo SN, Boussioutas A, Beer D, Giordano T, Mes-Masson A-M, Saad F, Bocklage T, Landrum L, Mannel R, Moore K, Moxley K, Postier R, Walker J, Zuna R, Feldman M, Valdivieso F, Dhir R, Luketich J, Pinero EMM, Quintero-Aguilo M, Carlotti CG, Santos JSD, Kemp R, Sankarankuty A, Tirapelli D, Catto J, Agnew K, Swisher E, Creaney J, Robinson B, Shelley CS, Godwin EM, Kendall S, Shipman C, Bradford C, Carey T, Haddad A, Moyer J, Peterson L, Prince M, Rozek L, Wolf G, Bowman R, Fong KM, Yang I, Korst R, Rathmell WK, Fantacone-Campbell JL, Hooke JA, Kovatich AJ, Shriver CD, DiPersio J, Drake B, Govindan R, Heath S, Ley T, Tine BV, Westervelt P, Rubin MA, Lee JI, Aredes ND, Mariamidze A, Stuart JM, Benz CC, Laird PW (2018) Cell-of-origin patterns dominate the molecular classification of 10,000 tumors from 33 types of cancer. Cell 173(2):291–304.e296. https://doi.org/10.1016/j.cell.2018.03.022

Hong TS, Wo JY, Borger DR, Yeap BY, McDonnell EI, Willers H, Blaszkowsky LS, Kwak EL, Allen JN, Clark JW, Tanguturi S, Goyal L, Murphy JE, Wolfgang JA, Drapek LC, Arellano RS, Mamon HJ, Mullen JT, Tanabe KK, Ferrone CR, Ryan DP, Iafrate AJ, DeLaney TF, Zhu AX (2017) Phase II study of proton-based stereotactic body radiation therapy for liver metastases: importance of tumor genotype. J Natl Cancer Inst 109(9). https://doi.org/10.1093/jnci/djx031

Hong TS, Wo JY-L, Ryan DP, Zheng H, Borger DR, Kwak EL, Allen JN, Berger DL, Rattner DW, Cusack JC, Gemma AJ, Mamon HJ, Eyler CE, Shellito PC, Zhu AX, Goyal L, Clark JW, Willers H, Haigis KM (2018) Phase Ib study of neoadjuvant chemoradiation (CRT) with midostaurin, 5-fluorouracil (5-FU) and radiation (XRT) for locally advanced rectal cancer:

sensitization of RAS mutant tumors. J Clin Oncol 36 (15_suppl):e15674–e15674. https://doi.org/10.1200/JCO.2018.36.15_suppl.e15674

Huang EH, Hynes MJ, Zhang T, Ginestier C, Dontu G, Appelman H, Fields JZ, Wicha MS, Boman BM (2009) Aldehyde dehydrogenase 1 is a marker for normal and malignant human colonic stem cells (SC) and tracks SC overpopulation during colon tumorigenesis. Cancer Res 69:3382–3389. https://doi.org/10.1158/0008-5472.CAN-08-4418

Huang Q, Li F, Liu X, Li W, Shi W, Liu FF, O'Sullivan B, He Z, Peng Y, Tan AC, Zhou L, Shen J, Han G, Wang XJ, Thorburn J, Thorburn A, Jimeno A, Raben D, Bedford JS, Li CY (2011) Caspase 3-mediated stimulation of tumor cell repopulation during cancer radiotherapy. Nat Med 17(7):860–866. https://doi.org/10.1038/nm.2385

Itoh K, Chiba T, Takahashi S, Ishii T, Igarashi K, Katoh Y, Oyake T, Hayashi N, Satoh K, Hatayama I, Yamamoto M, Nabeshima YI (1997) An Nrf2/Small Maf heterodimer mediates the induction of phase II detoxifying enzyme genes through antioxidant response elements. Biochem Biophys Res Commun 236(2):313–322. https://doi.org/10.1006/bbrc.1997.6943

Itoh K, Wakabayashi N, Katoh Y, Ishii T, Igarashi K, Engel JD, Yamamoto M (1999) Keap1 represses nuclear activation of antioxidant responsive elements by Nrf2 through binding to the amino-terminal Neh2 domain. Genes Dev 13(1):76–86

Jeong Y, Hoang NT, Lovejoy A, Stehr H, Newman AM, Gentles AJ, Kong W, Truong D, Martin S, Chaudhuri A, Heiser D, Zhou L, Say C, Carter JN, Hiniker SM, Loo BW, West RB, Beachy P, Alizadeh AA, Diehn M (2017) Role of KEAP1/NRF2 and TP53 mutations in lung squamous cell carcinoma development and radiation resistance. Cancer Discov 7(1):86–101. https://doi.org/10.1158/2159-8290.CD-16-0127

Jeong Y, Hellyer JA, Stehr H, Hoang NT, Niu X, Das M, Padda SK, Ramchandran K, Neal JW, Wakelee HA, Diehn M (2020) Role of KEAP1/NFE2L2 mutations in the chemotherapeutic response of non-small cell lung cancer patients. Clin Cancer Res 26(1):274–281. https://doi.org/10.1158/1078-0432.CCR-19-1237

Jethwa KR, Jang S, Mullikin TC, Harmsen WS, Petersen MM, Olivier KR, Park SS, Neben-Wittich MA, Hubbard JM, Sandhyavenu H, Whitaker TJ, Waltman LA, Kipp BR, Merrell KW, Haddock MG, Hallemeier CL (2020) Association of tumor genomic factors and efficacy for metastasis-directed stereotactic body radiotherapy for oligometastatic colorectal cancer. Radiother Oncol 146:29–36. https://doi.org/10.1016/j.radonc.2020.02.008

Johnson CR, Thames HD, Huang DT, Schmidt-Ullrich RK (1995) The tumor volume and clonogen number relationship: tumor control predictions based upon tumor volume estimates derived from computed tomography. Int J Radiat Oncol Biol Phys 33(2):281–287. https://doi.org/10.1016/0360-3016(95)00119-j

Jung J-W, Hwang S-Y, Hwang J-S, Oh E-S, Park S, Han I-O (2007) Ionising radiation induces changes associated with epithelial-mesenchymal transdifferentiation and increased cell motility of A549 lung epithelial cells. Eur J Cancer 43:1214–1224. https://doi.org/10.1016/J.EJCA.2007.01.034

Kamran SC, Lennerz JK, Margolis C, Li D, Reardon B, Wankowicz SA, Wo J, Willers H, Corcoran RB, Van Allen EM, Hong TS (2018) Genomic evolution and acquired resistance to preoperative chemoradiation therapy in rectal cancer. J Clin Oncol 36(Suppl 4S); abstr 613

Kamran SC, Lennerz JK, Margolis CA, Liu D, Reardon B, Wankowicz SA, Van Seventer EE, Tracy A, Wo JY, Carter SL, Willers H, Corcoran RB, Hong TS, Van Allen EM (2019) Integrative molecular characterization of resistance to neoadjuvant chemoradiation in rectal cancer. Clin Cancer Res 25(18):5561–5571. https://doi.org/10.1158/1078-0432.CCR-19-0908

Kim IA, Bae SS, Fernandes A, Wu J, Muschel RJ, McKenna WG, Birnbaum MJ, Bernhard EJ (2005) Selective inhibition of Ras, phosphoinositide 3 kinase, and Akt isoforms increases the radiosensitivity of human carcinoma cell lines. Cancer Res 65(17):7902–7910

Kirsch DG, Diehn M, Kesarwala AH, Maity A, Morgan MA, Schwarz JK, Bristow R, Demaria S, Eke I, Griffin RJ, Haas-Kogan D, Higgins GS, Kimmelman AC, Kimple RJ, Lombaert IM, Ma L, Marples B, Pajonk F, Park CC, Schaue D, Tran PT, Willers H, Wouters BG, Bernhard

EJ (2018) The future of radiobiology. J Natl Cancer Inst 110:329–340. https://doi.org/10.1093/jnci/djx231

Kitajima S, Ivanova E, Guo S, Yoshida R, Campisi M, Sundararaman SK, Tange S, Mitsuishi Y, Thai TC, Masuda S, Piel BP, Sholl LM, Kirschmeier PT, Paweletz CP, Watanabe H, Yajima M, Barbie DA (2019) Suppression of STING associated with LKB1 loss in KRAS-driven lung cancer. Cancer Discov 9(1):34–45. https://doi.org/10.1158/2159-8290.CD-18-0689

Kleiman LB, Krebs AM, Kim SY, Hong TS, Haigis KM (2013) Comparative analysis of radiosensitizers for K-RAS mutant rectal cancers. PLoS One 8(12):e82982

Kobayashi A, Kang MI, Okawa H, Ohtsuji M, Zenke Y, Chiba T, Igarashi K, Yamamoto M (2004) Oxidative stress sensor Keap1 functions as an adaptor for Cul3-based E3 ligase to regulate proteasomal degradation of Nrf2. Mol Cell Biol 24(16):7130–7139. https://doi.org/10.1128/MCB.24.16.7130-7139.2004

Krause M, Ostermann G, Petersen C, Yaromina A, Hessel F, Harstrick A, van der Kogel AJ, Thames HD, Baumann M (2005) Decreased repopulation as well as increased reoxygenation contribute to the improvement in local control after targeting of the EGFR by C225 during fractionated irradiation. Radiother Oncol 76(2):162–167

Krause M, Yaromina A, Eicheler W, Koch U, Baumann M (2011) Cancer stem cells: targets and potential biomarkers for radiotherapy. Clin Cancer Res 17(23):7224–7229

Krause M, Dubrovska A, Linge A, Baumann M (2017) Cancer stem cells: radioresistance, prediction of radiotherapy outcome and specific targets for combined treatments. Adv Drug Deliv Rev 109:63–73. https://doi.org/10.1016/J.ADDR.2016.02.002

Kriegs M, Gurtner K, Can Y, Brammer I, Rieckmann T, Oertel R, Wysocki M, Dorniok F, Gal A, Grob TJ, Laban S, Kasten-Pisula U, Petersen C, Baumann M, Krause M, Dikomey E (2015) Radiosensitization of NSCLC cells by EGFR inhibition is the result of an enhanced p53-dependent G1 arrest. Radiother Oncol 115(1):120–127. https://doi.org/10.1016/j.radonc.2015.02.018

Lagadec C, Vlashi E, Della Donna L, Dekmezian C, Pajonk F (2012) Radiation-induced reprogramming of breast cancer cells. Stem Cells (Dayton, Ohio) 30:833–844. https://doi.org/10.1002/stem.1058

Lee S, Lim M-J, Kim M-H, Yu C-H, Yun Y-S, Ahn J, Song J-Y (2012) An effective strategy for increasing the radiosensitivity of human lung cancer cells by blocking Nrf2-dependent antioxidant responses. Free Radic Biol Med 53(4):807–816. https://doi.org/10.1016/j.freeradbiomed.2012.05.038

Lin SH, Zhang J, Giri U, Stephan C, Sobieski M, Zhong L, Mason KA, Molkentine J, Thames HD, Yoo SS, Heymach JV (2014) A high content clonogenic survival drug screen identifies mek inhibitors as potent radiation sensitizers for KRAS mutant non-small-cell lung cancer. J Thorac Oncol 9(7):965–973. https://doi.org/10.1097/JTO.0000000000000199

Liu Q, Wang M, Kern AM, Khaled S, Han J, Yeap BY, Hong TS, Settleman J, Benes CH, Held KD, Efstathiou JA, Willers H (2015) Adapting a drug screening platform to discover associations of molecular targeted radiosensitizers with genomic biomarkers. Mol Cancer Res 13:713–720

Machtay M, Hsu C, Komaki R, Sause WT, Swann RS, Langer CJ, Byhardt RW, Curran WJ (2005) Effect of overall treatment time on outcomes after concurrent chemoradiation for locally advanced non-small-cell lung carcinoma: analysis of the Radiation Therapy Oncology Group (RTOG) experience. Int J Radiat Oncol Biol Phys 63(3):667–671. https://doi.org/10.1016/j.ijrobp.2005.03.037

Mak RH, Hermann G, Lewis JH, Aerts HJ, Baldini EH, Chen AB, Colson YL, Hacker FH, Kozono D, Wee JO, Chen YH, Catalano PJ, Wong KK, Sher DJ (2015) Outcomes by tumor histology and KRAS mutation status after lung stereotactic body radiation therapy for early-stage non-small-cell lung cancer. Clin Lung Cancer 16(1):24–32. https://doi.org/10.1016/j.cllc.2014.09.005

Mani SA, Guo W, Liao M-J, Eaton EN, Ayyanan A, Zhou AY, Brooks M, Reinhard F, Zhang CC, Shipitsin M, Campbell LL, Polyak K, Brisken C, Yang J, Weinberg RA (2008) The epithelial-mesenchymal transition generates cells with properties of stem cells. Cell 133:704–715. https://doi.org/10.1016/J.CELL.2008.03.027

Meade S, Sanghera P, McConkey C, Fowler J, Fountzilas G, Glaholm J, Hartley A (2013) Revising the radiobiological model of synchronous chemotherapy in head-and-neck cancer: a new analysis examining reduced weighting of accelerated repopulation. Int J Radiat Oncol Biol Phys 86(1):157–163. https://doi.org/10.1016/j.ijrobp.2012.11.023

Minjgee M, Toulany M, Kehlbach R, Giehl K, Rodemann HP (2011) K-RAS(V12) induces autocrine production of EGFR ligands and mediates radioresistance through EGFR-dependent Akt signaling and activation of DNA-PKcs. Int J Radiat Oncol Biol Phys 81(5):1506–1514

Moon BS, Jeong WJ, Park J, Kim TI, Min do S, Choi KY (2014) Role of oncogenic K-Ras in cancer stem cell activation by aberrant Wnt/beta-catenin signaling. J Natl Cancer Inst 106(2):djt373

Moore KN, Bauer TM, Falchook GS, Chowdhury S, Patel C, Neuwirth R, Enke A, Zohren F, Patel MR (2018) Phase I study of the investigational oral mTORC1/2 inhibitor sapanisertib (TAK-228): tolerability and food effects of a milled formulation in patients with advanced solid tumours. ESMO Open 3(2):e000291. https://doi.org/10.1136/esmoopen-2017-000291

Namani A, Matiur Rahaman M, Chen M, Tang X (2018) Gene-expression signature regulated by the KEAP1-NRF2-CUL3 axis is associated with a poor prognosis in head and neck squamous cell cancer. BMC Cancer 18:46. https://doi.org/10.1186/s12885-017-3907-z

Nguyen-Tan PF, Zhang Q, Ang KK, Weber RS, Rosenthal DI, Soulieres D, Kim H, Silverman C, Raben A, Galloway TJ, Fortin A, Gore E, Westra WH, Chung CH, Jordan RC, Gillison ML, List M, Le QT (2014) Randomized phase III trial to test accelerated versus standard fractionation in combination with concurrent cisplatin for head and neck carcinomas in the Radiation Therapy Oncology Group 0129 trial: long-term report of efficacy and toxicity. J Clin Oncol 32(34):3858–3866. https://doi.org/10.1200/JCO.2014.55.3925

O'Brien CA, Pollett A, Gallinger S, Dick JE (2007) A human colon cancer cell capable of initiating tumour growth in immunodeficient mice. Nature 445:106–110. https://doi.org/10.1038/nature05372

O'Cathail SM, Wu C-H, Lewis A, Holmes C, Hawkins MA, Maughan T (2019) A metagene of NRF2 expression is a prognostic biomarker in all stage colorectal cancer. Cancer Biol

Plo I, Laulier C, Gauthier L, Lebrun F, Calvo F, Lopez BS (2008) AKT1 inhibits homologous recombination by inducing cytoplasmic retention of BRCA1 and RAD51. Cancer Res 68(22):9404–9412

Ready N, Janne PA, Bogart J, Dipetrillo T, Garst J, Graziano S, Gu L, Wang X, Green MR, Vokes EE (2010) Chemoradiotherapy and gefitinib in stage III non-small cell lung cancer with epidermal growth factor receptor and KRAS mutation analysis: cancer and leukemia group B (CALEB) 30106, a CALGB-stratified phase II trial. J Thorac Oncol 5(9):1382–1390

Richman SD, Seymour MT, Chambers P, Elliott F, Daly CL, Meade AM, Taylor G, Barrett JH, Quirke P (2009) KRAS and BRAF mutations in advanced colorectal cancer are associated with poor prognosis but do not preclude benefit from oxaliplatin or irinotecan: results from the MRC FOCUS trial. J Clin Oncol 27(35):5931–5937. https://doi.org/10.1200/JCO.2009.22.4295

Robb R, Yang L, Shen C, Wolfe AR, Webb A, Zhang X, Vedaie M, Saji M, Jhiang S, Ringel MD, Williams TM (2019) Inhibiting BRAF oncogene-mediated radioresistance effectively radiosensitizes BRAF(V600E)-mutant thyroid cancer cells by constraining DNA double-strand break repair. Clin Cancer Res 25(15):4749–4760. https://doi.org/10.1158/1078-0432.CCR-18-3625

Romero R, Sayin VI, Davidson SM, Bauer MR, Singh SX, LeBoeuf SE, Karakousi TR, Ellis DC, Bhutkar A, Sanchez-Rivera FJ, Subbaraj L, Martinez B, Bronson RT, Prigge JR, Schmidt EE, Thomas CJ, Goparaju C, Davies A, Dolgalev I, Heguy A, Allaj V, Poirier JT, Moreira AL, Rudin CM, Pass HI, Vander Heiden MG, Jacks T, Papagiannakopoulos T (2017) Keap1 loss promotes Kras-driven lung cancer and results in dependence on glutaminolysis. Nat Med 23(11):1362–1368. https://doi.org/10.1038/nm.4407

Russo AL, Ryan DP, Borger DR, Wo JY, Szymonifka J, Liang WY, Kwak EL, Blaszkowsky LS, Clark JW, Allen JN, Zhu AX, Berger DL, Cusack JC, Mamon HJ, Haigis KM, Hong TS (2014) Mutational and clinical predictors of pathologic complete response in the treatment of locally advanced rectal cancer. J Gastrointest Cancer 45(1):34–39

Scott JG, Berglund A, Schell MJ, Mihaylov I, Fulp WJ, Yue B, Welsh E, Caudell JJ, Ahmed K, Strom TS, Mellon E, Venkat P, Johnstone P, Foekens J, Lee J, Moros E, Dalton WS, Eschrich SA, McLeod H, Harrison LB, Torres-Roca JF (2017) A genome-based model for adjusting radiotherapy dose (GARD): a retrospective, cohort-based study. Lancet Oncol 18(2):202–211. https://doi.org/10.1016/S1470-2045(16)30648-9

Seguin L, Kato S, Franovic A, Camargo MF, Lesperance J, Elliott KC, Yebra M, Mielgo A, Lowy AM, Husain H, Cascone T, Diao L, Wang J, Wistuba II, Heymach JV, Lippman SM, Desgrosellier JS, Anand S, Weis SM, Cheresh DA (2014) An integrin beta(3)-KRAS-RalB complex drives tumour stemness and resistance to EGFR inhibition. Nat Cell Biol 16(5):457–468

Seshacharyulu P, Baine MJ, Souchek JJ, Menning M, Kaur S, Yan Y, Ouellette MM, Jain M, Lin C, Batra SK (2017) Biological determinants of radioresistance and their remediation in pancreatic cancer. Biochim Biophys Acta Rev Cancer 1868(1):69–92. https://doi.org/10.1016/j.bbcan.2017.02.003

Shibata T, Ohta T, Tong KI, Kokubu A, Odogawa R, Tsuta K, Asamura H, Yamamoto M, Hirohashi S (2008) Cancer related mutations in NRF2 impair its recognition by Keap1-Cul3 E3 ligase and promote malignancy. Proc Natl Acad Sci U S A 105(36):13568–13573. https://doi.org/10.1073/pnas.0806268105

Shibata T, Saito S, Kokubu A, Suzuki T, Yamamoto M, Hirohashi S (2010) Global downstream pathway analysis reveals a dependence of oncogenic NF-E2–related factor 2 mutation on the mTOR growth signaling pathway. Cancer Res 70(22):9095–9105. https://doi.org/10.1158/0008-5472.CAN-10-0384

Simanshu DK, Nissley DV, McCormick F (2017) RAS proteins and their regulators in human disease. Cell 170(1):17–33. https://doi.org/10.1016/j.cell.2017.06.009

Singh SK, Hawkins C, Clarke ID, Squire JA, Bayani J, Hide T, Henkelman RM, Cusimano MD, Dirks PB (2004) Identification of human brain tumour initiating cells. Nature 432:396–401. https://doi.org/10.1038/nature03128

Singh A, Bodas M, Wakabayashi N, Bunz F, Biswal S (2010) Gain of Nrf2 function in non-small-cell lung cancer cells confers radioresistance. Antioxid Redox Signal 13(11):1627–1637. https://doi.org/10.1089/ars.2010.3219

Singh A, Venkannagari S, Oh KH, Zhang Y-Q, Rohde JM, Liu L, Nimmagadda S, Sudini K, Brimacombe KR, Gajghate S, Ma J, Wang A, Xu X, Shahane SA, Xia M, Woo J, Mensah GA, Wang Z, Ferrer M, Gabrielson E, Li Z, Rastinejad F, Shen M, Boxer MB, Biswal S (2016) Small molecule inhibitor of NRF2 selectively intervenes therapeutic resistance in KEAP1-deficient NSCLC tumors. ACS Chem Biol 11(11):3214–3225. https://doi.org/10.1021/acschembio.6b00651

Skoulidis F, Heymach JV (2019) Co-occurring genomic alterations in non-small-cell lung cancer biology and therapy. Nat Rev Cancer 19(9):495–509. https://doi.org/10.1038/s41568-019-0179-8

Skoulidis F, Byers LA, Diao L, Papadimitrakopoulou VA, Tong P, Izzo J, Behrens C, Kadara H, Parra ER, Canales JR, Zhang J, Giri U, Gudikote J, Cortez MA, Yang C, Fan Y, Peyton M, Girard L, Coombes KR, Toniatti C, Heffernan TP, Choi M, Frampton GM, Miller V, Weinstein JN, Herbst RS, Wong KK, Zhang J, Sharma P, Mills GB, Hong WK, Minna JD, Allison JP, Futreal A, Wang J, Wistuba II, Heymach JV (2015) Co-occurring genomic alterations define major subsets of KRAS-mutant lung adenocarcinoma with distinct biology, immune profiles, and therapeutic vulnerabilities. Cancer Discov 5(8):860–877. https://doi.org/10.1158/2159-8290.CD-14-1236

Skoulidis F, Goldberg ME, Greenawalt DM, Hellmann MD, Awad MM, Gainor JF, Schrock AB, Hartmaier RJ, Trabucco SE, Gay L, Ali SM, Elvin JA, Singal G, Ross JS, Fabrizio D, Szabo PM, Chang H, Sasson A, Srinivasan S, Kirov S, Szustakowski J, Vitazka P, Edwards R, Bufill JA, Sharma N, Ou SI, Peled N, Spigel DR, Rizvi H, Aguilar EJ, Carter BW, Erasmus J, Halpenny DF, Plodkowski AJ, Long NM, Nishino M, Denning WL, Galan-Cobo A, Hamdi H, Hirz T, Tong P, Wang J, Rodriguez-Canales J, Villalobos PA, Parra ER, Kalhor N, Sholl LM, Sauter JL, Jungbluth AA, Mino-Kenudson M, Azimi R, Elamin YY, Zhang J, Leonardi GC,

Jiang F, Wong KK, Lee JJ, Papadimitrakopoulou VA, Wistuba II, Miller VA, Frampton GM, Wolchok JD, Shaw AT, Janne PA, Stephens PJ, Rudin CM, Geese WJ, Albacker LA, Heymach JV (2018) STK11/LKB1 mutations and PD-1 inhibitor resistance in KRAS-mutant lung adeno-carcinoma. Cancer Discov 8(7):822–835. https://doi.org/10.1158/2159-8290.CD-18-0099

Soliman M, Yaromina A, Appold S, Zips D, Reiffenstuhl C, Schreiber A, Thames HD, Krause M, Baumann M (2013) GTV differentially impacts locoregional control of non-small cell lung cancer (NSCLC) after different fractionation schedules: subgroup analysis of the prospective randomized CHARTWEL trial. Radiother Oncol 106(3):299–304. https://doi.org/10.1016/j.radonc.2012.12.008

Stephen AG, Esposito D, Bagni RK, McCormick F (2014) Dragging ras back in the ring. Cancer Cell 25(3):272–281

Strom T, Hoffe SE, Fulp W, Frakes J, Coppola D, Springett GM, Malafa MP, Harris CL, Eschrich SA, Torres-Roca JF, Shridhar R (2015) Radiosensitivity index predicts for survival with adju-vant radiation in resectable pancreatic cancer. Radiother Oncol 117:159–164. https://doi.org/10.1016/j.radonc.2015.07.018

Sun X, Wang Q, Wang Y, Du L, Xu C, Liu Q (2016) Brusatol enhances the radiosensitivity of A549 cells by promoting ROS production and enhancing DNA damage. Int J Mol Sci 17(7):997. https://doi.org/10.3390/ijms17070997

Tang KJ, Constanzo JD, Venkateswaran N, Melegari M, Ilcheva M, Morales JC, Skoulidis F, Heymach JV, Boothman DA, Scaglioni PP (2016) Focal adhesion kinase regulates the DNA damage response and its inhibition radiosensitizes mutant KRAS lung cancer. Clin Cancer Res 22(23):5851–5863. https://doi.org/10.1158/1078-0432.CCR-15-2603

Tao Y, Zhang P, Frascogna V, Lecluse Y, Auperin A, Bourhis J, Deutsch E (2007) Enhancement of radiation response by inhibition of Aurora-a kinase using siRNA or a selective Aurora kinase inhibitor PHA680632 in p53-deficient cancer cells. Br J Cancer 97(12):1664–1672. https://doi.org/10.1038/sj.bjc.6604083

Theys J, Jutten B, Habets R, Paesmans K, Groot AJ, Lambin P, Wouters BG, Lammering G, Vooijs M (2011) E-cadherin loss associated with EMT promotes radioresistance in human tumor cells. Radiother Oncol 99:392–397. https://doi.org/10.1016/J.RADONC.2011.05.044

Torres-Roca JF (2012) A molecular assay of tumor radiosensitivity: a roadmap towards biology-based personalized radiation therapy. Pers Med 9:547–557. https://doi.org/10.2217/pme.12.55

Toulany M, Dittmann K, Kruger M, Baumann M, Rodemann HP (2005) Radioresistance of K-Ras mutated human tumor cells is mediated through EGFR-dependent activation of PI3K-AKT pathway. Radiother Oncol 76(2):143–150

Toulany M, Kasten-Pisula U, Brammer I, Wang S, Chen J, Dittmann K, Baumann M, Dikomey E, Rodemann HP (2006) Blockage of epidermal growth factor receptor-phosphatidylinositol 3-kinase-AKT signaling increases radiosensitivity of K-RAS mutated human tumor cells in vitro by affecting DNA repair. Clin Cancer Res 12(13):4119–4126

Toulany M, Dittmann K, Fehrenbacher B, Schaller M, Baumann M, Rodemann HP (2008) PI3K-Akt signaling regulates basal, but MAP-kinase signaling regulates radiation-induced XRCC1 expression in human tumor cells in vitro. DNA Repair (Amst) 7(10):1746–1756

Toulany M, Lee KJ, Fattah KR, Lin YF, Fehrenbacher B, Schaller M, Chen BP, Chen DJ, Rodemann HP (2012) Akt promotes post-irradiation survival of human tumor cells through initiation, progression, and termination of DNA-PKcs-dependent DNA double-strand break repair. Mol Cancer Res 10(7):945–957

Tsukamoto H, Shibata K, Kajiyama H, Terauchi M, Nawa A, Kikkawa F (2007) Irradiation-induced epithelial–mesenchymal transition (EMT) related to invasive potential in endometrial carcinoma cells. Gynecol Oncol 107:500–504. https://doi.org/10.1016/J.YGYNO.2007.08.058

Turrisi AT 3rd, Kim K, Blum R, Sause WT, Livingston RB, Komaki R, Wagner H, Aisner S, Johnson DH (1999) Twice-daily compared with once-daily thoracic radiotherapy in lim-ited small-cell lung cancer treated concurrently with cisplatin and etoposide. N Engl J Med 340(4):265–271

Vlashi E, Pajonk F (2015) Cancer stem cells, cancer cell plasticity and radiation therapy. Semin Cancer Biol 31:28–35. https://doi.org/10.1016/J.SEMCANCER.2014.07.001

Wang M, Kern AM, Hulskotter M, Greninger P, Singh A, Pan Y, Chowdhury D, Krause M, Baumann M, Benes CH, Efstathiou JA, Settleman J, Willers H (2014) EGFR-mediated chromatin condensation protects KRAS-mutant cancer cells against ionizing radiation. Cancer Res 74(10):2825–2834

Wang MT, Holderfield M, Galeas J, Delrosario R, To MD, Balmain A, McCormick F (2015) K-Ras promotes tumorigenicity through suppression of non-canonical Wnt Signaling. Cell 163(5):1237–1251. https://doi.org/10.1016/j.cell.2015.10.041

Wang M, Han J, Marcar L, Black J, Liu Q, Li X, Nagulapalli K, Sequist LV, Mak RH, Benes CH, Hong TS, Gurtner K, Krause M, Baumann M, Kang JX, Whetstine JR, Willers H (2017) Radiation resistance in KRAS-mutated lung cancer is enabled by stem-like properties mediated by an osteopontin-EGFR pathway. Cancer Res 77(8):2018–2028. https://doi.org/10.1158/0008-5472.CAN-16-0808

Wang Y, Li N, Jiang W, Deng W, Ye R, Xu C, Qiao Y, Sharma A, Zhang M, Hung MC, Lin SH (2018) Mutant LKB1 confers enhanced radiosensitization in combination with Trametinib in KRAS-mutant non-small cell lung cancer. Clin Cancer Res 24(22):5744–5756. https://doi.org/10.1158/1078-0432.CCR-18-1489

Werner-Wasik M, Swann RS, Bradley J, Graham M, Emami B, Purdy J, Sause W (2008) Increasing tumor volume is predictive of poor overall and progression-free survival: secondary analysis of the Radiation Therapy Oncology Group 93-11 phase I-II radiation dose-escalation study in patients with inoperable non-small-cell lung cancer. Int J Radiat Oncol Biol Phys 70(2):385–390. https://doi.org/10.1016/j.ijrobp.2007.06.034

Willers H, Held KD (2006) Introduction to clinical radiation biology. Hematol Oncol Clin North Am 20(1):1–24

Willers H, Azzoli CG, Santivasi WL, Xia F (2013) Basic mechanisms of therapeutic resistance to radiation and chemotherapy in lung cancer. Cancer J 19(3):200–207

Willers H, Keane FK, Kamran SC (2019) Toward a new framework for clinical radiation biology. Hematol Oncol Clin North Am 33(6):929–945. https://doi.org/10.1016/j.hoc.2019.07.001

Williams TM, Flecha AR, Keller P, Ram A, Karnak D, Galban S, Galban CJ, Ross BD, Lawrence TS, Rehemtulla A, Sebolt-Leopold J (2012) Cotargeting MAPK and PI3K signaling with concurrent radiotherapy as a strategy for the treatment of pancreatic cancer. Mol Cancer Ther 11(5):1193–1202

Winton T, Livingston R, Johnson D, Rigas J, Johnston M, Butts C, Cormier Y, Goss G, Inculet R, Vallieres E, Fry W, Bethune D, Ayoub J, Ding K, Seymour L, Graham B, Tsao MS, Gandara D, Kesler K, Demmy T, Shepherd J (2005) Vinorelbine plus cisplatin vs. observation in resected non-small-cell lung cancer. N Engl J Med 352(25):2589–2597

Withers HR, Taylor JM, Maciejewski B (1988) The hazard of accelerated tumor clonogen repopulation during radiotherapy. Acta Oncol 27(2):131–146. https://doi.org/10.3109/02841868809090333

Wurster S, Hennes F, Parplys AC, Seelbach JI, Mansour WY, Zielinski A, Petersen C, Clauditz TS, Munscher A, Friedl AA, Borgmann K (2016) PARP1 inhibition radiosensitizes HNSCC cells deficient in homologous recombination by disabling the DNA replication fork elongation response. Oncotarget 7(9):9732–9741. https://doi.org/10.18632/oncotarget.6947

Xiang T, Ohashi A, Huang Y, Pandita TK, Ludwig T, Powell SN, Yang Q (2008) Negative regulation of AKT activation by BRCA1. Cancer Res 68(24):10040–10044

Xu D, Allsop SA, Witherspoon SM, Snider JL, Yeh JJ, Fiordalisi JJ, White CD, Williams D, Cox AD, Baines AT (2011) The oncogenic kinase Pim-1 is modulated by K-Ras signaling and mediates transformed growth and radioresistance in human pancreatic ductal adenocarcinoma cells. Carcinogenesis 32(4):488–495

Yang H, Wang W, Zhang Y, Zhao J, Lin E, Gao J, He J (2011) The role of NF-E2-related factor 2 in predicting chemoresistance and prognosis in advanced non–small-cell lung cancer. Clin Lung Cancer 12(3):166–171. https://doi.org/10.1016/j.cllc.2011.03.012

Yard BD, Adams DJ, Chie EK, Tamayo P, Battaglia JS, Gopal P, Rogacki K, Pearson BE, Phillips J, Raymond DP, Pennell NA, Almeida F, Cheah JH, Clemons PA, Shamji A, Peacock CD, Schreiber SL, Hammerman PS, Abazeed ME (2016) A genetic basis for the variation in the vulnerability of cancer to DNA damage. Nat Commun 7:11428. https://doi.org/10.1038/ncomms11428

Yaromina A, Krause M, Thames H, Rosner A, Krause M, Hessel F, Grenman R, Zips D, Baumann M (2007) Pre-treatment number of clonogenic cells and their radiosensitivity are major determinants of local tumour control after fractionated irradiation. Radiother Oncol 83(3):304–310

Yin H, Glass J (2011) The phenotypic radiation resistance of CD44+/CD24(−or low) breast cancer cells is mediated through the enhanced activation of ATM signaling. PLoS One 6:e24080. https://doi.org/10.1371/journal.pone.0024080

Zhang X, Li X, Zhang N, Yang Q, Moran MS (2011) Low doses ionizing radiation enhances the invasiveness of breast cancer cells by inducing epithelial–mesenchymal transition. Biochem Biophys Res Commun 412:188–192. https://doi.org/10.1016/J.BBRC.2011.07.074

Zhang J, Jiao Q, Kong L, Yu J, Fang A, Li M, Yu J (2018) Nrf2 and Keap1 abnormalities in esophageal squamous cell carcinoma and association with the effect of chemoradiotherapy. Thoracic Cancer 9(6):726–735. https://doi.org/10.1111/1759-7714.12640

Chapter 5
Preclinical Strategies for Testing of Targeted Radiosensitizers

Steven H. Lin, Rui Ye, and Yifan Wang

Abstract Use of radiation for cancer therapy began shortly after the discovery of X-rays in 1895. Technological advances over the ensuing 120 years have enabled the development of sophisticated treatment systems, and radiation therapy remains an important component of cancer treatment, with more than 50% of all cancer patients receiving radiation therapy at some point in the course of the disease. In the 1960s and 1970s, combining chemotherapy with radiation was found to have synergistic anti-cancer effects for patients with advanced cancer. In more recent years, the advent of molecular biology has facilitated the development of specific drugs for molecular targets involved in neoplastic processes, giving rise to targeted therapy. Although the radiosensitization capabilities of some targeted agents have led to improved clinical outcomes in some cases, numerous clinical trials of targeted therapies with radiation have failed to demonstrate such improvements. One reason for this failure may be the use of poorly designed and reported preclinical studies as the rationale for undertaking large, expensive, and ultimately unsuccessful clinical trials. In this chapter, we introduce current preclinical screening methods for radiosensitizers, review current guidelines and recommendations for the standardization of preclinical studies, and discuss future opportunities in the era of precision radiation oncology.

Keywords Biomarkers · Clonogenic survival · Colony formation assay · DNA doube-strand breaks · Genetically engineered mouse models · High content screening · High-throughput screening · In vivo validation · Patient-derived xenografts · Preclinical models · Radioresistance · Radiosensitizers · Radiosensitivity · Screening

S. H. Lin (✉) · R. Ye · Y. Wang
Division of Radiation Oncology, Department of Radiation Oncology, MD Anderson Cancer Center, Houston, TX, USA
e-mail: SHLin@mdanderson.org

© Springer Nature Switzerland AG 2020
H. Willers, I. Eke (eds.), *Molecular Targeted Radiosensitizers*, Cancer Drug Discovery and Development, https://doi.org/10.1007/978-3-030-49701-9_5

1   Introduction

More than 50% of cancer patients receive radiation therapy, either alone or as a component of multimodality therapy, at some point in the course of the disease (Ahmed et al. 2016). Technological advancements in the planning and delivery of ionizing radiation have allowed ever-more precise and specific dose targeting to tumor tissues while minimizing the toxicity arising from exposure of nearby normal tissues to irradiation (Thariat et al. 2013; Lin et al. 2013). However, biologic factors such as the intrinsic and extrinsic radioresistance of tumors and inter- and intratumor heterogeneity (Orth et al. 2014) are barriers towards maximizing the effectiveness of radiation therapy. The realization in the 1960s and 1970s that cytotoxic chemotherapy could be combined with radiation therapy to enhance its effectiveness has clinically impacted nearly all tumor types, but also led to the realization that further augmentation of radiation therapy or chemoradiation could be possible (Begg et al. 2011). Much research in the following decades has identified cellular pathways involved in DNA repair, cell cycle checkpoints, oncogenic signaling, and metabolic pathways that could enhance the radiation response of tumors. Systematic studies of how to best combine agents that target these and other novel pathways with radiation therapy have been developed. In this chapter, we review current methods for preclinical testing of radiosensitizing targeted agents, existing guidelines, and recommendations as well as challenges and opportunities.

2   Preclinical Methods for Testing Targeted Radiosensitizers

The mechanisms of action of any potential radiosensitizer must be tested and validated preclinically, ideally with both in vitro and in vivo experiments. The most commonly used in vitro model system for testing the modulatory effects of radiosensitizers has been immortalized human cancer cell lines. The radiosensitivity of cell lines can be assessed with a large variety of different experimental assays, albeit the clonogenic cell survival assay, tested in 6-well plates or other vessel formats, remains the gold standard for analyzing both the radiosensitivity of tumors and normal cells as well as the potential of targeted agents to modify radiation effects in vitro (Stone et al. 2016; Kirsch et al. 2018).

Clonogenic or colony-formation assays measure the reproductive capability of an irradiated cell (Fig. 5.1a). This reflects clinical practice where it is the survival of the few cancer cells in patients, not the death of the many, that leads to recurrences months to years after therapy (Stone et al. 2016). Clonogenic assays are independent of the modes of cell death such as mitotic catastrophe, apoptosis, senescence, necrosis, or autophagy and the time intervals over which they occur. Lethally irradiated cells usually have prolonged cell cycles and may die after one or more cell divisions (Fig. 5.1b). Clonogenic assays allow time for elimination of lethally irradiated cells that are not capable of sustained proliferation. Therefore, short-term proliferation/viability endpoints that are based on modes of cell death, such as

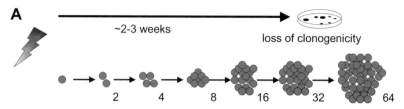

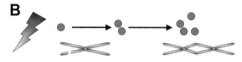

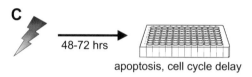

Fig. 5.1 Assessment of cell survival after treatment with ionizing radiation. (**a**) Colony formation assay tests the replicative potential of irradiated cells. (**b**) Lethally irradiated cells may experience cell cycle delay or divide one or more times before ceasing to proliferate. Because of this, short-term assays over 2–3 days are poorly suited to assess radiosensitivity/radioresistance of cells. (**c**) Short-term endpoints may reflect modes of cell death such as apoptosis

apoptosis assays, or cell cycle delays typically do not correlate well with clonogenic survival (Fig. 5.1c) (Brown and Wouters 1999).

Although clonogenic survival has the advantage of being able to account for radiation-related effects on cell growth, division, and proliferation (Franken et al. 2006), its relatively low-throughput limits the ability of this assay to identify novel radiosensitizers in unbiased screening studies. Therefore, surrogates for clonogenic assays that can be adapted for higher throughput studies, as described below, are greatly needed. It is important to note that even though short-term screening assays may not accurately measure cellular radiosensitivity or radioresistance, as defined though clonogenic survival, they may be able to capture the relative change in radiosensitivity that is caused by adding a radiosensitizer to irradiation in a given cell line.

2.1 High-Throughput In Vitro Screening Methods

In 1988, Alley and colleagues reported the feasibility of using 96-well plate microculture tetrazolium assays to measure short-term cell proliferation for drug screening (Alley et al. 1988). Since that time, several high-throughput screening studies designed specifically to identify radiosensitizers have been conducted, as summarized in Table 5.1, and are reviewed briefly below.

Lally and others described a colorimetric assay with 3-(4,5-dimethylthiazol-2-yl)-5-(3-carboxymethoxyphenyl)-2-(4-sulfophenyl)-2H-tetrazolium, inner salt [MTS]), to be used in 96-well plates to assess cellular survival in screens for novel radiosensitizers among 870 small molecule compounds (Lally et al. 2007). Both a glioma tumor cell line (U251) and a matched normal cell line (normal human astrocytes, or NHA) were used to identify 4′-bromo-3′-nitropropiophenone (NS-123), which radiosensitizes only glioma tumor cells but has limited toxicity for normal cell lines in response to a radiation dose of 4 Gy. The radiosensitizing effect of NS-123 was validated in vitro with an MTS assay of a colorectal cancer cell line (HT-29) and a lung cancer cell line (A549), and those results were further validated in vivo in zebrafish and nude mouse models.

Higgins and colleagues used DNA double-strand breaks (DSB), as quantified by γ-H2AX foci formation, as a surrogate for clonogenicity to screen 200 genes for their radiosensitizing effects (Higgins et al. 2010). By using a laryngeal cancer cell line (SQ20B) and a normal cell line (MRC5) irradiated with 4 Gy, POLQ was identified as a tumor-specific target for radiosensitization. The modulating effect of knocking down POLQ with small interfering RNA (siRNA) was further verified in standard clonogenic assays with a cervical cancer cell line (HeLa) and a bladder cancer cell line (T24) but were not reported to have been validated with in vivo models.

Lin et al. designed a novel high-content clonogenic survival assay system involving robotic cell seeding, drug dispensing, and automated imaging readouts of 96-well plates (Lin et al. 2014). This assay was used to screen 146 targeted agents in use in early-phase clinical trials. Of those agents, several were identified that potently sensitized the KRAS-mutated non-small cell lung cancer (NSCLC) cell lines H460 and A549 to a radiation dose of 2 Gy. MEK inhibitors were particularly effective for specifically sensitizing KRAS-mutated NSCLC cells to radiation. These results were validated with standard clonogenic assays and further validated in vivo by using a nude mouse xenograft model. These findings formed the basis of a phase I study, funded by a UM1 (CTEP9488) and a UT Southwest/MD Anderson Cancer Center Lung Cancer SPORE, to test a MEK1/2 inhibitor (trametinib) with chemoradiation therapy for patients with KRAS-mutated locally advanced NSCLC (NCT01912625). The radiosensitizing effect of trametinib was further shown by the same group to function only in cell lines with mutations in both KRAS and LKB1, based on an analysis of 8 cell lines, suggesting that a subset of radiosensitizing modulators may be genotype specific (Wang et al. 2018).

Goglia et al. described a high-throughput assay method based on detecting DSBs with fluorescence in 384-well plates to screen for DSB repair inhibitors that could function as novel radiosensitizers (Goglia et al. 2015). By using the red and green fluorescence protein reporter system, this method allows non-homologous end-joining repair and homologous recombination repair to be measured simultaneously in U2OS cells after treatment with a DSB-inducing ligand. They eventually were able to confirm the radiosensitizing effects of two drugs that were identified in the initial screen using standard clonogenic assays. Rather than a phenotype screen,

Table 5.1 Summary of high-throughput methods for screening novel radiosensitizers

Study	Surrogates	No. of agents tested	Cell line used	Tumor type	IR dose	Screen format	In vitro validation	In vivo validation	Normal tissue toxicity	Screening hits
Lally et al. (2007)	MTS assay	870 small-molecule compounds	U251	Glioma	4 Gy	96-well plate	MTS assay in two other cell lines (HT-29, A549)	Zebrafish embryo xenografts; nude mice xenografts	Limited toxicity to normal tissues was validated in vitro with NHA and in vivo with zebrafish and nude mice	4′-bromo-3′-nitropropiophenone (NS-123)
Higgins et al. (2010)	γ-H2AX foci quantification 24 hour after IR	siRNAs targeting 200 genes	SQ20B	Laryngeal	4 Gy	Not reported	Clonogenic assays in two other cell lines (HeLa, T24)	Not done	Limited toxicity to normal tissue was validated in vitro	POLQ
Lin et al. (2014)	High-content clonogenic assay	146 compounds	H460	Lung	2 Gy	96-well plate	Clonogenic assays in five other cell lines (A549, H2030, H1299, H661, EKVX)	Nude mice xenografts	Not done	MEK1/2 inhibitor (trametinib)
Goglia et al. (2015)	Double-strand break fluorescence-based assays	20,000 compounds	U2OS	Osteosarcoma	DSB-induced ligand	384-well plate	Clonogenic assays done in another cell line (T98G)	Not done	Not done	Benzamil and loperamide

(continued)

Table 5.1 (continued)

Study	Surrogates	No. of agents tested	Cell line used	Tumor type	IR dose	Screen format	In vitro validation	In vivo validation	Normal tissue toxicity	Screening hits
Tiwana et al. (2015)	Adapted clonogenic assay	siRNAs targeting 709 kinases	HeLa	Cervical	7 Gy	96-well plate	Clonogenic assays in two other cell lines (SQ20B, BT-549)	Not done	Limited toxicity to normal tissue was validated in vitro	TPK1
Liu et al. (2015)	Nucleic acid stain (syto60) quantification	18 targeted agents	32 cell lines	Lung, colorectal, genitourinary, and head and neck	2 Gy	96-well plate	Clonogenic assays in 25 cell lines	Not done	Not done	Everolimus and midostaurin

IR ionizing radiation, *MTS* tetrazolium salt, *NHA* normal human astrocytes

such as cell proliferation, cell death, or clonogenic survival which are biologic end-points based on multiple converging pathways, screens that assess the most proximal endpoints such as DNA damage or DNA foci formation could easily be automated and thereby enable the highest throughput screening of compounds. While such screens are highly sensitive, the sheer number of potential drugs that could be identified makes the task of subsequent validation much more difficult.

Tiwana and others used a 96-well high-throughput clonogenic survival assay for an siRNA screen targeting 709 kinases for novel radiosensitizers after a 7-Gy radiation dose (Tiwana et al. 2015). The most potent radiosensitizer among the candidates was one that targeted thiamin pyrophosphokinase 1 (TPK1). The radiosensitizing effect of TPK1 was validated by standard clonogenic survival assay in three cancer cell lines (HeLa, SQ20B, and BT-549) but not in normal cell lines.

Liu and colleagues adapted a high-throughput non-clonogenic drug screening platform on the basis of short-term cell proliferation/viability assays (3–5 days of incubation post-irradiation) (Liu et al. 2015). This format, tested on 32 cancer cell lines and 18 targeted drugs, was used to derive short-term radiosensitization factors at 2 Gy (SRF_{2Gy}), which were compared with standard dose enhancement factors (DEF) at a set survival fraction derived from clonogenic survival curves across doses from 2 to 8 Gy. The correlation between SRF_{2Gy} and DEF was associated with a sensitivity and specificity of more than 80% each. Drug-induced short-term radiosensitization was accompanied by changes in the mode of cell death such as senescence or apoptosis, thus providing a mechanistic basis for why short-term endpoints could predict radiosensitization in a clonogenic assay. Tumor genotype-dependent radiosensitization effects were observed, such as a KRAS-mutant specific effect of the multikinase inhibitor midostaurin.

2.2 In Vitro Validation

All "hits" in preclinical screening of candidate radiosensitizers should be validated using the gold standard clonogenic survival assay. At a minimum, in vitro validation testing should consist of at least two cell lines related to a cancer site of interest though higher cell line numbers have been suggested as well (Lin et al. 2013; Liu et al. 2015). Another important issue to consider is the reproducibility and robustness of the results as cell lines used in different labs derived from a same source stock could behave very differently. Tumor cell lines are known to undergo genetic drift through passages that may result in quite different phenotypes than their parental tumors (Stone et al. 2016). Moreover, the same cell line can undergo distinctly different clonal selection under different culture conditions (Ben-David et al. 2018). In one study, in the 27 different MCF7 strains that were identified, more than 75% of 321 tested anti-cancer drugs showed significant inconsistencies in their ability to inhibit proliferation in vitro. Hence, it is important to emphasize the importance of using validated cell lines from central resources like ATCC where quality controls are strictly enforced and limiting the number of passages used for any particular sets of experiments (e.g., at most 10 passages before a new batch is thawed out). Moreover, initial testing using a control drug with known sensitization properties could further ensure that in vitro conditions other than the passage number have not significantly deviated, before large-scale validation of drugs of unknown properties is done.

2.3   In Vivo Validation

In vivo validation of the effects of radiosensitizers is an important step in determining whether the tested agents can be translated robustly for clinical use. This is discussed in detail elsewhere in this volume and briefly reviewed below. For practical and economic reasons, nearly all in vivo validation is done using mouse systems although spontaneous canine cancer models have been used to a limited extent at specialized centers (Kunos and Coleman 2018). Second, for the same strain of animals, the company from which the animals are purchased from, and the facility at which the animals are being housed for experiments, can contribute to heterogeneity in drug response due to changes in the microbiota, which can significantly impact the immune system (Moore and Stanley 2016). Third, the impact of gender should be accounted for in the experiments. Lastly, studies should be powered sufficiently with appropriate number of animals per group in order to reach valid conclusions. Although no animal model can perfectly recapitulate human tumors, carefully designed animal model experiments can still provide invaluable insights on a candidate agent's mechanisms of action and radiation enhancement effects.

The most commonly used mouse models are ectopically or orthotopically implanted human or mouse cancer xenografts or genetically engineered mouse models (GEMMs). Depending on the context, each model has its own advantages and disadvantages and thus the choice of a specific model is crucial depending on the specific circumstances.

The most popular approach involves the transplantation of human xenografts into immunocompromised mice (Venditti 1981). A variety of xenograft materials can be used for preclinical screening, including human cell lines grown as monolayer on a dish and transplanted to the animals, from cell line-derived 3D spheroids or tumor organoids, or from patient-derived xenograft (PDX) models that have never been propagated in vitro. Human xenografts can either be heterotopically/ ectopically or orthotopically implanted. The prime advantage of using established human cell line xenograft models is the simplicity and throughput for use, but the relatively homogeneous cellular composition does not adequately account for the complexities of the tumor microenvironment. PDX models have the distinct advantage over other models in that they should recapitulate the genetic complexity and heterogeneity of the original tumor (Tentler et al. 2012). PDXs could also be more helpful for identifying potentially predictive biomarkers that can be quickly translated into clinical use (Pitts et al. 2010; Hidalgo et al. 2014). The key limitation of such models is the immunocompromised state that these tumors must be grown in.

Orthotopic models have been used to study the radiation enhancement effects in pancreatic, lung, breast, prostate, and brain tumors (Kahn et al. 2012). Unlike ectopic models, orthotopic models allow tumor cells to grow within stroma that most closely resemble the biology of the organ of origin, thereby better reflecting an agent's effects on stromal interaction, vascularization, and metabolism (Lawrence et al. 2013; Stone et al. 2016). Another advantage of orthotopic models is that local invasion and metastasis more closely reflect what is seen in humans. In addition to tumor size, another endpoint in orthotopic models often is survival time of the individual animals. The disadvantages of orthotopic models are their technical complexity and the time they require to establish (Bibby 2004).

GEMMs have been used to determine an agent's ability to prevent spontaneous tumor development and delay tumor progression (Hansen and Khanna 2004). The major advantage of GEMMs is their putative ability to recapitulate, at a molecular level, the progression of tumorigenesis in humans (Sharpless and DePinho 2006). These models also recapitulate most accurately human tumors since tumors that develop in specific organs within an immunocompetent host would not only allow testing the activity of specific agents and response biomarkers but would also allow assessment of tumor-stromal interactions and normal tissue toxicity simultaneously (Bristow et al. 2018; Hansen and Khanna 2004). However, major limitations of using GEMMs for these experiments are the length of time it takes to complete these experiments given the unpredictable growth rate, biological differences between murine tumors and human tumors may make GEMMs unreliable for assessing an agent's in vivo activity. Third, patent rights and regulations surrounding the use of GEMMs are limiting their use in preclinical testing (Hansen and Khanna 2004; Sharpless and DePinho 2006).

The tumor growth delay assay is most widely used for measuring the radiation enhancement effects of an agent (Kahn et al. 2012). In ectopic models, this assay involves subcutaneous implantation of tumor cells (of either human or murine origin) into mice, waiting for the tumors to grow to a specified size, and randomly assigning mice bearing tumors of similar size to control and treatment groups. Tumor growth is followed in all mice, and the difference between tumors in the control and treatment groups is the primary means of assessing the effectiveness of the candidate agent. The advantages of ectopic models include the simplicity of the implantation procedure, treatment delivery, and endpoint measurement, and their relatively low cost (Bristow et al. 2018). The major disadvantage of ectopic models is that they cannot account for the effects of the tested agent on the tumor microenvironment. Other, more costly measures include imaging-based measurements, such as computed tomographic or magnetic resonance imaging, which are needed for orthotopic models, or luminescence assays from luciferase expressing cell lines implanted ectopically or orthotopically.

2.4   Current Challenges to Translating Preclinical Screening Results to the Clinic

Although the past decades have seen rapid technological advances in radiation dose delivery, new insights on mechanisms underlying radiosensitivity and radioresistance, and expanding choices of experimental models, several obstacles still exist that complicate the efficient translation of preclinical results into clinical use and probably contribute to the high failure rates of clinical trials. These obstacles can be considered in two main categories: reliability and technical barriers. Regarding reliability, the high complexity and heterogeneity of both tumors and patients with cancer require that preclinical studies reflect those complexities and produce robust results before tested agents can be translated to clinical use (Begley and Ellis 2012). A key aspect of reproducibility in preclinical study is transparency. Stone and colleagues (Stone et al. 2016) critically analyzed 125 published preclinical studies testing the radiosensitization effects of 10 agents, focusing on methods, doses, dosing schedules, assays, measurement, data analysis, and conclusions. That analysis revealed that inadequate information and unclear reporting confounded the results of these studies in ways that made them difficult to interpret. Other groups have suggested that certain core aspects of preclinical testing should always be reported, including aspects of animal randomization, blinding, sample-size estimation, and data handling (Landis et al. 2012). Regarding technological barriers, most of the problems arise from the biological differences between animal models and humans. Although preclinical studies remain inadequate for addressing all the nuances and complexities of human physiology and cancer biology, we believe that, conducted appropriately, they are still a valuable tool to confirm mechanisms of action and radiation enhancement properties. This forms the basis for successful clinical translation of the most promising radiation/drug combinations (Fig. 5.2) (Bristow et al. 2018).

3   Existing Guidelines and Recommendations

To facilitate the preclinical development and translation of novel radiosensitizers, several organizations including the Cancer Therapy Evaluation Program (CTEP) and Radiation Research Program (RRP) of the National Cancer Institute in the United States (Coleman et al. 2014), the American Society for Radiation Oncology (ASTRO) (Wallner et al. 2014; Bristow et al. 2018), the Radiation Therapy Oncology Group (RTOG) (Lawrence et al. 2013), and the National Cancer Research Institute (NCRI) in the United Kingdom (Harrington et al. 2011) have acknowledged the challenges noted above and have proposed guidelines and recommendations for preclinical testing of potential radiosensitizing agents. Summarized in Table 5.2, these guidelines and recommendations have six main areas of focus: determination of agent activity; dose standardization; assessments of agent toxicity; in vitro validation; in vivo validation; and biomarker development.

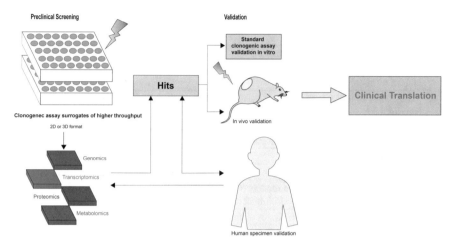

Fig. 5.2 Preclinical workflow for testing of targeted radiosensitizers (adapted from Bristow et al. (2018))

Table 5.2 Summary of current guidelines and recommendations

	Determination of agent activity
1.1	Agents of interest should enhance radiation effects through either synergistic or additive mechanisms but, if not, should at least have single-agent or combination activity with chemotherapy
1.2	Pharmacokinetics and pharmacodynamics of the agents should be tested
1.3	When generation of in vitro or in vivo preclinical data is not feasible, strong justification must be provided for the inability to perform these studies before a clinical study is proposed
1.4	A compendium of molecular pathways known to be important in the biological behavior of cancers that are routinely treated with radiation should be compiled for the agent of interest
1.5	The mechanisms of drug-radiation combinations should be thoroughly explored for spatial cooperation, cytotoxic enhancement, biological cooperation, temporal modulation, and normal tissue protection
	Dose standardization
2.1	Standard procedures with trackable radiation dosimetry, beam calibration, determination of the absorbed dose within the subject, and radiation source specification should be established
2.2	Fractionated radiation dose schedule resembling those used in clinical setting should be used
2.3	Radiation-radiosensitizer schedules should be both optimized for radiation-enhancing effects and for their transferability to the clinic
	Determination of agent toxicity to normal tissues
3.1	Possibilities for spatial cooperation and nonoverlapping toxicity in sparing normal tissues should be considered
3.2	Radioprotectors and mitigators should be investigated for further reducing normal tissue toxicity

(continued)

Table 5.2 (continued)

	In vitro validation
4.1	Clonogenic assay is the gold standard
4.2	Colorimetric assays of cell survival can be used as alternative approaches when cell lines fail to form colonies
4.3	The choice of tumor type is key; at least two cell lines from the same disease site should be required
4.4	The cell lines used should be fingerprinted and the passage number of the cell line should be the same across different experiments
	In vivo validation
5.1	Nude mice are preferable to test the effects of agents on human tumor intrinsic factors
5.2	Genetically engineered mouse models (GEMMs) are especially useful for testing agents that target the tumor microenvironment and normal tissues
5.3	Syngeneic models are preferable for testing agents that modulate immune components
5.4	Orthotopic models are useful for determining toxicity to normal tissues and tumor microenvironment effects
5.5	Statistical justification for the number of animals needed should be required
	Biomarker development
6.1	The development of radiation-enhancing agents should be prioritized when biomarker-based patient selection is available
6.2	Agents without validated predictive biomarkers available for clinical testing could be brought into clinical testing, but with the requirement for clear plans for concurrent preclinical research and clinical development of predictive biomarkers from pretreatment tissue specimens
6.3	Concurrent development of predictive biomarkers should be a priority during the preclinical and early clinical phases of testing followed by subsequent clinical validation. Clinical studies must mandate pretreatment tumor biopsy or serum collection, with strong consideration given to acquisition of serial tissue collection during early therapy and at the time of recurrence
6.4	Understanding the proper sequencing of combining targeted agents with radiation therapy is crucial before undertaking large clinical trials

3.1   Determination of Agent Activity

Comprehensive investigation of the mechanisms of action of novel radiosensitizers is an important prerequisite for their successful translation to the clinic. First proposed by Steel and Peckman and later refined by Bentzen and colleagues is the recommendation that mechanisms related to spatial cooperation, cytotoxic enhancement, biological cooperation, temporal modulation, and normal tissue protection for these agents should be exploited (Steel and Peckham 1979; Bentzen et al. 2007). Therefore, priority should be given to radiosensitizers with synergistic or additive effects, or at least those with single-agent or combination activity with chemotherapy that enhances local control and cytotoxicity to the tumor (Lin et al. 2013). The ability of the agent of interest to modulate molecular signaling pathways known to be important in biological responses of tumors routinely treated with radiation therapy should be investigated (Harrington et al. 2011). Another perspective that should be considered is the distribution of the agent in blood and tumor tissue. If the effects of irradiation impact a candidate agent's activity, that interaction could have important clinical consequences (Chen et al. 2017). Therefore, clarifying the potential pharmacokinetic, pharmacodynamic, and biochemical effects of the agent of interest would be useful for characterizing its radiation enhancement activities.

3.2 Dose Standardization

Guaranteeing the reproducibility of drug-radiation test studies requires that standard procedures be established for reporting radiation-related variables such as radiation dosimetry, radiation sources, radiation precision and accuracy, and detailed dose schedules (Ford and Deye 2016). A key aspect of translational preclinical radiation-related studies is to establish and use clinically relevant radiation doses and fractionation regimens, since for example DNA repair mechanisms after a single radiation dose and a multifractionated irradiation can be differentially impacting the efficacy of targeted drugs (Eke et al. 2020). The first step in this process is to establish universal standards and dosimetry centers that allow tracing and calibrating the radiation sources and doses for labs throughout the world (Desrosiers et al. 2013). Accomplishing this goal would require both central and institutional radiation-physics oversight of acceptance testing, commissioning, output calibration, and irradiation geometry dose specification (Yoshizumi et al. 2011; Kazi et al. 2014). Next, variations among radiation dosing schedules between studies can obscure the true sensitivity-modulating effects of the agents of interest. Therefore, testing and comparing different radiation doses and dosing schedules are recommended for both in vitro and in vivo studies. Another important perspective to consider is the sequence of the agent and the radiation. The importance of choosing drug-radiation schedules that are clinically practical and optimized for cytotoxic enhancement cannot be overstated. We recommend that special attention be paid to institutional radiation dosimetry programs that would report of all details of radiation geometry, radiation dose, and radiation-drug dosing schedules for preclinical screening tests.

3.3 Determining Toxicity of an Agent to Normal Tissues

Radiation is known to cause acute normal tissue toxicity, which results mostly from rapid cell death, and late normal tissue toxicity, which has been associated with irreversible vascular damage, fibrosis, atrophy, infertility, hormone deficiencies, and secondary malignancies (Liauw et al. 2013; Barnett et al. 2009). Thus, preclinical testing of candidate radiosensitizers must consider the potential side effects of those agents. Perhaps the easiest way to assess acute side effects is to test the cytotoxic effects of radiation combined with the radiosensitizer on immortalized normal cell lines of the same disease-site origin. However, given the biological differences between in vitro and in vivo systems, it may be more reliable to test radiation toxicity by using orthotopic syngeneic models or GEMMs. Another complementary approach would be the development of novel radioprotectors or mitigators. Radioprotectors are usually given before exposure to radiation, whereas mitigators are often given during or after the exposure to radiation (Moding et al. 2013). Regardless, research is needed to determine the specific molecular mechanisms of their normal tissue protection effects and to ensure their use would not mitigate the radiation enhancement effects of the radiosensitizers. We recommend that the toxicity of candidate radiosensitizers be tested preclinically in both in vitro and in vivo settings.

3.4 Biomarker Development

Bringing agents with established biomarkers into clinical tests with radiation requires some preclinical evidence of synergy with radiation therapy (Lin et al. 2013; Bristow et al. 2018). Some radiosensitizers may have much more profound radiation enhancement effects on tumors that have specific mutations. Therefore, preclinical development of biomarkers that are useful for patient selection, response classification, and resistance prediction could be another step towards increasing the likelihood of successfully translating preclinical results to clinical use (Morgan et al. 2014).

4   Opportunities

Although numerous challenges remain in translating preclinical findings on potential radiosensitizing agents into the clinic, we believe that, given the rapid technological advances in radiation delivery, genomics, proteomics, and metabolomics in the era of precision radiation medicine, unprecedented opportunities are available as well to reveal novel targets and mechanisms through the design of robust sophisticated preclinical studies. Key factors that should be reported for all future preclinical screening studies of novel radiosensitizers are summarized in Table 5.3.

Growing evidence suggests that immune checkpoint blockade (e.g., with inhibitors of CTLA-4 or PD-1/PD-L1) can re-sensitize tumor cells by normalizing the tumor vasculature and reversing tumor hypoxia (Wang et al. 2019). Thus, identifying novel radiosensitizers that can further enhance the effect of both radiation and immunotherapy to more effectively control tumors for longer periods is a focus of great interest. However, to date no efficient, unbiased methods have been developed to identify such agents mainly because of the time and technical complexities of screening studies done with GEMMs or orthotopic models. Therefore, novel screening methods or less costly humanized mouse models are greatly needed.

Table 5.3 Checklist of factors to report in preclinical screening studies

Core report factors	Screening	In vitro validation	In vivo validation
Cell lines	Cell line fingerprinting; cell line passage; culture conditions		
Assays	Initial cell number; assay length		
	Assay format	Rationale for using the assay if clonogenic assay cannot be done	Animal randomization
Radiation and drug delivery	Radiation dosimetry, dose and schedule; drug solvents used; drug concentrations and schedule; sequence of radiation and drug		
Measurement of endpoints	Raw data for all screening candidates	Standardized colony counting	Blinding; standardized tumor volume measurement
Sample estimation	Number of technical and biological replicates		
	Statistical cutoff for screening hits	Number of cell lines needed	Number of animals per group
Data analysis	Normalization method; statistical model; analysis software; error bars; raw data from which to replicate analytical results		

Recent decreases in the cost of next-generation sequencing will allow comprehensive genomic profiling of tumors treated with radiation. Techniques such as multiregion sequencing and single-cell sequencing offer the opportunity to visualize intratumor heterogeneity at unprecedented resolution, which will help not only to clarify the molecular responses of radiation-treated tumors but also to develop more personalized treatment plans for patients. Multi-omics studies that integrate the genomic, epigenomic, transcriptomic, proteomic, and metabolomic information would also be greatly useful for further elucidating mechanisms of radiosensitization and radioresistance. Finally, development of genome-editing techniques would increase the sophistication and efficiency of screening methods. For example, perturb-seq (Dixit et al. 2016) allows genetic perturbation on the single-cell level, which could be quite useful for identifying novel targets that control colony-formation ability. Another recently developed technique, sci-Plex, allows high-throughput screening of hundreds of chemical screens at the single-cell level within one experiment (Srivatsan et al. 2020). Techniques such as these will provide higher throughput and greater resolution that in turn will enable the robust identification of additional radiosensitizers that can be translated to the clinic.

References

Ahmed MM, Narendra A, Prasanna P, Coleman CN, Krishnan S (2016) Current insights in radiation combination therapies: influence of omics and novel targeted agents in defining new concepts in radiation biology and clinical radiation oncology. In: Seminars in radiation oncology. vol. 26, no. 4. WB Saunders Ltd, pp 251–253

Alley MC, Scudiero DA, Monks A, Hursey ML, Czerwinski MJ, Fine DL, Abbott BJ, Mayo JG, Shoemaker RH, Boyd MR (1988) Feasibility of drug screening with panels of human tumor cell lines using a microculture tetrazolium assay. Cancer Res 48(3):589–601

Barnett GC, West CM, Dunning AM, Elliott RM, Coles CE, Pharoah PD, Burnet NG (2009) Normal tissue reactions to radiotherapy: towards tailoring treatment dose by genotype. Nat Rev Cancer 9(2):134–142

Begg AC, Stewart FA, Vens C (2011) Strategies to improve radiotherapy with targeted drugs. Nat Rev Cancer 11(4):239–253

Begley CG, Ellis LM (2012) Raise standards for preclinical cancer research. Nature 483(7391):531–533

Ben-David U, Siranosian B, Ha G, Tang H, Oren Y, Hinohara K, Strathdee CA, Dempster J, Lyons NJ, Burns R, Nag A (2018) Genetic and transcriptional evolution alters cancer cell line drug response. Nature 560(7718):325–330

Bentzen SM, Harari PM, Bernier J (2007) Exploitable mechanisms for combining drugs with radiation: concepts, achievements and future directions. Nat Rev Clin Oncol 4(3):172

Bibby MC (2004) Orthotopic models of cancer for preclinical drug evaluation: advantages and disadvantages. Eur J Cancer 40(6):852–857

Bristow RG, Alexander B, Baumann M, Bratman SV, Brown JM, Camphausen K, Choyke P, Citrin D, Contessa JN, Dicker A, Kirsch DG (2018) Combining precision radiotherapy with molecular targeting and immunomodulatory agents: a guideline by the American Society for Radiation Oncology. Lancet Oncol 19(5):e240–e251

Brown JM, Wouters BG (1999) Apoptosis, p53, and tumor cell sensitivity to anticancer agents. Cancer Res 59(7):1391–1399

Chen YJ, Tsai TH, Wang LY, Hsieh CH (2017) Local radiotherapy affects drug pharmacokinetics—exploration of a neglected but significant uncertainty of cancer therapy. Technol Cancer Res Treat 16(6):705–716

Coleman CN, Lawrence TS, Kirsch DG (2014) Enhancing the efficacy of radiation therapy: premises, promises, and practicality. J Clin Oncol 32(26):2832

Desrosiers M, DeWerd L, Deye J, Lindsay P, Murphy MK, Mitch M, Macchiarini F, Stojadinovic S, Stone H (2013) The importance of dosimetry standardization in radiobiology. J R Natl Inst Standard Technol 118:403

Dixit A, Parnas O, Li B, Chen J, Fulco CP, Jerby-Arnon L, Marjanovic ND, Dionne D, Burks T, Raychowdhury R, Adamson B (2016) Perturb-Seq: dissecting molecular circuits with scalable single-cell RNA profiling of pooled genetic screens. Cell 167(7):1853–1866

Eke I, Zong D, Aryankalayil MJ, Sandfort V, Bylicky MA, Rath BH, Graves EE, Nussenzweig A, Coleman CN (2020) 53BP1/RIF1 signaling promotes cell survival after multifractionated radiotherapy. Nucleic Acids Res 48(3):1314–1326

Ford E, Deye J (2016) Current instrumentation and technologies in modern radiobiology research—opportunities and challenges. In: Seminars in radiation oncology, vol. 26, no. 4. WB Saunders, pp 349–355

Franken NA, Rodermond HM, Stap J, Haveman J, Van Bree C (2006) Clonogenic assay of cells in vitro. Nat Protocol 1(5):2315

Goglia AG, Delsite R, Luz AN, Shahbazian D, Salem AF, Sundaram RK, Chiaravalli J, Hendrikx PJ, Wilshire JA, Jasin M, Kluger HM (2015) Identification of novel radiosensitizers in a high-throughput, cell-based screen for DSB repair inhibitors. Mol Cancer Ther 14(2):326–342

Hansen K, Khanna C (2004) Spontaneous and genetically engineered animal models: use in preclinical cancer drug development. Eur J Cancer 40(6):858–880

Harrington KJ, Billingham LJ, Brunner TB, Burnet NG, Chan CS, Hoskin P, Mackay RI, Maughan TS, Macdougall J, McKenna WG, Nutting CM (2011) Guidelines for preclinical and early phase clinical assessment of novel radiosensitisers. Br J Cancer 105(5):628–639

Hidalgo M, Amant F, Biankin AV, Budinská E, Byrne AT, Caldas C, Clarke RB, de Jong S, Jonkers J, Mælandsmo GM, Roman-Roman S (2014) Patient-derived xenograft models: an emerging platform for translational cancer research. Cancer Discov 4(9):998–1013

Higgins GS, Prevo R, Lee YF, Helleday T, Muschel RJ, Taylor S, Yoshimura M, Hickson ID, Bernhard EJ, McKenna WG (2010) A small interfering RNA screen of genes involved in

DNA repair identifies tumor-specific radiosensitization by POLQ knockdown. Cancer Res 70(7):2984–2993

Kahn J, Tofilon PJ, Camphausen K (2012) Preclinical models in radiation oncology. Radiat Oncol 7(1):223

Kazi AM, MacVittie TJ, Lasio G, Lu W, Prado KL (2014) The MCART radiation physics core: the quest for radiation dosimetry standardization. Health Phys 106(1):97

Kirsch DG, Diehn M, Kesarwala AH, Maity A, Morgan MA, Schwarz JK, Bristow R et al (2018) The future of radiobiology. J Natl Cancer Inst 110(4):329–340

Kunos CA, Coleman CN (2018) Current and future initiatives for radiation oncology at the National Cancer Institute in the era of precision medicine. Int J Radiat Oncol Biol Phys 102(1):18–25

Lally BE, Geiger GA, Kridel S, Arcury-Quandt AE, Robbins ME, Kock ND, Wheeler K, Peddi P, Georgakilas A, Kao GD, Koumenis C (2007) Identification and biological evaluation of a novel and potent small molecule radiation sensitizer via an unbiased screen of a chemical library. Cancer Res 67(18):8791–8799

Landis SC, Amara SG, Asadullah K, Austin CP, Blumenstein R, Bradley EW, Crystal RG, Darnell RB, Ferrante RJ, Fillit H, Finkelstein R (2012) A call for transparent reporting to optimize the predictive value of preclinical research. Nature 490(7419):187–191

Lawrence YR, Vikram B, Dignam JJ, Chakravarti A, Machtay M, Freidlin B, Takebe N, Curran WJ Jr, Bentzen SM, Okunieff P, Coleman CN (2013) NCI–RTOG translational program strategic guidelines for the early-stage development of radiosensitizers. J Natl Cancer Inst 105(1):11–24

Liauw SL, Connell PP, Weichselbaum RR (2013) New paradigms and future challenges in radiation oncology: an update of biological targets and technology. Sci Transl Med 5(173):173sr2–173sr2

Lin SH, George TJ, Ben-Josef E, Bradley J, Choe KS, Edelman MJ, Guha C, Krishnan S, Lawrence TS, Le QT, Lu B (2013) Opportunities and challenges in the era of molecularly targeted agents and radiation therapy. J Natl Cancer Inst 105(10):686–693

Lin SH, Zhang J, Giri U, Stephan C, Sobieski M, Zhong L, Mason KA, Molkentine J, Thames HD, Yoo SS, Heymach JV (2014) A high content clonogenic survival drug screen identifies MEK inhibitors as potent radiation sensitizers for KRAS mutant non–small-cell lung cancer. J Thorac Oncol 9(7):965–973

Liu Q, Wang M, Kern AM, Khaled S, Han J, Yeap BY, Hong TS, Settleman J, Benes CH, Held KD, Efstathiou JA, Willers H (2015) Adapting a drug screening platform to discover associations of molecular targeted radiosensitizers with genomic biomarkers. Mol Cancer Res 13(4):713–720

Moding EJ, Kastan MB, Kirsch DG (2013) Strategies for optimizing the response of cancer and normal tissues to radiation. Nat Rev Drug Discov 12(7):526–542

Moore RJ, Stanley D (2016) Experimental design considerations in microbiota/inflammation studies. Clin Transl Immunol 5(7):e92

Morgan MA, Parsels LA, Maybaum J, Lawrence TS (2014) Improving the efficacy of chemoradiation with targeted agents. Cancer Discov 4(3):280–291

Orth M, Lauber K, Niyazi M, Friedl AA, Li M, Maihöfer C, Schüttrumpf L, Ernst A, Niemöller OM, Belka C (2014) Current concepts in clinical radiation oncology. Radiat Environ Biophys 53(1):1–29

Pitts TM, Tan AC, Kulikowski GN, Tentler JJ, Brown AM, Flanigan SA, Leong S, Coldren CD, Hirsch FR, Varella-Garcia M, Korch C (2010) Development of an integrated genomic classifier for a novel agent in colorectal cancer: approach to individualized therapy in early development. Clin Cancer Res 16(12):3193–3204

Sharpless NE, DePinho RA (2006) The mighty mouse: genetically engineered mouse models in cancer drug development. Nat Rev Drug Discov 5(9):741–754

Srivatsan SR, McFaline-Figueroa JL, Ramani V, Saunders L, Cao J, Packer J, Pliner HA, Jackson DL, Daza RM, Christiansen L, Zhang F (2020) Massively multiplex chemical transcriptomics at single-cell resolution. Science 367(6473):45–51

Steel GG, Peckham MJ (1979) Exploitable mechanisms in combined radiotherapy-chemotherapy: the concept of additivity. Int J Radiat Oncol Biol Phys 5(1):85–91

Stone HB, Bernhard EJ, Coleman CN, Deye J, Capala J, Mitchell JB, Brown JM (2016) Preclinical data on efficacy of 10 drug-radiation combinations: evaluations, concerns, and recommendations. Transl Oncol 9(1):46–56

Tentler JJ, Tan AC, Weekes CD, Jimeno A, Leong S, Pitts TM, Arcaroli JJ, Messersmith WA, Eckhardt SG (2012) Patient-derived tumour xenografts as models for oncology drug development. Nat Rev Clin Oncol 9(6):338

Thariat J, Hannoun-Levi JM, Myint AS, Vuong T, Gérard JP (2013) Past, present, and future of radiotherapy for the benefit of patients. Nat Rev Clin Oncol 10(1):52

Tiwana GS, Prevo R, Buffa FM, Yu S, Ebner DV, Howarth A, Folkes LK, Budwal B, Chu KY, Durrant L, Muschel RJ (2015) Identification of vitamin B1 metabolism as a tumor-specific radiosensitizing pathway using a high-throughput colony formation screen. Oncotarget 6(8):5978

Venditti JM (1981) Preclinical drug development: rationale and methods. Semin Oncol 8(4):349–361

Wallner PE, Anscher MS, Barker CA, Bassetti M, Bristow RG, Cha YI, Dicker AP, Formenti SC, Graves EE, Hahn SM, Hei TK (2014) Current status and recommendations for the future of research, teaching, and testing in the biological sciences of radiation oncology: report of the American Society for Radiation Oncology Cancer Biology/Radiation Biology Task Force, executive summary. Int J Radiat Oncol Biol Phys 88(1):11–17

Wang Y, Li N, Jiang W, Deng W, Ye R, Xu C, Qiao Y, Sharma A, Zhang M, Hung MC, Lin SH (2018) Mutant LKB1 confers enhanced radiosensitization in combination with Trametinib in KRAS-mutant non–small cell lung cancer. Clin Cancer Res 24(22):5744–5756

Wang Y, Liu ZG, Yuan H, Deng W, Li J, Huang Y, Kim BY, Story MD, Jiang W (2019) The reciprocity between radiotherapy and cancer immunotherapy. Clin Cancer Res 25(6):1709–1717

Yoshizumi T, Brady SL, Robbins ME, Bourland JD (2011) Specific issues in small animal dosimetry and irradiator calibration. Int J Radiat Biol 87(10):1001–1010

Chapter 6
3D Radiation Biology for Identifying Radiosensitizers

Anne Vehlow, Sara Sofia Deville, and Nils Cordes

Abstract The development and clinical implementation of novel therapeutics for the improvement of cancer patient survival is based on innovative and reproducible translational research. Despite extensive efforts from large-scale preclinical initiatives, many approaches fail to translate from bench to bedside. In the past decade, three-dimensional (3D) cell culture systems have gained increasing attention for overcoming challenges to clinical translation due to their apparent advantages in providing more physiological and predictive information on cellular behavior. This chapter discusses the characteristic properties of 3D cell culture systems in comparison with conventional two-dimensional (2D) monolayer cultures with particular focus on the cellular response to radio- and chemotherapy.

Keywords 2D cell culture · 3D cell culture · Adhesome · AKT · Cell adhesion-mediated radioresistance · Cellular adhesion · EGFR · Ex-vivo cultures · Extracellular matrix · Focal adhesion kinase · Integrins · Organoid · Radiation biology · Radioresistance · Spheroid · Tumoroid

A. Vehlow
National Center for Tumor Diseases Dresden, Dresden, Germany

OncoRay—National Center for Radiation Research in Oncology, Technische Universität Dresden, Dresden, Germany
e-mail: anne.vehlow@nct-dresden.de

S. S. Deville · N. Cordes (✉)
OncoRay—National Center for Radiation Research in Oncology, Technische Universität Dresden, Dresden, Germany
e-mail: sarasofia.deville@OncoRay.de; nils.cordes@OncoRay.de

© Springer Nature Switzerland AG 2020
H. Willers, I. Eke (eds.), *Molecular Targeted Radiosensitizers*, Cancer Drug Discovery and Development, https://doi.org/10.1007/978-3-030-49701-9_6

1   Introduction

During the past century, radiation therapy has technically evolved as a highly pre-cise cancer treatment modality and is often delivered in combination with surgery and chemotherapy as standard of care for about 50% of cancer patients worldwide (Delaney et al. 2005). As tumors are equipped with a heterogeneous and dynamic ability to resist and adapt to these cytotoxic treatments, a patient- and tumor-tailored combination of radiation with molecular targeted agents and chemotherapy will be required to eventually take big steps in improving therapy outcome in the future (Bristow et al. 2018; Sharma et al. 2016). The basics for the development and therapeutic implementation of such individualized radiosensitizers are the identifi-cation and preclinical evaluation of specific genetic, epigenetic, transcriptional, pro-teomic, and kinomic inter- as well as intratumoral variations that can be targeted to make tumors more susceptible to irradiation while limiting normal tissue toxicities (Bentzen et al. 2007; Morris and Harari 2014). Currently, these factors are being assessed by large-scale screening initiatives in a variety of cancer entities and are of crucial value not only for radiation biology research (Bailey et al. 2018; Corces et al. 2018; Raphael et al. 2017; The Cancer Genome Atlas Network et al. 2015; The Cancer Genome Atlas Network et al. 2012; The Cancer Genome Atlas Research Network et al. 2008). In addition to such intrinsic tumor cell aberrations, interac-tions of tumor cells with components of the microenvironment greatly modulate the tumor response to therapy and represent key targets for individualized multimodal treatment strategies (Kirsch et al. 2018; McGee et al. 2019; Vehlow et al. 2016).

The prime example of a clinically implemented and approved radiosensitizing approach is the targeting of the epidermal growth factor receptor (EGFR) in patients with head and neck squamous cell carcinomas (HNSCC) (Bonner et al. 2006, 2010). In this tumor entity, the EGFR is highly expressed in about 90% of the cases and correlates with a decreased response to radiation therapy, an increased recurrence and poor clinical outcome (Ang et al. 2002; Bonner et al. 2000; Rubin Grandis et al. 1998). Initial preclinical studies suggested a radiosensitizing effect of EGFR target-ing (Bonner et al. 1994; Huang et al. 1999; Mendelsohn 1997), a result that success-fully translated from bench to bedside and highlight the radiosensitizing potential of molecular targeted agents.

As increasing numbers of potential anti-cancer drugs are being discovered and enter drug development pipelines, the number of agents progressing from launch to entry into phase I trials remains below 0.1% (Dowden and Munro 2019). There is an urgent need to advance translatability of identified preclinical approaches, as the main cause for the failure of more than 50% of novel therapeutics in late stage clini-cal trials is the lack of efficacy (Harrison 2016). In part, these failures relate to the design and execution of experimental approaches. In radiation biology, two-dimensionally (2D) grown tumor cell cultures routinely serve for the characteriza-tion of targeted and non-targeted effects of ionizing irradiation and the identification of potential radiosensitizers. As these assays study cells under unnatural growth conditions, results may be compromised with regard to the response of cells to irra-

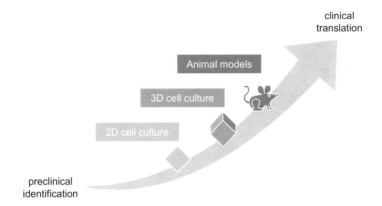

Fig. 6.1 3D cell culture in radiation biology. 3D cell culture bridges the gap between traditional 2D cell culture and preclinical animal studies during progression of any given radiosensitizer from preclinical identification to clinical translation

diation as well as chemotherapy (Coleman et al. 2016; Stone et al. 2016). The implementation of three-dimensional (3D) cell culture systems in preclinical radiation biology research bridges the gap to preclinical animal studies and represents one substantial and robust progress towards improved bench to bedside translation (Fig. 6.1) (Eke and Cordes 2011b). 3D cell cultures incorporate essential extracellular cues, such as the extracellular matrix (ECM), soluble factors and other cells, and have so far provided a much-improved understanding of the tumor cell response to radiotherapy (Eke and Cordes 2011b). Thus, it is not surprising that the implementation of 3D cell culture systems for drug discovery is indispensable and has gained enormous importance. This chapter discusses the characteristic properties of 3D cell culture with particular focus on the underlying mechanisms of the cellular radiation response and the identification of radiosensitizers.

2   Characteristics of 2D and 3D Cell Culture

Cell-based assays assessing radiobiological endpoints, such as the reproductive integrity of tumor cells and their DNA double-strand break (DSB) repair capacity, are essential tools for the identification of novel radiosensitizers. In fact, most theories and conclusions on the radiobiological effects of ionizing radiation over the past century are based on the results of 2D cell culture assays. Growing normal and malignant cells as 2D monolayer cultures is a generally accepted, fast, and cost-effective method to observe cellular behavior on flat and inflexible substrates, such as polystyrene plastic or glass surfaces (Fig. 6.2). Thus, it is not surprising that the 2D clonogenic (or colony formation) assay represents the current gold standard in radiation biology research. This assay assesses the replicative potential of cultured cells following irradiation, often in combination with chemotherapeutics and molecular targeted agents and serves the identification of novel radiosensitizers.

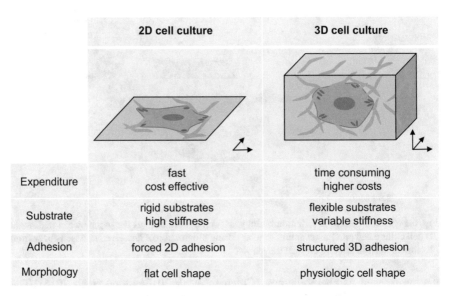

Fig. 6.2 Comparison of 2D and 3D cell culture. Simplified schemes and associated characteristics of cells grown as 2D and 3D cultures

However, 2D cell cultures have several limitations, one of which is the lack of a structural 3D organization enabling ECM adhesion, cell–cell communication, and growth factor signaling (Fig. 6.2). Due to these restrictions, 2D-grown cells display unnatural growth kinetics, compromised cellular functions and behavior, and data from such tests are frequently misleading and non-predictive (Cukierman et al. 2001; Pampaloni et al. 2007).

In recent years, tremendous effort has focused on the development and implementation of 3D cell culture models mimicking tissue-specific microarchitecture, since a physiologic cellular function requires the precise reproduction of the dominating microenvironmental conditions (Pampaloni et al. 2007; Schmeichel and Bissell 2003). In comparison to 2D cell culture, growing cells in a physiologic 3D environment is marginally more time, cost, and labor consuming but provides functional flexibility and adaptability (Fig. 6.2). Additionally, 3D cell cultures allow the growth of cells in their physical shape and provide improved cell–ECM and cell–cell contacts with profound functional impact on, for example, intracellular signaling networks, cell survival, cell proliferation as well as radiosensitivity (Abbott 2003; Cukierman et al. 2002; Eke and Cordes 2011b). Several different approaches to 3D cell culture exist (Breslin and O'Driscoll 2013; Edmondson et al. 2014; Eke et al. 2016; Friedrich et al. 2009; Pampaloni et al. 2007) (Fig. 6.3), such as the growth of single or multicellular monocultures and cocultures. These include:

1. Cells in solution or as hanging drops
2. ECM-based biological scaffolds and synthetic materials
3. Microfluidic cell culture systems
4. Agitation-based systems

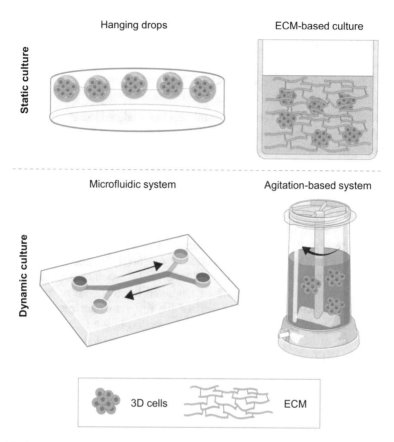

Fig. 6.3 3D cell culture technologies. Schematic representation of different approaches to 3D monocultures including static cultures such as hanging drops and ECM-based cell culture and dynamic microfluidic systems and agitation-based cultures. Created with BioRender

While most of these 3D cell culture methods do not completely reproduce physiological in vivo growth conditions, they do mimic the cellular microenvironment and incorporate both spatial organization and specific functional cues similarly found in tissues and organs. Therefore, it is not surprising that cellular functions can be different in 2D compared to 3D growth conditions. After all, cells grow embedded in 3D ECM in all organs, tissues as well as in tumors, and the functions of cells within these complex systems depend on their interactions with cellular and noncellular factors within the microenvironment. Consequently, 3D cell culture systems will certainly improve the functional relevance and the predictive power of cell-based screens and are invaluable tools for the identification of therapeutic drugs and radiosensitizers.

3 The Influence of 3D Growth Conditions on Tumor Cell Radiosensitivity

3.1 The Impact of the ECM on Radioresistance

The use of 3D ECM-based cell culture models in radiation biology research during the past two decades has particularly highlighted the critical impact of biochemical and biophysical ECM features for the cellular therapy response (Eke and Cordes 2011b). As a 3D structural, non-cellular component of all tissues, the ECM is essential for all cellular functions and the maintenance of tissue integrity and homeostasis during development as well as cancer progression (Bonnans et al. 2014; Muncie and Weaver 2018; Pickup et al. 2014). Embedded in hydrated gel-like structures made of proteoglycans, around 300 ECM proteins form the core matrisome together with a large number of ECM-modifying enzymes, ECM-binding growth factors, and ECM-associated proteins (Hynes and Naba 2012; Naba et al. 2012). Different ECM types exist, such as the basement membrane or the matrix found in interstitial connective tissue, and these consist of tissue-specific quantities and specialized arrangements of the different matrisome components (Hynes and Naba 2012). Eventually, the key function of the ECM lies within this great diversity of ECM components, allowing integration of signals from multiple transmembrane ECM and growth factor receptors to regulate all cellular functions such as cell survival, differentiation, and cell migration in both healthy and malignant cell types.

Apart from essential functions in development and physiology, a large body of evidence demonstrates the importance of the ECM in modulating therapy sensitivity. In this regard, the terms "cell adhesion-mediated radioresistance" (CAM-RR) and "cell adhesion-mediated drug resistance" (CAM-DR) describe the increase in tumor cell radio- and chemoresistance upon exposure of normal and malignant cells to ECM proteins (Cordes and Meineke 2003; Damiano et al. 1999; Hazlehurst et al. 2000; Sandfort et al. 2007). Especially, the radioresistance of lung, breast and pancreatic carcinoma, glioblastoma, and melanoma is greatly enhanced by adhesion to ECM proteins such as fibronectin, laminin, and collagen (Cordes and Beinke 2004; Cordes et al. 2003a, b; Cordes and Meineke 2003; Kraus et al. 2002). This relationship further expands to hematopoietic malignancies and even normal cells, which are more radioresistant when bound to ECM (Damiano et al. 2001; Estrugo et al. 2007; Hess et al. 2007).

While these examples highlight the importance of cellular adhesion to ECM under 2D cell culture conditions, many studies characterize the radiation response of 3D ECM-based cell cultures. At present, there is considerable data to indicate that the response of 3D cell cultures to external stress, such as exposure to ionizing radiation, better reflects the physiological cellular response than 2D monolayer cultures (Ahmed et al. 2013; Eke and Cordes 2011a; Eke et al. 2015a; Nam et al. 2010; Zschenker et al. 2012). This discordance is driven by the lack of important key parameters required for the functional communication of cells with their environment. In particular, 2D cell cultures lack dimensionality and mechanical linkage of cellular ECM adhesion receptors and nuclear chromatin remodeling, which strongly influences cell morphology, gene and protein expression, signal transduction as well as therapy sensitivity (Eke et al. 2012a, 2013; Fernandez-Fuente et al. 2014; Hehlgans et al. 2012; Storch and Cordes 2012; Zschenker et al. 2012). Thus, it is easy to imagine that the identification and development of many radiosensitizers critically depend on the cell culture modalities, which need adjustment to reflect physiological cell functions.

3.2   Radioresistance Elicited by Integrins and the Adhesome

Crosstalk of cells with ECM substrates occurs through different cell adhesion molecules that regulate all cell fate decisions throughout development (Buck and Horwitz 1987). Amongst these, the integrin family of heterodimeric transmembrane receptors are by far the most investigated ECM adhesion molecules (Humphries et al. 2006; Hynes 2002). In total, 24 possible alpha and beta (α/β) integrin pairs mediate adhesion to specific ECM proteins in focalized cell surface adhesions, provide mechanical anchorage, and transmit signals in a bidirectional manner (Calderwood 2004; Geiger and Yamada 2011; Humphries et al. 2006). Intracellularly, integrins connect to the adhesome, a myriad of adapter and cytoplasmic signaling proteins that regulate survival, cell proliferation, and differentiation as well as cell motility (Geiger and Zaidel-Bar 2012; Zaidel-Bar et al. 2007).

A substantial amount of studies has focused on the integrin family of heterodimeric transmembrane receptors and their associated signaling networks as mediators of radioresistance owing to a frequently altered expression in various tumor entities (Dickreuter and Cordes 2017; Hamidi and Ivaska 2018; Vehlow et al. 2016). Especially integrin receptors containing the $\beta1$ subunit and their downstream signaling mediators are well-characterized anti-cancer targets (Barkan and Chambers 2011; Blandin et al. 2015; Cordes and Park 2007; Nam et al. 2009). In 3D-grown HNSCC cells, $\beta1$ integrin targeting reduces clonogenic radiation survival by affecting the repair of DSBs (Ahmed et al. 2018; Dickreuter et al. 2016; Eke et al. 2012a, b). In addition, combined targeting of $\beta1$ integrin and the EGFR appears to be a promising approach to overcome therapy resistance of HNSCC in vitro and in vivo (Eke et al. 2015b). Similar results exist for 3D-grown breast carcinoma cells where $\beta1$ integrin inhibition reduces cellular resistance to apoptosis by downregulating AKT signaling (Nam et al. 2010; Park et al. 2008). In contrast, inhibition of $\beta1$ integrin in glioblastoma activates pro-survival bypass mechanisms that counteract therapeutic benefit but reduces 3D glioblastoma cell invasion (Eke et al. 2012c; Vehlow et al. 2017).

Downstream of $\beta1$ integrin, the focal adhesion kinase (FAK) is a central determinant of radiation survival of many tumor entities by mediating integrin as well as growth factor triggered signaling events (Hehlgans et al. 2012; Mantoni et al. 2011; Skinner et al. 2016; Sulzmaier et al. 2014). Inhibition of FAK enhances cellular radiosensitivity of HNSCC by deactivating AKT and MEK1/2 signaling and inducing apoptosis (Hehlgans et al. 2009, 2012). Amongst numerous other adhesome components, the adapter protein Particularly Interesting New Cysteine-Histidine-rich 1 (PINCH1) promotes cell survival upon treatment with ionizing radiation by perpetuating AKT1 activity (Eke et al. 2010). Intriguingly, in HNSCC cells refractory to β1 integrin and EGFR inhibition, targeting of mTOR and KEAP1 may promote radiosensitization (Klapproth et al. 2018). Taken together, by mimicking physiological growth conditions, 3D cell cultures have significantly contributed to our understanding of the tumor therapy response and effectively support the identification of potent radiosensitizers.

4 The Potential of 3D Multicellular Culture Systems in Radiation Biology

In recent years, microphysiological systems such as organoids and tumoroids as well as organotypic tissue slices cultures have emerged as additional approaches to mimic 3D organ and tumor complexity. These culture models retain cell interactions amongst different cell types and tissue components outperforming the simple architecture of 3D monocultures for high-throughput and more translational readouts (Fig. 6.4). This section discusses the advantages and challenges of the current organoids and organotypic tissue slices models in the context of radiation biology.

4.1 Implementation of Tumoroid Models in Radiation Biology

Defined as a simplified and downsized organ generated in a 3D culture system, an organoid shows realistic microanatomy, architecture, and functionality. Organoids can be generated from cells derived from primary tissues (e.g., esophagus, stomach, intestine, colon, liver, pancreas, and prostate), embryonic stem cells or induced pluripotent stem cells, which have the ability to differentiate, self-organize, and grow in 3D culture systems (Fatehullah et al. 2016) (Fig. 6.4). Sato and colleagues successfully established the first interstitial organoids growing in a stem cell niche containing laminin-rich ECM supplemented with specific endogenous growth factors (Sato et al. 2009). These organoids comprised the different intestinal compartments composed of stem, progenitor, and differentiated cell types recapitulating the in vivo tissue architecture (Sato et al. 2009). Subsequently, the organoid system has been extended to generate organoids of tissues from different anatomical sites such as colon, stomach, and liver (Fatehullah et al. 2016).

Especially in cancer research, the implementation of tumor-derived organoids, the so-called tumoroids, has gained increasing interest for the screening of the tumor treatment response. In contrast to normal tissue-derived organoids, patient-

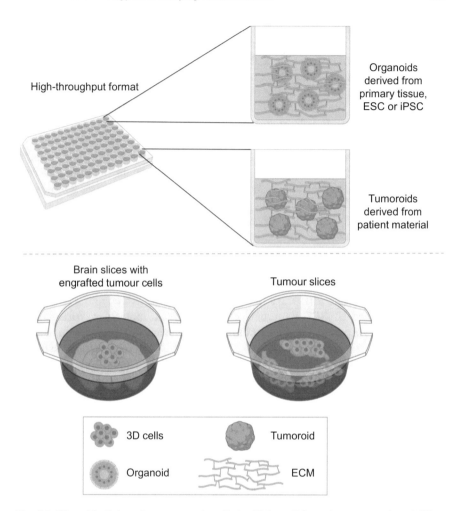

Fig. 6.4 3D multicellular culture systems in radiation biology. Schematic representation of different approaches to multicellular 3D cultures. Upper part: Organoids are derived from primary tissue, embryonic stem cells (EPC), or induced pluripotent stem cells (iPSC). Tumoroids are derived from patient material. Both organoids and tumoroids are adaptable to high-throughput screening systems. Lower part: Organotypic brain slices with engrafted tumor cells and tumor slice cultured on membrane inserts. Created with BioRender

derived tumor material is used to generate a complex tumor culture system that preserves the phenotypic and genotypic properties of the corresponding primary tumor (Drost and Clevers 2018). The successful culture of patient-derived tumoroids has been reported in a variety of tumor entities such as gastrointestinal cancer (Vlachogiannis et al. 2018), pancreatic cancer (Boj et al. 2015; Huang et al. 2015; Seino et al. 2018), HNSCC (Driehuis et al. 2019a; Tanaka et al. 2018), breast cancer (Sachs et al. 2018), and hepatic cancer (Broutier et al. 2017). Tumoroid culture models are powerful tools for preclinical applications such as drug screening and treatment individualization, because a single piece of primary tumor allows the generation of several sets of tumoroids with highly conserved tumor heterogeneity. While it was shown that genetic and histological features of tumoroid mutational profiles and architecture show high similarity to parental tumors independently of early passages, the maintenance of tumoroid heterogeneity at later passages is still a matter of debate (van de Wetering et al. 2015; Weeber et al. 2017). It remains to be determined how exactly culture conditions influence proliferation, adaptation, and clonal selectivity as well as therapy response of the different tumoroid models.

A small number of studies have employed patient-derived tumoroids for individualized chemoradiation screening and emphasized the applicability of tumoroid systems to radiobiological studies. Ganesh and colleagues established a biorepository of tumoroids from patients with primary, metastatic, or recurrent rectal cancer, which maintained molecular features, specific architectural and cytological subtleties and mutational profiles of the parental tumors (Ganesh et al. 2019). Radiation and chemotherapy response of these tumoroids significantly correlated with the respective clinical responses of the individual patients, indicating comparability between patient-derived tumoroids and the tumors from which they were derived (Ganesh et al. 2019). By optimizing specific growth conditions, Clevers' group established HNSCC tumoroids with genetic and molecular characteristics comparable to the parental tumors for the investigation and characterization of treatment sensitizers (Driehuis et al. 2019a). These HNSCC tumoroids responded differently to the various standard treatment regimens such as chemotherapy, ionizing radiation and targeted drugs, emphasizing the potential of tumoroids for personalized management of HNSCC and the identification of alternative therapeutic approaches and radiosensitizers (Driehuis et al. 2019a).

The success of generating tumoroids might be subject to the tumor entity and specific microenvironmental requirements. For example, the generation of tumoroids from glioblastoma is limited by a poor growth rate, as glioblastoma frequently fail to adapt to 3D culture conditions due to their complex physiological environment within the human brain (Drost and Clevers 2018). An alternative 3D model approach for glioblastoma is the culture as neurospheres or spheroids in suspension (Caragher et al. 2019), which sometimes fail to represent the parental tumor. Hubert and co-workers successfully established patient-derived glioblastoma tumoroids, which showed improved recapitulation of the characteristic infiltrative phenotype relative to patient-derived neurospheres (Hubert et al. 2016). Orthotopic xenograft models derived from these tumoroids displayed a single-cell infiltrative phenotype and diffuse tumor growth pattern comparative to the parental tumors (Hubert et al. 2016). Nevertheless, establishment of glioblastoma tumoroids requires around 6 months, challenging their practicality as a model system for radiation biology research and the identification of radiosensitizers for such an aggressive tumor entity as glioblastoma.

Different studies emphasize the applicability of tumoroid systems in radiobiological research as well as individualized screening of treatment sensitivity. Hubrecht Organoid Technology (https://hub4organoids.eu/) is a biorepository platform maintaining a diverse collection of patient-derived tumoroids and the related genetic and molecular profiles as well as the treatment outcome of the donors. Tumoroids expanded within this platform are clinically relevant in cancer research and drug development (Weeber et al. 2017). In the future, using tumoroids in radiation biology research will be greatly beneficial in many ways, such as patient stratification and outcome prediction based on tumoroid responses. With the known genetic and molecular characteristics of tumoroids, more predictive models of the therapy response might be developed, assisting physicians in the decision-making process.

4.2   Ex Vivo Tissue Cultures in Radiation Biology

While the dissociation of tumor cells from tumor tissue is a necessary step for producing 3D cell cultures as well as tumoroids, this process generates selective pressure, exerting cellular adaptability and loss of tumor heterogeneity due to the outgrowth of specific subsets of tumor cells. An approach to overcome the selective pressure is the ex vivo culture of tumor slices without the intermediate cell dissociation step (Fig. 6.4). Such 3D organotypic tumor cultures are advantageous over other 3D culture models as they maintain the ultrastructural tumor architecture and functionality, tumor heterogeneity and stromal interactions, which often influence tumor behavior and the therapy response (Misra et al. 2019; Sivakumar et al. 2019). In addition, Sivakumar et al. characterized the composition of immune cells in organotypic tumor slices derived from transgenic mouse breast, pancreatic, colon, and melanoma models as well as human hepatic tumors. The authors identified similar immune cell compositions between organotypic slices and the tumor counterparts providing a platform for immuno-oncology and drug discovery screens (Sivakumar et al. 2019). Furthermore, the usage of organotypic slice cultures can be extended to normal tissues such as lung, small intestine, colon, brain, and aorta, which can be employed for the simultaneous assessment of several functional readouts, such as cellular interactions or endocrine/paracrine signaling loops (Shamir and Ewald 2014).

To generate these slices, tumor materials from patients or experimental rodent models are cut to pieces with thicknesses ranging between 100 and 500 μm depending on the tumor density using a tissue slicer or vibratome. Tissue slices are often cultured on polytetrafluoroethylene or polycarbonate membrane inserts, creating an air–liquid interface culture environment for thorough tissue oxygenation. Since the administration of drugs relies on diffusion, an optimization of tumor slice thickness is required to achieve a homogeneous distribution. In general, the tumor slice culture does not require cost-intensive consumables and expertise, thus facilitating establishment and accessibility. However, an optimized media composition and culture condition is required for the culture of particular tumor entities. While tumor slices cultures are employable for a wide spectrum of applications such as drug screening tests and other functional endpoints, its usage is limited to short-term studies due to the shorter lifetime of the tissues relative to the conventional cell culture systems or tumoroids. Although a single tumor slice might be divided into multiple technical replicates, it is likely that the analysis of multiple-subclones distributed within a single tumor fosters heterogeneity in the experimental readout. Therefore, this cell culture system might be considered a low-throughput technique with limited use in personalized medicine. However, even with these limitations, the organotypic culture system is a useful model for radiation biology studies in preclinical and basic research.

Historically, organotypic slice culture was developed in 1981 using rodent brains for physiological and pharmacological studies on morphologically identified nerve cells (Gahwiler 1981). Since this technique has been particularly optimized for brain slice culture, it is not surprising that glioblastoma slice cultures are most commonly used. While the histopathological features of glioblastoma slices relative to the parental tumors could be preserved up to 16 days without any significant alteration (Merz et al. 2013), rodent-derived normal brain slices are co-cultured with glioblastoma cells in many cases to study pathological interactions, proliferation, apoptosis, migration, and invasion changes upon different treatments (Marques-Torrejon et al. 2018; Pencheva et al. 2017). In a preclinical study, Merz and colleagues used patient-derived glioblastoma slices to study the treatment response of the tumors to irradiation and temozolomide chemotherapy. In line with the clinical observation that some patients show different susceptibility to cancer therapies, glioblastoma slices also displayed differential responses to the treatments (Merz et al. 2013).

Pancreatic ductal adenocarcinoma (PDAC) possesses a unique and complex microenvironment, which is related to a poor treatment response and therapy resistance. In a recent study, tumor slices generated from a small cohort of patients with PDAC were tested for histology, stromal compositions, and response to cytotoxic agents. Tumor slices treated with staurosporine, gemcitabine, or cisplatin exerted proportional cytotoxic effects determined by cell viability, tumor cell number, proliferation, and apoptosis markers (Lim et al. 2018). Therefore, testing cytotoxic drugs and combinational treatments in PDAC tumor slices might be more clinically relevant than the conventional 2D culture systems. Additionally, HNSCC and breast cancer tumor slices have been implemented for short-term and long-term cultures, respectively (Donnadieu et al. 2016; Naipal et al. 2016). The data revealed a conserved heterogeneity of the tumor and clonal sensitivity to targeted therapies. In both studies, individual tumor responses to anti-cancer drugs were highly different from patient to patient, indicating that this culture technique is a representative model for treatment personalization. Taken together, these studies suggest organotypic slice cultures as powerful tools to explore treatment responsiveness of individual tumors.

4.3   Analytical Endpoints of Tumoroid and Organotypic Slice Cultures

Tumoroids as well as organotypic slice cultures hold a great potential as models for the establishment of predictive and prognostic assays, particularly treatment individualization. It is feasible that such predictive approaches are executed simultaneously with the patient's disease management, supporting physicians in the treatment decision. Additionally, these more complex cell culture models are also adaptable to high-throughput preclinical studies and identification of novel therapeutic targets (Shamir and Ewald 2014). Even though these two cell culture systems are distinctively different in practice, the complementary analytical assays are relatively similar. Table 6.1 summarizes frequently used analytical endpoints for radiation biology studies using tumoroid and organotypic slice culture modalities.

Determination of cell viability in organotypic tumor slices and tumoroids is a common approach to assess the dynamic response to cytotoxic agents. Common viability assays indirectly measure cell survival through quantification of cellular metabolic activity based on enzyme activity (MTT assay), presence of ATP (CellTiter-Glo 3D reagent), and cellular reducing environment (PrestoBlue assay) (Driehuis et al. 2019a, b; Ganesh et al. 2019; Vaira et al. 2010). However, due to cellular heterogeneity within organotypic tumor slices the readouts from cell viability-type assays might be inaccurate in comparison to tumoroids. In this regard, measurements of cells undergoing apoptosis offer a more specific readout. Detection of DNA fragments generated during apoptosis (TUNEL assay) or immunohistochemical staining of cleaved caspase-3 and annexin V combined with hematoxylin and eosin staining (H&E) can be performed to obtain the number of early and late apoptotic cells as well as necrosis. These methods offer a more accurate estimate of apoptotic cell death and the possibility to differentiate cell swelling, necrosis and nuclear pyknosis/karyolysis/karyorrhexis (Naipal et al. 2016). The growth rate of tumoroids, e.g., tumoroid enlargement, number of tumoroids, and number of cells within tumoroids, can be microscopically quantified (Driehuis et al. 2019a, b). In contrast, it is more difficult to determine the growth rate in organotypic tumor slices. Here, only single or combinatory immunohistochemical staining for common proliferation markers such as Ki-67, Edu, and phospho-histone 3 can be used to assess tumor growth (Driehuis et al. 2019a, b; Ganesh et al. 2019).

Since radiation and cytotoxic agents severely damage DNA, one of the most prominently evaluated endpoints to determine the cellular response is the analysis of DNA breaks and the DNA damage response. While several assays for DNA damage analysis are available, the immunohistological staining of DNA single-strand breaks (SSB) or DSB biomarkers such as XRCC1 (SSB), 53BP1, and γ-H2AX (DSB) has been proven most sensitive and quantifiable in tumoroids and organotypic tumor slices. Furthermore, the observation of DNA damage repair provides essential information about the tumor intrinsic radiation sensitivity. Estimates of DNA damage repair in patient-derived rectal tumoroids demonstrated inter-patient heterogeneity, suggesting the assay and the model are clinically relevant (Ganesh

Table 6.1 Overview of analytical assays for radiation biology studies

Assay	Readout	Description	Quantification
CellTiter-Glo assay	Cell viability	Determination of the number of viable cells in culture based on the amount of ATP	Luminescence
MTT	Cell viability	NAD(P)H-dependent cellular oxidoreductase enzymes are capable of reducing the tetrazolium dye MTT 3-(4,5-dimethylthiazol-2-yl)-2,5-diphenyltetrazolium bromide to its insoluble formazan	Colorimetric
PrestoBlue	Cell viability	Cell permeable resazurin-based solution that is modified by the reducing environment of the viable cell by changing its color	Fluorescence absorbance
TUNEL assay	Apoptosis	Terminal deoxynucleotidyl transferase (TdT) dUTP nick end labeling (TUNEL) is a method for detecting DNA fragments by labeling the 3′-hydroxyl termini in DNA double-strand breaks generated during apoptosis by the incorporation of biotinylated nucleotides through TdT enzymes	Colorimetric
Cleaved caspase 3 immunostaining	Apoptosis	During apoptosis, caspase 3 is cleaved and degrades multiple cellular proteins and DNA fragments in cells	Microscopy Flow cytometry
AnnexinV staining	Apoptosis	AnnexinV situated on the outer leaflet of the plasma membrane is a mark of apoptosis in early/late apoptotic and necrotic cells	Microscopy Flow cytometry
Beta-galactosidase staining	Senescence	Beta-galactosidase is a hydrolase enzyme that catalyzes the hydrolysis of β-galactosides into monosaccharides during senescence	Microscopy Flow cytometry
H&E immune-histochemistry	Necrosis	Hematoxylin and eosin (H&E) is a basic staining for nuclei and cytoplasm to examine cell types and tissue structure	Microscopy
Ki-67 immuno-histochemistry	Proliferation	Ki-67 is a nuclear protein which is associated with cellular proliferation	Microscopy
DDR immuno-fluorescence	DNA double-strand breaks (DSB)	Immunostaining of DNA damage response (DDR) proteins, such as γ-H2AX, 53BP1 for the quantification of residual damage	Microscopy

et al. 2019). In addition, a variety of molecular biological analytical approaches, such as analysis of DNA, RNA, and protein expression, epigenomic and post-translational modification, are compatible with the complex culture systems, allowing deep investigation of ongoing signaling events and even therapy resistance mechanism (Driehuis et al. 2019b).

5 Conclusions and Perspective

In conclusion, 3D cell culture technologies are promising tools for the identification of radiosensitizers by bridging the gap between standard 2D monocultures and animal models. Today, a large body of data demonstrates that 3D cell culture systems reflect the physiological microenvironment to a far greater extent than traditional 2D cell cultures. Especially, cell adhesion to the ECM and its fundamental consequences for signal transduction profoundly influences tumor cell behavior, in general, and therapy sensitivity, in particular, and is underestimated in 2D cellular systems. There is no doubt that 3D cell culture systems are powerful applications for drug discovery, cell biology, cancer, and radiation biology research. In the future, optimization and validation of the different culture modalities are warranted to improve the reproducibility and standardization of 3D cell culture models with excellent biological relevance.

References

Abbott A (2003) Cell culture: biology's new dimension. Nature 424:870–872

Ahmed KM, Zhang H, Park CC (2013) NF-kappaB regulates radioresistance mediated by beta1-integrin in three-dimensional culture of breast cancer cells. Cancer Res 73:3737–3748

Ahmed KM, Pandita RK, Singh DK, Hunt CR, Pandita TK (2018) Beta1-integrin impacts Rad51 stability and DNA double-strand break repair by homologous recombination. Mol Cell Biol 38(9):e00672–e00617

Ang KK, Berkey BA, Tu X, Zhang HZ, Katz R, Hammond EH, Fu KK, Milas L (2002) Impact of epidermal growth factor receptor expression on survival and pattern of relapse in patients with advanced head and neck carcinoma. Cancer Res 62:7350–7356

Bailey MH, Tokheim C, Porta-Pardo E, Sengupta S, Bertrand D, Weerasinghe A, Colaprico A, Wendl MC, Kim J, Reardon B et al (2018) Comprehensive characterization of cancer driver genes and mutations. Cell 173:371–385.e318

Barkan D, Chambers AF (2011) Beta1-integrin: a potential therapeutic target in the battle against cancer recurrence. Clin Cancer Res 17:7219–7223

Bentzen SM, Harari PM, Bernier J (2007) Exploitable mechanisms for combining drugs with radiation: concepts, achievements and future directions. Nat Clin Pract Oncol 4:172–180

Blandin AF, Renner G, Lehmann M, Lelong-Rebel I, Martin S, Dontenwill M (2015) Beta1 integrins as therapeutic targets to disrupt hallmarks of cancer. Front Pharmacol 6:279

Boj SF, Hwang CI, Baker LA, Chio II, Engle DD, Corbo V, Jager M, Ponz-Sarvise M, Tiriac H, Spector MS et al (2015) Organoid models of human and mouse ductal pancreatic cancer. Cell 160:324–338

Bonnans C, Chou J, Werb Z (2014) Remodelling the extracellular matrix in development and disease. Nat Rev Mol Cell Biol 15:786–801

Bonner JA, Maihle NJ, Folven BR, Christianson TJ, Spain K (1994) The interaction of epidermal growth factor and radiation in human head and neck squamous cell carcinoma cell lines with vastly different radiosensitivities. Int J Radiat Oncol Biol Phys 29:243–247

Bonner JA, Raisch KP, Trummell HQ, Robert F, Meredith RF, Spencer SA, Buchsbaum DJ, Saleh MN, Stackhouse MA, LoBuglio AF et al (2000) Enhanced apoptosis with combination C225/radiation treatment serves as the impetus for clinical investigation in head and neck cancers. J Clin Oncol 18:47S–53S

Bonner JA, Harari PM, Giralt J, Azarnia N, Shin DM, Cohen RB, Jones CU, Sur R, Raben D, Jassem J et al (2006) Radiotherapy plus cetuximab for squamous-cell carcinoma of the head and neck. N Engl J Med 354:567–578

Bonner JA, Harari PM, Giralt J, Cohen RB, Jones CU, Sur RK, Raben D, Baselga J, Spencer SA, Zhu J et al (2010) Radiotherapy plus cetuximab for locoregionally advanced head and neck cancer: 5-year survival data from a phase 3 randomised trial, and relation between cetuximab-induced rash and survival. Lancet Oncol 11:21–28

Breslin S, O'Driscoll L (2013) Three-dimensional cell culture: the missing link in drug discovery. Drug Discov Today 18:240–249

Bristow RG, Alexander B, Baumann M, Bratman SV, Brown JM, Camphausen K, Choyke P, Citrin D, Contessa JN, Dicker A et al (2018) Combining precision radiotherapy with molecular targeting and immunomodulatory agents: a guideline by the American Society for Radiation Oncology. Lancet Oncol 19:e240–e251

Broutier L, Mastrogiovanni G, Verstegen MM, Francies HE, Gavarro LM, Bradshaw CR, Allen GE, Arnes-Benito R, Sidorova O, Gaspersz MP et al (2017) Human primary liver cancer-derived organoid cultures for disease modeling and drug screening. Nat Med 23:1424–1435

Buck CA, Horwitz AF (1987) Cell surface receptors for extracellular matrix molecules. Annu Rev Cell Biol 3:179–205

Calderwood DA (2004) Integrin activation. J Cell Sci 117:657–666

Caragher S, Chalmers AJ, Gomez-Roman N (2019) Glioblastoma's next top model: novel culture systems for brain cancer radiotherapy research. Cancers (Basel) 11:44

Coleman CN, Higgins GS, Brown JM, Baumann M, Kirsch DG, Willers H, Prasanna PG, Dewhirst MW, Bernhard EJ, Ahmed MM (2016) Improving the predictive value of preclinical studies in support of radiotherapy clinical trials. Clin Cancer Res 22:3138–3147

Corces MR, Granja JM, Shams S, Louie BH, Seoane JA, Zhou W, Silva TC, Groeneveld C, Wong CK, Cho SW et al (2018) The chromatin accessibility landscape of primary human cancers. Science 362:eaav1898

Cordes N, Beinke C (2004) Fibronectin alters cell survival and intracellular signaling of confluent A549 cultures after irradiation. Cancer Biol Ther 3:47–53

Cordes N, Meineke V (2003) Cell adhesion-mediated radioresistance (CAM-RR). Extracellular matrix-dependent improvement of cell survival in human tumor and normal cells in vitro. Strahlenther Onkol 179:337–344

Cordes N, Park CC (2007) Beta1 integrin as a molecular therapeutic target. Int J Radiat Biol 83:753–760

Cordes N, Blaese MA, Plasswilm L, Rodemann HP, Van Beuningen D (2003a) Fibronectin and laminin increase resistance to ionizing radiation and the cytotoxic drug Ukrain in human tumour and normal cells in vitro. Int J Radiat Biol 79:709–720

Cordes N, Hansmeier B, Beinke C, Meineke V, van Beuningen D (2003b) Irradiation differentially affects substratum-dependent survival, adhesion, and invasion of glioblastoma cell lines. Br J Cancer 89:2122–2132

Cukierman E, Pankov R, Stevens DR, Yamada KM (2001) Taking cell-matrix adhesions to the third dimension. Science 294:1708–1712

Cukierman E, Pankov R, Yamada KM (2002) Cell interactions with three-dimensional matrices. Curr Opin Cell Biol 14:633–639

Damiano JS, Cress AE, Hazlehurst LA, Shtil AA, Dalton WS (1999) Cell adhesion mediated drug resistance (CAM-DR): role of integrins and resistance to apoptosis in human myeloma cell lines. Blood 93:1658–1667

Damiano JS, Hazlehurst LA, Dalton WS (2001) Cell adhesion-mediated drug resistance (CAM-DR) protects the K562 chronic myelogenous leukemia cell line from apoptosis induced by BCR/ABL inhibition, cytotoxic drugs, and gamma-irradiation. Leukemia 15:1232–1239

Delaney G, Jacob S, Featherstone C, Barton M (2005) The role of radiotherapy in cancer treatment: estimating optimal utilization from a review of evidence-based clinical guidelines. Cancer 104:1129–1137

Dickreuter E, Cordes N (2017) The cancer cell adhesion resistome: mechanisms, targeting and translational approaches. Biol Chem 398:721–735

Dickreuter E, Eke I, Krause M, Borgmann K, van Vugt MA, Cordes N (2016) Targeting of beta1 integrins impairs DNA repair for radiosensitization of head and neck cancer cells. Oncogene 35:1353–1362

Donnadieu J, Lachaier E, Peria M, Saidak Z, Dakpe S, Ikoli JF, Chauffert B, Page C, Galmiche A (2016) Short-term culture of tumour slices reveals the heterogeneous sensitivity of human head and neck squamous cell carcinoma to targeted therapies. BMC Cancer 16:273

Dowden H, Munro J (2019) Trends in clinical success rates and therapeutic focus. Nat Rev Drug Discov 18:495–496

Driehuis E, Kolders S, Spelier S, Lohmussaar K, Willems SM, Devriese LA, de Bree R, de Ruiter EJ, Korving J, Begthel H et al (2019a) Oral mucosal organoids as a potential platform for personalized cancer therapy. Cancer Discov 9:852–871

Driehuis E, van Hoeck A, Moore K, Kolders S, Francies HE, Gulersonmez MC, Stigter ECA, Burgering B, Geurts V, Gracanin A et al (2019b) Pancreatic cancer organoids recapitulate disease and allow personalized drug screening. Proc Natl Acad Sci U S A 116:26580

Drost J, Clevers H (2018) Organoids in cancer research. Nat Rev Cancer 18:407–418

Edmondson R, Broglie JJ, Adcock AF, Yang LJ (2014) Three-dimensional cell culture systems and their applications in drug discovery and cell-based biosensors. Assay Drug Dev Technol 12:207–218

Eke I, Cordes N (2011a) Dual targeting of EGFR and focal adhesion kinase in 3D grown HNSCC cell cultures. Radiother Oncol 99:279–286

Eke I, Cordes N (2011b) Radiobiology goes 3D: how ECM and cell morphology impact on cell survival after irradiation. Radiother Oncol 99:271–278

Eke I, Koch U, Hehlgans S, Sandfort V, Stanchi F, Zips D, Baumann M, Shevchenko A, Pilarsky C, Haase M et al (2010) PINCH1 regulates Akt1 activation and enhances radioresistance by inhibiting PP1alpha. J Clin Invest 120:2516–2527

Eke I, Deuse Y, Hehlgans S, Gurtner K, Krause M, Baumann M, Shevchenko A, Sandfort V, Cordes N (2012a) Beta(1)integrin/FAK/cortactin signaling is essential for human head and neck cancer resistance to radiotherapy. J Clin Invest 122:1529–1540

Eke I, Dickreuter E, Cordes N (2012b) Enhanced radiosensitivity of head and neck squamous cell carcinoma cells by beta1 integrin inhibition. Radiother Oncol 104:235–242

Eke I, Storch K, Kastner I, Vehlow A, Faethe C, Mueller-Klieser W, Taucher-Scholz G, Temme A, Schackert G, Cordes N (2012c) Three-dimensional invasion of human glioblastoma cells remains unchanged by X-ray and carbon ion irradiation in vitro. Int J Radiat Oncol Biol Phys 84:e515–e523

Eke I, Schneider L, Forster C, Zips D, Kunz-Schughart LA, Cordes N (2013) EGFR/JIP-4/JNK2 signaling attenuates cetuximab-mediated radiosensitization of squamous cell carcinoma cells. Cancer Res 73:297–306

Eke I, Hehlgans S, Zong Y, Cordes N (2015a) Comprehensive analysis of signal transduction in three-dimensional ECM-based tumor cell cultures. J Biol Methods 2:e31

Eke I, Zscheppang K, Dickreuter E, Hickmann L, Mazzeo E, Unger K, Krause M, Cordes N (2015b) Simultaneous beta1 integrin-EGFR targeting and radiosensitization of human head and neck cancer. J Natl Cancer Inst 107

Eke I, Hehlgans S, Sandfort V, Cordes N (2016) 3D matrix-based cell cultures: automated analysis of tumor cell survival and proliferation. Int J Oncol 48:313–321

Estrugo D, Fischer A, Hess F, Scherthan H, Belka C, Cordes N (2007) Ligand bound beta1 integrins inhibit procaspase-8 for mediating cell adhesion-mediated drug and radiation resistance in human leukemia cells. PLoS One 2:e269

Fatehullah A, Tan SH, Barker N (2016) Organoids as an in vitro model of human development and disease. Nat Cell Biol 18:246–254

Fernandez-Fuente G, Mollinedo P, Grande L, Vazquez-Barquero A, Fernandez-Luna JL (2014) Culture dimensionality influences the resistance of glioblastoma stem-like cells to multikinase inhibitors. Mol Cancer Ther 13:1664–1672

Friedrich J, Seidel C, Ebner R, Kunz-Schughart LA (2009) Spheroid-based drug screen: considerations and practical approach. Nat Protoc 4:309–324

Gahwiler BH (1981) Organotypic monolayer cultures of nervous tissue. J Neurosci Methods 4:329–342

Ganesh K, Wu C, O'Rourke KP, Szeglin BC, Zheng Y, Sauve CG, Adileh M, Wasserman I, Marco MR, Kim AS et al (2019) A rectal cancer organoid platform to study individual responses to chemoradiation. Nat Med 25:1607–1614

Geiger B, Yamada KM (2011) Molecular architecture and function of matrix adhesions. Cold Spring Harb Perspect Biol 3:a005033

Geiger T, Zaidel-Bar R (2012) Opening the floodgates: proteomics and the integrin adhesome. Curr Opin Cell Biol 24:562–568

Hamidi H, Ivaska J (2018) Every step of the way: integrins in cancer progression and metastasis. Nat Rev Cancer 18:533–548

Harrison RK (2016) Phase II and phase III failures: 2013-2015. Nat Rev Drug Discov 15:817–818

Hazlehurst LA, Damiano JS, Buyuksal I, Pledger WJ, Dalton WS (2000) Adhesion to fibronectin via beta1 integrins regulates p27kip1 levels and contributes to cell adhesion mediated drug resistance (CAM-DR). Oncogene 19:4319–4327

Hehlgans S, Lange I, Eke I, Cordes N (2009) 3D cell cultures of human head and neck squamous cell carcinoma cells are radiosensitized by the focal adhesion kinase inhibitor TAE226. Radiother Oncol 92:371–378

Hehlgans S, Eke I, Cordes N (2012) Targeting FAK radiosensitizes 3-dimensional grown human HNSCC cells through reduced Akt1 and MEK1/2 signaling. Int J Radiat Oncol Biol Phys 83:e669–e676

Hess F, Estrugo D, Fischer A, Belka C, Cordes N (2007) Integrin-linked kinase interacts with caspase-9 and -8 in an adhesion-dependent manner for promoting radiation-induced apoptosis in human leukemia cells. Oncogene 26:1372–1384

Huang SM, Bock JM, Harari PM (1999) Epidermal growth factor receptor blockade with C225 modulates proliferation, apoptosis, and radiosensitivity in squamous cell carcinomas of the head and neck. Cancer Res 59:1935–1940

Huang L, Holtzinger A, Jagan I, BeGora M, Lohse I, Ngai N, Nostro C, Wang R, Muthuswamy LB, Crawford HC et al (2015) Ductal pancreatic cancer modeling and drug screening using human pluripotent stem cell- and patient-derived tumor organoids. Nat Med 21:1364–1371

Hubert CG, Rivera M, Spangler LC, Wu Q, Mack SC, Prager BC, Couce M, McLendon RE, Sloan AE, Rich JN (2016) A three-dimensional organoid culture system derived from human glioblastomas recapitulates the hypoxic gradients and cancer stem cell heterogeneity of tumors found in vivo. Cancer Res 76:2465–2477

Humphries JD, Byron A, Humphries MJ (2006) Integrin ligands at a glance. J Cell Sci 119:3901–3903

Hynes RO (2002) Integrins: bidirectional, allosteric signaling machines. Cell 110:673–687

Hynes RO, Naba A (2012) Overview of the matrisome—an inventory of extracellular matrix constituents and functions. Cold Spring Harb Perspect Biol 4:a004903

Kirsch DG, Diehn M, Kesarwala AH, Maity A, Morgan MA, Schwarz JK, Bristow R, Demaria S, Eke I, Griffin RJ et al (2018) The future of radiobiology. J Natl Cancer Inst 110:329–340

Klapproth E, Dickreuter E, Zakrzewski F, Seifert M, Petzold A, Dahl A, Schrock E, Klink B, Cordes N (2018) Whole exome sequencing identifies mTOR and KEAP1 as potential targets for radiosensitization of HNSCC cells refractory to EGFR and beta1 integrin inhibition. Oncotarget 9:18099–18114

Kraus AC, Ferber I, Bachmann SO, Specht H, Wimmel A, Gross MW, Schlegel J, Suske G, Schuermann M (2002) In vitro chemo- and radio-resistance in small cell lung cancer correlates with cell adhesion and constitutive activation of AKT and MAP kinase pathways. Oncogene 21:8683–8695

Lim CY, Chang JH, Lee WS, Lee KM, Yoon YC, Kim J, Park IY (2018) Organotypic slice cultures of pancreatic ductal adenocarcinoma preserve the tumor microenvironment and provide a platform for drug response. Pancreatology 18:913–927

Mantoni TS, Lunardi S, Al-Assar O, Masamune A, Brunner TB (2011) Pancreatic stellate cells radioprotect pancreatic cancer cells through beta1-integrin signaling. Cancer Res 71:3453–3458

Marques-Torrejon MA, Gangoso E, Pollard SM (2018) Modelling glioblastoma tumour-host cell interactions using adult brain organotypic slice co-culture. Dis Model Mech 11:dmm031435

McGee HM, Jiang D, Soto-Pantoja DR, Nevler A, Giaccia AJ, Woodward WA (2019) Targeting the tumor microenvironment in radiation oncology: proceedings from the 2018 ASTRO-AACR research workshop. Clin Cancer Res 25:2969–2974

Mendelsohn J (1997) Epidermal growth factor receptor inhibition by a monoclonal antibody as anticancer therapy. Clin Cancer Res 3:2703–2707

Merz F, Gaunitz F, Dehghani F, Renner C, Meixensberger J, Gutenberg A, Giese A, Schopow K, Hellwig C, Schafer M et al (2013) Organotypic slice cultures of human glioblastoma reveal different susceptibilities to treatments. Neuro Oncol 15:670–681

Misra S, Moro CF, Del Chiaro M, Pouso S, Sebestyen A, Lohr M, Bjornstedt M, Verbeke CS (2019) Ex vivo organotypic culture system of precision-cut slices of human pancreatic ductal adenocarcinoma. Sci Rep 9:2133

Morris ZS, Harari PM (2014) Interaction of radiation therapy with molecular targeted agents. J Clin Oncol 32:2886–2893

Muncie JM, Weaver VM (2018) The physical and biochemical properties of the extracellular matrix regulate cell fate. Curr Top Dev Biol 130:1–37

Naba A, Clauser KR, Hoersch S, Liu H, Carr SA, Hynes RO (2012) The matrisome: in silico definition and in vivo characterization by proteomics of normal and tumor extracellular matrices. Mol Cell Proteomics 11(M111):014647

Naipal KA, Verkaik NS, Sanchez H, van Deurzen CH, den Bakker MA, Hoeijmakers JH, Kanaar R, Vreeswijk MP, Jager A, van Gent DC (2016) Tumor slice culture system to assess drug response of primary breast cancer. BMC Cancer 16:78

Nam JM, Chung Y, Hsu HC, Park CC (2009) Beta1 integrin targeting to enhance radiation therapy. Int J Radiat Biol 85:923–928

Nam JM, Onodera Y, Bissell MJ, Park CC (2010) Breast cancer cells in three-dimensional culture display an enhanced radioresponse after coordinate targeting of integrin alpha5beta1 and fibronectin. Cancer Res 70:5238–5248

Pampaloni F, Reynaud EG, Stelzer EH (2007) The third dimension bridges the gap between cell culture and live tissue. Nat Rev Mol Cell Biol 8:839–845

Park CC, Zhang HJ, Yao ES, Park CJ, Bissell MJ (2008) Beta1 integrin inhibition dramatically enhances radiotherapy efficacy in human breast cancer xenografts. Cancer Res 68:4398–4405

Pencheva N, de Gooijer MC, Vis DJ, Wessels LFA, Wurdinger T, van Tellingen O, Bernards R (2017) Identification of a druggable pathway controlling glioblastoma invasiveness. Cell Rep 20:48–60

Pickup MW, Mouw JK, Weaver VM (2014) The extracellular matrix modulates the hallmarks of cancer. EMBO Rep 15:1243–1253

Raphael BJ, Hruban RH, Aguirre AJ, Moffitt RA, Yeh JJ, Stewart C, Robertson AG, Cherniack AD, Gupta M, Getz G et al (2017) Integrated genomic characterization of pancreatic ductal adenocarcinoma. Cancer Cell 32:185–203.e113

Rubin Grandis J, Melhem MF, Gooding WE, Day R, Holst VA, Wagener MM, Drenning SD, Tweardy DJ (1998) Levels of TGF-alpha and EGFR protein in head and neck squamous cell carcinoma and patient survival. J Natl Cancer Inst 90:824–832

Sachs N, de Ligt J, Kopper O, Gogola E, Bounova G, Weeber F, Balgobind AV, Wind K, Gracanin A, Begthel H et al (2018) A living biobank of breast cancer organoids captures disease heterogeneity. Cell 172:373–386.e10

Sandfort V, Koch U, Cordes N (2007) Cell adhesion-mediated radioresistance revisited. Int J Radiat Biol 83:727–732

Sato T, Vries RG, Snippert HJ, van de Wetering M, Barker N, Stange DE, van Es JH, Abo A, Kujala P, Peters PJ et al (2009) Single Lgr5 stem cells build crypt-villus structures in vitro without a mesenchymal niche. Nature 459:262–265

Schmeichel KL, Bissell MJ (2003) Modeling tissue-specific signaling and organ function in three dimensions. J Cell Sci 116:2377–2388

Seino T, Kawasaki S, Shimokawa M, Tamagawa H, Toshimitsu K, Fujii M, Ohta Y, Matano M, Nanki K, Kawasaki K et al (2018) Human pancreatic tumor organoids reveal loss of stem cell niche factor dependence during disease progression. Cell Stem Cell 22:454–467.e56

Shamir ER, Ewald AJ (2014) Three-dimensional organotypic culture: experimental models of mammalian biology and disease. Nat Rev Mol Cell Biol 15:647–664

Sharma RA, Plummer R, Stock JK, Greenhalgh TA, Ataman O, Kelly S, Clay R, Adams RA, Baird RD, Billingham L et al (2016) Clinical development of new drug-radiotherapy combinations. Nat Rev Clin Oncol 13:627–642

Sivakumar R, Chan M, Shin JS, Nishida-Aoki N, Kenerson HL, Elemento O, Beltran H, Yeung R, Gujral TS (2019) Organotypic tumor slice cultures provide a versatile platform for immuno-oncology and drug discovery. Oncoimmunology 8:e1670019

Skinner HD, Giri U, Yang L, Woo SH, Story MD, Pickering CR, Byers LA, Williams MD, El-Naggar A, Wang J et al (2016) Proteomic profiling identifies PTK2/FAK as a driver of radioresistance in HPV-negative head and neck cancer. Clin Cancer Res 22:4643–4650

Stone HB, Bernhard EJ, Coleman CN, Deye J, Capala J, Mitchell JB, Brown JM (2016) Preclinical data on efficacy of 10 drug-radiation combinations: evaluations, concerns, and recommendations. Transl Oncol 9:46–56

Storch K, Cordes N (2012) Focal adhesion-chromatin linkage controls tumor cell resistance to radio- and chemotherapy. Chemother Res Pract 2012:319287

Sulzmaier FJ, Jean C, Schlaepfer DD (2014) FAK in cancer: mechanistic findings and clinical applications. Nat Rev Cancer 14:598–610

Tanaka N, Osman AA, Takahashi Y, Lindemann A, Patel AA, Zhao M, Takahashi H, Myers JN (2018) Head and neck cancer organoids established by modification of the CTOS method can be used to predict in vivo drug sensitivity. Oral Oncol 87:49–57

The Cancer Genome Atlas Network, Muzny DM, Bainbridge MN, Chang K, Dinh HH, Drummond JA, Fowler G, Kovar CL, Lewis LR, Morgan MB et al (2012) Comprehensive molecular characterization of human colon and rectal cancer. Nature 487:330

The Cancer Genome Atlas Network, Lawrence MS, Sougnez C, Lichtenstein L, Cibulskis K, Lander E, Gabriel SB, Getz G, Ally A, Balasundaram M et al (2015) Comprehensive genomic characterization of head and neck squamous cell carcinomas. Nature 517:576

The Cancer Genome Atlas Research Network, McLendon R, Friedman A, Bigner D, Van Meir EG, Brat DJ, Mastrogianakis GM, Olson JJ, Mikkelsen T, Lehman N et al (2008) Comprehensive genomic characterization defines human glioblastoma genes and core pathways. Nature 455:1061

Vaira V, Fedele G, Pyne S, Fasoli E, Zadra G, Bailey D, Snyder E, Faversani A, Coggi G, Flavin R et al (2010) Preclinical model of organotypic culture for pharmacodynamic profiling of human tumors. Proc Natl Acad Sci U S A 107:8352–8356

van de Wetering M, Francies HE, Francis JM, Bounova G, Iorio F, Pronk A, van Houdt W, van Gorp J, Taylor-Weiner A, Kester L et al (2015) Prospective derivation of a living organoid biobank of colorectal cancer patients. Cell 161:933–945

Vehlow A, Storch K, Matzke D, Cordes N (2016) Molecular targeting of Integrins and integrin-associated signaling networks in radiation oncology. Recent Results Cancer Res 198:89–106

Vehlow A, Klapproth E, Storch K, Dickreuter E, Seifert M, Dietrich A, Butof R, Temme A, Cordes N (2017) Adhesion- and stress-related adaptation of glioma radiochemoresistance is circumvented by beta1 integrin/JNK co-targeting. Oncotarget 8:49224–49237

Vlachogiannis G, Hedayat S, Vatsiou A, Jamin Y, Fernandez-Mateos J, Khan K, Lampis A, Eason K, Huntingford I, Burke R et al (2018) Patient-derived organoids model treatment response of metastatic gastrointestinal cancers. Science 359:920–926

Weeber F, Ooft SN, Dijkstra KK, Voest EE (2017) Tumor organoids as a pre-clinical cancer model for drug discovery. Cell Chem Biol 24:1092–1100

Zaidel-Bar R, Itzkovitz S, Ma'ayan A, Iyengar R, Geiger B (2007) Functional atlas of the integrin adhesome. Nat Cell Biol 9:858–867

Zschenker O, Streichert T, Hehlgans S, Cordes N (2012) Genome-wide gene expression analysis in cancer cells reveals 3D growth to affect ECM and processes associated with cell adhesion but not DNA repair. PLoS One 7:e34279

Chapter 7
Preclinical In Vivo Evaluation of Novel Radiosensitizers by Local Tumor Control Experiments

Karolin Schneider, Nadja Ebert, Ina Kurth, and Michael Baumann

Abstract Over the past several years, significant technological and biological progress has been made in radiation oncology with focus on the development of new treatment schemes to target tumors more precisely and increase the susceptibility of tumor cells to radiation therapy. It is essential that new treatment concepts are first appropriately evaluated and validated in preclinical settings before they are translated into the clinic. In vivo models are the most valid model systems for preclinical investigations, as they best resemble the physiological complexity needed for translational studies. For the preclinical evaluation of promising radiosensitizers, relevant clinical endpoints should be defined in order to draw the correct conclusions for clinical translation. In addition, the appropriate preclinical model should be considered (patient-derived, cell line-derived, transgenic, etc.). Local tumor control is the endpoint of choice for preclinical assessments of the efficacy of new combination treatments in radiation oncology for curative radiation-based treatment strategies. Local tumor control takes into account the potential presence

K. Schneider · I. Kurth
German Cancer Research Center (DKFZ), Heidelberg, Germany
e-mail: karolin.schneider@dkfz.de; ina.kurth@dkfz.de

N. Ebert
German Cancer Research Center (DKFZ), Heidelberg, Germany

OncoRay – National Center for Radiation Research in Oncology, Faculty of Medicine and University Hospital Carl Gustav Carus, Technische Universität Dresden, Helmholtz-Zentrum Dresden – Rossendorf, Dresden, Germany
e-mail: nadja.ebert@dkfz.de

M. Baumann (✉)
German Cancer Research Center (DKFZ), Heidelberg, Germany

OncoRay – National Center for Radiation Research in Oncology, Faculty of Medicine and University Hospital Carl Gustav Carus, Technische Universität Dresden, Helmholtz-Zentrum Dresden – Rossendorf, Dresden, Germany

Department of Radiotherapy and Radiation Oncology, Faculty of Medicine and University Hospital Carl Gustav Carus, Technische Universität Dresden, Dresden, Germany
e-mail: michael.baumann@dkfz.de

© Springer Nature Switzerland AG 2020
H. Willers, I. Eke (eds.), *Molecular Targeted Radiosensitizers*, Cancer Drug Discovery and Development, https://doi.org/10.1007/978-3-030-49701-9_7

of cancer stem cells that may lead to recurrence after treatment. In addition to the correct tumor model and the clinical endpoint, other factors such as tumor heterogeneity, clinically relevant treatment regimens, and the presence of predictive biomarkers must be considered to reliably evaluate novel radiosensitizers.

Keywords Cancer stem cells · Heterotopic model · Local tumor control · NSG mice · NRG mice · Nude mice · Orthotopic model · Radiation dose · Radiosensitization · Scid mice · Sensitizer enhancement ratio · Tumor control dose · Tumor growth delay · Tumor heterogeneity · Tumor volume · Xenografts

1 Introduction

Radiation therapy (RT), together with surgery, drug treatment, and increasingly immunotherapy is a mainstay of today's cancer treatment arsenal. Approximately 50% of all cancer patients receive RT alone or in combination with systemic therapy during their course of disease (Barton et al. 2014; Borras et al. 2015).

Over the past years, significant progress has been made in radiation oncology, including advances in technology, image guidance, and biological understanding of mechanisms underlying radioresistance of tumors or pathogenesis of radiation-induced normal tissue reactions (Baumann et al. 2016; Stewart and Dorr 2009). These advances do not only provide opportunities to further improve the precision of radiation delivery, they also allow the development of novel and more specific treatments that target mainly tumor cells by increasing their sensitivity to RT.

There exists a considerable need for new anti-cancer drugs in radiation/multi-modal treatment strategies because local tumor control and cancer cure rates are still often insufficient after RT alone or in combination with standard cytotoxic drugs. To take a historical example, the loco-regional control rate of head and neck cancer of 27% with RT alone in the 1980s increased to more than 80% in the 2010s when RT was optimized in terms of dose–time–fractionation and combined with cisplatin and nimorazole (data from randomized DAHANCA studies, reviewed in Baumann et al. (2016)). Part of this improvement can certainly be allocated to improved RT techniques and stage migration. However, overall these results of a series of randomized trials show a clear benefit of improving RT based on biology in terms of fractionation and combination with radiosensitizers, one of which is a cytotoxic drug and the other a hypoxic cell radiosensitizer. A host of other studies on combined modality treatments corroborate this conclusion (Seiwert et al. 2007; Grégoire et al. 2019).

For the development of new drugs and their implementation into clinical settings including RT, solid preclinical evidence regarding dose, treatment effect and toxicity tests are indispensable. In vitro models allow to address fundamental questions like cellular and molecular pathways of drug–tumor cell interaction, necessary drug concentrations, and they provide first ideas on efficacy and toxic effects. In the in vitro setting, it is also possible to test and evaluate a drug and radiation interaction in terms of cell survival after single dose or fractionated irradiation with or without drug administration (Coleman et al. 2016). However, in vitro models have important limitations. The most important of these is that neither the complexity of tumors nor their interaction with the local microenvironment and with systemic influences by the host can be reliably studied. Tumors are a highly heterogeneous composition of different types of malignant and host cells and tissues. It can be assumed that the tumor cell population in any given tumor consists of a number of (clonal) subpopulations with different mutational burdens and epigenetic modifications which are constantly adapting to or being selected by their local microenvironment. This complexity cannot be reproduced by today's 2D or 3D cell culture systems which limits the potential of in vitro experiments for translation of results into the clinical setting. Furthermore, typical cell culture systems are neither able to model tumor host interactions regarding treatment effect (e.g., immune response) nor to evaluate the effects on tumor and normal tissues at the same time in the same model.

For the time being, animal models are therefore more suitable and more valid preclinical systems to generate the complexity needed for preclinical translational studies in the areas of RT and radiosensitization. In comparison to clinical translational studies, animal models remain important since they allow for a greater insight into treatment responses. For example, in vivo investigations in animals have the potential to provide large and meaningful data sets on treatment modulation for a single tumor model, while in clinical studies only one event can usually be scored for an individual tumor. Thus, while clinical studies measure almost always population effects, deeper insight into the response of individual tumors may be gained by preclinical in vivo experiments. Another argument is based on the ever increasing number of newly discovered potential molecular targets and newly developed radiosensitizing agents, making it difficult if not impossible to test all of them in clinical studies. Preclinical experiments can help to select the most promising candidates for further drug development and, at a later stage of the translational pipeline, for clinical trials.

Very promising developments have been made in radiosensitization strategies for human tumors (Higgins et al. 2015; Stone et al. 2016; Bristow et al. 2018; Kirsch et al. 2018). For example, since radiation-induced DNA double-strand breaks (DSB) are repaired by the cellular repair machinery, proteins in the DNA damage response (DDR) and DNA repair have a high potential as molecular targets for enhancing the effect of radiation on tumors (Russo et al. 2009; Khan et al. 2010; Fokas et al. 2012b; Biddlestone-Thorpe et al. 2013; Pospisilova et al. 2017; Durant et al. 2018; Laird et al. 2018; Bochum et al. 2018). Targeting signal transduction associated with radioresistance, for example, via the epidermal growth factor receptor (EGFR), has been demonstrated to be able to radiosensitize tumors (Ang et al. 2002, 2004; Baumann and Krause 2004; Krause et al. 2009; Gurtner et al. 2011, 2014; Koi et al. 2017). Tumor hypoxia is a long known obstacle for effective radiation treatment and diverse promising approaches to target hypoxic tumor areas for radiosensitization have been investigated (Nordsmark and Overgaard 2004; Overgaard 2011). For example, tumor hypoxia reduction by inhibition of mitochondrial oxidative phosphorylation (OXPHOS) (Ashton et al. 2018), increase of tumor oxygen level by reduction of oxygen consumption (e.g., metformin) (Lin and Maity 2015; Koritzinsky 2015) or by re-establishing normal vascularization within the tumor (Fokas et al. 2012a). Furthermore, oxygen mimetic drugs like nimorazole act as radiosensitizers (Overgaard et al. 1982, 1991; Metwally et al. 2014).

An emerging field of potential radiosensitizing agents, which currently attracts much attention, is to target the immune system in the context of RT (Burnette et al. 2012; Sharabi et al. 2015; Twyman-Saint Victor et al. 2015; Bristow et al. 2018; Rekers et al. 2018; Pitroda et al. 2019; Lambin et al. 2019). However, like all other radiosensitizing drugs, immune-based optimization of RT needs to be evaluated in terms of therapeutic gain: In preclinical experiments and clinical studies, the potential of immunotherapy combined with RT should improve local control of tumors but without increasing normal tissue toxicity, which might eventually enable radiation dose reduction without compromising local tumor control (Weichselbaum et al. 2017; Lambin et al. 2019).

2   Tumor Models In Vivo

2.1   Heterotopic Mouse Models

The use of small animals in preclinical oncology studies is an essential element and an important bridge for translation of experimental in vitro data to clinical application. Animal models represent the tumor integrated in a living organism, allowing a better investigation of tumor development, growth, treatment-induced reduction, and relapse, but also angiogenesis, metabolism, hypoxia, metastasis, immune, and normal tissue effects.

The most frequently used animals for scientific purposes are mice. The choice of the proper mouse and tumor model depends on the research question and aim and requires careful consideration and planning (Gengenbacher et al. 2017).

In the heterotopic (ectopic) model, the transplantation site differs from the original organ of the transplanted tumors. Most often, subcutaneous or intramuscular sites are chosen. Common practice involves injection of tumor cells or insertion of tumor pieces into the back, the flank, or the hind leg of the mouse. This approach has several advantages such as easy tumor transplantation and simple tumor size monitoring by external caliper measurements. Additionally, the transplanted tumors do not impair any organ function. The spatial separation between the tumor (to be treated) and healthy organs (to be spared) facilitates the use of relatively simple irradiation techniques which can be scaled to large cohorts of animals (Baumann et al. 2012). Heterotopic tumor models in irradiation studies allow robust assessments of tumor volume changes over time, which is the basis for determination of tumor growth delay and permanent local tumor control (Baumann et al. 2012).

Nevertheless, heterotopic models by definition cannot fully recapitulate a physiological tumor microenvironment, which is characterized by the interplay of the different intra-tumoral cell populations with body site-specific normal tissues and systemic components. This limits the ability to investigate normal tissue interactions, tumor invasion, and metastatic spread.

2.2 Orthotopic Mouse Models

In orthotopic models, tumor cells or pieces are transplanted into the original anatomical site of the mice. These models are more difficult to establish than heterotopic tumors (Bibby 2004). Due to the difficulty in accessing the involved organ, tumor monitoring is usually dependent on imaging approaches such as optical imaging, CT, and MRI (Wang et al. 2015; Aktar et al. 2019). In addition, because of the location of tumors in organs such as lung, brain, pancreas, or liver, these models may influence the well-being of the host animals already at small tumor volumes. Thus, imaging usually needs to be performed frequently before, during, and after RT. In addition, treatment usually necessitates advanced radiation techniques with precise image-guided planning, accurate positioning of the mouse, and appropriate collimator settings shielding organs at risk (Lewis et al. 2002; Kagadis et al. 2010; Verhaegen et al. 2011; Tillner et al. 2014). In recent years, small imaging and radiation device platforms have been developed. These devices commonly consist of a shielded cabinet with isocentric treatment tables, 360° movable X-ray tubes, various collimators and flat-panel detectors, and include advanced 3D planning software (Tillner et al. 2016).

The increased investment of time and equipment for orthotopic models, as compared to heterotopic models, enables investigations into tumor interactions with the original tissue environment, invasion into surrounding normal tissues, and metastatic spread. Orthotopic tumors may reflect radiation response and systemic reactions of human tumors better than heterotopic subcutaneous tumors (Bibby 2004).

2.3 Immunocompromised Mouse Strains

Although cell line-derived tumors (cell line-derived xenografts, CDX) are most commonly used in preclinical studies and can reveal important information about the efficacy of RT alone and combined with novel drugs, they are limited by several important differences compared to primary human tumors. For example, CDXs, which have been passaged for a long time show differences in tissue architecture and microenvironment, less genetic heterogeneity and altered gene expression compared to the tumor origin (Gillet et al. 2011; Day et al. 2015). Patient-derived xenografts (PDX) harbor more intact tumor samples, which were obtained directly from patients. PDX may more reliably predict treatment response of the initial tumor and are used in parallel to clinical trials for individual evaluation of therapeutic options and for screening of different drug candidates (Tentler et al. 2012; Clohessy and Pandolfi 2015; Gao et al. 2015; Lai et al. 2017). However, PDX studies are costly, logistically difficult, for example, with regard to strongly varying engraftment rates, limited passaging number, and availability of tumor material (Gengenbacher et al. 2017; Byrne et al. 2017; Meehan et al. 2017). Typically, in heterotopic or orthotopic xenograft models, human material is transplanted into immunocompromised mice to avoid the rejection of the introduced human material by the murine organism. Immune-compromised mouse strains with different disruptions in the functionality of innate and adaptive immune compartments are available (Shultz et al. 2007; Belizário 2009).

2.3.1 Nude Mice

Nude mice with a *Foxn1* gene mutation are athymic and T-lymphocyte deficient (Flanagan 1966). Athymic nude mice are used in more than 55% of tumor studies with immunocompromised animals (Gengenbacher et al. 2017). They are suitable for xenotransplantation experiments of a variety of solid tumors (Fogh et al. 1977) and are used for combined treatment evaluations and drug resistance studies (Szadvari et al. 2016). Due to the long life span of athymic nude mice (up to 2 years under specific pathogen free conditions) and their low risk for distant metastasis, they are particularly beneficial for long-term tumor follow-up experiments. Importantly, B-lymphocytes and innate immune compartments such as granulocytes, macrophages, and natural killer (NK) cells are functional in athymic nude mice. This needs to be considered when interpreting tumor engraftment rate, growth, and treatment response.

2.3.2 Scid Mice

The hirsute scid (Severe Combined Immunodeficiency, *Pkrdc^{scid/scid}*) mouse strain is fully T- and B-lymphocyte deficient (Bosma et al. 1983). However, a spontaneous production of sporadic mature lymphocytes is possible and the innate immune system is intact (Bosma et al. 1988; Carroll and Bosma 1988). With a NOD (non-obese diabetic) mouse strain background, scid mice have also defective NK cells, macrophages, and dendritic cells (NOD/scid, Shultz et al. 1995). NOD/scid mice are suitable for a variety of human xenografts such as breast, brain, and spleen tumors (Singh et al. 2004; Beckhove et al. 2003; Greiner et al. 1995) and, importantly, also for the engraftment of hematopoietic cancer cell lines (Greiner et al. 1998).

2.3.3 NSG Mice

In addition, mice with an *IL-2Rγ* (IL-2 receptor gamma) mutation completely lack NK cells and have a highly deficient T- and B-lymphocyte development (DiSanto et al. 1995). Thus, a highly immunodeficient mouse model results from the combination of the *IL-2Rγ*$^{-/-}$ and *Pkrdc*$^{scid/scid}$ mutations on a NOD strain background (Ito et al. 2002). These hybrid mice, the so-called NSG (NOD scid gamma) mice, are particularly utilized for transplantation of human tumors (Bankert et al. 2002) and more broadly, of human tissues, cells, bone marrow, and peripheral blood with the aim to develop a humanized mouse model (Ishikawa et al. 2005; Shultz et al. 2005). The tumor engraftment rate in NSG mice is higher compared to NOD/scid mice (Ito et al. 2002; Agliano et al. 2008) and the required cell number for tumor initiation is very low (towards one single cell (Quintana et al. 2008)). However, the *Pkrdc*$^{scid/scid}$ mutation causes defects in DSB repair (Fulop and Phillips 1990; Chang et al. 1993). NOD/scid and NSG mice are therefore not adequate for studies of radiation response and testing of radiosensitizers because DSB repair defects significantly increase normal tissue radiosensitivity.

2.3.4 NRG Mice

NRG (NOD/Rag$^{1/2null}$/IL-2Rγ$^{-/-}$) mice harbor *Rag1/2*^{null} mutation, which causes T- and B-lymphocyte depletion (like the *Pkrdc*$^{scid/scid}$ mutation), but does not impair DNA repair. NRG mice may engraft hematopoietic progenitors, blood cells, and extremely poorly outgrowing tumor cells (Shultz et al. 2003; Maykel et al. 2014). In contrast to NSG mice, they have a higher radioresistance, which is similar to athymic nude mice. This fact makes NRG mice more adequate for RT studies with clinical relevant doses (Barve et al. 2018). However, NSG and NRG mice have a relatively short life span (8–9 month), which makes long-term tumor follow-up unfeasible.

Overall, a disadvantage of human xenografts (CDX, PDX) is that they require immunocompromised models, which impedes investigation of the role and response of the immune system. However, human-derived tumors reflect at least in some aspects the response of patients' tumors to RT and combined treatments. A very important advantage is the availability of human pharmaceuticals that can be directly used to treat human xenograft tumors. The advantages are reflected by the extensive use of CDX and PDX in 89% of preclinical studies (Gengenbacher et al. 2017).

2.4   *Immunocompetent Mouse Models*

Syngeneic models are based on immunocompetent mice. Tumors result either from transplantation of samples with the same genetic background (allograft) or from induction by environmental agents, such as chemicals, UV radiation, ionizing radiation, pathogens, or by the introduction of genetic drivers via viral vectors or plasmid DNA (Kemp 2015; Galuschka et al. 2017).

Tumor induction by environmental cancer-causing agents leads to de novo carcinogenesis and enables the investigation of preventive actions and risk factors. For example, in very early mouse studies, UV radiation (1920s), and X-rays (1930s) were confirmed to cause skin cancer, and the interaction of carcinogenic chemicals with DNA was discovered in the 1960s, all of which led to important prevention strategies in humans (Kemp 2015). Since the 1990s, exposure with carcinogenic agents has been applied to genetically engineered mouse models (GEMM), in order to explore the intertwined actions between environmental factors and genetic predisposition in cancer development (Kemp 2015). However, due to the long latency of tumorigenesis and high heterogeneity, environmentally induced tumor models are only used in 6% of cancer studies (Gengenbacher et al. 2017).

Syngeneic tumors can furthermore be induced by injection of oncogenes. For example, a retroviral vector derived from avian leucosis virus subgroup A (ALV-A) was used to transfer and express exogenous oncogenes in murine neuronal stem cells in order to induce brain tumors (Holland 2000). These murine tumors strongly resembled the histopathology of human glioblastoma in 60% of the mice. This syngeneic model is suitable to test new drugs in combination with RT for brain tumors (Hambardzumyan et al. 2009).

Instead of introducing genetic material into locally restricted regions of the murine organism before/during each experiment, GEMMs receive genetic modifications already at the stage of the fertilized oocyte, the 8-cell stage embryo, or via targeted embryonic stem cells injected into the blastocyst (Lampreht Tratar et al. 2018). Genetic modifications can be restricted to somatic cells (non-germline GEMM, e.g., by CRISPR/Cas9 genome editing) or included in the germline (germline GEMM, e.g., by knockout/knock-in of genes) (Kersten et al. 2017). GEMMs can harbor dominant oncogenes, carry mutations in tumor suppressor genes, or more recently, carry human cancer-related mutations, which enable a controlled de novo tumorigenesis and autochthonous disease progression (Donehower et al. 1992; Gengenbacher et al. 2017; Kersten et al. 2017). GEMMs may help to identify genetic markers to predict therapy response or resistance, to screen for novel radiosensitizers, and to validate them (Singh et al. 2012; Kersten et al. 2017).

These models have the advantage of a natural tumor development and interaction between tumor and immune compartments. Twenty-seven percent of tumor model studies included GEMMs (Gengenbacher et al. 2017).

2.5   Model Considerations for Drug/Radiation Studies

Since GEMMs express only the murine homologue of a desired human target, the main drawback for this model is that the observed responses to (new) treatments are restricted to the murine biology (Teicher 2006). As is true for all mouse models, the metabolism of a new drug in GEMMs may differ from humans. This has to be considered when interpreting results and translation into the human organism.

Orthotopic PDXs, which have been passaged in vivo, represent important models that can produce results with relevance for clinical trials (Lawrence et al. 2013). The use of PDX models complementary to other preclinical models with a well-defined genetic background are beneficial for drug response studies (Tentler et al. 2012). The aim of novel combinatory drugs is to widen the therapeutic window of RT, that is to improve the anti-tumor effect compared to the standard treatment without increasing normal tissue toxicity. To facilitate preclinical translational studies, it is therefore indispensable to advance also normal tissue models to investigate treatment-related toxicity (Moses and Kummermehr 1986; Dörr 1998). In order to estimate the gain for the therapeutic ratio and to evaluate the risk-benefit relation, normal tissue effects should be surveyed during the investigation of novel treatments (Lehnert and el-Khatib 1989; Liao et al. 1995; Herrmann et al. 1997; Stewart and Dorr 2009).

The term "sensitizer enhancement ratio" (SER) describes the increased effect of a combined treatment of RT with a radiosensitizer compared to RT alone. It needs to be ensured that the SER of the normal tissue is smaller than the SER of the tumor before a new treatment combination can be moved to clinical studies (Harrington et al. 2011).

Overall, it is important to realize that each tumor or mouse model has its limitations and benefits. What all of the tumor models have in common is that they constantly need to be developed further, to be enhanced and refined (Day et al. 2015). Importantly, specific experiments require the appropriate model according to the study aim and endpoints.

3   Experimental Endpoints

Preclinical studies using laboratory animals require detailed planning. Depending on the exact scientific question to be answered, different animal and tumor models are advantageous (vide supra) and different endpoints are in use.

3.1 Tumor Volume-Based Endpoints

In preclinical experiments on tumors using radiation, most commonly volume-based endpoints, such as tumor regression or progression and tumor growth delay, are utilized. The tumor volume is repeatedly measured before, during, and after treatment. In subcutaneous (s.c.) tumors, the measurements are usually performed using calipers while in orthotopic tumors often advanced imaging techniques are needed (Zips 2019). An individual tumor growth curve over time is generated as basis for further analysis. It is important to note that this growth curve reflects the average of the dynamics of all cell populations present in the tumor and usually does not allow to differentiate between different cell populations (e.g., tumor cells versus infiltrating cells of the immune system) or between cell production and cell loss (e.g., into necrosis). Furthermore, effects of treatment on tumor volume are influenced by many factors including the capability of the murine organism to remove dead cells, the formation of edema, or invasion of normal cells into the tumor (Baumann et al. 2012). Finally, tumor volume-dependent endpoints reflect the effect of a treatment on the bulk of tumor cells and not the effect on tumor cells that are able to form a recurrence or to metastasize, i.e., cancer stem cells (CSC) or clonogenic cells.

The most basic parameter is tumor regression, which simply compares the volume of a tumor at a given time during or after treatment to the volume at start of treatment. In contrast, tumor growth delay (GD) reveals more information by comparing the time needed for treated versus control tumors to reach a specified volume. For radiation alone, due to a greater inactivation of CSCs (or clonogenic precursor cells with a high capacity to divide), GD increases with increasing radiation dose (Baumann et al. 2003). However, this relationship may be obscured by adding drugs. Evaluation of GD at several dose levels, for example, by using GD per Gy, allows to some extent to estimate whether the effect of a drug combined with radiation is limited to the bulk of non-stem tumor cells or is also enhancing inactivation of CSCs (Baumann et al. 2003, 2008; Krause et al. 2007). The endpoint of tumor GD is suitable for initial drug screenings, "proof-of-concept" studies, investigation of mechanistic actions, and evaluation of non-curative treatments (Baumann et al. 2012; Coleman et al. 2016). However, standard GD experiments fail to assess treatment efficacy against CSCs as GD only measures bulk tumor killing.

3.2 Local Tumor Control Assay

Since evidence has accumulated over the past years that CSCs may be dormant, are cycling slower, exhibit a higher DNA damage repair capacity, and overall can be more treatment resistant than the bulk of tumor cells, it is important to use preclinical assays able to measure effects of treatment on CSCs and not just on the bulk of tumor cells (Reya et al. 2001; Bao et al. 2006; Clarke and Fuller 2006; Baumann et al. 2008; Peitzsch et al. 2019).

Permanent local tumor control after RT depends on the inactivation of all CSCs in the radiation field by the treatment or by host factors. Therefore, radiation local control assays are suitable to functionally assess the effect of a given treatment or combination of treatments on inactivation of CSCs (Krause et al. 2006; Baumann et al. 2008).

For local tumor control experiments, tumor bearing mice are treated with graded dose levels of either radiation alone or radiation plus a novel drug. After the end of the treatment, the mice are observed until no or almost no new tumor recurrences occur anymore. A dose–response curve is established from the rates of tumor control probability (TCP) per dose level (Zips 2019) (Fig. 7.1). The more a dose–response curve is shifted towards lower doses, the higher is the overall radiation sensitivity of a tumor type.

The simplest experimental design is to give one standard radiation treatment at one dose level and to compare this to the same radiation treatment plus a novel drug. Local tumor control is then plotted as function of the time after treatment in a Kaplan–Meier diagram and gives evidence for an altered response effect with the combined treatment (Fig. 7.2).

The limitation of Kaplan–Meier curves is that only the combined effect of one radiation dose level plus the drug can be derived. It cannot, or only under assumptions, be estimated how a modified radiation dose would change the treatment response. Therefore, even in this simple setting it is useful to add at least a second radiation dose level to gain some insight of the importance of the efficacy of the combined treatment to enhance tumor control in comparison to an increase of radiation dose alone.

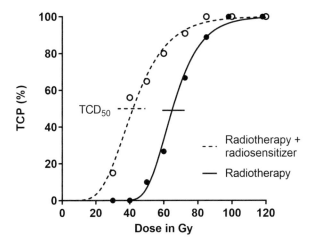

Fig. 7.1 Theoretical dose–response curves according to the observed local tumor control rates (symbols) for two different treatment groups: radiation therapy alone and combined treatment (e.g., radiation plus radiosensitizer). Error bars represent the 95% CI for the TCD_{50} (tumor control dose 50%) value. TCP, tumor control probability

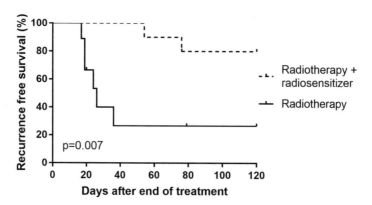

Fig. 7.2 Theoretical Kaplan–Meier survival curve for a fractionated radiation regimen with or without a radiosensitizer

In contrast, the dose–response curve in a "TCD_{50}" (tumor control dose 50%) experiment provides a quantitative description of the tumor control probability at different dose levels and enables to calculate radiation dose needed to cure 50% of the mice (Zips 2019). The dose modifying factor (DMF), which is calculated from the TCD_{50} values of different dose–response curves, represents the decrease in radiation dose after adding a drug to reach the same tumor control probability compared to RT alone (Zips 2019). From this comparison, the radiation dose level within the combined treatment needed to achieve the same TCD_{50} as for RT alone can easily be estimated.

Additional information can be gained from the steepness of dose–response curves in TCD_{50} experiments. The steeper a dose–response curve, the smaller is the radiation dose range for a broad range of tumor control probability and the smaller is usually the heterogeneity of response. For example, for a very steep dose–response relationship only a minimal increase of radiation dose may greatly increase tumor control probability. This is also true for dose-normal tissue toxicity curves in effective dose 50% (ED_{50}) experiments. On the other hand, there is a risk of a significant reduction of local tumor control if the radiation dose is only slightly decreased. For tumor types with flat dose–response curves, the dose range to decrease the tumor control probability is much larger. This allows for a radiation dose reduction in preclinical studies with combined treatment strategies without major local tumor control reduction, which may be compensated by the drug given concurrently. If a drug added to RT increases the steepness of the dose–response curve while shifting the curve to the left compared to RT alone, this can be taken as indication that on a CSC level the drug has decreased the inter-tumoral heterogeneity of one or more important factors contributing to radioresistance.

TCD_{50} experiments are more time- as well as cost-intensive compared to tumor volume or GD investigations and require higher numbers of laboratory mice (Baumann et al. 2012; Coleman et al. 2016). However, this experimental design is important and appropriate for preclinical validation of novel sensitizing treatments in radiation oncology since clinical studies have shown similarly shaped curves for local tumor control in patients (Zips 2019).

Combined treatment studies have shown that these two endpoints, tumor GD and local tumor control, not always produce congruent results (Budach et al. 1993; Baumann et al. 2003, 2008; Krause et al. 2007; Gurtner et al. 2014). Only tumor local control can predict tumor cure since it measures CSC inactivation. Just one surviving CSC, if not inactivated by the host, can lead to a local tumor relapse. This makes TCD_{50} assays very sensitive and valuable for preclinical assessments of the efficacy of new combination treatments to enhance curative radiation-based treatment strategies (Krause et al. 2006).

4   Tumor Heterogeneity

Clinical studies have demonstrated inter-tumoral heterogeneity in CSC numbers, hypoxia, and other factors that influence response to radiation treatment, which leads to a different treatment success in patients with the same tumor entity (Baumann et al. 2008).

This inter-tumoral heterogeneity in (radiation) treatment response is also found in preclinical models (Yaromina et al. 2007; Gurtner et al. 2011, 2014) (Fig. 7.3). This phenomenon may cause a risk of overestimating the therapeutic potential of a new radiosensitizer if only well-responding tumor models are used for testing (Zips et al. 2005). Consequently, inter-tumor heterogeneity should be simulated in local tumor control experiments by the investigation of a panel of different tumor models in order to obtain insight into the heterogeneity of response (Yaromina et al. 2006, 2007; Gurtner et al. 2014). Living tumor biobanks, i.e., collections of CDXs and PDXs, provide a broad spectrum of heterogeneity (Gao et al. 2015; Bruna et al. 2016). Regular molecular profiling of the investigated tumors is needed to ensure preservation of relevant tumor characteristics through passaging and to conserve the heterogeneity of the biobank (Cassidy et al. 2015; Bristow et al. 2018). Establishing living tumor biobanks is complex, cost-, space-, and time-intensive in terms of mouse numbers, housing, care taking personal, tumor biology validation, and prolonged experimental time span for the development of new radiosensitizers.

Fig. 7.3 Tumor control probability for ten different heterotopic human head and neck squamous cell carcinomas illustrates the heterogeneity of dose–response relationships. The red curve represents the composite dose–response relationship of all tumor xenografts (redrawn from Baumann and Krause 2009 in Molls et al. (eds))

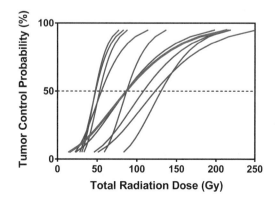

However, this will enable large-scale screening for suitable radiosensitizers and improve the transferability of in vivo therapy responses to patient tumor response (Gao et al. 2015). In order to minimize costs and efforts for individual working groups, laboratories may be well advised to collaborate and share tumor banks. This requires standard operating procedures and strict quality control (Coleman et al. 2016). Another practical approach to minimize animal numbers is to perform an initial screening of GD effects of a new drug or to conduct restricted TCD_{50} experiments and select suitable tumor models, which are then further investigated in more extensive local tumor control experiments.

In parallel, the development of predictive biomarkers for stratification of patients according to their heterogeneous tumor characteristics is of emerging importance. Single biomarkers or sets of biomarkers such as gene expression profiles (Baumann et al. 2016; Bristow et al. 2018) can help to identify radioresistant tumors and predict response to treatment strategies with novel radiosensitizers. For example, in patients with head and neck squamous cell carcinoma, HPV/p16 status and the CSC marker CD44 were shown to be predictive of local tumor control (Linge et al. 2016). Biomarker development can be realized in mouse models from large xenograft biobanks, which reflect the heterogeneity of individual tumors.

5 Clinically Relevant Treatment Schedules

Proof-of-concept in vivo experiments may provide preliminary evidence for the potential treatment success of a novel radiosensitizer. However, additional preclinical studies under conditions that are as close as possible to clinical settings are indispensable.

Clinically relevant radiation schedules include fractionated RT instead of single fraction irradiation (Harrington et al. 2011). It is important to apply fractionated or split radiation doses in mouse studies since tumor effects are different after fractionated RT with regard to biological factors such as tumor cell repopulation, reoxygenation, and development of necrosis (Hessel et al. 2004a, b; Baumann and Krause 2004; Krause et al. 2005; Eicheler et al. 2005; Yaromina et al. 2007). The schedule of a combined treatment with RT has been shown to influence the treatment outcome as well: radiosensitizers might be administered prior to RT (neoadjuvant), during the course of RT (concomitant) or only after radiation treatment has been completed (adjuvant) (Zips et al. 2003). Radiation dose levels and doses per fraction should also be kept in the range of clinical use in preclinical trials. The same is true for novel drugs, which need to be tested in vivo in clinically achievable dosage and administration forms (Lawrence et al. 2013).

In many cases, human tumors are not only treated with RT, but with concurrent RT and chemotherapy (chemoradiation). In preclinical models of those tumor entities in which chemoradiation is standard of care, chemotherapy should also be included in the preclinical treatment schedule for the development of additional radiosensitizers. The optimal approach, although resource-demanding, is to test RT alone, standard chemoradiation alone, RT plus novel sensitizer, and standard chemoradiation plus novel sensitizer. If this is not possible, it is recommended to use at least a control group with the clinical standard treatment in comparison to the new combined treatment.

6   Summary and Conclusions

Different experimental model systems and endpoints are suitable for specific questions regarding a potential new radiosensitizer. Growth delay assays reveal interactions of the new radiosensitizer with radiation treatment, the tumor microenvironment, and the whole organism in vivo (Coleman et al. 2016). Tumor control dose (TCD_{50}) experiments are necessary for consideration of CSCs in order to evaluate whether the new radiosensitizer in combination with the standard radiation treatment has curative potential or only a palliative effect (persistence of CSCs that could give rise to a recurrence).

Normal tissue toxicity needs to be assessed in appropriate models, and the risk-benefit ratio associated with the new radiosensitizer must be weighed. With normal toxicity mouse models it needs to be ensured that the SER of the normal tissue is smaller than the SER of the tumor before a new treatment combination can be moved to clinical studies (Harrington et al. 2011).

In parallel to the testing of novel radiosensitizers, it is crucial to develop biomarkers that represent tumor characteristics and predict the sensitivity or resistance of individual tumors to the combined treatment and consequently their treatment response. The ultimate objective is to select the proper radiosensitizer for each individual patient according to an integrated model of therapy response that includes predictive biomarkers. Treatment adaptations may not only include intensification of RT by combination with novel drugs in situations where local tumor control is poor but also de-escalation of the standard dose of RT when combined with an effective radiosensitizer, which could result in reduced radiation-induced toxicity to the normal tissue.

In conclusion, in vivo experiments on tumor models will remain indispensable for the development of novel radiosensitizers and chemoradiosensitizers for radiation oncology. These experiments need to be expertly designed according to the specific scientific question and the hypothesis addressed. Deliberate choices of the most appropriate tumor/mouse model and the experimental endpoint need to be made. The design of such studies should consider inter-tumoral heterogeneity, including biomarker assessment, as well as a clinically relevant dosing of RT to achieve a suitable preclinical body of data for further optimization and clinical translation of the most promising novel candidate drugs.

Acknowledgement   We thank Carol Bacchus-Wermke for her editorial contribution.

References

Agliano A, Martin-Padura I, Mancuso P, Marighetti P, Rabascio C, Pruneri G, Shultz LD, Bertolini F (2008) Human acute leukemia cells injected in NOD/LtSz-scid/IL-2Rgamma null mice generate a faster and more efficient disease compared to other NOD/scid-related strains. Int J Cancer 123(9):2222–2227. https://doi.org/10.1002/ijc.23772

Aktar R, Dietrich A, Tillner F, Kotb S, Lock S, Willers H, Baumann M, Krause M, Butof R (2019) Pre-clinical imaging for establishment and comparison of orthotopic non-small cell lung carcinoma: in search for models reflecting clinical scenarios. Br J Radiol 92(1095):20180539. https://doi.org/10.1259/bjr.20180539

Ang KK, Andratschke NH, Milas L (2004) Epidermal growth factor receptor and response of head-and-neck carcinoma to therapy. Int J Radiat Oncol Biol Phys 58(3):959–965. https://doi.org/10.1016/j.ijrobp.2003.07.010

Ang KK, Berkey BA, Tu X, Zhang HZ, Katz R, Hammond EH, Fu KK, Milas L (2002) Impact of epidermal growth factor receptor expression on survival and pattern of relapse in patients with advanced head and neck carcinoma. Cancer Res 62(24):7350–7356

Ashton TM, McKenna WG, Kunz-Schughart LA, Higgins GS (2018) Oxidative phosphorylation as an emerging target in cancer therapy. Clin Cancer Res 24(11):2482–2490. https://doi.org/10.1158/1078-0432.CCR-17-3070

Bankert RB, Hess SD, Egilmez NK (2002) SCID mouse models to study human cancer pathogenesis and approaches to therapy: potential, limitations, and future directions. Front Biosci 7:c44–c62

Bao S, Wu Q, McLendon RE, Hao Y, Shi Q, Hjelmeland AB, Dewhirst MW, Bigner DD, Rich JN (2006) Glioma stem cells promote radioresistance by preferential activation of the DNA damage response. Nature 444(7120):756–760. https://doi.org/10.1038/nature05236

Barton MB, Jacob S, Shafiq J, Wong K, Thompson SR, Hanna TP, Delaney GP (2014) Estimating the demand for radiotherapy from the evidence: a review of changes from 2003 to 2012. Radiother Oncol 112(1):140–144. https://doi.org/10.1016/j.radonc.2014.03.024

Barve A, Casson L, Krem M, Wunderlich M, Mulloy JC, Beverly LJ (2018) Comparative utility of NRG and NRGS mice for the study of normal hematopoiesis, leukemogenesis, and therapeutic response. Exp Hematol 67:18–31. https://doi.org/10.1016/j.exphem.2018.08.004

Baumann M, Krause M (2004) Targeting the epidermal growth factor receptor in radiotherapy: radiobiological mechanisms, preclinical and clinical results. Radiother Oncol 72(3):257–266. https://doi.org/10.1016/j.radonc.2004.07.007

Baumann M, Krause M (2009) Tumor Biology's impact on clinical cure rates. In: Molls M, Vaupel P, Nieder C, Anscher MS (eds) The impact of tumor biology on cancer treatment and multidisciplinary strategies. Springer

Baumann M, Krause M, Hill R (2008) Exploring the role of cancer stem cells in radioresistance. Nat Rev Cancer 8(7):545–554. https://doi.org/10.1038/nrc2419

Baumann M, Krause M, Overgaard J, Debus J, Bentzen SM, Daartz J, Richter C, Zips D, Bortfeld T (2016) Radiation oncology in the era of precision medicine. Nat Rev Cancer 16(4):234–249. https://doi.org/10.1038/nrc.2016.18

Baumann M, Krause M, Zips D, Eicheler W, Dorfler A, Ahrens J, Petersen C, Bruchner K, Hilberg F (2003) Selective inhibition of the epidermal growth factor receptor tyrosine kinase by BIBX1382BS and the improvement of growth delay, but not local control, after fractionated irradiation in human FaDu squamous cell carcinoma in the nude mouse. Int J Radiat Biol 79(7):547–559. https://doi.org/10.1080/0955300031000112839

Baumann M, Zips D, Krause M (2012) Experimental tumor therapy. Strahlenther Onkol 188(Suppl 3):291–294. https://doi.org/10.1007/s00066-012-0201-5

Beckhove P, Schutz F, Diel IJ, Solomayer EF, Bastert G, Foerster J, Feuerer M, Bai L, Sinn HP, Umansky V, Schirrmacher V (2003) Efficient engraftment of human primary breast cancer transplants in nonconditioned NOD/Scid mice. Int J Cancer 105(4):444–453. https://doi.org/10.1002/ijc.11125

Belizário JE (2009) Immunodeficient mouse models: an overview. Open Immunol J 2:79–85

Bibby MC (2004) Orthotopic models of cancer for preclinical drug evaluation: advantages and disadvantages. Eur J Cancer 40(6):852–857. https://doi.org/10.1016/j.ejca.2003.11.021

Biddlestone-Thorpe L, Sajjad M, Rosenberg E, Beckta JM, Valerie NC, Tokarz M, Adams BR, Wagner AF, Khalil A, Gilfor D, Golding SE, Deb S, Temesi DG, Lau A, O'Connor MJ, Choe KS, Parada LF, Lim SK, Mukhopadhyay ND, Valerie K (2013) ATM kinase inhibition preferentially sensitizes p53-mutant glioma to ionizing radiation. Clin Cancer Res 19(12):3189–3200. https://doi.org/10.1158/1078-0432.CCR-12-3408

Bochum S, Berger S, Martens UM (2018) Olaparib. Recent Results Cancer Res 211:217–233. https://doi.org/10.1007/978-3-319-91442-8_15

Borras JM, Lievens Y, Dunscombe P, Coffey M, Malicki J, Corral J, Gasparotto C, Defourny N, Barton M, Verhoeven R, van Eycken L, Primic-Zakelj M, Trojanowski M, Strojan P, Grau C (2015) The optimal utilization proportion of external beam radiotherapy in European countries: an ESTRO-HERO analysis. Radiother Oncol 116(1):38–44. https://doi.org/10.1016/j.radonc.2015.04.018

Bosma GC, Custer RP, Bosma MJ (1983) A severe combined immunodeficiency mutation in the mouse. Nature 301(5900):527–530

Bosma GC, Fried M, Custer RP, Carroll A, Gibson DM, Bosma MJ (1988) Evidence of functional lymphocytes in some (leaky) scid mice. J Exp Med 167(3):1016–1033. https://doi.org/10.1084/jem.167.3.1016

Bristow RG, Alexander B, Baumann M, Bratman SV, Brown JM, Camphausen K, Choyke P, Citrin D, Contessa JN, Dicker A, Kirsch DG, Krause M, Le QT, Milosevic M, Morris ZS, Sarkaria JN, Sondel PM, Tran PT, Wilson GD, Willers H, Wong RKS, Harari PM (2018) Combining precision radiotherapy with molecular targeting and immunomodulatory agents: a guideline by the American Society for Radiation Oncology. Lancet Oncol 19(5):e240–e251. https://doi.org/10.1016/S1470-2045(18)30096-2

Bruna A, Rueda OM, Greenwood W, Batra AS, Callari M, Batra RN, Pogrebniak K, Sandoval J, Cassidy JW, Tufegdzic-Vidakovic A, Sammut SJ, Jones L, Provenzano E, Baird R, Eirew P, Hadfield J, Eldridge M, McLaren-Douglas A, Barthorpe A, Lightfoot H, O'Connor MJ, Gray J, Cortes J, Baselga J, Marangoni E, Welm AL, Aparicio S, Serra V, Garnett MJ, Caldas C (2016) A biobank of breast cancer explants with preserved intra-tumor heterogeneity to screen anticancer compounds. Cell 167(1):260–274. e222. https://doi.org/10.1016/j.cell.2016.08.041

Budach W, Budach V, Stuschke M, Dinges S, Sack H (1993) The TCD50 and regrowth delay assay in human tumor xenografts: differences and implications. Int J Radiat Oncol Biol Phys 25(2):259–268. https://doi.org/10.1016/0360-3016(93)90347-x

Burnette B, Fu YX, Weichselbaum RR (2012) The confluence of radiotherapy and immunotherapy. Front Oncol 2:143. https://doi.org/10.3389/fonc.2012.00143

Byrne AT, Alferez DG, Amant F, Annibali D, Arribas J, Biankin AV, Bruna A, Budinska E, Caldas C, Chang DK, Clarke RB, Clevers H, Coukos G, Dangles-Marie V, Eckhardt SG, Gonzalez-Suarez E, Hermans E, Hidalgo M, Jarzabek MA, de Jong S, Jonkers J, Kemper K, Lanfrancone L, Maelandsmo GM, Marangoni E, Marine JC, Medico E, Norum JH, Palmer HG, Peeper DS, Pelicci PG, Piris-Gimenez A, Roman-Roman S, Rueda OM, Seoane J, Serra V, Soucek L, Vanhecke D, Villanueva A, Vinolo E, Bertotti A, Trusolino L (2017) Interrogating open issues in cancer precision medicine with patient-derived xenografts. Nat Rev Cancer 17(4):254–268. https://doi.org/10.1038/nrc.2016.140

Carroll AM, Bosma MJ (1988) Detection and characterization of functional T cells in mice with severe combined immune deficiency. Eur J Immunol 18(12):1965–1971. https://doi.org/10.1002/eji.1830181215

Cassidy JW, Caldas C, Bruna A (2015) Maintaining tumor heterogeneity in patient-derived tumor xenografts. Cancer Res 75(15):2963–2968. https://doi.org/10.1158/0008-5472.CAN-15-0727

Chang C, Biedermann KA, Mezzina M, Brown JM (1993) Characterization of the DNA double strand break repair defect in scid mice. Cancer Res 53(6):1244–1248

Clarke MF, Fuller M (2006) Stem cells and cancer: two faces of eve. Cell 124(6):1111–1115. https://doi.org/10.1016/j.cell.2006.03.011

Clohessy JG, Pandolfi PP (2015) Mouse hospital and co-clinical trial project—from bench to bedside. Nat Rev Clin Oncol 12(8):491–498. https://doi.org/10.1038/nrclinonc.2015.62

Coleman CN, Higgins GS, Brown JM, Baumann M, Kirsch DG, Willers H, Prasanna PG, Dewhirst MW, Bernhard EJ, Ahmed MM (2016) Improving the predictive value of preclinical studies in support of radiotherapy clinical trials. Clin Cancer Res 22(13):3138–3147. https://doi.org/10.1158/1078-0432.CCR-16-0069

Day CP, Merlino G, Van Dyke T (2015) Preclinical mouse cancer models: a maze of opportunities and challenges. Cell 163(1):39–53. https://doi.org/10.1016/j.cell.2015.08.068

DiSanto JP, Muller W, Guy-Grand D, Fischer A, Rajewsky K (1995) Lymphoid development in mice with a targeted deletion of the interleukin 2 receptor gamma chain. Proc Natl Acad Sci U S A 92(2):377–381. https://doi.org/10.1073/pnas.92.2.377

Donehower LA, Harvey M, Slagle BL, McArthur MJ, Montgomery CA Jr, Butel JS, Bradley A (1992) Mice deficient for p53 are developmentally normal but susceptible to spontaneous tumours. Nature 356(6366):215–221. https://doi.org/10.1038/356215a0

Dörr W (1998) Radiobiological models of normal tissue reactions. Strahlenther Onkol 174:4–7

Durant ST, Zheng L, Wang Y, Chen K, Zhang L, Zhang T, Yang Z, Riches L, Trinidad AG, Fok JHL, Hunt T, Pike KG, Wilson J, Smith A, Colclough N, Reddy VP, Sykes A, Janefeldt A, Johnstrom P, Varnas K, Takano A, Ling S, Orme J, Stott J, Roberts C, Barrett I, Jones G, Roudier M, Pierce A, Allen J, Kahn J, Sule A, Karlin J, Cronin A, Chapman M, Valerie K, Illingworth R, Pass M (2018) The brain-penetrant clinical ATM inhibitor AZD1390 radiosensitizes and improves survival of preclinical brain tumor models. Sci Adv 4(6):eaat1719. https://doi.org/10.1126/sciadv.aat1719

Eicheler W, Krause M, Hessel F, Zips D, Baumann M (2005) Kinetics of EGFR expression during fractionated irradiation varies between different human squamous cell carcinoma lines in nude mice. Radiother Oncol 76(2):151–156. https://doi.org/10.1016/j.radonc.2005.06.033

Flanagan SP (1966) 'Nude', a new hairless gene with pleiotropic effects in the mouse. Genet Res 8(3):295–309

Fogh J, Fogh JM, Orfeo T (1977) One hundred and twenty-seven cultured human tumor cell lines producing tumors in nude mice. J Natl Cancer Inst 59(1):221–226. https://doi.org/10.1093/jnci/59.1.221

Fokas E, im JH, Hill S, Yameen S, Stratford M, Beech J, Hackl W, Maira SM, Bernhard EJ, McKenna WG, Muschel RJ (2012a) Dual inhibition of the PI3K/mTOR pathway increases tumor radiosensitivity by normalizing tumor vasculature. Cancer Res 72(1):239–248. https://doi.org/10.1158/0008-5472.CAN-11-2263

Fokas E, Prevo R, Pollard JR, Reaper PM, Charlton PA, Cornelissen B, Vallis KA, Hammond EM, Olcina MM, Gillies McKenna W, Muschel RJ, Brunner TB (2012b) Targeting ATR in vivo using the novel inhibitor VE-822 results in selective sensitization of pancreatic tumors to radiation. Cell Death Dis 3:e441. https://doi.org/10.1038/cddis.2012.181

Fulop GM, Phillips RA (1990) The scid mutation in mice causes a general defect in DNA repair. Nature 347(6292):479–482. https://doi.org/10.1038/347479a0

Galuschka C, Proynova R, Roth B, Augustin HG, Muller-Decker K (2017) Models in translational oncology: a public resource database for preclinical cancer research. Cancer Res 77(10):2557–2563. https://doi.org/10.1158/0008-5472.CAN-16-3099

Gao H, Korn JM, Ferretti S, Monahan JE, Wang Y, Singh M, Zhang C, Schnell C, Yang G, Zhang Y, Balbin OA, Barbe S, Cai H, Casey F, Chatterjee S, Chiang DY, Chuai S, Cogan SM, Collins SD, Dammassa E, Ebel N, Embry M, Green J, Kauffmann A, Kowal C, Leary RJ, Lehar J, Liang Y, Loo A, Lorenzana E, Robert McDonald E 3rd, ME ML, Merkin J, Meyer R, Naylor TL, Patawaran M, Reddy A, Roelli C, Ruddy DA, Salangsang F, Santacroce F, Singh AP, Tang Y, Tinetto W, Tobler S, Velazquez R, Venkatesan K, Von Arx F, Wang HQ, Wang Z, Wiesmann M, Wyss D, Xu F, Bitter

H, Atadja P, Lees E, Hofmann F, Li E, Keen N, Cozens R, Jensen MR, Pryer NK, Williams JA, Sellers WR (2015) High-throughput screening using patient-derived tumor xenografts to predict clinical trial drug response. Nat Med 21(11):1318–1325. https://doi.org/10.1038/nm.3954

Gengenbacher N, Singhal M, Augustin HG (2017) Preclinical mouse solid tumour models: status quo, challenges and perspectives. Nat Rev Cancer 17(12):751–765. https://doi.org/10.1038/nrc.2017.92

Gillet JP, Calcagno AM, Varma S, Marino M, Green LJ, Vora MI, Patel C, Orina JN, Eliseeva TA, Singal V, Padmanabhan R, Davidson B, Ganapathi R, Sood AK, Rueda BR, Ambudkar SV, Gottesman MM (2011) Redefining the relevance of established cancer cell lines to the study of mechanisms of clinical anti-cancer drug resistance. Proc Natl Acad Sci U S A 108(46):18708–18713. https://doi.org/10.1073/pnas.1111840108

Grégoire V, Machiels J-P, Baumann M (2019) Combined radiotherapy and chemotherapy. In: Joiner MC, van der Kogel AJ (eds) Basic clinical radiobiology vol 5, pp 217–229

Greiner DL, Hesselton RA, Shultz LD (1998) SCID mouse models of human stem cell engraftment. Stem Cells 16(3):166–177. https://doi.org/10.1002/stem.160166

Greiner DL, Shultz LD, Yates J, Appel MC, Perdrizet G, Hesselton RM, Schweitzer I, Beamer WG, Shultz KL, Pelsue SC et al (1995) Improved engraftment of human spleen cells in NOD/LtSz-scid/scid mice as compared with C.B-17-scid/scid mice. Am J Pathol 146(4):888–902

Gurtner K, Deuse Y, Butof R, Schaal K, Eicheler W, Oertel R, Grenman R, Thames H, Yaromina A, Baumann M, Krause M (2011) Diverse effects of combined radiotherapy and EGFR inhibition with antibodies or TK inhibitors on local tumour control and correlation with EGFR gene expression. Radiother Oncol 99(3):323–330. https://doi.org/10.1016/j.radonc.2011.05.035

Gurtner K, Ebert N, Pfitzmann D, Eicheler W, Zips D, Baumann M, Krause M (2014) Effect of combined irradiation and EGFR/Erb-B inhibition with BIBW 2992 on proliferation and tumour cure in cell lines and xenografts. Radiat Oncol 9:261. https://doi.org/10.1186/s13014-014-0261-z

Hambardzumyan D, Amankulor NM, Helmy KY, Becher OJ, Holland EC (2009) Modeling adult gliomas using RCAS/t-va technology. Transl Oncol 2(2):89–95. https://doi.org/10.1593/tlo.09100

Harrington KJ, Billingham LJ, Brunner TB, Burnet NG, Chan CS, Hoskin P, Mackay RI, Maughan TS, Macdougall J, McKenna WG, Nutting CM, Oliver A, Plummer R, Stratford IJ, Illidge T (2011) Guidelines for preclinical and early phase clinical assessment of novel radiosensitisers. Br J Cancer 105(5):628–639. https://doi.org/10.1038/bjc.2011.240

Herrmann T, Baumann M, Voigtmann L, Knorr A (1997) Effect of irradiated volume on lung damage in pigs. Radiother Oncol 44(1):35–40. https://doi.org/10.1016/s0167-8140(97)01930-0

Hessel F, Krause M, Helm A, Petersen C, Grenman R, Thames HD, Baumann M (2004a) Differentiation status of human squamous cell carcinoma xenografts does not appear to correlate with the repopulation capacity of clonogenic tumour cells during fractionated irradiation. Int J Radiat Biol 80(10):719–727. https://doi.org/10.1080/095530003400017812

Hessel F, Krause M, Petersen C, Horcsoki M, Klinger T, Zips D, Thames HD, Baumann M (2004b) Repopulation of moderately well-differentiated and keratinizing GL human squamous cell carcinomas growing in nude mice. Int J Radiat Oncol Biol Phys 58(2):510–518. https://doi.org/10.1016/j.ijrobp.2003.09.065

Higgins GS, O'Cathail SM, Muschel RJ, McKenna WG (2015) Drug radiotherapy combinations: review of previous failures and reasons for future optimism. Cancer Treat Rev 41(2):105–113. https://doi.org/10.1016/j.ctrv.2014.12.012

Holland EC (2000) A mouse model for glioma: biology, pathology, and therapeutic opportunities. Toxicol Pathol 28(1):171–177. https://doi.org/10.1177/019262330002800122

Ishikawa F, Yasukawa M, Lyons B, Yoshida S, Miyamoto T, Yoshimoto G, Watanabe T, Akashi K, Shultz LD, Harada M (2005) Development of functional human blood and immune systems in NOD/SCID/IL2 receptor {gamma} chain(null) mice. Blood 106(5):1565–1573. https://doi.org/10.1182/blood-2005-02-0516

Ito M, Hiramatsu H, Kobayashi K, Suzue K, Kawahata M, Hioki K, Ueyama Y, Koyanagi Y, Sugamura K, Tsuji K, Heike T, Nakahata T (2002) NOD/SCID/gamma(c)(null) mouse: an excellent recipient mouse model for engraftment of human cells. Blood 100(9):3175–3182. https://doi.org/10.1182/blood-2001-12-0207

Kagadis GC, Loudos G, Katsanos K, Langer SG, Nikiforidis GC (2010) In vivo small animal imaging: current status and future prospects. Med Phys 37(12):6421–6442. https://doi.org/10.1118/1.3515456

Kemp CJ (2015) Animal models of chemical carcinogenesis: driving breakthroughs in cancer research for 100 years. Cold Spring Harb Protoc 2015(10):865–874. https://doi.org/10.1101/pdb.top069906

Kersten K, de Visser KE, van Miltenburg MH, Jonkers J (2017) Genetically engineered mouse models in oncology research and cancer medicine. EMBO Mol Med 9(2):137–153. https://doi.org/10.15252/emmm.201606857

Khan K, Araki K, Wang D, Li G, Li X, Zhang J, Xu W, Hoover RK, Lauter S, O'Malley B Jr, Lapidus RG, Li D (2010) Head and neck cancer radiosensitization by the novel poly(ADP-ribose) polymerase inhibitor GPI-15427. Head Neck 32(3):381–391. https://doi.org/10.1002/hed.21195

Kirsch DG, Diehn M, Kesarwala AH, Maity A, Morgan MA, Schwarz JK, Bristow R, Demaria S, Eke I, Griffin RJ, Haas-Kogan D, Higgins GS, Kimmelman AC, Kimple RJ, Lombaert IM, Ma L, Marples B, Pajonk F, Park CC, Schaue D, Tran PT, Willers H, Wouters BG, Bernhard EJ (2018) The future of radiobiology. J Natl Cancer Inst 110(4):329–340. https://doi.org/10.1093/jnci/djx231

Koi L, Lock S, Linge A, Thurow C, Hering S, Baumann M, Krause M, Gurtner K (2017) EGFR-amplification plus gene expression profiling predicts response to combined radiotherapy with EGFR-inhibition: a preclinical trial in 10 HNSCC-tumour-xenograft models. Radiother Oncol 124(3):496–503. https://doi.org/10.1016/j.radonc.2017.07.009

Koritzinsky M (2015) Metformin: a novel biological modifier of tumor response to radiation therapy. Int J Radiat Oncol Biol Phys 93(2):454–464. https://doi.org/10.1016/j.ijrobp.2015.06.003

Krause M, Gurtner K, Deuse Y, Baumann M (2009) Heterogeneity of tumour response to combined radiotherapy and EGFR inhibitors: differences between antibodies and TK inhibitors. Int J Radiat Biol 85(11):943–954. https://doi.org/10.3109/09553000903232835

Krause M, Prager J, Zhou X, Yaromina A, Dorfler A, Eicheler W, Baumann M (2007) EGFR-TK inhibition before radiotherapy reduces tumour volume but does not improve local control: differential response of cancer stem cells and nontumourigenic cells? Radiother Oncol 83(3):316–325. https://doi.org/10.1016/j.radonc.2007.04.014

Krause M, Schutze C, Petersen C, Pimentel N, Hessel F, Harstrick A, Baumann M (2005) Different classes of EGFR inhibitors may have different potential to improve local tumour control after fractionated irradiation: a study on C225 in FaDu hSCC. Radiother Oncol 74(2):109–115. https://doi.org/10.1016/j.radonc.2004.10.011

Krause M, Zips D, Thames HD, Kummermehr J, Baumann M (2006) Preclinical evaluation of molecular-targeted anticancer agents for radiotherapy. Radiother Oncol 80(2):112–122. https://doi.org/10.1016/j.radonc.2006.07.017

Lai Y, Wei X, Lin S, Qin L, Cheng L, Li P (2017) Current status and perspectives of patient-derived xenograft models in cancer research. J Hematol Oncol 10(1):106. https://doi.org/10.1186/s13045-017-0470-7

Laird JH, Lok BH, Ma J, Bell A, de Stanchina E, Poirier JT, Rudin CM (2018) Talazoparib is a potent Radiosensitizer in small cell lung cancer cell lines and xenografts. Clin Cancer Res 24(20):5143–5152. https://doi.org/10.1158/1078-0432.CCR-18-0401

Lambin P, Lieverse R, Baumann M, Ebert N (2019) Will immunotherapy really change radiotherapy? Lancet Oncol 20(12):1642–1644. https://doi.org/10.1016/S1470-2045(19)30682-5

Lampreht Tratar U, Horvat S, Cemazar M (2018) Transgenic mouse models in cancer research. Front Oncol 8:268. https://doi.org/10.3389/fonc.2018.00268

Lawrence YR, Vikram B, Dignam JJ, Chakravarti A, Machtay M, Freidlin B, Takebe N, Curran WJ Jr, Bentzen SM, Okunieff P, Coleman CN, Dicker AP (2013) NCI-RTOG translational program strategic guidelines for the early-stage development of radiosensitizers. J Natl Cancer Inst 105(1):11–24. https://doi.org/10.1093/jnci/djs472

Lehnert S, el-Khatib E (1989) The use of CT densitometry in the assessment of radiation-induced damage to the rat lung: a comparison with other endpoints. Int J Radiat Oncol Biol Phys 16(1):117–124. https://doi.org/10.1016/0360-3016(89)90018-7

Lewis JS, Achilefu S, Garbow JR, Laforest R, Welch MJ (2002) Small animal imaging. Current technology and perspectives for oncological imaging. Eur J Cancer 38(16):2173–2188. https://doi.org/10.1016/s0959-8049(02)00394-5

Liao ZX, Travis EL, Tucker SL (1995) Damage and morbidity from pneumonitis after irradiation of partial volumes of mouse lung. Int J Radiat Oncol Biol Phys 32(5):1359–1370. https://doi.org/10.1016/0360-3016(94)00660-D

Lin A, Maity A (2015) Molecular pathways: a novel approach to targeting hypoxia and improving radiotherapy efficacy via reduction in oxygen demand. Clin Cancer Res 21(9):1995–2000. https://doi.org/10.1158/1078-0432.CCR-14-0858

Linge A, Lohaus F, Lock S, Nowak A, Gudziol V, Valentini C, von Neubeck C, Jutz M, Tinhofer I, Budach V, Sak A, Stuschke M, Balermpas P, Rodel C, Grosu AL, Abdollahi A, Debus J, Ganswindt U, Belka C, Pigorsch S, Combs SE, Monnich D, Zips D, Buchholz F, Aust DE, Baretton GB, Thames HD, Dubrovska A, Alsner J, Overgaard J, Krause M, Baumann M, Dktk ROG (2016) HPV status, cancer stem cell marker expression, hypoxia gene signatures and tumour volume identify good prognosis subgroups in patients with HNSCC after primary radio-chemotherapy: a multicentre retrospective study of the German Cancer Consortium Radiation Oncology Group (DKTK-ROG). Radiother Oncol 121(3):364–373. https://doi.org/10.1016/j.radonc.2016.11.008

Maykel J, Liu JH, Li H, Shultz LD, Greiner DL, Houghton J (2014) NOD-scidIl2rg (tm1Wjl) and NOD-Rag1 (null) Il2rg (tm1Wjl) : a model for stromal cell-tumor cell interaction for human colon cancer. Dig Dis Sci 59(6):1169–1179. https://doi.org/10.1007/s10620-014-3168-5

Meehan TF, Conte N, Goldstein T, Inghirami G, Murakami MA, Brabetz S, Gu Z, Wiser JA, Dunn P, Begley DA, Krupke DM, Bertotti A, Bruna A, Brush MH, Byrne AT, Caldas C, Christie AL, Clark DA, Dowst H, Dry JR, Doroshow JH, Duchamp O, Evrard YA, Ferretti S, Frese KK, Goodwin NC, Greenawalt D, Haendel MA, Hermans E, Houghton PJ, Jonkers J, Kemper K, Khor TO, Lewis MT, Lloyd KCK, Mason J, Medico E, Neuhauser SB, Olson JM, Peeper DS, Rueda OM, Seong JK, Trusolino L, Vinolo E, Wechsler-Reya RJ, Weinstock DM, Welm A, Weroha SJ, Amant F, Pfister SM, Kool M, Parkinson H, Butte AJ, Bult CJ (2017) PDX-MI: minimal information for patient-derived tumor xenograft models. Cancer Res 77(21):e62–e66. https://doi.org/10.1158/0008-5472.CAN-17-0582

Metwally MA, Frederiksen KD, Overgaard J (2014) Compliance and toxicity of the hypoxic radio-sensitizer nimorazole in the treatment of patients with head and neck squamous cell carcinoma (HNSCC). Acta Oncol 53(5):654–661. https://doi.org/10.3109/0284186X.2013.864050

Moses R, Kummermehr J (1986) Radiation response of the mouse tongue epithelium. Br J Cancer Suppl 7:12–15

Nordsmark M, Overgaard J (2004) Tumor hypoxia is independent of hemoglobin and prognostic for loco-regional tumor control after primary radiotherapy in advanced head and neck cancer. Acta Oncol 43(4):396–403. https://doi.org/10.1080/02841860410026189

Overgaard J (2011) Hypoxic modification of radiotherapy in squamous cell carcinoma of the head and neck—a systematic review and meta-analysis. Radiother Oncol 100(1):22–32. https://doi.org/10.1016/j.radonc.2011.03.004

Overgaard J, Overgaard M, Nielsen OS, Pedersen AK, Timothy AR (1982) A comparative investigation of nimorazole and misonidazole as hypoxic radiosensitizers in a C3H mammary carcinoma in vivo. Br J Cancer 46(6):904–911. https://doi.org/10.1038/bjc.1982.300

Overgaard J, Sand Hansen H, Lindelov B, Overgaard M, Jorgensen K, Rasmusson B, Berthelsen A (1991) Nimorazole as a hypoxic radiosensitizer in the treatment of supraglottic larynx and pharynx carcinoma. First report from the Danish Head and Neck Cancer Study (DAHANCA) protocol 5-85. Radiother Oncol 20(Suppl 1):143–149. https://doi.org/10.1016/0167-8140(91)90202-r

Peitzsch C, Kurth I, Ebert N, Dubrovska A, Baumann M (2019) Cancer stem cells in radiation response: current views and future perspectives in radiation oncology. Int J Radiat Biol 95(7):900–911. https://doi.org/10.1080/09553002.2019.1589023

Pitroda SP, Chmura SJ, Weichselbaum RR (2019) Integration of radiotherapy and immunotherapy for treatment of oligometastases. Lancet Oncol 20(8):e434–e442. https://doi.org/10.1016/S1470-2045(19)30157-3

Pospisilova M, Seifrtova M, Rezacova M (2017) Small molecule inhibitors of DNA-PK for tumor sensitization to anticancer therapy. J Physiol Pharmacol 68(3):337–344

Quintana E, Shackleton M, Sabel MS, Fullen DR, Johnson TM, Morrison SJ (2008) Efficient tumour formation by single human melanoma cells. Nature 456(7222):593–598. https://doi.org/10.1038/nature07567

Rekers NH, Olivo Pimentel V, Yaromina A, Lieuwes NG, Biemans R, Zegers CML, Germeraad WTV, Van Limbergen EJ, Neri D, Dubois LJ, Lambin P (2018) The immunocytokine L19-IL2: an interplay between radiotherapy and long-lasting systemic anti-tumour immune responses. Onco Targets Ther 7(4):e1414119. https://doi.org/10.1080/2162402X.2017.1414119

Reya T, Morrison SJ, Clarke MF, Weissman IL (2001) Stem cells, cancer, and cancer stem cells. Nature 414(6859):105–111. https://doi.org/10.1038/35102167

Russo AL, Kwon HC, Burgan WE, Carter D, Beam K, Weizheng X, Zhang J, Slusher BS, Chakravarti A, Tofilon PJ, Camphausen K (2009) In vitro and in vivo radiosensitization of glioblastoma cells by the poly (ADP-ribose) polymerase inhibitor E7016. Clin Cancer Res 15(2):607–612. https://doi.org/10.1158/1078-0432.CCR-08-2079

Seiwert TY, Salama JK, Vokes EE (2007) The concurrent chemoradiation paradigm—general principles. Nat Clin Pract Oncol 4(2):86–100. https://doi.org/10.1038/ncponc0714

Sharabi AB, Lim M, DeWeese TL, Drake CG (2015) Radiation and checkpoint blockade immunotherapy: radiosensitisation and potential mechanisms of synergy. Lancet Oncol 16(13):e498–e509. https://doi.org/10.1016/S1470-2045(15)00007-8

Shultz LD, Banuelos S, Lyons B, Samuels R, Burzenski L, Gott B, Lang P, Leif J, Appel M, Rossini A, Greiner DL (2003) NOD/LtSz-Rag1nullPfpnull mice: a new model system with increased levels of human peripheral leukocyte and hematopoietic stem-cell engraftment. Transplantation 76(7):1036–1042. https://doi.org/10.1097/01.TP.0000083041.44829.2C

Shultz LD, Ishikawa F, Greiner DL (2007) Humanized mice in translational biomedical research. Nat Rev Immunol 7(2):118–130. https://doi.org/10.1038/nri2017

Shultz LD, Lyons BL, Burzenski LM, Gott B, Chen X, Chaleff S, Kotb M, Gillies SD, King M, Mangada J, Greiner DL, Handgretinger R (2005) Human lymphoid and myeloid cell development in NOD/LtSz-scid IL2R gamma null mice engrafted with mobilized human hemopoietic stem cells. J Immunol 174(10):6477–6489. https://doi.org/10.4049/jimmunol.174.10.6477

Shultz LD, Schweitzer PA, Christianson SW, Gott B, Schweitzer IB, Tennent B, McKenna S, Mobraaten L, Rajan TV, Greiner DL et al (1995) Multiple defects in innate and adaptive immunologic function in NOD/LtSz-scid mice. J Immunol 154(1):180–191

Singh M, Murriel CL, Johnson L (2012) Genetically engineered mouse models: closing the gap between preclinical data and trial outcomes. Cancer Res 72(11):2695–2700. https://doi.org/10.1158/0008-5472.CAN-11-2786

Singh SK, Hawkins C, Clarke ID, Squire JA, Bayani J, Hide T, Henkelman RM, Cusimano MD, Dirks PB (2004) Identification of human brain tumour initiating cells. Nature 432(7015):396–401. https://doi.org/10.1038/nature03128

Stewart FA, Dorr W (2009) Milestones in normal tissue radiation biology over the past 50 years: from clonogenic cell survival to cytokine networks and back to stem cell recovery. Int J Radiat Biol 85(7):574–586. https://doi.org/10.1080/09553000902985136

Stone HB, Bernhard EJ, Coleman CN, Deye J, Capala J, Mitchell JB, Brown JM (2016) Preclinical data on efficacy of 10 drug-radiation combinations: evaluations, concerns, and recommendations. Transl Oncol 9(1):46–56. https://doi.org/10.1016/j.tranon.2016.01.002

Szadvari I, Krizanova O, Babula P (2016) Athymic nude mice as an experimental model for cancer treatment. Physiol Res 65(Supplementum 4):S441–S453

Teicher BA (2006) Tumor models for efficacy determination. Mol Cancer Ther 5(10):2435–2443. https://doi.org/10.1158/1535-7163.MCT-06-0391

Tentler JJ, Tan AC, Weekes CD, Jimeno A, Leong S, Pitts TM, Arcaroli JJ, Messersmith WA, Eckhardt SG (2012) Patient-derived tumour xenografts as models for oncology drug development. Nat Rev Clin Oncol 9(6):338–350. https://doi.org/10.1038/nrclinonc.2012.61

Tillner F, Thute P, Bütof R, Krause M, Enghardt W (2014) Pre-clinical research in small animals using radiotherapy technology—a bidirectional translational approach. Z Med Phys 24:335

Tillner F, Thute P, Löck S, Dietrich A, Fursov A, Haase R, Lukas M, Rimarzig B, Sobiella M, Krause M, Baumann M, Bütof R, Enghardt W (2016) Precise image-guided irradiation of small animals: a flexible non-profit platform. Phys Med Biol 61(8):3084–3108. https://doi.org/10.1088/0031-9155/61/8/3084

Twyman-Saint Victor C, Rech AJ, Maity A, Rengan R, Pauken KE, Stelekati E, Benci JL, Xu B, Dada H, Odorizzi PM, Herati RS, Mansfield KD, Patsch D, Amaravadi RK, Schuchter LM, Ishwaran H, Mick R, Pryma DA, Xu X, Feldman MD, Gangadhar TC, Hahn SM, Wherry EJ, Vonderheide RH, Minn AJ (2015) Radiation and dual checkpoint blockade activate non-redundant immune mechanisms in cancer. Nature 520(7547):373–377. https://doi.org/10.1038/nature14292

Verhaegen F, Granton P, Tryggestad E (2011) Small animal radiotherapy research platforms. Phys Med Biol 56(12):R55–R83. https://doi.org/10.1088/0031-9155/56/12/R01

Wang Y, Tseng JC, Sun Y, Beck AH, Kung AL (2015) Noninvasive imaging of tumor burden and molecular pathways in mouse models of cancer. Cold Spring Harb Protoc 2015(2):135–144. https://doi.org/10.1101/pdb.top069930

Weichselbaum RR, Liang H, Deng L, Fu YX (2017) Radiotherapy and immunotherapy: a beneficial liaison? Nat Rev Clin Oncol 14(6):365–379. https://doi.org/10.1038/nrclinonc.2016.211

Yaromina A, Krause M, Thames H, Rosner A, Krause M, Hessel F, Grenman R, Zips D, Baumann M (2007) Pre-treatment number of clonogenic cells and their radiosensitivity are major determinants of local tumour control after fractionated irradiation. Radiother Oncol 83(3):304–310. https://doi.org/10.1016/j.radonc.2007.04.020

Yaromina A, Zips D, Thames HD, Eicheler W, Krause M, Rosner A, Haase M, Petersen C, Raleigh JA, Quennet V, Walenta S, Mueller-Klieser W, Baumann M (2006) Pimonidazole labelling and response to fractionated irradiation of five human squamous cell carcinoma (hSCC) lines in nude mice: the need for a multivariate approach in biomarker studies. Radiother Oncol 81(2):122–129. https://doi.org/10.1016/j.radonc.2006.08.010

Zips D (2019) Tumor growth and response to radiation. In: Joiner MC, van der Kogel AJ (eds) Basic clinical radiobiology, vol 5. CRC Press Taylor&Francis Group, pp 81–98

Zips D, Krause M, Hessel F, Westphal J, Bruchner K, Eicheler W, Dorfler A, Grenman R, Petersen C, Haberey M, Baumann M (2003) Experimental study on different combination schedules of VEGF-receptor inhibitor PTK787/ZK222584 and fractionated irradiation. Anticancer Res 23(5A):3869–3876

Zips D, Thames HD, Baumann M (2005) New anticancer agents: in vitro and in vivo evaluation. In Vivo 19(1):1–7

Chapter 8
Genetically Engineered Mouse Models for Studying Radiation Biology and Radiosensitizers

Warren Floyd, Hsuan-Cheng Kuo, Jonathon E. Himes, Rutulkumar Patel, and David G. Kirsch

Abstract Genetically engineered mouse models (GEMMs) are powerful research tools that have improved our understanding of cancer and enabled the identification of novel targets for the radiosensitization of human cancer. The use of GEMMs in cancer has evolved significantly since early models of organism-wide oncogene knock-in and tumor suppressor knock-out mice. Advances in recombinase technology have enabled the development of GEMMs with site- and tissue-specific genetic manipulation and temporal control of multiple genetic alterations. There are multiple advantages to using GEMMs to study radiation biology when compared to in vitro or transplant in vivo models. First, they provide a robust platform for the study of normal tissue injury generated by treatment with radiation therapy and radiosensitizers. Second, tumors develop in a native microenvironment, which preserves the stromal and vascular compartments. Third, they allow precise spatial and temporal control of multiple genetic alterations, allowing scientists to dissect the effect of specific genetic mutations on tumor development and radiation response. Finally, these mice have an intact immune system that co-evolves with tumor formation, which is critical to evaluating combined radiation therapy and immunotherapy. Here we review current approaches to mouse modeling for the study of radiation biology and radiosensitizers.

Keywords ATM · Abscopal effect · Cardiac toxicity · Cre-LoxP · CRISPR-Cas9 · Dual recombinase · Gastrointestinal syndrome · Genetically engineered mouse models · Immunocompetent · Immunotherapy · Normal tissue response · p53 · Radiation biology · shRNA · Tumor microenvironment

W. Floyd · H.-C. Kuo · J. E. Himes · R. Patel · D. G. Kirsch (✉)
Department of Radiation Oncology, Duke University Medical Center, Durham, NC, USA
e-mail: david.kirsch@duke.edu

© Springer Nature Switzerland AG 2020
H. Willers, I. Eke (eds.), *Molecular Targeted Radiosensitizers*, Cancer Drug Discovery and Development, https://doi.org/10.1007/978-3-030-49701-9_8

161

1   Introduction

Cancer is a prehistoric disease dating back to ancient Egyptian and Greek civilization, where it was mostly treated by radical surgery with minimal success leading to the death of many patients. However, significant advances have been made since then, especially in terms of understanding and treating the disease. Over the centuries, important discoveries have provided key insights into biological and pathological features of cancers that spurred the development of effective therapies. A major breakthrough came late after 1895, when the discovery of X-rays and gamma-rays changed our approach to cancer treatment and ushered in the era of studying radiation biology. In the field of pharmacological intervention, a major breakthrough came after the Second World War, with the discovery of cytotoxic anticancer drugs leading to the birth of chemotherapy for the treatment of various cancers. Since the 1950s, the cornerstone of cancer treatment has included surgery, radiation, and chemotherapy (Rius and Lyko 2012). Although in the past decade immunotherapy has been added as an additional pillar of cancer therapy, cancer remains the second leading cause of death with over 8.2 million cancer deaths worldwide in 2012 (Ferlay et al. 2015). High incidence rates of cancer are due in part to an increasing population with a longer average life span, while overall reductions in mortality rates are likely associated with early diagnosis and the evolution of targeted drug therapies, such as selective kinase inhibitors, monoclonal antibodies, and immune checkpoint inhibitors. Despite many ongoing challenges, from a historical perspective there has been continuous progress in the prevention, detection, and treatment of cancer.

Radiation therapy remains one of the primary modalities for the treatment of human cancer. In fact, approximately 50% of human cancers are treated by radiation therapy with either palliative or curative intent (Moding et al. 2013). Rapid advances in physics and computing have led to significant technological development in the field of radiation oncology which has dramatically increased the efficacy of radiation therapy for multiple cancer types. There is a significant opportunity for further advancement of the field of radiation oncology via improved understanding of the radiation biology of human cancer and development of targeted radiosensitizers that increase the therapeutic index of radiation treatment. To make further advances in radiation therapy, GEMMs provide a powerful tool for preclinical radiation biology research (Coleman et al. 2016).

An ideal tumor model for the study of radiation biology and radiosensitizers in vivo should satisfy several key criteria. First, the tumor model should present with the same histopathological features that are used to diagnose the human cancer in the same anatomical location as its human counterpart. Second, the tumor model should develop in the native tumor microenvironment, including stroma and vasculature that develop in a manner as similar to human cancers as possible. This point is especially important, as multiple researchers have demonstrated the importance of hypoxia and stromal composition in radiation response (Horsman and Overgaard 2016). Third, the tumor model should allow single or multiple genetic manipulations that are relevant to human cancer to be spatially and temporally controlled. This allows for reproducibility and flexibility in experimental design, greatly increasing the number of experimental questions that can be asked using the model. Finally, the model should have a native and intact immune system that has co-evolved with the cancer during tumor development. This most closely models the co-evolution of human tumors with the immune system and allows for evaluation of immunomodulatory therapies alone or in concert with radiation therapy. Human xenografts grown in immunodeficient mice and mouse cancers transplanted into syngeneic mice are frequently used in research because of their relative ease of use and low cost. Despite these advantages and their usefulness to answer specific scientific questions, transplant systems fail to fulfill many of the criteria of an ideal in vivo model of human cancer for studying radiation biology listed above. In contrast, GEMMs meet all of these requirements and enable the study of multiple critical determinants of radiosensitizer efficacy with tools that allow precise spatial and temporal control of genetic manipulations.

In this chapter, we will discuss the principle of the most popular genetic engineering technologies used to generate GEMMs, including Cre recombinase, the dual recombinase system, and the CRISPR-Cas9 system. We will provide recent examples of how these technologies have been applied at the intersection of cancer and radiation biology research. Next, we will highlight how GEMMs are used to study radiation biology in the fields of immuno-oncology and normal tissue radiation injury, which are exciting areas of study that are crucial for the development and evaluation of novel radiosensitizers. Finally, we will outline important considerations in the design and execution of experiments involving GEMMs.

2   GEMMs: Cre-Loxp System

Prior to the development of GEMMs, researchers used immunocompetent and immunodeficient mice with implanted syngeneic and xenograft tumors, respectively. Tumor implants are made subcutaneously or orthotopically to study drug or radiation response in animal models. These models are widely used even today to investigate drug toxicity, efficacy, and potency in part due to the reasonable cost of the experiments. However, such models may fail to fully recapitulate important aspects of human cancer in terms of the genetic versatility, histological and immunological characteristics, and organ-specific microenvironment. Many studies have shown that cancer evolves under the influence of a native microenvironment, including interactions with immune and stromal cells. Because of this, xenografts and syngeneic mouse models of cancer have natural limitations. In the late 1980s, the first GEMMs (also known as transgenic mouse model) were produced by genetically expressing a dominant oncogene in the germline of the mouse from a tissue-specific promoter (Stewart et al. 1984). Since then, advances in engineering the mouse genome have enabled the development of GEMMs. One of the most popular strategies for conditional genetic manipulation is to generate GEMMs using the Cre-LoxP system adapted from bacteriophage (Kirsch 2011).

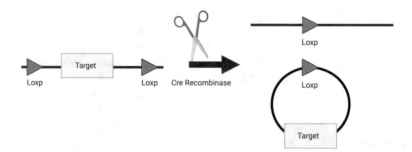

Fig. 8.1 Schematic showing how the Cre-LoxP system deletes a target DNA sequence. DNA flanked by loxP sites (triangles) remains intact until encountering Cre recombinase. Cre recombinase recognizes the loxP sites and drives their recombination, which deletes the target DNA flanked by the loxP sites

Cre recombinase is a protein that recognizes a short DNA sequence annotated as loxP. Cre does not exist in mouse or human genomes unless introduced by genetic engineering. When two loxP sites are engineered to flank both ends of a genomic sequence, Cre expression leads to the deletion of the intervening sequence of DNA, leaving only one loxP site behind (Fig. 8.1). After loxP flanked genetic sequences are introduced into the germline of genetically engineered mice, they can be bred with other conditional mutant mice so that Cre can initiate cancer driven by multiple genetic events. One of the most common applications of this technology has been to flank a critical portion of a gene with loxP sites so that, upon exposure to Cre recombinase, the gene is deleted so that its functional impact can be tested. This technology can also be used to induce gene expression. In this scenario, a gene or oncogene is preceded by a loxP-STOP-loxP sequence (LSL; STOP cassette flanked by two loxP sites). The STOP cassette will prevent expression of the downstream oncogene, but upon Cre recombinase expression the STOP cassette will be removed and the downstream gene will be expressed (Jackson et al. 2001). Another strength of this technology is that it allows targeted gene deletion or expression in a specific cell type. To achieve this, a transgenic mouse can be generated to express Cre recombinase from a cell type-specific promoter, which can be crossed with mice harboring conditional alleles flanked by loxP sites termed floxed alleles (Branda and Dymecki 2004). In the compound mutant mice, only cells where the promoter drives expression of Cre recombinase will undergo Cre-mediated recombination of the floxed alleles. A modified version of Cre recombinase, CreERT2, provides additional temporal control of gene manipulations. CreERT2 is a fusion protein that brings together Cre and a mutant estrogen receptor T2. In its basal state, CreERT2 is inactive in the cytoplasm and does not recombine genomic sequences. In the presence of 4-hydroxy-tamoxifen CreERT2 translocates into the nucleus where it recombines the loxP flanked DNA. Therefore, Cre-ERT2 allows researchers to control the timing of Cre-mediated recombination.

Over the past two decades, the Cre-LoxP system has been used to generate tissue or cell type-specific knock-outs and/or activate oncogenes or reporter genes in primary mouse models of human cancers. A key advantage of this system is that it can be used to make a conditional knock-out such that the gene is ablated only after a critical developmental phase. This technique allows researchers command over spatial (tissue/cell-specific) and/or temporal (time-specific) control of the gene of interest. Depending upon orientation of the loxP sequence, it causes deletion (both sequences oriented in the same direction), inversion (both sequences oriented in opposite direction), or translocation (both sequences located on different chromosome/DNA fragment) of a targeted gene. The production of GEMMs are traditionally time-consuming and costly, but widely used in preclinical settings due to close recapitulation of human disease in mice.

To date, several GEMMs of cancer have been created using the Cre-LoxP system utilizing either tissue-specific or inducible Cre expression. Many studies have used the Cre-LoxP system to knock-out tumor suppressor genes in order to study cancer initiation and progression, for instance, deletion of *Apc* in the intestinal epithelium (Clarke 2005), *Brca1*, *Brca2*, *Pten*, *Smad4*, or *Tp53* in mammary epithelium cells (Xu et al. 1999; Jonkers et al. 2001; Li et al. 2002; Li et al. 2003), and *NF1* in the endothelial cells (Gitler et al. 2004). Apart from knocking out tumor suppressor genes to generate primary mouse models of cancer, the Cre-LoxP system can achieve spatial and temporal activation of oncogenes. Many human cancers occur due to the activation of different oncogenes, but activating mutations of *RAS* oncogenes or *RAS* downstream target genes are involved in roughly one-third of all human cancers. Activation of *KRAS* occurs more frequently in human cancers compared to the other two members of the RAS family (*NRAS* and *HRAS*). In fact, oncogenic *KRAS* activation has been found in many human cancers, including a high prevalence in pancreatic carcinomas, colon carcinomas, and lung carcinomas (Rodenhuis et al. 1988; Bos et al. 1987). The mutant version of *Kras* (*Kras*[G12V]) was first expressed in lung epithelial cells to generate a primary mouse model of lung cancer (Meuwissen et al. 2001). In this model, the *Kras*[G12V] transgene contained an active Beta-actin promoter, followed by floxed GFP (green fluorescent protein flanked by two loxP sites), and then a cDNA for *Kras*[G12V]. Therefore, constitutive expression of mutant *Kras*[G12V] can only be achieved by removal of the floxed GFP via Cre-mediated recombination. In this study, researchers expressed Cre by directly injecting an adenovirus carrying Cre recombinase into the trachea (Fig. 8.2), which infected the lung epithelium to give rise to pulmonary adenocarcinomas within 9–13 weeks. Similar approaches have been used to express other tumor suppressors and oncogenes to study cancer in mouse models.

The Cre-LoxP system has been widely used for the simultaneous manipulation of multiple genes in mice to recapitulate mutations found human cancers. These primary mouse models of cancer can be employed to study radiation biology. For example, GEMMs of primary non-small cell lung cancer with different initiating mutations (*Tp53* vs. *Ink4a/Arf* deletion) have revealed that genetic differences in tumors influence tumor growth delay after radiation therapy (Perez et al. 2013). A spatially and temporally restricted mouse model of soft tissue sarcoma driven by *Kras*[G12D] and *Tp53* (Kirsch et al. 2007) has been utilized to study radiation response (Moding et al. 2014). The role of hypoxia-inducible factor 1-alpha (HIF-1α) in radiation response was investigated in a primary model of soft tissue sarcoma generated by Cre-LoxP system to demonstrate that HIF-1α signaling contributes to radiation resistance (Zhang et al. 2015). In addition, deletion of *Atm* in either tumor cells or endothelial cells was used to clarify the distinct role of each population in tumor

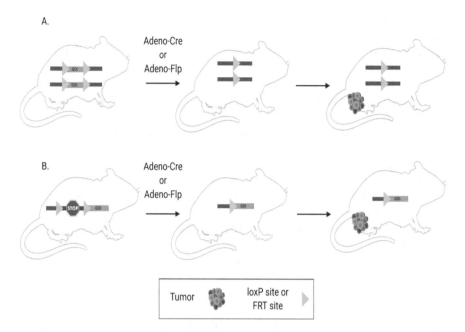

Fig. 8.2 The Cre-LoxP system. Injection of adenovirus that expresses either Cre or Flp recombinase allows for precise spatial and temporal control of genetic mutations in vivo. Upon expression of the recombinase, loxP or frt flanked tumor suppressors genes are deleted, enabling tumor development (**a**). The expression of a recombinase also can enable deletion of a loxP or frt flanked STOP cassette preceding an oncogene, resulting in increased oncogene expression and tumor development (**b**)

response to radiotherapy (Moding et al. 2015, 2014; Torok et al. 2019). These studies demonstrated that radiosensitizing the tumor vasculature can enhance tumor growth delay after radiation therapy, but radiosensitizing the tumor cells is required to enhance local control (Castle and Kirsch 2019). Furthermore, these primary mouse models can be imaged using small animal micro-CT or other imaging techniques to quantify tumor response to radiation therapy alone or in combination with systemic therapy (Kirsch et al. 2010a; Ashton et al. 2018). In summary, the application of Cre recombinase to activate oncogenes and delete tumor suppressor genes in mice has facilitated the generation of primary mouse models of human cancers, which can not only be used to study tumorigenesis, but can also be used to investigate tumor response to radiation therapy and to test radiosensitizers.

3   GEMMs: Dual Recombinase System

GEMMs are excellent models of human cancer in part because they contain a mix of native stromal cells, immune cells, and tumor cells that co-evolve as the tumor grows and responds to therapy. The use of GEMMs can therefore facilitate the study

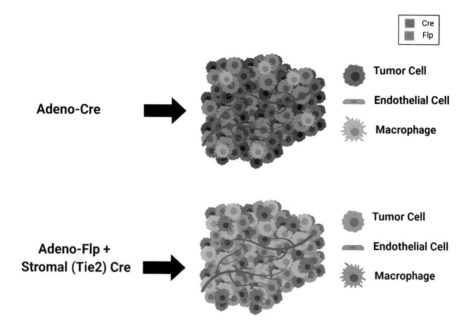

Fig. 8.3 Using the Dual Recombinase System to Study Cancer Cell and Stromal Components of Tumors. In the above model, Cre-mediated genetic alteration is denoted by purple, while green coloration represents FlpO recombinase-mediated genetic alteration. (**a**) Use of virally delivered Cre allows for generation of tumor cells (purple) in a spatially and temporally controlled manner. Other cellular components, such as endothelial cells and macrophages (red), do not undergo any genetic manipulation with this approach. (**b**) The use of a dual recombinase system allows for both the generation of tumor cells with precisely controlled genetic mutations and for different specific genetic alterations of other cell types, such as macrophages and endothelial cells. In this example, FlpO recombinase expressed from the adenovirus drives deletion of tumor suppressors and activates oncogenes in tumor initiating cells (green) by recombining FRT sites, while Cre expressed by the Tie2 promoter in transgenic mice deletes a separate gene in endothelial cells and macrophages (purple) by recombining loxP sites

of how each of these tumor components contributes to radiation response and treatment with radiosensitizers. GEMMs in which tumors are initiated by Cre recombinase are not optimally suited for genetic experiments to study how stromal and immune cells mediate radiation response in vivo. As discussed above, Cre can induce driver mutations in oncogenes and tumor suppressors to initiate cancer. These recombination events are restricted to a single time point and limit the target of genetic alterations to cancer cells (Fig. 8.3, top). However, Cre recombinase cannot simultaneously be used to mutate different genes specifically in stromal cell populations. To simultaneously initiate primary tumors by mutating one group of genes in tumor cells while mutating other genes in stromal cells, a second recombinase is required. To meet this need, the Flp/FRT recombinase system can be employed together with the Cre/LoxP recombinase system for dual recombinase technology (Lee et al. 2012b). By optimizing Flp which comes from yeast for activity in mammalian cells (FlpO), recombination of Frt flanked DNA by FlpO will occur in a manner analogous to Cre-mediated recombination of loxP flanked DNA (Fig. 8.1) (Sadowski 1995). By combining these two systems, researchers are able to generate multiple distinct mutations in more than one cell type (Fig. 8.3, bottom). In addition, this dual recombinase system can also be employed within the same cell type for sequential mutagenesis with precise temporal control (Van Mater et al. 2015). These expanded capabilities have allowed for experiments that not only dissect the contribution of various cell types to tumor development and radiation response, but also to determine how specific genetic mutations that occur at differing time points during tumor development affect tumor response.

Dual recombinase models have facilitated numerous discoveries that inform the development of radiosensitizers for the treatment of human cancer. For example, conditional Ataxia Telangectasia Mutated (*ATM*) deletion was used to determine the cellular targets in the radiation field that mediate tumor radiation response (Sarkaria and Eshleman 2001). ATM, is a serine threonine kinase and a promising target for radiosensitizers, which is recruited to double-stranded DNA breaks and coordinates DNA damage response via phosphorylation of multiple downstream targets. Patients with homozygous mutations in this gene show hypersensitivity to radiation, which has led to interest in the development of drugs that can radiosensitize tumors through the pharmacological inhibition of ATM function (Raleigh and Haas-Kogan 2013). Deletion of *ATM* radiosensitizes specific normal tissues, such as the intestine, in vivo (Barlow et al. 1996). Dual recombinase technology was applied to the important question of whether the response of tumors to single high-dose radiation was mediated through stromal cells such as endothelial cells, or via increased radiation-induced cell death of the tumor cells themselves. To address this question, we generated GEMMs of sarcoma with *Atm* deletion in either endothelial cells or tumor cells. By radiosensitizing different cell types (endothelial cell vs. tumor cell) in each model, we dissected how each of these cellular compartments contributed to tumor response following high single dose radiation therapy (Moding et al. 2014). To conduct these experiments, an FlpO recombinase was injected intramuscularly into the mouse hindlimb to drive deletion of a conditional FRTed allele for both copies of p53 (p53 $^{FRT/FRT}$). The FlpO recombinase also drove recombination of an FRT flanked stop codon preceding oncogenic *Kras*. Upon recombination the STOP cassette was excised, allowing for expression of the oncogenic *Kras*^{G12D}. About 60–90 days after intramuscular injection of adenoviral FlpO, a sarcoma formed in the mouse hindlimb. One experimental arm of sarcoma bearing mice also expressed Cre recombinase specifically in endothelial cells (VE Cadherin Cre), which deleted conditional floxed alleles of both copies of *Atm* (*Atm*$^{Fl/Fl}$). Mice with these additional conditional mutants were therefore dual recombinase mice, where hindlimb sarcomas formed via FlpO Recombinase and endothelial cell-specific *Atm* was deleted via Cre recombinase. Using these *Kras*$^{FSF-G12D;}$ p53$^{Frt/Frt;}$ VE-Cadherin Cre *Atm*$^{Fl/Fl}$; dual recombinase mice (Table 8.1) we showed that *Atm* deletion in endothelial cells specifically radiosensitized proliferating endothelial cells within tumors, but not in quiescent endothelial such as in the heart following stereotactic body radiation therapy (SBRT) (Moding et al. 2014). This genetic experiment suggests that radiosensitizers that inhibit ATM

Table 8.1 Application of dual recombinase technology for deletion of *Atm* in GEMMs

Genotype	Kras$^{FSF\,G12D}$p53$^{Frt/Frt}$ VE-Cadherin-Cre; Atm$^{Fl/+}$		Kras$^{FSF\,G12D}$p53$^{Frt/Frt}$ VE-Cadherin-Cre; Atm$^{Fl/+}$	
	Tumor parenchyma	Endothelial cells	Tumor parenchyma	Endothelial cells
No Cre; no FLPo				
+FLP (adenoviral delivery)	Mutant Kras, p53 null	No change	Mutant Kras, p53 null	No change
+Cre (driven by VE-Cadherin promoter)	No change	Express Cre; One Atm allele retained	No change	Express Cre; Both Atm alleles deleted

function may increase the therapeutic index of radiation therapy. Further experiments, however, demonstrated that *Atm* deletion in proliferating endothelial cells did not result in an increase in local tumor control after radiation (Moding et al. 2015). Taken together, these findings clarified that endothelial cell death can mediate growth delay following high-dose radiation therapy, but tumor cell death rather than endothelial cell death is rate-limiting for local control. Similar results were obtained by applying dual recombinase technology in a GEMM of lung adenocarcinoma. These conclusions were only possible because of the use of a dual recombinase GEMMs, demonstrating how this tool can empower radiation biology research.

Dual recombinase technology provides a robust platform to study of the intersecting fields of cancer immunology and radiation biology. Using dual recombinase technology, mouse models can be developed whereby specific populations of immune cells in the tumor are targeted with conditional mutations. This enables stepwise examination of how each immune component contributes to radiation response and to observed abscopal effects. This application is particularly important given the growing interest in the synergy of radiation therapy and radiosensitizers with the immune response for the treatment of cancer. Finally, dual recombinase technology can be used to achieve precise temporal control of the order of mutations within a cancer. This facilitates improved understanding of how sequential mutagenesis of oncogenes and tumor suppressors within cancer can alter tumor development and treatment response. An example of this type of dual recombinase approach is a GEMM in which conditional *Tp53* floxed alleles are combined with a tamoxifen-activated CreER expressed from the ubiquitous Rosa26 promoter and an FRTed STOP cassette preceding oncogenic *Kras*^{G12D}. Upon injection of adenoviral FlpO, the STOP cassette is excised, leading to expression of Kras^{G12D}. Then, tamoxifen can be injected, activating CRE-ER to delete both copies of p53 before, after, or at the same time as expression of oncogenic *Kras* (Van Mater et al. 2015). This system was used to study how the timing of gene mutations and muscle injury impacts sarcoma development (Van Mater et al. 2018). Understanding how the order of deletion of key tumor suppressors and activation of oncogenes affects tumor development and therapeutic response may lead to important insights that will inform therapeutic strategies for the application of radiosensitizers.

Dual recombinase technology provides the flexibility and precision necessary to dissect the complex interplay of specific cell types in tumor response to radiation therapy. Because these models allow close examination of native stroma and intact immune systems, they are a particularly powerful GEMM. As cancer biology and radiation biology increasingly focus on complex questions such as immune-tumor co-evolution and the epigenetic interplay between stroma and tumor microenvironments, dual recombinase models can be used to develop strategies for radiosensitizers that can be applied to improve outcomes for cancer patients.

4   GEMMs: CRISPR-Cas9

Despite the many advantages of GEMMs initiated by site-specific recombinases, one significant drawback is the high cost and prolonged period of breeding needed to generate mice with the appropriate number of loxP or frt flanked alleles. This has limited the use of traditional GEMMs for some applications such as the rapid screening of mutant alleles on radiation response and as a preclinical platform to test radiosensitizers. However, the application of the cluster regularly interspaced short palindromic repeats (CRISPR)-Cas9 system to create of GEMMs of cancer in a more rapid and inexpensive manner can overcome this limitation for the application of GEMMs to study radiation biology and to test radiosensitizers in primary tumor models.

CRISPR was first discovered in *E. coli* by Ishino et al. in 1987 (Ishino et al. 1987). The function of CRISPR was unknown at the time, but three separate groups revealed that CRISPR functions as a part of an adaptive prokaryotic immune system termed CRISPR-associated system or Cas (Bolotin et al. 2005; Mojica et al. 2005; van der Oost et al. 2009). Subsequently, researchers modified the bacterial adaptive immune system to become a genome editing tool that revolutionized the field of molecular biology (Jinek et al. 2012; Cho et al. 2013; Mali et al. 2013). Many scientists are using CRISPR-Cas9 to identify and understand mechanisms of genetic diseases, to develop animal disease models, and to edit the genome for advanced gene therapy.

Creating a DNA double-strand break (DSB) in the host genome at a precise location is the ultimate goal of the CRISPR-Cas9 system. CRISPR-Cas9 is comprised of two central components, a universal DNA endonuclease (Cas9 protein, most commonly derived from *Streptococcus Pyogenes* known as SpCas9) and a custom designed single-stranded guide RNA (sgRNA). CRISPR-Cas9 specificity depends on identifying two distinct sequences present in the genome of interest: a trinucleotide sequence called the proto-spacer adjacent motif (PAM) recognized by the originating species of Cas9 (e.g., "NGG" for SpCas9) and a 17–20 nucleotide sequence upstream of PAM that is recognized by the custom sgRNA. Therefore, the PAM serves as an initial recognition signal for the CRISPR-Cas9 complex in the host genome, while the sgRNA is designed to complement a specific DNA sequence (17–20 nucleotides) in the genome upstream of the PAM. Once introduced into the cell, the CRISPR-

Cas9 complex enters into the nucleus and rapidly scans the host genome. When it locates the PAM sequence, it checks for a complementary DNA sequence in the host genome that matches the custom sgRNA. If a match exists between the sgRNA and the host DNA sequence, then sgRNA will anneal to the host DNA sequence to form a DNA-RNA hybrid. Remarkably, this scanning process can identify one unique site in the host genome out of 2.7 billion base pairs. After finding a suitable match, Cas9 undergoes conformational changes to activate endonuclease activity and create a DSB 3–4 bases upstream of the PAM in the host DNA.

Notably, DSBs naturally occur in cells and are rapidly recognized and repaired by either non-homologous end joining (NHEJ) or homologous recombination (HR) depending upon the cell-cycle phase. During NHEJ, the broken ends of the DNA are chewed back in a process also known as DNA-end resection, before they are patched back together. This process most often leads to the addition or removal of one or more base pairs, which may produce a non-functional protein (Fig. 8.4). If cells are in S or G2 phase, HR usually occurs to correct DSBs by utilizing the sister chromatid as a repair template and seals the break without introducing any insertions or deletions (indels). Therefore, CRISPR-Cas9 introduced DNA breaks may form functional or non-functional protein depending upon the cell-cycle phase and the DNA repair process utilized by the cell. Scientists have taken advantage of this feature of CRISPR to introduce precisely targeted mutations to mutate genes in cancer cells in vitro and to mutate genes in animals in vivo to initiate tumorigenesis. Importantly, the HR pathway can be used to incorporate a specific mutation or DNA fragment into the host genome during double-strand break repair if an exogenous "donor" DNA template is introduced at the time as Cas9 expression (Fig. 8.4). Because the CRISPR-Cas9 system avoids the need for protein engineering to target the endonuclease to a specific DNA site and instead relies on the design of synthetic sgRNAs that recognize specific DNA sites of interest, this process dramatically reduces the time and cost associated with gene editing.

In cancer research, the CRISPR-Cas9 system has been rapidly adopted for applications such as genetic screening, DNA sequence barcoding, genome editing to generate oncogenic alterations in cell culture, creating organoid cancer models, and directly modifying the genome of somatic cells in adult mice to generate different cancers. CRISPR-Cas9 technology has two major advantages to generate primary mouse models of cancer: (1) it directly uses somatic cells, avoiding a lengthy process of genetic manipulation of embryonic stem (ES) cells, ES cell selection, injection into blastocysts, implantation into pseudopregnant female, and breeding and (2) multiple genetic manipulations can be achieved at the same time, allowing for a faster and less expensive process. This strategy was first used by Tyler Jacks' laboratory to target *Pten* and *Tp53* tumor suppressor genes in the liver of wild-type mice for tumor generation (Xue et al. 2014). Around the same time, several other laboratories successfully generated cancer mouse models by using a CRISPR-Cas9 approach to modify somatic genes (Sanchez-Rivera et al. 2014; Platt et al. 2014; Maddalo et al. 2014). Since then, the technology has been used to modify somatic genes in order to generate mouse models of different cancers, such as lung cancer (Blasco et al. 2014), breast cancer (Annunziato et al. 2016), brain cancer (Zuckermann

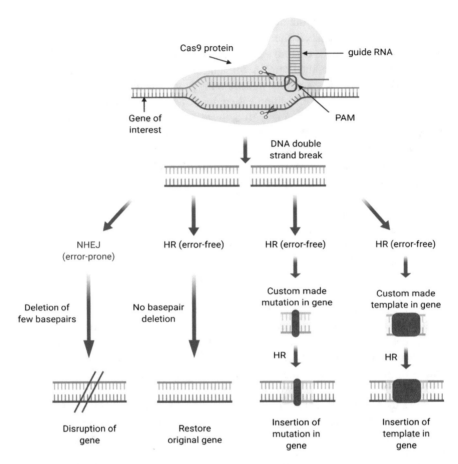

Fig. 8.4 CRISPR Cas9. Schematic representation of possible outcomes of CRISPR-Cas9-driven DNA double-strand breaks. Non-homologous end joining (NHEJ) leads to error-prone DNA double-strand break repair causing random deletion or insertion of nucleotide(s) in the gene of interest. Homologous recombination (HR) leads to error-free DNA double-stand break repair, but by providing a DNA template, it can be utilized to incorporate a mutation or a foreign DNA fragment into a gene of interest

et al. 2015), pancreatic cancer (Chiou et al. 2015), leukemias (Heckl et al. 2014), and sarcomas (Huang et al. 2017). The discovery of CRISPR-Cas9 changed the way we model human cancers in mice. In fact, radiation biologists are using CRISPR-driven next-generation mouse modeling approaches to understand acute and chronic radiation effects on normal tissues, radiation-induced tumorigenesis, and optimizing radiation therapy. CRISPR-based screening approaches have been used to identify radioresistant and radiosensitive genetic and epigenetic components (Adamson et al. 2012; Floyd et al. 2013). In vivo CRISPR technology has been used to rapidly generate mouse model of high-grade FUS-CHOP-driven sarcomas to study tumor radiation response (Chen et al. 2019). Despite the versatility and ease of use of

CRISPR/Cas9, the system does have limitations. First, it requires a unique PAM sequence for targeting, which may not be located at a site of interest. Second, off-target effects or large deletions are possible. Third, precise gene editing via HR in none proliferating cells is inefficient. Finally, the system sequence is too large to easily incorporate into adeno-associated virus, which is the preferred viral vector for many applications of human gene therapy. Scientists are currently working to address many of these shortcomings by discovering new classes and engineered variants of Cas9 proteins (Ran et al. 2015). CRISPR-Cas9 technology is still in its infancy and the near future will bring more uses for basic and translational cancer research.

5 Using GEMMs to Study Normal Tissue Response to Radiation

The development of GEMMs for the study of radiation biology has opened up new fields of research that are essential to the identification and development of highly efficacious radiosensitizers. One key consideration when evaluating the promise of a radiosensitizer is its therapeutic index, or the relative effect of the drug to target (cancer) cells relative to its effect on normal tissue. When radiation therapy is applied to tumors, it can cause injury to the adjacent normal tissue within the radiation field. Newer radiation technology has improved precision of targeting lesions, but the dose of radiation that can be safely administered to a tumor is still often limited by the potential for radiation-induced injury to adjacent normal tissue. Because of the complexity of normal tissue responses to radiation, a cancer model that preserves a normal immune system and native anatomical location of the tumor is highly desirable.

Although the effects of radiation on a specific cell type can be examined by using in vitro cell culture systems, this system does not recapitulate what happens in the human body, where there are complex tissue architectures, temporal variations due to circulation, and interactions among various cell populations. Different tissues exhibit different responses to radiation. Some tissues are inherently more sensitive to radiation-induced injury due to high basal proliferation rates. For example, whole body irradiation can cause anemia, bleeding, and abnormal immune functions due to impaired fitness and viability of hematopoietic cells. Another example is radiation injury to the gastrointestinal tract. Radiation may cause disruption of the integrity of intestinal mucosa, leading to nausea, vomiting, diarrhea, dehydration, infection, or even death. The quality of life for patients with cancer is determined by not only control of their tumors but also the function of normal tissues affected by radiation treatment. Given that clinical advancements have enabled better outcomes for cancer patients, it is anticipated that the number of patients living with radiation therapy-associated late effects will increase in the future. Cancer survivors may develop symptoms associated with previous radiation exposure months to years following treatment. Therefore, as researchers develop radiosensitizers in an attempt to boost the efficacy of radiation therapy, it is important to understand whether these drugs enhance acute and late radiation injury to normal tissues.

GEMMs provide multiple ways of manipulating gene expression to study radiation biology. For example, mouse models equipped with (1) loss of function or (2) gain of function of a particular gene allow researchers to investigate the contribution of the gene to radiation-induced cellular responses and tissue changes (Walrath et al. 2010). Germline knock-out creates a mouse with complete loss of the gene throughout the entire animal. Knock-down models can diminish expression of the gene via short hairpin RNA (shRNA). As for gain of function, transgenic mouse models harbor engineered gene sequences inserted into the mouse genome. The engineered sequences can be foreign (from human or other organisms), or they can be an extra copy of a particular mouse gene, which allows investigation of the dosage effect. In addition to changing the levels of wild-type gene dosage, knock-in of a modified gene sequence at its endogenous gene locus provides a platform for the dissection of the function of specific genes in radiation injury. The sequence of the gene can be modified to render the gene constitutively active, truncated, or dysfunctional. In addition to abolishing, diminishing, or increasing the gene function by engineering a loss or gain quantitatively, introducing mutations at specific sites within the gene enables identification of critical amino acid residues that regulate radiation response. Situated at its native locus, the expression of knock-in mutants is regulated in a similar, if not the same, way to its wild-type version.

The modifications of the gene can be controlled conditionally and temporally. For example, tools such as Cre-LoxP system enable spatial control to confine gene modifications to a specific cell population. As described about in using the Cre-LoxP system to generate cancer, once Cre recombines DNA to activate gene expression or delete a gene, this is a permanent change to the genome in this cell and all of its progeny. Other systems are needed to temporally and reversibly control gene expression. For example, by adapting the way antibiotics regulate gene transcription in bacteria, researchers developed tetracycline-regulated systems to utilize a transactivator protein that responds to tetracycline (or its derivatives, such as doxycycline) by binding to a promoter sequence called a tetracycline response element (TRE). If a gene is preceded by a TRE sequence, then the transcription of the gene is controlled by the transactivator. Depending on the design of the transactivator protein, tetracycline either prevents the binding of the protein to TRE or permits the binding to TRE. The Tet-On system exploits the fact that reverse tetracycline-controlled transactivator (rtTA) only binds to TRE only in the presence of doxycycline. Thus, temporal control of gene expression is achieved by administering doxycycline to allow binding of rtTA to TRE. The binding induces transcription of the gene downstream of TRE, and it is reversible after doxycycline withdrawal. This system can also be adapted to knock-down the expression of a gene by inserting an shRNA downstream of the TRE (Fig. 8.5). In this scenario, administering doxycycline causes rtTA to bind to the TRE to activate expression of shRNA, which in turn diminishes the expression of its target gene. Because discontinuing treatment with doxycycline, the effects on gene expression are reversible and limited for a specific time. Therefore, the Tet-On system can be applied in combination with

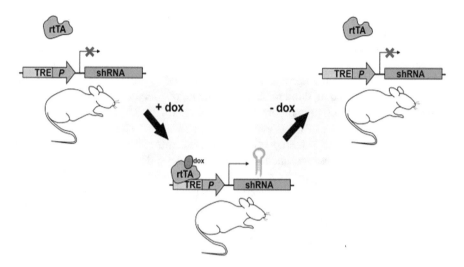

Fig. 8.5 A Tet-ON GEMM. A tetracycline responsive element (TRE) precedes a promoter and shRNA targeting a gene of interest. In the absence of doxycycline, a tetracycline analogue, the reverse tetracycline-controlled transactivator (rtTA) is not bound to the TRE and thus does not activate expression of the shRNA (left). Administration of doxycycline allows formation of a doxycycline-rtTA complex, which is now able to bind and activate the TRE. This in turn allows expression of the shRNA and knock-down of the gene of interest (middle). Upon withdrawal of doxycycline, the rtTA loses affinity for the TRE (right). The TRE is therefore no longer activated and shRNA expression is halted, allowing for restoration of normal expression of the target gene

radiation treatments to simulates clinical scenarios and provide insight for developing radiation modulators.

GEMMs can also be used to identify certain cell populations that regulate the pathological response to radiation. For example, cell-specific promotor-regulated expression of a fluorescence protein can be used to label cells expressing in which the specific promotor is active (Bouabe and Okkenhaug 2013; Walrath et al. 2010). Expression of the fluorescence protein or other reporters under the control of the Cre-LoxP system can limit expression of the reporter to cells expressing Cre and their progeny (Fig. 8.2) (Walrath et al. 2010). Therefore, this technology can be applied to examine the cell lineages that regulate radiation response. In radiation biology, lineage tracing (i.e., labeling cells and their progeny with a reporter gene) facilitates the understanding of how cells that survive radiation regenerate and re-establish the integrity of the tissue architecture/functions following radiation injury.

5.1   Example: Using GEMMs to Study how p53 Regulates Hematopoietic Response to Radiation

Radiation creates lesions in the genome and results in the activation of the DNA damage response (Jackson and Bartek 2009), which in many cell types is regulated by activation of p53. P53 is a multifunctional protein and a well-known transcription factor (Bieging et al. 2014). As an important tumor suppressor protein, p53 is frequently deleted or dysfunctional in mouse tumor models and in human cancers while most of the normal cells retain functional p53 protein. Because the radiation field is often a mixture of cells with different p53 status, how p53-controlled pathways affect the response of a heterogeneous group of cells to radiation is an important question. It is known that, upon radiation treatment, p53 mediates apoptotic death in hematopoietic stem and progenitor cells (Pant et al. 2012). Radiation toxicity to the hematopoietic system can be alleviated when p53 is lost (Kirsch et al. 2010b). However, inhibiting p53 therapeutically is concerning because p53 possesses important tumor suppression functions. While it is possible to ameliorate radiation-induced hematopoietic injury by suppressing p53, whether or not this will enhance the risk of developing radiation-induced cancers is unclear. There have been multiple examples of using GEMMs to study p53 in radiation biology research. While p53 germline knock-out mice are susceptible to radiation-induced lymphomas, it was unknown if p53-mediated acute DNA damage responses were required for suppressing radiation-induced lymphomagenesis. Research by Christophorou et al. demonstrated the effects of temporary restoration of p53 function in animals lacking p53 expression on radiation-induced tumorigenesis by using a mouse model with inducible expression of p53ER fusion protein (Christophorou et al. 2006). The p53ER mice were functionally p53 knock-out until administration of 4-hydroxytamoxifen, which bound to and activated the fusion protein (Fig. 8.6). When p53 was temporarily restored concurrent with radiation treatments, it induced p53-dependent apoptosis in radiosensitive tissues but this did not protect against radiation-induced lymphomagenesis when compared with mice without p53 restoration. However, p53 restoration beginning 8 days after irradiation resulted in significantly delayed lymphomagenesis (Christophorou et al. 2006). Hinkal et al. used tamoxifen to temporally control the deletion of both p53 alleles either before, concurrent with, or after irradiation treatment (Hinkal et al. 2009). Irrespective of the time points when the permanent p53 deletion was induced, there was no significant difference in the latency of the development of radiation-induced lymphoma.

We utilized the Tet-On system and shRNA knock-down technology to study the effects of temporary p53 knock-down on radiation-induced lymphomagenesis (Lee et al. 2015). Mice harboring ubiquitous rtTA transgene and TRE-controlled shRNA transgene expressed shRNA against p53 upon doxycycline treatments. Doxycycline was given concurrently with the regimen of fractionated total-body irradiation. Afterward, the mice were returned to a regular diet (doxycycline withdrawal). This constituted a temporary knock-down of p53 in the animals to mimic the clinical setting whereby normal tissue expressing wild-type p53 is exposed to a p53 inhibitor during radiation to limit hematopoietic toxicity. We investigated if mice were protected from acute hematopoietic injury and if radiation-induced lymphomagenesis was impacted by the temporary suppression of p53 through shRNA induction. Apoptotic death of hematopoietic stem and progenitor cells was significantly decreased by temporary p53 knock-down. Surprisingly, lymphoma-free survival significantly improved in mice with temporary reduction of p53 levels during total-body irradiation (TBI). Bone marrow transplant studies in irradiated recipient mice demonstrated that transplanted irradiated hematopoietic stem and progenitor cells

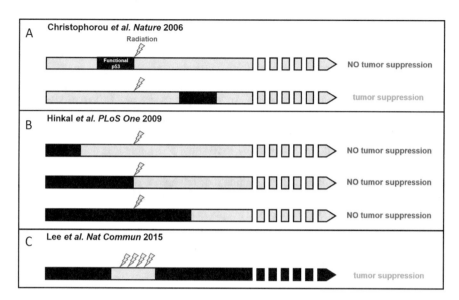

Fig. 8.6 Schematic of three mouse models investigating p53's control of radiation-induced tumorigenesis. (**a**) Christophorou et al. (Christophorou et al. 2006) induced p53 restoration in p53-deficient mice either during or after radiation. While tamoxifen-induced p53 restoration during radiation did not protect mice from radiation-induced tumorigenesis, delayed p53 restoration conferred tumor suppression. (**b**) Hinkal et al. (Hinkal et al. 2009) induced p53 deletion by tamoxifen before, concurrent with, or after radiation. Regardless of the time of deletion, there was no significant difference in mouse survival. (**c**) Lee et al. (Lee et al. 2015) induced temporary p53 blockade during radiation treatments. Temporary decrease of p53 levels resulted in the suppression of radiation-induced lymphomagenesis

with temporary p53 knock-down prevented radiation-induced thymic lymphomas compared to cells with normal p53 levels. This indicated that temporary p53 knock-down during TBI prevented radiation-induced lymphomagenesis in a non-cell-autonomous manner, supporting a model where bone marrow cells with low p53 levels survive radiation and compete with preexisting tumor initiating cells to prevent lymphomagenesis. In this example, the GEMM serves as a platform for studying the impact of temporary knock-down of a therapeutic target during radiation. This facilitates an understanding of whether an intervention could diminish acute radiation injury and also prevent long-term radiation-induced carcinogenesis thereby improving patient survival and quality of life.

5.2   Example: Using GEMMs to Study Radiation-Induced Gastrointestinal (GI) Syndrome

Another example of the use of GEMMs to study normal tissue response to radiation therapy is found in research on the intestine. The intestine is a complex structure composed of cell populations with distinct functions. Radiation therapy administered to the abdomen or pelvis inevitably delivers radiation dose to the intestines and can cause unwanted acute side effects and long-term toxicity. While mice exposed to total-body irradiation may develop acute hematopoietic syndrome manifested as bleeding, neutropenia, and death, mice that receive high-dose irradiation develop radiation-induced gastrointestinal syndrome and may die from disruption of intestinal tissue integrity within 5–10 days (Williams et al. 2010). We have utilized intestinal epithelium-specific Cre (Villin-Cre) to examine the role of p53 and the pathway of intrinsic apoptosis in the radiation-induced GI syndrome (Kirsch et al. 2010b). When a floxed (flanked by loxP sites) p53 allele was deleted in intestinal epithelial cells, p53 FL/− mice were significantly more sensitized to radiation-induced GI syndrome than p53 FL/+ mice that retained a p53 allele. Interestingly, we found that when the intrinsic apoptosis was abrogated (by deletion Bak1 and Bax) there was a decrease in apoptotic events in the intestinal epithelium; however, there was no protection against radiation-induced gastrointestinal syndrome. Therefore, these results indicated that p53 protected the intestine from radiation injury independent of apoptosis.

5.3   Example: Using GEMMs to Study Radiation-Induced Heart Injury

When radiation therapy is administered to the chest, the heart may also be exposed to radiation. It has been found that left-sided breast cancer patients can develop radiation-associated cardiovascular disease years after radiation therapy (Roychoudhuri et al. 2007). Endothelial cells are one of the main cell populations that maintain the structure and function of the cardiovascular system. We previously utilized Cre/-LoxP systems to delete p53 specifically in endothelial cells and found that p53 in endothelial cells protects mice from developing radiation-induced cardiac injury (Lee et al. 2012a). When p53 was deleted in the endothelial cells, mice developed multifocal myocardial necrosis. The heart also displayed decreased micro-vessel density, vascular permeability, and elevated hypoxia.

The advantages of using GEMMs in radiation research include the maintenance of native organ structure and easier genetic manipulation of specific cell populations in a temporally and/or spatially controlled fashion. Unlike in vitro systems, GEMMs allow various simulations of clinical treatment regimens and modalities, which include radiation, chemotherapy, surgery, diet control, imaging, and other monitoring approaches. Additionally, GEMMs enable long-term monitoring of late effects induced by radiation and dissection of the critical components contributing to the control of radiation injury. In the search for radiosensitizers for different cancers, it is important to investigate not only the efficacy of tumor control but also the impact on normal tissues to understand whether a therapeutic window exists. This knowledge may be exploited in utilizing radiosensitizers in clinical trials to maximize local control while minimizing the risk of developing short-term toxicity and long-term effects following radiotherapy combined with the radiosensitizer.

6 GEMMs at the Intersection of Radiation Biology and Immuno-Oncology

Another area of study where GEMMs provide strong advantages is the intersection of radiation biology and immuno-oncology. Many of the effects of radiation therapy are thought to be mediated through the immune system (Grassberger et al. 2019). In fact, several immunomodulatory agents have the potential to act synergistically with radiation (Lhuillier et al. 2019). There is therefore significant interest in the development of radiosensitizers that can modulate the immune system and thereby improve patient outcomes. While mouse tumors transplanted into syngeneic mice and human xenograft tumors in immunodeficient mice provide practical and fiscal advantages for preclinical studies of radiation therapy, GEMMs offer key features that make them ideal for studying how radiation therapy interacts with novel immunotherapies. These features include the native tumor microenvironment and an intact immune system that co-evolved with the cancer throughout tumor development. In contrast, xenograft models in immunodeficient mice lack a functioning immune system. Although transplanted murine models do have intact immune systems, tumor cell injection artificially activates the immune system in ways that can impact the response of tumors to radiation therapy and immunotherapy (Crittenden et al. 2018). Conversely, cancers are initiated in GEMMs by inducing mutations in tumor initiating cells that eventually result in autochthonous tumors. According to the theory of cancer immunoediting, the immune system co-evolves with these tumor cells and their progeny so that tumor outgrowth occurs only after tumor cell immune escape (Ribatti 2017). Because GEMMs capture this natural pathologic process, they provide a good platform for studies in radiation therapy and immunotherapy. One potential limitation of GEMMs for immunotherapy studies is that these tumor models have a relatively low tumor mutational burden (Huang et al. 2017). Therefore, adapting GEMMs to increase tumor mutational burden through the use of chemical carcinogens (Lee et al. 2019) or other approaches is an important direction for future research of radiation and immunotherapy.

Immune checkpoint inhibitors have been approved for the treatment of many cancers because they improve the survival of a subset of patients across multiple tumor types (Hodi et al. 2010; Thomas 2011; Reck et al. 2016). Particularly, immune checkpoint inhibitors targeting programmed cell death protein 1 (PD-1), ligand to PD-1 (PD-L1), and cytotoxic T-lymphocyte-associated protein 4 (CTLA-4) have proven effective in a minority of patients with metastatic disease. Immune checkpoints function normally to prevent excessive and prolonged inflammation after antigen exposure, but cancer cells utilize these inhibitory mechanisms to evade immunity by exhausting tumor-specific cytotoxic T cell responses (Fig. 8.7). Other

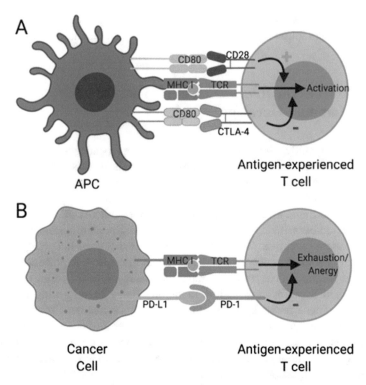

Fig. 8.7 Cancer cells utilize immune checkpoint inhibitors to induce T cell exhaustion and/or anergy. Normally, CTLA-4 and PD-1 function as inhibitory mechanisms to immune over activation. (**a**) CTLA-4 expression is induced upon initial antigen experience of T cells and is proportional to antigen affinity. This is essential for promoting a consistent immune response given the wide affinity ranges of MHC-presented antigens. (**b**) PD-1 expression occurs in activated T cells and enables control of T cell activity at the site of inflammation through binding of PD-1 ligands, such as PD-L1. Some cancer cells are capable of agonizing these immune checkpoint receptors to induce T cell exhaustion and/or anergy. This represents one mechanism of immune evasion for tumors. *APC* antigen presenting cell, *TCR* T cell receptor

avenues of cancer immunotherapy currently being investigated include cytokine therapies (IL-2, interferon, GM-CSF, TGF-ß) and immunostimulatory receptor agonists (TLR-4, TLR-7, anti-OX40, anti-GITR) intended to promote tumor-specific inflammation (Kang et al. 2016; Bristow et al. 2018).

While immunotherapy has demonstrated promise as a cancer therapy, it currently exhibits efficacy in only subsets of patients. Tumors with low mutational loads, few tumor-specific antigens, and a resulting lower immunogenicity have been reported as less responsive to checkpoint blockade. Additionally, high PD-L1 levels on tumor cells have been associated with increased response to PD-1 blockade (Aguilar et al. 2019; Reck et al. 2016). Yet, other potential biomarkers of immunotherapy efficacy remain poorly defined. Furthermore, several technical challenges currently hinder efficient preclinical research into immunotherapy. Many preclinical studies in transplant mouse models have demonstrated impressive efficacy of immune checkpoint inhibitors combined with radiation therapy (Twyman-Saint Victor et al. 2015). However, subsequent clinical trials have not reflected the same degree of benefit in patient populations (Luke et al. 2018; Maity et al. 2018) possibly due to increased tumor diversity or long-term immune system-tumor coevolution. This inconsistency demonstrates a major shortcoming of transplant models for studying the immune response to cancer treated with immunotherapy and radiation therapy.

The involvement of the immune system to radiation therapy effectiveness has long been suspected. In 1953, a phenomenon termed the abscopal effect was reported in patients receiving local radiation therapy (Siva et al. 2015). The abscopal effect is a systemic tumor-specific immune response leading to multi-site tumor size reduction, which has been reported in a very small number of patients following single-site tumor irradiation. This phenomenon as well as a contrary effect of radiation-induced distant secondary tumor growth have been observed in various animal models. Regardless, the systemic responses observed following tumor-specific irradiation and cell killing clearly suggests that the immune system has the potential to mediate radiation effects. Furthermore, data from transplant tumor models suggest a role for cytotoxic T cells, helper T cells, and natural killer cells in tumor response to radiation therapy (Formenti and Demaria 2009). With the widespread adoption of immunotherapies in clinical medicine, case reports of abscopal responses increased and preclinical combination immunotherapy and radiation therapy studies in transplant models demonstrated the abscopal effect (Wisdom et al. 2018; Dewan et al. 2009). These findings suggest that tumor irradiation has the potential to enhance the systemic effectiveness of immunotherapy. In other words, combination immunotherapy and radiation therapy may act as an in situ tumor vaccine. Irradiation of the tumor can enhance antitumor immunity through several mechanisms including direct tumor cell killing with subsequent tumor-specific antigen expression by antigen presenting cells (APC), proinflammatory cytokine induction, killing of immune regulatory cells (Tregs), and tumor architecture alteration allowing for increased immune cell penetration of the tumor (Demaria et al. 2005a). Several preclinical studies have demonstrated a cooperative effect of radiation and immunotherapy in transplant tumor models (Dovedi et al. 2017; Demaria et al. 2005b; Belcaid et al. 2014; Morris et al. 2016). Additionally, early clinical trials have noted acceptable safety profiles following immunotherapy and radiation therapy (Golden et al. 2015; Seung et al. 2012).

Many recent cancer studies of radiation therapy, immunotherapy, and the immune system have been conducted using GEMMs as a preclinical model. Wisdom et al. demonstrated that neutrophils mediate radiation resistance and could be targeted to radiosensitize tumors (Wisdom et al. 2019). The GEMM used in this study contained several key genetic factors: (1) activation of oncogenic $Kras^{G12D}$ and $Trp53$ knock-out both initiated through FlpO recombinase to induce sarcomagenesis, and (2) neutrophil depletion through $MRP8^{Cre}$-mediated transcription of diphtheria toxin. Similarly, natural killer (NK) cells have been identified as important antitumor components of the immune system through both innate and adaptive immune mechanisms (Guillerey et al. 2016). Using a GEMM of lung adenocarcinoma,

Schmidt et al. showed that induced expression of activating NK cell ligands leading to stimulation promoted NK-mediated antitumor responses (Schmidt et al. 2019). This GEMM contained: (1) oncogenic $Kras^{G12D}$ and $Trp53$ knock-out both initiated through Cre recombinase to induce tumorigenesis, and (2) lentivirus-delivered doxycycline-dependent expression of the murine cytomegalovirus protein m157, which is capable of specifically stimulating NK cells. The cGMP–AMP synthase (cGAS)–stimulator of interferon genes (STING) pathway is a key component of both the innate and adaptive immune systems through sensing cytosolic DNA. Furthermore, activation of this pathway has been associated with both antitumor and protumor responses (Ng et al. 2018). Ahn et al. used a GEMM to demonstrate that inflammation-driven carcinogenesis is mediated through the STING pathway. In this study, a STING−/− GEMM was shown to resist 7,12-dimethylbenz(a) anthracene (DMBA)-induced tumorigenesis when compared to wild-type controls (Ahn et al. 2017). These three examples demonstrate the broad utility of GEMMs for studies of the immune system in autochthonous tumors.

7 Practical Considerations for GEMM Experimental Planning

Unfortunately, the success rate for the translation of preclinical studies to positive clinical trials is low in biomedical research including trials in radiation oncology (Liu et al. 2013; Hackam and Redelmeier 2006; Landis et al. 2012). This may be in part due to limitations of preclinical studies, such as the use of sub-optimal murine models. Ideally, tumor models will closely resemble the key characteristics of the analogous human cancer including genetic driver mutations, histology, and the tumor microenvironment (Castle et al. 2017). Mouse transplant models in syngeneic mice or patient-derived xenografts (PDX) in immunodeficient mice are popular preclinical models in oncology research due to their relatively low cost and short timeframe for generating tumors and for conducting the experiments. While GEMMs with autochthonous primary tumors require more resources and usually take longer to develop, they do possess major advantages including a natural tumor microenvironment and intact immune system (Kirsch et al. 2018). These features are particularly vital components for studies employing radiation therapy and immunotherapy. Furthermore, using recombinase technologies, GEMMs can address mechanistic questions involving treatment responses. With the continued advancement of CRISPR technologies (Huang et al. 2017), the cost and time to generate tumors with GEMMs will decrease so that they can be more widely used for preclinical studies.

When designing preclinical experiments in GEMMs, many factors must be considered and optimal controls used to generate the most reliable results. Given the genetic variability that exists between mice of the same strain, such as C57 BL/6 mice, littermate controls should always be used rather than wild-type mice of the same strain in an effort to minimize genetic differences between study groups. In radiation studies, contemporaneous control groups should be irradiated to account for fluctuations in radiation source due to differences in X-ray tube or calibration over time. Housing animals of different study groups in the same cage (i.e., cage-matched controls) reduces the effects of variable stressors and the microbiome between groups. Animal sex may also impact results in both drug and radiation studies. In fact, many examples exist of sex either influencing drug effectiveness or having variable side effects for males and females (Parekh et al. 2011). Indeed, we have observed that the effectiveness of a mitigator or total-body irradiation (Lee et al. 2014) is dependent on sex and mouse strain (Daniel et al. 2019). While sex-specific effects of radiation are still poorly understood, several studies suggest different metabolic responses may influence the hematopoietic acute radiation syndrome (Jones et al. 2019; Tonorezos et al. 2012).

Additionally, Stone et al. reviewed studies of ten preclinical drug–radiation combinations in an attempt to discern best practices for preclinical trial design and reporting with the maximum potential for reproducibility and adequately informing clinical trial design (Stone et al. 2016). One major concern raised by this review involved the scientific rigor of experiments. Stone et al. reported only 12% of the reviewed studies claimed reproducibility of their findings, the majority of studies were un-blinded, and power calculations were often absent. Specific to radiation biology, many of the studies failed to report radiation source, energy, dose, and calibration. To ensure reliable and reproducible results across preclinical studies, describing these details of radiation delivery in the methods section are essential for all in vivo studies.

8 Conclusion

Here we reviewed the applications of mouse models in preclinical radiation biology research. We introduced fundamental concepts of mouse modeling and summarized several technologies for mouse modeling including site-specific recombinases, shRNA, and CRISPR/Cas9. We demonstrated the utility of these technologies and mouse modeling in radiation biology research by highlighting several publications that used GEMMs in preclinical research on radiation-induced carcinogenesis, normal tissue radiation injury, the in vivo targets of radiation in tumors, and the development of immunotherapies that synergize with radiation therapy. Despite the important contributions GEMMs have made in radiation research, these and next-generation mouse models are poised to reveal additional insights in the future. Experiments performed in robust in vivo systems, such as GEMMs, will continue to play an important role in making discoveries in radiation research. GEMMs of cancer are powerful tools for investigating the cell-autonomous and non-cell-autonomous mechanisms that contribute to normal and tumor tissue response to radiation. We anticipate that increased adoption of GEMMs in radiation biology research will not only lead to important new knowledge but also increase the predictive value of preclinical research to accelerate clinical translation of radiosensitizers to improve outcomes for patients treated with radiation therapy.

Acknowledgements We thank Andrea Daniel for providing constructive feedback on this chapter.

References

Adamson B, Smogorzewska A, Sigoillot FD, King RW, Elledge SJ (2012) A genome-wide homologous recombination screen identifies the RNA-binding protein RBMX as a component of the DNA-damage response. Nat Cell Biol 14:318–328

Aguilar EJ, Ricciuti B, Gainor JF, Kehl KL, Kravets S, Dahlberg S, Nishino M, Sholl LM, Adeni A, Subegdjo S, Khosrowjerdi S, Peterson RI, Digumarthy S, Liu C, Sauter J, Rizvi H, Arbour KC, Carter BW, Heymach JV, Altan M, Hellmann MD, Awad MM (2019) Outcomes to first-line pembrolizumab in patients with non-small cell lung cancer and very high PD-L1 expression. Ann Oncol 30:1653

Ahn R, Sabourin V, Bolt AM, Hebert S, Totten S, De Jay N, Festa MC, Young YK, Im YK, Pawson T, Koromilas AE, Muller WJ, Mann KK, Kleinman CL, Ursini-Siegel J (2017) The Shc1 adaptor simultaneously balances Stat1 and Stat3 activity to promote breast cancer immune suppression. Nat Commun 8:14638

Annunziato S, Kas SM, Nethe M, Yucel H, Del Bravo J, Pritchard C, Bin Ali R, van Gerwen B, Siteur B, Drenth AP, Schut E, van de Ven M, Boelens MC, Klarenbeek S, Huijbers IJ, van Miltenburg MH, Jonkers J (2016) Modeling invasive lobular breast carcinoma by CRISPR/Cas9-mediated somatic genome editing of the mammary gland. Genes Dev 30:1470–1480

Ashton JR, Castle KD, Qi Y, Kirsch DG, West JL, Badea CT (2018) Dual-energy CT imaging of tumor liposome delivery after gold nanoparticle-augmented radiation therapy. Theranostics 8:1782–1797

Barlow C, Hirotsune S, Paylor R, Liyanage M, Eckhaus M, Collins F, Shiloh Y, Crawley JN, Ried T, Tagle D, Wynshaw-Boris A (1996) Atm-deficient mice: a paradigm of ataxia telangiectasia. Cell 86:159–171

Belcaid Z, Phallen JA, Zeng J, See AP, Mathios D, Gottschalk C, Nicholas S, Kellett M, Ruzevick J, Jackson C, Albesiano E, Durham NM, Ye X, Tran PT, Tyler B, Wong JW, Brem H, Pardoll DM, Drake CG, Lim M (2014) Focal radiation therapy combined with 4-1BB activation and CTLA-4 blockade yields long-term survival and a protective antigen-specific memory response in a murine glioma model. PLoS One 9:e101764

Bieging KT, Mello SS, Attardi LD (2014) Unravelling mechanisms of p53-mediated tumour suppression. Nat Rev Cancer 14:359–370

Blasco RB, Karaca E, Ambrogio C, Cheong TC, Karayol E, Minero VG, Voena C, Chiarle R (2014) Simple and rapid in vivo generation of chromosomal rearrangements using CRISPR/Cas9 technology. Cell Rep 9:1219–1227

Bolotin A, Quinquis B, Sorokin A, Ehrlich SD (2005) Clustered regularly interspaced short palindrome repeats (CRISPRs) have spacers of extrachromosomal origin. Microbiology 151:2551–2561

Bos JL, Fearon ER, Hamilton SR, Verlaan-de Vries M, van Boom JH, van der Eb AJ, Vogelstein B (1987) Prevalence of ras gene mutations in human colorectal cancers. Nature 327:293–297

Bouabe H, Okkenhaug K (2013) A protocol for construction of gene targeting vectors and generation of homologous recombinant embryonic stem cells. Methods Mol Biol 1064:337–354

Branda CS, Dymecki SM (2004) Talking about a revolution: the impact of site-specific recombinases on genetic analyses in mice. Dev Cell 6:7–28

Bristow RG, Alexander B, Baumann M, Bratman SV, Brown JM, Camphausen K, Choyke P, Citrin D, Contessa JN, Dicker A, Kirsch DG, Krause M, Le QT, Milosevic M, Morris ZS, Sarkaria JN, Sondel PM, Tran PT, Wilson GD, Willers H, Wong RKS, Harari PM (2018) Combining precision radiotherapy with molecular targeting and immunomodulatory agents: a guideline by the American Society for Radiation Oncology. Lancet Oncol 19:e240–ee51

Castle KD, Chen M, Wisdom AJ, Kirsch DG (2017) Genetically engineered mouse models for studying radiation biology. Transl Cancer Res 6:S900–SS13

Castle KD, Kirsch DG (2019) Establishing the impact of vascular damage on tumor response to high-dose radiation therapy. Cancer Res 79:5685

Chen M, Xu ES, Leisenring NH, Cardona DM, Luo L, Ma Y, Ventura A, Kirsch DG (2019) The fusion oncogene FUS-CHOP drives sarcomagenesis of high-grade spindle cell sarcomas in mice. Sarcoma 2019:1340261

Chiou SH, Winters IP, Wang J, Naranjo S, Dudgeon C, Tamburini FB, Brady JJ, Yang D, Gruner BM, Chuang CH, Caswell DR, Zeng H, Chu P, Kim GE, Carpizo DR, Kim SK, Winslow MM (2015) Pancreatic cancer modeling using retrograde viral vector delivery and in vivo CRISPR/Cas9-mediated somatic genome editing. Genes Dev 29:1576–1585

Cho SW, Kim S, Kim JM, Kim JS (2013) Targeted genome engineering in human cells with the Cas9 RNA-guided endonuclease. Nat Biotechnol 31:230–232

Christophorou MA, Ringshausen I, Finch AJ, Swigart LB, Evan GI (2006) The pathological response to DNA damage does not contribute to p53-mediated tumour suppression. Nature 443:214–217

Clarke AR (2005) Studying the consequences of immediate loss of gene function in the intestine: APC. Biochem Soc Trans 33:665–666

Coleman CN, Higgins GS, Brown JM, Baumann M, Kirsch DG, Willers H, Prasanna PG, Dewhirst MW, Bernhard EJ, Ahmed MM (2016) Improving the predictive value of preclinical studies in support of radiotherapy clinical trials. Clin Cancer Res 22:3138–3147

Crittenden MR, Zebertavage L, Kramer G, Bambina S, Friedman D, Troesch V, Blair T, Baird JR, Alice A, Gough MJ (2018) Tumor cure by radiation therapy and checkpoint inhibitors depends on pre-existing immunity. Sci Rep 8:7012

Daniel AR, Lee CL, Oh P, Luo L, Ma Y, Kirsch DG (2019) Inhibiting glycogen synthase kinase-3 mitigates the hematopoietic acute radiation syndrome in a sex and strain dependent manner in mice. Health Phys. https://doi.org/10.1097/HP.0000000000001243

Demaria S, Bhardwaj N, McBride WH, Formenti SC (2005a) Combining radiotherapy and immunotherapy: a revived partnership. Int J Radiat Oncol Biol Phys 63:655–666

Demaria S, Kawashima N, Yang AM, Devitt ML, Babb JS, Allison JP, Formenti SC (2005b) Immune-mediated inhibition of metastases after treatment with local radiation and CTLA-4 blockade in a mouse model of breast cancer. Clin Cancer Res 11:728–734

Dewan MZ, Galloway AE, Kawashima N, Dewyngaert JK, Babb JS, Formenti SC, Demaria S (2009) Fractionated but not single-dose radiotherapy induces an immune-mediated abscopal effect when combined with anti-CTLA-4 antibody. Clin Cancer Res 15:5379–5388

Dovedi SJ, Cheadle EJ, Popple AL, Poon E, Morrow M, Stewart R, Yusko EC, Sanders CM, Vignali M, Emerson RO, Robins HS, Wilkinson RW, Honeychurch J, Illidge TM (2017) Fractionated radiation therapy stimulates antitumor immunity mediated by both resident and infiltrating polyclonal T-cell populations when combined with PD-1 blockade. Clin Cancer Res 23:5514–5526

Ferlay J, Soerjomataram I, Dikshit R, Eser S, Mathers C, Rebelo M, Parkin DM, Forman D, Bray F (2015) Cancer incidence and mortality worldwide: sources, methods and major patterns in GLOBOCAN 2012. Int J Cancer 136:E359–E386

Floyd SR, Pacold ME, Huang Q, Clarke SM, Lam FC, Cannell IG, Bryson BD, Rameseder J, Lee MJ, Blake EJ, Fydrych A, Ho R, Greenberger BA, Chen GC, Maffa A, Del Rosario AM, Root DE, Carpenter AE, Hahn WC, Sabatini DM, Chen CC, White FM, Bradner JE, Yaffe MB (2013) The bromodomain protein Brd4 insulates chromatin from DNA damage signalling. Nature 498:246–250

Formenti SC, Demaria S (2009) Systemic effects of local radiotherapy. Lancet Oncol 10:718–726

Gitler AD, Kong Y, Choi JK, Zhu Y, Pear WS, Epstein JA (2004) Tie2-Cre-induced inactivation of a conditional mutant Nf1 allele in mouse results in a myeloproliferative disorder that models juvenile myelomonocytic leukemia. Pediatr Res 55:581–584

Golden EB, Chhabra A, Chachoua A, Adams S, Donach M, Fenton-Kerimian M, Friedman K, Ponzo F, Babb JS, Goldberg J, Demaria S, Formenti SC (2015) Local radiotherapy and granulocyte-macrophage colony-stimulating factor to generate abscopal responses in patients with metastatic solid tumours: a proof-of-principle trial. Lancet Oncol 16:795–803

Grassberger C, Ellsworth SG, Wilks MQ, Keane FK, Loeffler JS (2019) Assessing the interactions between radiotherapy and antitumour immunity. Nat Rev Clin Oncol 16:729

Guillerey C, Huntington ND, Smyth MJ (2016) Targeting natural killer cells in cancer immunotherapy. Nat Immunol 17:1025–1036

Hackam DG, Redelmeier DA (2006) Translation of research evidence from animals to humans. JAMA 296:1731–1732

Heckl D, Kowalczyk MS, Yudovich D, Belizaire R, Puram RV, McConkey ME, Thielke A, Aster JC, Regev A, Ebert BL (2014) Generation of mouse models of myeloid malignancy with combinatorial genetic lesions using CRISPR-Cas9 genome editing. Nat Biotechnol 32:941–946

Hinkal G, Parikh N, Donehower LA (2009) Timed somatic deletion of p53 in mice reveals age-associated differences in tumor progression. PLoS One 4:e6654

Hodi FS, O'Day SJ, McDermott DF, Weber RW, Sosman JA, Haanen JB, Gonzalez R, Robert C, Schadendorf D, Hassel JC, Akerley W, van den Eertwegh AJ, Lutzky J, Lorigan P, Vaubel JM, Linette GP, Hogg D, Ottensmeier CH, Lebbe C, Peschel C, Quirt I, Clark JI, Wolchok JD, Weber JS, Tian J, Yellin MJ, Nichol GM, Hoos A, Urba WJ (2010) Improved survival with ipilimumab in patients with metastatic melanoma. N Engl J Med 363:711–723

Horsman MR, Overgaard J (2016) The impact of hypoxia and its modification of the outcome of radiotherapy. J Radiat Res 57(Suppl 1):i90–i98

Huang J, Chen M, Whitley MJ, Kuo HC, Xu ES, Walens A, Mowery YM, Van Mater D, Eward WC, Cardona DM, Luo L, Ma Y, Lopez OM, Nelson CE, Robinson-Hamm JN, Reddy A, Dave SS, Gersbach CA, Dodd RD, Kirsch DG (2017) Generation and comparison of CRISPR-Cas9 and Cre-mediated genetically engineered mouse models of sarcoma. Nat Commun 8:15999

Ishino Y, Shinagawa H, Makino K, Amemura M, Nakata A (1987) Nucleotide sequence of the iap gene, responsible for alkaline phosphatase isozyme conversion in Escherichia coli, and identification of the gene product. J Bacteriol 169:5429–5433

Jackson EL, Willis N, Mercer K, Bronson RT, Crowley D, Montoya R, Jacks T, Tuveson DA (2001) Analysis of lung tumor initiation and progression using conditional expression of oncogenic K-ras. Genes Dev 15:3243–3248

Jackson SP, Bartek J (2009) The DNA-damage response in human biology and disease. Nature 461:1071–1078

Jinek M, Chylinski K, Fonfara I, Hauer M, Doudna JA, Charpentier E (2012) A programmable dual-RNA-guided DNA endonuclease in adaptive bacterial immunity. Science 337:816–821

Jones JW, Alloush J, Sellamuthu R, Chua HL, MacVittie TJ, Orschell CM, Kane MA (2019) Effect of sex on biomarker response in a mouse model of the hematopoietic acute radiation syndrome. Health Phys 116:484–502

Jonkers J, Meuwissen R, van der Gulden H, Peterse H, van der Valk M, Berns A (2001) Synergistic tumor suppressor activity of BRCA2 and p53 in a conditional mouse model for breast cancer. Nat Genet 29:418–425

Kang X, Kim J, Deng M, John S, Chen H, Wu G, Phan H, Zhang CC (2016) Inhibitory leukocyte immunoglobulin-like receptors: immune checkpoint proteins and tumor sustaining factors. Cell Cycle 15:25–40

Kirsch DG (2011) Using genetically engineered mice for radiation research. Radiat Res 176:275–279

Kirsch DG, Diehn M, Kesarwala AH, Maity A, Morgan MA, Schwarz JK, Bristow R, Demaria S, Eke I, Griffin RJ, Haas-Kogan D, Higgins GS, Kimmelman AC, Kimple RJ, Lombaert IM, Ma

L, Marples B, Pajonk F, Park CC, Schaue D, Tran PT, Willers H, Wouters BG, Bernhard EJ (2018) The future of radiobiology. J Natl Cancer Inst 110:329–340

Kirsch DG, Dinulescu DM, Miller JB, Grimm J, Santiago PM, Young NP, Nielsen GP, Quade BJ, Chaber CJ, Schultz CP, Takeuchi O, Bronson RT, Crowley D, Korsmeyer SJ, Yoon SS, Hornicek FJ, Weissleder R, Jacks T (2007) A spatially and temporally restricted mouse model of soft tissue sarcoma. Nat Med 13:992–997

Kirsch DG, Grimm J, Guimaraes AR, Wojtkiewicz GR, Perez BA, Santiago PM, Anthony NK, Forbes T, Doppke K, Weissleder R, Jacks T (2010a) Imaging primary lung cancers in mice to study radiation biology. Int J Radiat Oncol Biol Phys 76:973–977

Kirsch DG, Santiago PM, di Tomaso E, Sullivan JM, Hou WS, Dayton T, Jeffords LB, Sodha P, Mercer KL, Cohen R, Takeuchi O, Korsmeyer SJ, Bronson RT, Kim CF, Haigis KM, Jain RK, Jacks T (2010b) p53 controls radiation-induced gastrointestinal syndrome in mice independent of apoptosis. Science 327:593–596

Landis SC, Amara SG, Asadullah K, Austin CP, Blumenstein R, Bradley EW, Crystal RG, Darnell RB, Ferrante RJ, Fillit H, Finkelstein R, Fisher M, Gendelman HE, Golub RM, Goudreau JL, Gross RA, Gubitz AK, Hesterlee SE, Howells DW, Huguenard J, Kelner K, Koroshetz W, Krainc D, Lazic SE, Levine MS, Macleod MR, McCall JM, Moxley RT 3rd, Narasimhan K, Noble LJ, Perrin S, Porter JD, Steward O, Unger E, Utz U, Silberberg SD (2012) A call for transparent reporting to optimize the predictive value of preclinical research. Nature 490:187–191

Lee CL, Castle KD, Moding EJ, Blum JM, Williams N, Luo L, Ma Y, Borst LB, Kim Y, Kirsch DG (2015) Acute DNA damage activates the tumour suppressor p53 to promote radiation-induced lymphoma. Nat Commun 6:8477

Lee CL, Lento WE, Castle KD, Chao NJ, Kirsch DG (2014) Inhibiting glycogen synthase kinase-3 mitigates the hematopoietic acute radiation syndrome in mice. Radiat Res 181:445–451

Lee CL, Moding EJ, Cuneo KC, Li Y, Sullivan JM, Mao L, Washington I, Jeffords LB, Rodrigues RC, Ma Y, Das S, Kontos CD, Kim Y, Rockman HA, Kirsch DG (2012a) p53 functions in endothelial cells to prevent radiation-induced myocardial injury in mice. Sci Signal 5:ra52

Lee CL, Moding EJ, Huang X, Li Y, Woodlief LZ, Rodrigues RC, Ma Y, Kirsch DG (2012b) Generation of primary tumors with Flp recombinase in FRT-flanked p53 mice. Dis Model Mech 5:397–402

Lee CL, Mowery YM, Daniel AR, Zhang D, Sibley AB, Delaney JR, Wisdom AJ, Qin X, Wang X, Caraballo I, Gresham J, Luo L, Van Mater D, Owzar K, Kirsch DG (2019) Mutational landscape in genetically engineered, carcinogen-induced, and radiation-induced mouse sarcoma. JCI Insight 4:128698

Lhuillier C, Rudqvist NP, Elemento O, Formenti SC, Demaria S (2019) Radiation therapy and anti-tumor immunity: exposing immunogenic mutations to the immune system. Genome Med 11:40

Li G, Robinson GW, Lesche R, Martinez-Diaz H, Jiang Z, Rozengurt N, Wagner KU, Wu DC, Lane TF, Liu X, Hennighausen L, Wu H (2002) Conditional loss of PTEN leads to precocious development and neoplasia in the mammary gland. Development 129:4159–4170

Li W, Qiao W, Chen L, Xu X, Yang X, Li D, Li C, Brodie SG, Meguid MM, Hennighausen L, Deng CX (2003) Squamous cell carcinoma and mammary abscess formation through squamous metaplasia in Smad4/Dpc4 conditional knockout mice. Development 130:6143–6153

Liu, F. F., participants workshop, P. Okunieff, E. J. Bernhard, H. B. Stone, S. Yoo, C. N. Coleman, B. Vikram, M. Brown, J. Buatti, and C. Guha. 2013. 'Lessons learned from radiation oncology clinical trials', Clin Cancer Res, 19: 6089–6100

Luke JJ, Lemons JM, Karrison TG, Pitroda SP, Melotek JM, Zha Y, Al-Hallaq HA, Arina A, Khodarev NN, Janisch L, Chang P, Patel JD, Fleming GF, Moroney J, Sharma MR, White JR, Ratain MJ, Gajewski TF, Weichselbaum RR, Chmura SJ (2018) Safety and clinical activity of pembrolizumab and multisite stereotactic body radiotherapy in patients with advanced solid Tumors. J Clin Oncol 36:1611–1618

Maddalo D, Manchado E, Concepcion CP, Bonetti C, Vidigal JA, Han YC, Ogrodowski P, Crippa A, Rekhtman N, de Stanchina E, Lowe SW, Ventura A (2014) In vivo engineering of oncogenic chromosomal rearrangements with the CRISPR/Cas9 system. Nature 516:423–427

Maity A, Mick R, Huang AC, George SM, Farwell MD, Lukens JN, Berman AT, Mitchell TC, Bauml J, Schuchter LM, O'Hara M, Lin LL, Demichele A, Christodouleas JP, Haas NB, Patsch DM, Hahn SM, Minn AJ, Wherry EJ, Vonderheide RH (2018) A phase I trial of pembrolizumab with hypofractionated radiotherapy in patients with metastatic solid tumours. Br J Cancer 119:1200–1207

Mali P, Aach J, Stranges PB, Esvelt KM, Moosburner M, Kosuri S, Yang L, Church GM (2013) CAS9 transcriptional activators for target specificity screening and paired nickases for cooperative genome engineering. Nat Biotechnol 31:833–838

Meuwissen R, Linn SC, van der Valk M, Mooi WJ, Berns A (2001) Mouse model for lung tumorigenesis through Cre/lox controlled sporadic activation of the K-Ras oncogene. Oncogene 20:6551–6558

Moding EJ, Castle KD, Perez BA, Oh P, Min HD, Norris H, Ma Y, Cardona DM, Lee CL, Kirsch DG (2015) Tumor cells, but not endothelial cells, mediate eradication of primary sarcomas by stereotactic body radiation therapy. Sci Transl Med 7:278ra34

Moding EJ, Kastan MB, Kirsch DG (2013) Strategies for optimizing the response of cancer and normal tissues to radiation. Nat Rev Drug Discov 12:526–542

Moding EJ, Lee CL, Castle KD, Oh P, Mao L, Zha S, Min HD, Ma Y, Das S, Kirsch DG (2014) Atm deletion with dual recombinase technology preferentially radiosensitizes tumor endothelium. J Clin Invest 124:3325–3338

Mojica FJ, Diez-Villasenor C, Garcia-Martinez J, Soria E (2005) Intervening sequences of regularly spaced prokaryotic repeats derive from foreign genetic elements. J Mol Evol 60:174–182

Morris ZS, Guy EI, Francis DM, Gressett MM, Werner LR, Carmichael LL, Yang RK, Armstrong EA, Huang S, Navid F, Gillies SD, Korman A, Hank JA, Rakhmilevich AL, Harari PM, Sondel PM (2016) In situ tumor vaccination by combining local radiation and tumor-specific antibody or immunocytokine treatments. Cancer Res 76:3929–3941

Ng KW, Marshall EA, Bell JC, Lam WL (2018) cGAS-STING and cancer: dichotomous roles in tumor immunity and development. Trends Immunol 39:44–54

Pant V, Quintas-Cardama A, Lozano G (2012) The p53 pathway in hematopoiesis: lessons from mouse models, implications for humans. Blood 120:5118–5127

Parekh A, Fadiran EO, Uhl K, Throckmorton DC (2011) Adverse effects in women: implications for drug development and regulatory policies. Expert Rev Clin Pharmacol 4:453–466

Perez BA, Ghafoori AP, Lee CL, Johnston SM, Li Y, Moroshek JG, Ma Y, Mukherjee S, Kim Y, Badea CT, Kirsch DG (2013) Assessing the radiation response of lung cancer with different gene mutations using genetically engineered mice. Front Oncol 3:72

Platt RJ, Chen S, Zhou Y, Yim MJ, Swiech L, Kempton HR, Dahlman JE, Parnas O, Eisenhaure TM, Jovanovic M, Graham DB, Jhunjhunwala S, Heidenreich M, Xavier RJ, Langer R, Anderson DG, Hacohen N, Regev A, Feng G, Sharp PA, Zhang F (2014) CRISPR-Cas9 knockin mice for genome editing and cancer modeling. Cell 159:440–455

Raleigh DR, Haas-Kogan DA (2013) Molecular targets and mechanisms of radiosensitization using DNA damage response pathways. Future Oncol 9:219–233

Ran FA, Cong L, Yan WX, Scott DA, Gootenberg JS, Kriz AJ, Zetsche B, Shalem O, Wu X, Makarova KS, Koonin EV, Sharp PA, Zhang F (2015) In vivo genome editing using Staphylococcus aureus Cas9. Nature 520:186–191

Reck M, Rodriguez-Abreu D, Robinson AG, Hui R, Csoszi T, Fulop A, Gottfried M, Peled N, Tafreshi A, Cuffe S, O'Brien M, Rao S, Hotta K, Leiby MA, Lubiniecki GM, Shentu Y, Rangwala R, Brahmer JR, Keynote-Investigators (2016) Pembrolizumab versus chemotherapy for PD-L1-positive non-small-cell lung cancer. N Engl J Med 375:1823–1833

Ribatti D (2017) Sales for anti-angiogenic drugs. Oncotarget 8:38080–38081

Rius M, Lyko F (2012) Epigenetic cancer therapy: rationales, targets and drugs. Oncogene 31:4257–4265

Rodenhuis S, Slebos RJ, Boot AJ, Evers SG, Mooi WJ, Wagenaar SS, van Bodegom PC, Bos JL (1988) Incidence and possible clinical significance of K-ras oncogene activation in adenocarcinoma of the human lung. Cancer Res 48:5738–5741

Roychoudhuri R, Robinson D, Putcha V, Cuzick J, Darby S, Moller H (2007) Increased cardiovascular mortality more than fifteen years after radiotherapy for breast cancer: a population-based study. BMC Cancer 7:9

Sadowski PD (1995) The Flp recombinase of the 2-microns plasmid of Saccharomyces cerevisiae. Prog Nucleic Acid Res Mol Biol 51:53–91

Sanchez-Rivera FJ, Papagiannakopoulos T, Romero R, Tammela T, Bauer MR, Bhutkar A, Joshi NS, Subbaraj L, Bronson RT, Xue W, Jacks T (2014) Rapid modelling of cooperating genetic events in cancer through somatic genome editing. Nature 516:428–431

Sarkaria JN, Eshleman JS (2001) ATM as a target for novel radiosensitizers. Semin Radiat Oncol 11:316–327

Schmidt L, Eskiocak B, Kohn R, Dang C, Joshi NS, DuPage M, Lee DY, Jacks T (2019) Enhanced adaptive immune responses in lung adenocarcinoma through natural killer cell stimulation. Proc Natl Acad Sci U S A 116:17460–17469

Seung SK, Curti BD, Crittenden M, Walker E, Coffey T, Siebert JC, Miller W, Payne R, Glenn L, Bageac A, Urba WJ (2012) Phase 1 study of stereotactic body radiotherapy and interleukin-2—tumor and immunological responses. Sci Transl Med 4:137ra74

Siva S, MacManus MP, Martin RF, Martin OA (2015) Abscopal effects of radiation therapy: a clinical review for the radiobiologist. Cancer Lett 356:82–90

Stewart TA, Pattengale PK, Leder P (1984) Spontaneous mammary adenocarcinomas in transgenic mice that carry and express MTV/myc fusion genes. Cell 38:627–637

Stone HB, Bernhard EJ, Coleman CN, Deye J, Capala J, Mitchell JB, Brown JM (2016) Preclinical data on efficacy of 10 drug-radiation combinations: evaluations, concerns, and recommendations. Transl Oncol 9:46–56

Thomas JM (2011) Sentinel-lymph-node biopsy for cutaneous melanoma. N Engl J Med 365:569–570. author reply 71

Tonorezos ES, Vega GL, Sklar CA, Chou JF, Moskowitz CS, Mo Q, Church TS, Ross R, Janiszewski PM, Oeffinger KC (2012) Adipokines, body fatness, and insulin resistance among survivors of childhood leukemia. Pediatr Blood Cancer 58:31–36

Torok JA, Oh P, Castle KD, Reinsvold M, Ma Y, Luo L, Lee CL, Kirsch DG (2019) Deletion of Atm in tumor but not endothelial cells improves radiation response in a primary mouse model of lung adenocarcinoma. Cancer Res 79:773–782

Twyman-Saint Victor C, Rech AJ, Maity A, Rengan R, Pauken KE, Stelekati E, Benci JL, Xu B, Dada H, Odorizzi PM, Herati RS, Mansfield KD, Patsch D, Amaravadi RK, Schuchter LM, Ishwaran H, Mick R, Pryma DA, Xu X, Feldman MD, Gangadhar TC, Hahn SM, Wherry EJ, Vonderheide RH, Minn AJ (2015) Radiation and dual checkpoint blockade activate nonredundant immune mechanisms in cancer. Nature 520:373–377

van der Oost J, Jore MM, Westra ER, Lundgren M, Brouns SJ (2009) CRISPR-based adaptive and heritable immunity in prokaryotes. Trends Biochem Sci 34:401–407

Van Mater D, Ano L, Blum JM, Webster MT, Huang W, Williams N, Ma Y, Cardona DM, Fan CM, Kirsch DG (2015) Acute tissue injury activates satellite cells and promotes sarcoma formation via the HGF/c-MET signaling pathway. Cancer Res 75:605–614

Van Mater D, Xu E, Reddy A, Ano L, Sachdeva M, Huang W, Williams N, Ma Y, Love C, Happ L, Dave S, Kirsch DG (2018) Injury promotes sarcoma development in a genetically and temporally restricted manner. JCI Insight 3:123687

Walrath JC, Hawes JJ, Van Dyke T, Reilly KM (2010) Genetically engineered mouse models in cancer research. Adv Cancer Res 106:113–164

Williams JP, Johnston CJ, Finkelstein JN (2010) Treatment for radiation-induced pulmonary late effects: spoiled for choice or looking in the wrong direction? Curr Drug Targets 11:1386–1394

Wisdom AJ, Hong CS, Lin AJ, Xiang Y, Cooper DE, Zhang J, Xu ES, Kuo HC, Mowery YM, Carpenter DJ, Kadakia KT, Himes JE, Luo L, Ma Y, Williams N, Cardona DM, Haldar M,

Diao Y, Markovina S, Schwarz JK, Kirsch DG (2019) Neutrophils promote tumor resistance to radiation therapy. Proc Natl Acad Sci U S A 116:18584–18589

Wisdom AJ, Mowery YM, Riedel RF, Kirsch DG (2018) Rationale and emerging strategies for immune checkpoint blockade in soft tissue sarcoma. Cancer 124:3819–3829

Xu X, Wagner KU, Larson D, Weaver Z, Li C, Ried T, Hennighausen L, Wynshaw-Boris A, Deng CX (1999) Conditional mutation of Brca1 in mammary epithelial cells results in blunted ductal morphogenesis and tumour formation. Nat Genet 22:37–43

Xue W, Chen S, Yin H, Tammela T, Papagiannakopoulos T, Joshi NS, Cai W, Yang G, Bronson R, Crowley DG, Zhang F, Anderson DG, Sharp PA, Jacks T (2014) CRISPR-mediated direct mutation of cancer genes in the mouse liver. Nature 514:380–384

Zhang M, Qiu Q, Li Z, Sachdeva M, Min H, Cardona DM, DeLaney TF, Han T, Ma Y, Luo L, Ilkayeva OR, Lui K, Nichols AG, Newgard CB, Kastan MB, Rathmell JC, Dewhirst MW, Kirsch DG (2015) HIF-1 alpha regulates the response of primary sarcomas to radiation therapy through a cell autonomous mechanism. Radiat Res 183:594–609

Zuckermann M, Hovestadt V, Knobbe-Thomsen CB, Zapatka M, Northcott PA, Schramm K, Belic J, Jones DT, Tschida B, Moriarity B, Largaespada D, Roussel MF, Korshunov A, Reifenberger G, Pfister SM, Lichter P, Kawauchi D, Gronych J (2015) Somatic CRISPR/Cas9-mediated tumour suppressor disruption enables versatile brain tumour modelling. Nat Commun 6:7391

Chapter 9
Targeting the DNA Damage Response for Radiosensitization

Matthew T. McMillan, Theodore S. Lawrence, and Meredith A. Morgan

Abstract Radiation is a DNA-damaging agent that exerts its lethal anti-tumoral effects predominately by inducing DNA double-strand breaks. Tumor cells can evade radiation-induced cell death through upregulating elements of the DNA damage response (DDR) that promote DNA repair and cell cycle checkpoint activation. These critical mediators include PARP1, WEE1, DNA-PK, ATM, ATR, and CHK1. Agents that inhibit these components of the DDR can act as radiosensitizers that enhance tumor cell killing. In this chapter, we discuss actionable DDR targets and their role in radiosensitization. This includes detailing their normal physiological roles, mechanisms for radiosensitization, immunomodulatory properties, clinical trials, and mechanistically based rational treatment combinations.

Keywords Alternative end-joining · ATM · ATR · Cell cycle checkpoints · CHK1 · DNA damage response · DNA-dependent protein kinase · DNA double-strand breaks · DNA replication fork · Homologous recombination repair · Non-homologous end joining · p53 · Poly (ADP-ribose) polymerase · Radiosensitization · Single-strand annealing · WEE1

1 Introduction

DNA damage is omnipresent and exists as a by-product of endogenous and/or exogenous stressors. Consequently, cells have evolved a complex molecular infrastructure—the DNA damage response (DDR)—for detecting and repairing DNA damage as needed. When DNA damage is detected, cell cycle checkpoints (G_1, intra-S, or G_2) are activated to prevent propagation of cells with a damaged DNA template (Reichert et al. 2016) (Fig. 9.1). This activation induces cell cycle

M. T. McMillan · T. S. Lawrence · M. A. Morgan (✉)
Department of Radiation Oncology, University of Michigan Medical School, Ann Arbor, MI, USA
e-mail: mmccrack@med.umich.edu

© Springer Nature Switzerland AG 2020
H. Willers, I. Eke (eds.), *Molecular Targeted Radiosensitizers*, Cancer Drug Discovery and Development, https://doi.org/10.1007/978-3-030-49701-9_9

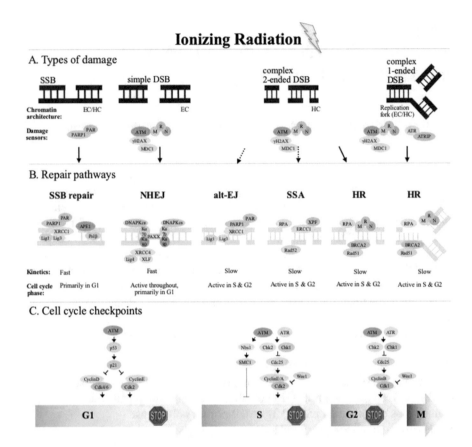

Fig. 9.1 The effects of radiation-induced DNA damage. (**a**) Major types of radiation-induced DNA damage with respective DNA damage sensor proteins are illustrated. Radiation induces single-strand breaks (SSB) either directly or indirectly as intermediates of base excision repair. Simple double-strand breaks (DSB) involve two broken DNA ends in close proximity and occur in euchromatin (EC). Complex DSBs involve two broken DNA ends (i.e., 2-ended DSB) in proximity to additional DNA damage (e.g., crosslinks, SSBs) or within heterochromatin (HC), or a DSB within a replication fork (1-ended DSB). (**b**) SSBs and simple DSBs are repaired with fast kinetics by SSB repair and non-homologous end joining (NHEJ) pathways, respectively. Alternative end-joining (alt-EJ) and single-strand annealing (SSA) are slow, compensatory repair pathways activated when DNA-PKcs is absent or when NHEJ/HR attempt, but fail, to complete repair. Alt-EJ and SSA likely contributes to repair of complex 2-ended DSBs. Homologous recombination (HR) operates under slow kinetics and is partly responsible for repair of complex 2-ended DSBs and exclusively responsible for repair of 1-ended DSBs. These repair pathways function in a cell cycle-dependent manner, as illustrated. (**c**) Cell cycle checkpoints are activated in response to DNA damage to prevent propagation of cells with damaged DNA and to permit time for DNA repair. The major checkpoints include those occurring in G1, S, and G2. While ATM activation is the initial response to radiation-induced DNA DSBs, ATR is subsequently activated and contributes to a sustained cell cycle checkpoint response. Dashed lines represent incompletely understood pathways. Other abbreviations: ATRIP, ATR-interacting protein; MRN, Mre11-Rad50-Nbs1

arrest, permitting coordination of DNA repair machinery to the site of damage and the restitution of DNA integrity; cells with extensive or irreparable DNA damage undergo mitotic cell death, senescence, or apoptosis.

Ataxia-telangiectasia mutated (ATM) kinase is the apical kinase responsible for inducing each of the cell cycle checkpoint pathways. Cells with damaged DNA in G_1 avoid replication of a damaged DNA template by arresting at the G_1-S interface through ATM-dependent activation of p53 and p21. Cells that sustain DNA damage in S phase transiently arrest through activation of checkpoint kinase (CHK) 2, which leads to the inhibition of cyclin-dependent kinase (CDK) 2. Lastly, the G_2 checkpoint delays the progression of cells with damaged DNA into mitosis by activating CHK1, resulting in inhibition of the mitotic cyclin CDK1.

DNA damage most commonly presents as single-strand breaks (SSB); however, the less frequent double-strand breaks (DSB) are more lethal, so DDR-associated therapeutics targeting the signaling and repair mechanisms associated with DSBs are preferred. An initial response to DNA DSBs is ATM-mediated phosphorylation of H2AX, which forms multiprotein complexes (i.e., foci) at DSBs to promote the recruitment of additional ATM molecules and other repair factors. In mammalian cells, there are several pathways available for the repair of DNA DSBs: non-homologous end joining (NHEJ), homologous recombination repair (HRR), alternative end-joining (alt-EJ) repair, or single-strand annealing (SSA).

NHEJ repairs the majority of radiation-induced DNA DSBs, and in addition to functioning as the predominate DSB repair mechanism in the G_1 phase, it is also active in all other phases of the cell cycle. NHEJ is notable for being fast and highly efficient because it is able to catalyze simple rejoining reactions between DNA ends with no sequence homology. Although mutagenic, its rapid kinetics are important for preserving genomic integrity, including the suppression of chromosomal translocations (Ceccaldi et al. 2016a). A major pharmacological target for inhibiting NHEJ repair is DNA-dependent protein kinase (DNA-PK); the kinase activity of DNA-PK is required for the activation of several NHEJ effector proteins including the DNA-PKcs catalytic subunit (DNA-PKcs) itself.

HRR is a relatively slow, yet highly accurate repair process owing to its requirement for extensive end resection and homologous DNA sequences. Consequently, HRR preferentially operates during the S and G_2 phases of the cell cycle when sister chromatids are present to facilitate DSB repair. Notable proteins involved in HRR are BRCA1, BRCA2, PALB2, and RAD51. Similar to HRR, alt-EJ repair also occurs during the S and G_2 phases of the cell cycle. Although it anneals at microhomologies, it often harms genomic integrity through causing chromosomal translocations and mutagenic rearrangements. Key distinguishing features for alt-EJ repair are its lack of requirement of core NHEJ proteins, such as DNA-PKcs and its dependence on poly (ADP-ribose) polymerase (PARP) 1 and DNA polymerase Θ (POLQ). SSA requires more extensive DNA end resection than alt-EJ; however, one copy of the repeat and the intervening sequence between repeats are deleted in the repair process, leading to the loss of genetic information. The inhibition of HRR upregulates RAD52-mediated SSA activity, and loss of RAD52 function is synthetically lethal with the deficiency of some HRR factors (i.e., BRCA1, BRCA2, PALB2).

DDR inhibitors were initially developed as monotherapy to therapeutically exploit synthetic lethality interactions. The underlying premise for these interactions is that replication stress, genomic instability, or other DDR defects present in tumor cells—but absent in normal cells—represent actionable vulnerabilities that can be targeted with DDR inhibitors. The concept of synthetic lethality was clinically validated using PARP1/2 inhibitors in patients with *BRCA1/2* mutations (i.e., HRR deficiency) (Farmer et al. 2005). Beyond PARP, small-molecule inhibitors targeting other key mediators of DNA repair and replication, such as WEE1, DNA-PK, ATM, ATR, and CHK1, are now being tested both as single agents and in combination with DNA-damaging agents for a wide variety of indications.

Radiation is an attractive DNA-damaging agent to combine with DDR inhibitors given its spatial selectivity. In addition, many DDR inhibitors can promote tumor cell-selective radiosensitization due to the molecular characteristics of tumor cells including defects in the G_1 checkpoint (e.g., p53, p21, Rb), genomic instability, oncogene-induced replication stress (*KRAS*), and other DDR defects (Morgan and Lawrence 2015). Advancements in biomarker assays and improved access to next-generation sequencing have led to the identification of biomarkers predictive of improved clinical responses to combinations of radiation therapy (RT) and various DDR inhibitors. In this chapter, we discuss the major drug classes of DDR inhibitors; this includes delving into the normal physiological roles of their targets and the mechanisms for their radiosensitization and immunomodulation. We will also discuss clinical trials, rational treatment combinations for optimizing radiosensitization in the clinic, and future directions.

2 General Principles Linking the DDR and Anti-Tumoral Immunity

It is becoming increasingly apparent that a critical component of DDR inhibitor-induced radiosensitization is immunomodulation. Each DDR target is characterized by unique immunomodulatory properties; however, some fundamental aspects are shared and a preliminary introduction to their general role is critical for developing rational treatment combinations.

RT promotes antigenicity through damaging DNA and disrupting genomic integrity. If a tumor cell survives this insult, loss of normal DNA repair fidelity through DDR inhibition may increase the tumor mutational burden, which could lead to neoantigen production (promoting microbial mimicry) and enhanced T cell activity (Mouw et al. 2017). In addition, RT causes the release of endogenous adjuvants (e.g., single-strand DNA, ssDNA; double-strand DNA, dsDNA) into the cytosol, leading to the activation of cytosolic pattern recognition receptors (PRR) (e.g., cyclic GMP-AMP synthase [cGAS]) (Galluzzi et al. 2017). These PRRs generate a

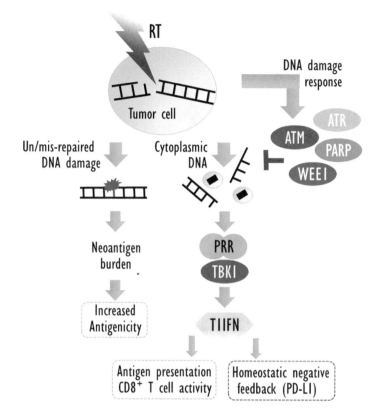

Fig. 9.2 Linking radiotherapy and DNA damage response inhibitors to anti-tumoral immunity. Radiation causes both SSBs and DSBs in nuclear DNA which can result in increased mutational and neoantigen burden (left) as well as accumulation of ssDNA, dsDNA, or micronuclei in the cytoplasm of cells (right). Defects in DDR proteins can further enhance this process resulting in a greater mutational/neoantigen burden and further increases in both nuclear DNA damage and cytoplasmic DNA. Cytoplasmic DNA is sensed by pattern recognition receptor (PRR) pathways such as cGAS/STING/TBK1 that activate type I interferon (T1IFN) production. Collectively, neoantigens and cytoplasmic DNA promote anti-tumor immunity but may also activate negative feedback mechanisms such as programmed death-ligand 1 (PD-L1) expression

signaling cascade which sets off a series of events promoting antigen-specific adaptive immunity. Furthermore, targeting the DDR appears to potentiate the activation of these immune pathways (Fig. 9.2).

One proposed mechanism asserts that when RT-induced DNA DSBs are not repaired due to inhibited or defective DDR proteins, mitotic mis-segregation of RT-damaged acentric chromosomes leads to the generation of micronuclei; these micronuclei often have defective nuclear lamina organization leading to DNA release into the cytosol and activation of innate immune signaling through cGAS PRRs (Hatch et al. 2013). Induction of the cGAS-stimulator of interferon genes (STING) pathway leads to TBK1 activation and type I interferon (T1IFN) production. T1IFN's positive immune modulatory effects include promoting the maturation and antigen presentation of dendritic cells as well as the recruitment and effector function of memory CD8$^+$ T cells. T1IFN also stimulates negative feedback mechanisms such as tumor cell programmed death-ligan 1 (PD-L1) expression. These immune regulatory functions of DDR inhibitors and RT may be leveraged therapeutically to improve immunotherapy efficacy and will be discussed in this chapter.

3 Common DDR Targets

3.1 PARP1/2

PARP1/2 enzymes play key roles in the DDR as both DNA damage sensors and signal transducers. These proteins detect DNA SSBs and DSBs, recruit DNA repair effectors, and stabilize replication forks during repair (Pommier et al. 2016) (Fig. 9.1). Upon generation of a DNA SSB, PARP1/2 binds to the DNA lesion and utilizes nicotinamide adenine dinucleotide (NAD$^+$) to add PAR chains to histones, chromatin-associated proteins, and itself (i.e., auto-PARylation) (Pommier et al. 2016). This post-translational modification leads to chromatin relaxation, recruitment of DNA repair proteins (e.g., XRCC1), and PARP1/2 dissociation with cumulative auto-PARylation.

The canonical model for PARP1/2 inhibitor monotherapy efficacy is based on two linked mechanisms: (i) catalytic inhibition of PARylation and (ii) PARP trapping. All clinical PARP inhibitors address the first mechanism by sharing a nicotinamide moiety that competes with the enzyme cofactor, NAD$^+$, for binding to the catalytic domain of PARP1/2 (Lord and Ashworth 2017). However, PARP inhibitors with equal catalytic inhibition potency can vary greatly in terms of their PARP-trapping abilities. The relative size and rigidity of the PARP inhibitor appears to play a role in its cytotoxic potency and the ability to trap PARP on DNA. Of the current clinically available PARP inhibitors, the smallest—veliparib—demonstrates the least PARP-trapping activity, while the more rigid and bulky, talazoparib, has the most potent PARP-trapping activity (talazoparib > niraparib > rucaparib = olaparib > > veliparib) (Pommier et al. 2016). Notably, the trapping ability of a PARP inhibitor reflects its cytotoxic potency as monotherapy. In the setting of PARP trapping, PARP is unable to dissociate from the DNA SSB, resulting in the accumulation of unrepaired DNA SSBs and stalled replication forks. In replicating cells, these SSBs convert to DSBs, which require HRR; herein lies the conventional rationale for using PARP inhibitor in the setting of homologous recombination-deficient (HRD) tumors.

The possibility of using PARP inhibitors in HRD tumors to achieve synthetic lethality was first reported in 2005 (Bryant et al. 2005; Farmer et al. 2005). It was shown that *BRCA*-mutant tumor cells were up to 1000 times more sensitive to PARP inhibitors than *BRCA*-wild type cells. Both BRCA1 and BRCA2 proteins are vital for HRR, which is a conservative, high-fidelity mechanism of DNA repair (Morgan and Lawrence 2015). When cells become HRD (e.g., *BRCA1/2* mutation) in the context of PARP inhibition, lower fidelity mechanisms, such as deregulated NHEJ and single-strand annealing, predominate. Upregulation of non-conservative repair pathways in HRD tumor cells treated with PARP inhibitors has been shown to lead to increased genomic instability and cytotoxicity (Patel et al. 2011). Consistent with this finding, restoration of HRR in BRCA1-deficient cells by 53BP1 deletion leads to reduced genomic instability following PARP inhibition and consequently insensitivity to PARP inhibition (Bunting et al. 2010).

Recently, alternative mechanisms for PARP inhibitor efficacy have been reported that contradict the established construct (Maya-Mendoza et al. 2018; Caron et al. 2019). One study demonstrated that PARP inhibitors *increase* the speed of fork elongation and do not cause fork stalling, which is in contrast to the accepted model in which PARP inhibitors induce fork stalling and collapse (Maya-Mendoza et al. 2018). This finding was reproduced using PARP inhibitors with both the strongest (talazoparib) and weakest (veliparib) trapping abilities. Furthermore, these findings are consistent with the increased replication velocity observed in pancreatic cancer cells treated with olaparib (Fig. 9.3). Mechanistically, PARylation and p21 modulate fork progression in a process regulated by PARP1 and p53 proteins. PARylation acts as a sensor of replication stress; therefore, in the setting of PARP inhibition,

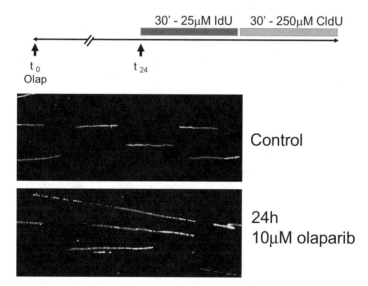

Fig. 9.3 Increased replication velocity in response to PARP inhibitor treatment as assessed by DNA fiber combing. Representative DNA fiber images from MiaPaCa2 cells treated with 10 µM olaparib for 24 h. Replication fork speed is calculated for individual forks labelled with an IdU track flanked by a single CldU track. Mean replication forks speeds were 1.0 ± 0.02 kb/min and 1.5 ± 0.05 kb/min for control and 10 mM olaparib, respectively. Increased fork speed following olaparib treatment can be visualized by the increased fiber length. Figure provided by Dr. Leslie A. Parsels (University of Michigan)

DNA lesions that would normally induce fork arrest—to allow time for repair—remain unrecognized by replication machinery.

Other mechanisms for PARP inhibitor efficacy relate to its role in immunomodulation. Preclinical studies have demonstrated that PARP inhibitors lead to an accumulation of cytosolic dsDNA, thereby activating the cGAS-STING-TBK1-IRF3 innate immune pathway and inducing T1IFN production. This results in increased infiltration by immune cells and enhanced functionality of CD8$^+$ T cells and natural killer cells (Ding et al. 2018; Shen et al. 2019). This promising PARP inhibitor-induced anti-tumoral activity is blunted, however, through adaptive (Minn 2015) and intrinsic (Jiao et al. 2017) upregulation of PD-L1. Fortunately, it appears that targeting this homeostatic negative feedback mechanism through immune checkpoint blockade (ICB) potentiates the efficacy of PARP inhibitors (Jiao et al. 2017; Ding et al. 2018; Shen et al. 2019).

The effectiveness of PARP inhibitors as radiosensitizers has been thoroughly investigated in numerous preclinical studies with median enhancement ratios varying from 1.3 to 1.5 (Lesueur et al. 2017). While the efficacy of PARP inhibitor monotherapy largely depends upon an "HRDness" phenotype, its radiosensitization capacity appears to be driven more by replication stress and PARP trapping, with more potent trapping agents associated with greater radiosensitization (Bridges et al. 2014; Laird et al. 2018). This does not, however, minimize the significance of a tumor's HRDness in PARP inhibitor-induced radiosensitization; lower concentrations of PARP inhibitor can be used for HRD tumors (Lesueur et al. 2017). Furthermore, PARP1 is a critical regulator of DNA end resection of RT-induced DNA DSBs; inhibition of PARP promotes HRR, deregulated NHEJ, and hyperresected DSBs (Caron et al. 2019). Therefore, PARP inhibitor-induced radiosensitization in some HRD tumors also acts by producing DSBs that must be repaired through deregulated NHEJ, creating genomic instability and cytotoxicity (Patel et al. 2011; Caron et al. 2019). Notably, DSB hyperresection is dependent on functional DNA resection machinery; therefore, this phenotype would be observed in BRCA2-deficient cells but not in BRCA1-deficient cells (Caron et al. 2019).

There are numerous ongoing clinical trials combining PARP1/2 inhibitors with RT or chemo-RT (Table 9.1). A recent phase I study showed that olaparib may be safely combined with concurrent cetuximab and RT for patients with smoking-related locally advanced head and neck squamous cell carcinoma (HNSCC) (Karam et al. 2018). The maximum tolerated dose (MTD) of olaparib was 50 mg BID; however, the recommended phase 2 dose (RP2D) was 25 mg BID since increased mucositis and dermatitis were observed primarily above 25 mg BID. Dose-limiting toxicities (DLT) were assessed over a 10-week period; they were observed in three (19%) patients (Grade (G) 4 dermatitis, $n = 2$; G3 nausea/vomiting, $n = 1$). G3-4 lymphopenia occurred in three (19%) patients. The 2-year overall survival (OS) rate of 72% in the trial was favorable compared to the expected OS rate of 60% in HNSCC patients with a heavy smoking history (Ang et al. 2010).

A phase I multicenter study evaluated veliparib and concurrent RT for 30 patients with inflammatory or locally recurrent breast cancer after complete surgical resection (Jagsi et al. 2018). Only five (16.7%) patients experienced a DLT within

Table 9.1 Select ongoing clinical trials combining DNA damage response (DDR) inhibitors with radiation

Target	DDRi	Chemotherapy/biologic agent	RT details	Clinical Setting	Phase	Clinical trial identifier
PARP	Veliparib (concurrent)	mFOLFOX (pre-RT); capecitabine or pembro (concurrent)	50.4 Gy/5 weeks	LA rectal ca	II	NCT02921256
PARP	Niraparib (concurrent)	Carboplatin and paclitaxel (induction)	Definitive	Met cervical ca	I/II	NCT03644342
PARP	Olaparib (concurrent, maintenance)	TMZ (concurrent, maintenance)	60 Gy/30 fx/6 weeks	Unresectable GBM	I/IIa	NCT03212742
PARP	Niraparib (concurrent)	GnRH agonist (concurrent)	6–9 weeks	Prostate ca at high risk for recurrence	II	NCT04037254
PARP	Veliparib (concurrent, maintenance)	TMZ (maintenance)	30 fx/6–7 weeks	High-grade gliomas (H3 K27M and BRAF WT)	II	NCT03581292
PARP	Olaparib (concurrent)	None	6 weeks	Inflammatory breast ca w/ out distant mets	II	NCT03598257
WEE1	Adavosertib (concurrent)	TMZ (concurrent, maintenance)	30 fx/6 weeks	GBM	I	NCT01849146
WEE1	Adavosertib (concurrent)	Cisplatin (concurrent)	70 Gy/35 fx/7 weeks	LA HNSCC	I	NCT02585973
WEE1	Adavosertib (concurrent)	Cisplatin (concurrent)	30 fx/6 weeks	HNSCC	I	NCT03028766
WEE1	Adavosertib (concurrent)	None	30 fx/6 weeks	DIPG	I	NCT01922076
WEE1	Adavosertib (concurrent)	Cisplatin (concurrent)	45 Gy/25 fx/5 weeks	Cervical, vaginal, uterine ca	I	NCT03345784
DNA-PK	M3814 (concurrent)	Avelumab (concurrent)	30 Gy/10 fx/2 weeks	Advanced solid tumors/ mets	I	NCT03724890
DNA-PK	M3814 (concurrent)	Capecitabine (concurrent)	50 Gy/25 fx/5 weeks	LA rectal ca	I/II	NCT03770689

(continued)

Table 9.1 (continued)

Target	DDRi	Chemotherapy/biologic agent	RT details	Clinical Setting	Phase	Clinical trial identifier
DNA-PK	M3814 (concurrent)	Cisplatin (concurrent)	66 Gy/33 fx/7 weeks	Advanced solid tumors/mets	I	NCT02516813
ATM	M3541 (concurrent)	None	30 Gy/10 fx/2 weeks	Solid tumors	I	NCT03225105
ATM	AZD1390 (pre-RT, concurrent, post-RT)	None	A: 35 Gy/10 fx/2 weeks B: 30 Gy/10 fx/2 weeks C: 60 Gy/30 fx/6 weeks	A: Recurrent GBM B: Brain mets (WBRT) C: Primary GBM	I	NCT03423628
ATR	M6620 (18-30 h after first RT)	None	15 fx/3 weeks	NSCLC brain mets (WBRT)	I	NCT02589522
ATR	M6620 (start on day −7)	Cisplatin (concurrent)	35 fx/7 weeks	LA HPV (−) HNSCC	I	NCT02567422
ATR	AZD6738 (concurrent)	None	20 Gy/10 fx/2 weeks or 30 Gy/15 fx/3 weeks	Solid tumors refractory to conventional tx	I	NCT02223923

10 weeks from RT initiation; four were moist desquamation and one was neutropenia. Although severe acute toxicity did not exceed 30% at even the highest dose, nearly half of the surviving patients demonstrated G3 adverse events at 3 years. Of the 30 patients, 15 experienced disease control failures during the 3 years of follow-up and 13 died.

One of the most common tumor types demonstrating HRDness is pancreatic cancer (Heeke et al. 2018). A phase I study of 30 patients with locally advanced pancreatic cancer combined veliparib with concurrent chemo-RT (Tuli et al. 2019). The MTD of veliparib was 40 mg BID with gemcitabine 400 mg/m^2 and hypofractionated RT (36 Gy in 15 fractions). DLTs were monitored for 6 weeks and 16 were detected in 12 (40%) patients; the most common DLT was lymphopenia ($n = 10$). Notably, 25 (83.3%) patients experienced G3/4 lymphopenia. Median progression-free survival (PFS) and OS for all 30 patients was 9.8 and 14.6 months, respectively. Median OS for DDR pathway gene-altered- and DDR-intact patients was 19 and 14 months, respectively. The most commonly mutated DDR gene was *ARID1A* ($n = 4$). Loss of *ARID1A* impairs both checkpoint activation and the repair of DSBs, which sensitizes cells to DSB-inducing treatments such as PARP inhibitors and RT (Shen et al. 2015).

PARP inhibitors appear to confer promise as a radiosensitizing strategy for numerous malignancies; however, there are several important considerations for future trials testing PARP inhibitor treatment combinations. First, the toxicity profile varies significantly depending on both the site being investigated and the other agents used concurrently with PARP inhibitors. In particular, combining PARP inhibitors with chemotherapy has been problematic owing to substantial toxicity—predominately myelosuppression—requiring dose reductions and treatment delays, even in the absence of RT (Dréan et al. 2016; Pilié et al. 2019).

Additionally, because the toxicity profile of radiosensitizing agents appears to depend on the body site treated and the dose of RT delivered, disease site-specific phase I testing will be necessary to identify unique DLTs for the various combinations of PARP inhibitors, chemotherapy, and RT. For example, due to skin-related DLTs in head and neck (i.e., dermatitis, mucositis) and breast (i.e., moist desquamation) cancers, the RP2D is 25 mg BID for olaparib and 50 mg BID for veliparib, respectively. Conversely, the RP2D is 400 mg BID for rectal cancer concurrent with chemo-RT. Another consideration with the combination of PARP inhibitors and RT will be the neutralization of immunosuppressive negative feedback mechanisms such as upregulation of PD-L1 expression.

Lastly, identifying biomarkers for response to PARP inhibitor-induced radiosensitization will be important to target patients who will derive the most benefit from aggressive combination therapies (Table 9.2). Beyond germline or somatic *BRCA1/2* status, other markers of HRDness include high levels of genomic instability via global loss of heterozygosity and telomeric-allelic imbalances (Abkevich et al. 2012; Watkins et al. 2014). Other non-*BRCA* HRDness mutations include ARID1A deficiency, BAP1 deficiency, loss of CDK12 function, IDH1 mutations, and FEN1 mutations (Hanzlikova et al. 2018; Pilié et al. 2019). In addition to pursuing exploratory biomarker analysis during clinical trials, it will be

Table 9.2 Biomarkers associated with sensitivity to DNA damage response (DDR) inhibitors

Target	DDR inhibitor	Biomarker(s)
PARP	Talazoparib, Niraparib, Rucaparib, Olaparib, Veliparib	*BRCA1/2* mutations *RAD51* mutations *PALB2* mutations ARID1A deficiency BAP1 deficiency Loss of CDK12 function *IDH1/2* mutations *FEN1* mutations *ATM* mutations Loss of *Rb* Loss of heterozygosity Large-scale translocations Telomeric-allelic imbalances BET deficiency Elevated tumoral levels of PARP1, SLFN11, E-cadherin RPA exhaustion Histological phenotype of neuroendocrine differentiation
WEE1	Adavosertib (i.e., AZD1775)	*P53* mutations *BRCA1/2* mutations *FANC* mutations *KRAS* mutations *cMYC* mutations *SETD2* mutations CDKN2A deficiency RB1 deficiency Amplifications of *CCNE1*, *MYC*, *MYCL*, or *MYCN* Elevated levels of EZH2 H3K36me3 deficiency
DNA-PK	M3814	*P53* mutations HRD (particularly in the setting of high-LET RT)
ATM	M3541, AZD1390	*P53* mutations
ATR	AZD6738, M6620	*P53* mutations *BRCA1/2* mutations *RAD51* mutations *ATM* mutations *ARID1A* mutations MDM2 overexpression Rb loss of function cMYC or cyclin E1 amplification
CHK1	Prexasertib	*P53* mutations *KRAS* mutations

vital to move beyond a *BRCA1/2*-centric view of DDR biomarkers and investigate and a broader HRDness phenotype when attempting to identify patients who will respond to PARP inhibitors and other DDR inhibitors.

3.2 WEE1

WEE1 is a protein kinase with an important regulatory role in the cellular response to DNA damage (Fig. 9.1). It catalyzes the inhibitory phosphorylation of CDK1/2, thereby activating the G_2-M checkpoint and causing cell cycle arrest (Pilié et al. 2019). In addition, through negative regulation of CDK1/2, it prevents aberrant origin firing, nucleotide pool depletion, and replication stress (Beck et al. 2012; Krajewska et al. 2013). Furthermore, WEE1 promotes HRR (Krajewska et al. 2013; Karnak et al. 2014). Given WEE1's role as a critical mediator of the cellular response to DNA damage, it is a logical target for treatment strategies combining WEE1 inhibition with DNA-damaging agents such as RT and chemotherapy.

Adavosertib (i.e., AZD1775) is a first-in-class WEE1 inhibitor and the only WEE1 inhibitor currently in clinical development (Pilié et al. 2019). Preclinically, adavosertib is an effective radiosensitizer, particularly in the setting of chemo-RT (Kausar et al. 2015). Mechanistically, adavosertib abrogates the G_2-M checkpoint (Sarcar et al. 2011; Kausar et al. 2015), which enhances cancer cell death by forcing cells into mitosis with DNA damage leading to mitotic catastrophe and cell death. This is a tumor cell-selective mechanism given that the majority of cancers lack a G_1 checkpoint due to *TP53* mutation and therefore rely mainly on the G_2 checkpoint for cell cycle arrest upon DNA damage (Table 9.2). In addition to cell cycle effects, adavosertib induces DNA replication stress which is a key determinant of sensitization to RT and chemotherapy (Beck et al. 2012; Cuneo et al. 2016; Parsels et al. 2018b). Replication stress offers yet another potential tumor cell-selective mechanism given that oncogenic mutations in cancer, in particular *KRAS* or *cMYC* mutation, cause an increase in the baseline levels of replication stress making cancer cells especially vulnerable to agents which further exacerbate replication stress like those which target WEE1 (Kotsantis et al. 2018).

In addition to the effects of WEE1 inhibition on DNA, emerging evidence suggests that WEE1 inhibition may also have beneficial effects on anti-tumor immunity. WEE1 blockade by adavosertib has been shown to fully revert the resistance of (pancreatic) cancer cells undergoing epithelial-to-mesenchymal transition (EMT) to lysis by both antigen-specific T cells and natural killer cells (Hamilton et al. 2014). By reconstituting CDK1 activity, adavosertib improves immune-mediated attack of mesenchymal-like tumor cells by restoring CDK1-mediated nuclear lamin phosphorylation and consequently caspase-mediated apoptosis. Consistent with these studies, adavosertib was shown to promote anti-tumoral immunity through activation of CDK1 and abrogation of the G_2/M checkpoint, which otherwise protected cancer cells from immune-mediated cell death induced by cytotoxic T lymphocyte-derived granzyme B and TNFα (Sun et al.

2018; Patel et al. 2019). Furthermore, these anti-tumor immune effects of adavosertib are also associated with increased sensitivity to anti-PD-1 ICB, marked by increased antigen-specific T lymphocyte killing of tumor cells following treatment with adavosertib in combination with RT (Patel et al. 2019).

Second only to PARP inhibitors, adavosertib represents the most mature of the DDR inhibitors in the context of development as a radiosensitizer. A recently completed phase I study evaluated adavosertib in combination with RT and full-dose gemcitabine for 34 patients with locally advanced pancreatic cancer (Cuneo et al. 2019). The study's median OS finding of 21.7 months compares favorably with that of patients treated in the LAP07 trial (11.9–13.6 months), which had similar eligibility criteria and used gemcitabine (Hammel et al. 2016). Adavosertib was also well tolerated with only eight (24%) patients experiencing DLTs within the first 15 weeks of therapy; half of the DLTs were due to fatigue ($n = 2$) or anorexia/nausea ($n = 2$). Interestingly, the MTD of adavosertib (150 mg) with gemcitabine and concurrent RT was only slightly lower than the previously reported MTD with dual adavosertib and gemcitabine therapy (175 mg) (Cuneo et al. 2019). Numerous other active clinical trials are actively investigating the treatment combination of adavosertib plus RT with or without chemotherapy (Table 9.1).

3.3   DNA-PKcs

DNA-PKcs is a critical enzyme for NHEJ, which is the predominant repair mechanism for RT-induced DSBs (Fig. 9.1) (Willers et al. 2004; Morgan and Lawrence 2015). Following recognition of DSBs, NHEJ begins with the stabilization of free DNA ends mediated by binding of the KU70/80 heterodimers and subsequent recruitment of DNA-PKcs; 53BP1 and KU70/80 prevent DNA resection. NHEJ proceeds in a DNA-PK-dependent manner with recruitment of other downstream core NHEJ proteins including XRCC4, LIG4, XLF, and PAXX, which together mediate alignment and ligation of DNA ends. NHEJ likely represents the a priori DSB repair mechanism as other DSB repair pathways only occur following initial attempts to repair by NHEJ (Kakarougkas and Jeggo 2014).

Cells deficient in DNA-PKcs have significantly impaired DSB repair capacity and are markedly radiosensitive. This has been demonstrated both in vitro and in vivo using small-molecule DNA-PKcs inhibitors across a variety of cancer cell lines (Zhao et al. 2006; Shaheen et al. 2011; Li et al. 2012; Ciszewski et al. 2014; Timme et al. 2018; Sun et al. 2019). The exquisite radiosensitization conferred by DNA-PKcs inhibitors naturally prompts concerns regarding enhanced normal tissue toxicity. However, preclinical studies have demonstrated that DNA-PKcs inhibitors appear to operate as classic radiosensitizers since they cause minimal cytotoxicity to normal tissues outside of the irradiated target volume (Zhao et al. 2006; Shaheen et al. 2011; Ciszewski et al. 2014; Timme et al. 2018). Furthermore, a recent study assessed the DNA-PKcs inhibitor, VX-984, in combination with RT in two orthotopic glioblastoma multiforme (GBM) models and found no excessive weight loss or skin toxicity in the RT field in mice receiving combination therapy. Additionally, in the setting of minimal normal tissue toxicity, these mice derived a significant survival benefit from DNA-PKcs inhibitor plus RT (Timme et al. 2018). Finally, *TP53* mutation, a common discriminator between tumor and normal cells, is a determinant of radiosensitization by the DNA-PKcs inhibitor M3814, as *TP53*-deficient tumor cells are preferentially radiosensitized by M3814 compared to their isogenic *TP53* wild type counterparts (Table 9.2) (Sun et al. 2019).

Recent studies have evaluated the immunomodulatory role of DNA-PKcs inhibitor treatment in the setting of RT (Harding et al. 2017; Sun et al. 2018; Carr et al. 2019). While RT alone caused micronuclei formation in irradiated *TP53*-wild type MCF10A and prostate epithelial cells, inhibition of DNA-PKcs in combination with RT resulted in a diminished level of micronuclei despite the presence of elevated levels of DNA DSBs. Attenuated micronuclei formation following DNA-PKcs inhibition was associated with decreased innate immunity, a finding attributed to G_1 cell cycle arrest and consequently reduced mitotic mis-segregation leading to reduced micronuclei formation (Harding et al. 2017). It is reasonable to speculate from these data that inhibition of DNA-PKcs in *TP53*-mutant cancer cells—which lack a functional G_1 checkpoint—might increase radiation-induced micronuclei formation and hence innate immunity. This is supported by a recent study which showed that in response to RT, DNA-PKcs inhibition increased micronuclei formation resulting in a STING-driven inflammatory response, associated with expression of cytokines, chemokines, and PD-L1, as well as increased sensitivity to ICB (Carr et al. 2019). It is unclear, however, whether an intact G_2 checkpoint might protect *TP53*-mutant cancer cells from mitotic mis-segregation and micronuclei formation given that in some *TP53*-mutant models, DNA-PK inhibition reduces RT-induced micronuclei formation (Fig. 9.4).

Promising preclinical work with the DNA-PKcs inhibitor, M3814, has led to three active clinical trials investigating its radiosensitizing efficacy (Table 9.1). Preliminary anti-tumor activity was recently reported by one of the studies (Van Triest et al. 2018). In this phase Ia trial, involving 16 patients with tumors or

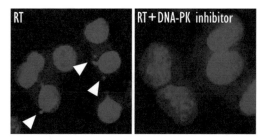

Fig. 9.4 Micronuclei following treatment with RT and DNA-PK inhibitor. Panc1 human pancreatic cancer cells were treated with 8 Gy +/− DNA-PK inhibitor (M3814). Three days after treatment, cells were fixed and stained with DAPI. Micronuclei located on the outside of the nucleus are indicated. Radiation-induced micronuclei generation was inhibited by DNA-PK inhibitor treatment. Image provided by Drs. Qiang Zhang and Weiwei Wang, University of Michigan

metastases in the head and neck or thoracic regions, M3814 was combined with palliative RT (30 Gy in ten fractions). Four DLTs were reported, three of which were G3 mucositis lasting >7 days. All patients with DLTs recovered without sequelae. Preliminary efficacy was reported via in-field response: One patient with a pathologic complete response, four with partial responses, seven with stable disease, three had not been evaluated, and one was not evaluable. The second arm of the phase Ia study is actively accruing patients for M3814 in combination with definitive fractionated RT (66-70 Gy in 33-35 fractions) and cisplatin (Van Triest et al. 2018). Only one of three active clinical trials using M3814 plus RT is using ICB to account for interferon-mediated PD-L1 upregulation (NCT03724890).

3.4 ATM

Ataxia telangiectasia mutated (ATM) is an apical kinase that plays a critical role in the detection, signaling, and repair of RT-induced DNA DSBs (Fig. 9.1). ATM is recruited to sites of DSBs via the MRE11-RAD50-NBS1 (MRN) complex, where it is activated by trans-autophosphorylation at Ser1981 (Bakkenist and Kastan 2003). ATM also phosphorylates the histone protein H2AX, which forms foci at DNA DSBs to promote the recruitment of additional ATM molecules and other repair factors (Blackford and Jackson 2017). The particular set of DDR proteins assembled— promoting either NHEJ or HRR—is biased by the phase of the cell cycle and the presence of homologous sister chromatid DNA. Two other important ATM target proteins—CHK2 and p53—provide the link to cell cycle checkpoints and apoptosis. The net result of ATM activation is the downstream activation of p53, leading to the transcription of the CDK inhibitor, p21, and the activation of CHK2, resulting in degradation of the CDC25 phosphatases, CDK-cyclin complex inactivation, and cell cycle arrest (DeVita Jr. et al. 2018).

The mechanisms for ATM inhibitor-induced radiosensitization have been explored extensively. In line with ATM's role as a regulator of cell cycle progression, *TP53*-mutant cells are preferentially radiosensitized by ATM inhibition (Table 9.2) (Biddlestone-Thorpe et al. 2013; Durant et al. 2018). Preclinical mechanistic studies have demonstrated that ATM inhibitors combined with RT cause cell cycle checkpoint abrogation, gross genomic instability, micronuclei formation, and apoptosis (Durant et al. 2018). These sequelae play a major role in the anti-tumoral immunostimulatory effects of ATM inhibitors. In vivo models of pancreatic cancer have shown that ATM inhibition induces TBK1 activation and T1IFN production, which is further enhanced by RT (Zhang et al. 2019). The increased interferon signaling that accompanies ATM inhibition also results in increased PD-L1 expression. Consequently, combination therapy with ATM inhibition plus RT sensitizes tumor cells to PD-L1 blockade.

Despite extensive preclinical testing of ATM as a therapeutic target for radiosensitization, and, more recently as an immune modulator, the clinical experience with ATM inhibition is limited. Currently, there are two ATM inhibitors

(M3541, AZD1390) in the early stages of clinical development as radiosensitizers (Table 9.1). In a phase I study, M3541 is being combined with palliative RT (i.e., 30 Gy in ten fractions) in patients with solid tumors (NCT03225105). In another phase I study, AZD1390 is being combined with RT for patients with various brain malignancies (NCT03423528).

3.5 ATR

Similar to the role of ATM in the cellular response to DSBs, ataxia telangiectasia Rad3-related (ATR) is an initiating kinase in the DDR to a variety of types of DNA damage including SSBs and replication stress. While ATR is also important for DSB repair, it is activated by a much wider range of genotoxic stresses compared to other related members of the PIKK family (e.g., ATM, DNA-PK) (Blackford and Jackson 2017). ATR is recruited to RPA-coated ssDNA by its stable binding partner ATR-interacting protein (ATRIP) and activated by topoisomerase binding partner 1 (TOPBP1) or Ewing's tumor-associated antigen 1 (ETAA1) (Kumagai et al. 2006; Haahr et al. 2016). Subsequently, ATR signaling leads to the phosphorylation and activation of CHK1 (Fig. 9.1). Activated CHK1 phosphorylates CDC25 and triggers its cytoplasmic sequestration and inactivation (Morgan and Lawrence 2015). In the absence of CDC25 phosphatase activity, CDK1 remains bound by inhibitory phosphorylation, resulting in G_2 arrest. This critical regulatory mechanism for the intra-S and G_2 checkpoints allows time for DNA repair in order to avoid premature mitotic entry and mitotic catastrophe after DNA damage; furthermore, if the damage is beyond repair, this allows for activation of apoptotic or senescent pathways (Blackford and Jackson 2017). Other important regulatory roles for ATR include slowing replication origin firing (Toledo et al. 2013), promoting replication fork repair (e.g., for DNA interstrand crosslinks) (Ceccaldi et al. 2016b), and managing nucleotide availability (Buisson et al. 2015).

ATR's crucial role in DDR signaling makes it an attractive target for radiosensitization. In order to identify tumors most likely to demonstrate ATR inhibitor-induced preferential radiosensitization, it is important to identify molecular features that increase dependence on ATR in the cellular response to DNA damage. Such features include loss of G_1 cell cycle checkpoint control resulting from mutations in *TP53*, as well as *MDM2* gain, and *RB* loss (Table 9.2). These molecular alterations increase reliance on ATR-mediated intra-S and G_2-M checkpoints following DNA damage (Reaper et al. 2011; Kwok et al. 2016; Tu et al. 2018). Other attractive targets for ATR inhibitors are tumors with high levels of oncogene-induced replication stress resulting from amplification of *MYC* or *CCNE1* encoding cyclin E1. These alterations drive cells to enter S phase, even in the presence of RT-induced ssDNA breaks, which can result in replication fork stalling (Halazonetis et al. 2008). In the setting of ATR inhibition, stalled replication forks might collapse, resulting in replication-associated DNA DSBs and cell death. Another subgroup of tumors that might be particularly susceptible to ATR inhibitors are those with functional deficiencies in HRR (Table 9.2). The absence or inhibition of HRR results in increased replication stress and ATR-mediated signaling; consequentially, ATR inhibition has been shown to preferentially target HRD cells (Krajewska et al. 2015). However, other studies in ovarian, colorectal, and triple-negative breast cancer have shown that ATR broadly sensitizes tumor cells to DNA-damaging agents, regardless of HRR status (Huntoon et al. 2013; Dillon et al. 2017; Tu et al. 2018).

An example of a tumor type that meets many of these criteria for sensitivity to ATR inhibitors is triple-negative breast cancer (TNBC). These tumors are often characterized by loss of G_1 checkpoint control, oncogene-induced replication stress, and HRR deficiency (Turner et al. 2004; Cancer Genome Atlas Network 2012; Nik-Zainal et al. 2016). In a recent study of TNBC, patient-derived tumor xenografts (PDX)—generated prospectively as part of the neoadjuvant BEAUTY trial—showed that surgical specimens with both chemosensitive and chemoresistant residual disease were highly radiosensitized following ATR inhibition (Tu et al. 2018). Moreover, ATR inhibition demonstrated greater radiosensitization of TNBC over normal cells within the irradiated target volume, and it showed little single-agent cytotoxicity at the dose required for radiosensitization outside of the irradiated target volume.

Another tumor type that appears to demonstrate preferential radiosensitization with ATR inhibitors is non-small cell lung carcinoma (NSCLC) (Dunne et al. 2017). Considering the widespread prevalence of stereotactic body RT (SBRT) for early-stage NSCLC, a preclinical study evaluated the impact of RT dose and fractionation on synergy with ATR inhibition (Dunne et al. 2017). The combination ATR inhibitor with fractionated RT (4 Gy x 3) was superior to single-dose (12 Gy) RT for tumor growth inhibition. Furthermore, radiosensitization by the ATR inhibitor was tumor cell selective as toxicity was not observed in relevant normal tissue (i.e., lung fibrosis).

One of the major mechanisms for ATR inhibitor-induced radiosensitization is G_2 checkpoint abrogation leading to mitotic catastrophe with acentric micronuclei formation (Dillon et al. 2017) leading to a robust immune response in immunocompetent hosts (Dillon et al. 2019). As previously described, this process involves activation of the cGAS-STING-TBK1-IRF3-NFκB signal transduction pathway, which activates innate immunity and subsequently adaptive immunity. ATR inhibitor plus RT produces a gene expression signature matching a T1IFN/T2IFN response, with upregulation of genes that play a role in PRR detection of nucleic acids (Dillon et al. 2019). These changes following ATR inhibitor-induced radiosensitization lead to significant elevations in cytokine and chemokine activity with increasing antigen presentation and immune infiltration.

The importance of ATR inhibitor as an immune modulator was assessed in a recent study by Vendetti and colleagues, which demonstrated that ATR inhibitor-induced radiosensitization is CD8[+] T cell-dependent for some tumors (Vendetti et al. 2018). This was observed in a syngeneic CT26 colorectal carcinoma mouse model and in a GEMM of *Kras*[G12D]/*Twist1* lung adenocarcinoma. The study showed that the ATR inhibitor, AZD6738, blocked PD-L1 upregulation on tumor cells and dramatically decreased the number of immunosuppressive tumor-infiltrating T-regulatory cells (T_{regs}). In these tumor models, ATR inhibition not only potentiated the cytotoxic effects of RT, but also acted as an immune stimulant by increasing the immunogenicity of the tumor microenvironment.

The preclinical success of ATR inhibitors in combination with RT has motivated several phase I clinical trials (Table 9.1). PATRIOT is an ongoing three-part trial assessing the feasibly and safety of the ATR inhibitor, AZD6738, as a single agent and in combination with different schedules of RT (NCT02223923) (Dillon et al. 2018). Another ATR inhibitor, M6620, will be combined with cisplatin to assess sensitization to chemoradiation in locally advanced HNSCC (NCT02567422, Table 9.1). In addition to acting as a robust radiosensitizer, ATR inhibitor has also been shown to synergize with cisplatin (Vendetti et al. 2015), which is likely due to ATR's role in replication fork repair. As a result, this study combines all three treatment modalities in an attempt to optimize anti-tumoral synergy. In addition, M6620 is being investigated in combination with whole-brain RT for patients with NSCLC brain metastases (NCT02589522).

3.6 CHK1

Checkpoint kinase 1 (CHK1) plays a central role in both S phase and G_2 checkpoints (Fig. 9.1). It is activated in an ATR-dependent manner in response to either DNA damage or replication stress (Morgan and Lawrence 2015). Subsequently, CHK1 phosphorylates and inhibits CDC25A/C proteins, resulting in activation of the intra-S and G_2 checkpoints (Sørensen and Syljuåsen 2012). Additional CHK1 functions include promoting HRR (Sørensen et al. 2005), stabilizing stalled replication forks (Syljuåsen et al. 2005), and preventing excess origin firing. Through these actions, CHK1 facilitates cellular recovery from DNA damage and alleviates replication stress (Petermann et al. 2010). Thus, impairment of the DDR through CHK1 inhibition renders cells more sensitive to DNA damage.

In the preclinical setting, CHK1 inhibitors preferentially radiosensitize *TP53*-mutant cancers (Table 9.2) (Morgan et al. 2010). This is partly due to abrogation of the G_2 checkpoint by CHK1 inhibitors, which is particularly deleterious in *TP53*-mutant cancers that lack a functional G_1 checkpoint. Additionally, the ability of CHK1 inhibitors to inhibit HRR (Morgan et al. 2010; Engelke et al. 2013) may also play a significant role in their selective radiosensitization, as *TP53*-mutant cancer cells are more likely than normal cells to rely on HRR for DSB repair due to their inability to arrest in G_1 where NHEJ is the dominant DSB repair mechanism. Cell cycle-independent HRR preference in *TP53*-mutant cells has been reported as well. Moreover, CHK1 inhibitors cause DNA damage in replicating cells (Forment et al. 2011; Thompson et al. 2012), which could disproportionately affect tumor cells relative to normal cells based on their high fraction of cycling cells and elevated levels of endogenous DNA damage due to genetic aberrations (Sørensen and Syljuåsen 2012).

CHK1 inhibitor-induced preferential radiosensitization of tumor cells relative to normal cells has been demonstrated in pancreatic cancer (Morgan et al. 2010; Engelke et al. 2013) and HNSCC (Zeng et al. 2017). In addition to the mechanisms detailed above, tumor cell-selective radiosensitization by CHK1 inhibitors could also be due to the aberrant activity of oncogenes such as of *KRAS* which is especially relevant in pancreatic cancer and causes replication stress, genomic instability, endogenous DNA damage, and an increased reliance on DDR pathways such as those mediated by ATR/CHK1 (Table 9.2) (Morgan and Lawrence 2015). Studies have shown that CHK1 inhibitors confers greater radiosensitization in isogenic *KRAS*-mutant vs. *KRAS*-wild type cancer cells (Morgan et al. 2014) (Dinkelborg et al. 2019).

Although certain KRAS variants have been found in HNSCC (Weidhaas et al. 2017), preferential radiosensitization for this tumor type is also likely related to the significant upregulation of CHK1 and CHK2 phosphoproteins at baseline in HNSCC compared to normal surrounding tissue (Frederick et al. 2011). Upregulation of DDR elements—in this case cell cycle checkpoint proteins—is possibly a mechanism of resistance that can be exploited through CHK1 inhibition. In one study of HNSCC, CHK1 inhibition with prexasertib plus RT was comparable to anti-EGFR therapy plus RT (Zeng et al. 2017).

Despite their success in the preclinical setting, the clinical development of CHK1 inhibitors has been slowed by cardiac toxicities and off-target effects of earlier agents (AZD7762, rabusertib, MK-8776) (Pilié et al. 2019). Currently, there is one clinical trial evaluating CHK1 inhibition as a radiosensitization strategy for locally advanced HNSCC (NCT02555644). This phase I study is combining the second-generation CHK1-selective inhibitor, prexasertib, with concurrent intensity-modulated RT (IMRT) plus either cisplatin or cetuximab. The study recently completed recruitment, but no results have been posted.

The major molecular characteristics associated with the tumor cell selectivity of CHK1 inhibitor-mediated radiosensitization, such as mutations in *TP53* and *KRAS*, make the treatment combinations of CHK1 inhibition plus RT attractive for a wide variety of malignancies. In addition, CHK1 inhibition also appears to have a role in augmenting anti-PD-L1 therapy through promoting cytotoxic T lymphocyte tumor infiltration and activation (Sen et al. 2019). Due to the unfortunate history of off-target effects during clinical testing with early CHK1 inhibitors, it is likely that the outcome of the most recent prexasertib clinical trial will be a major determinant in the future of this drug class in the setting of RT.

4   DDR Inhibitor Combinations with RT

Strategic combinations of DDR inhibitors have the potential to overcome acquired resistance to DDR inhibitor monotherapy and induce synthetic lethality. Furthermore, preclinical work has demonstrated that DDR inhibitor combinations can induce profound radiosensitization. In preclinical tumor models, combining PARP inhibitors and WEE1 inhibitors is an effective radiosensitization strategy for both pancreatic cancer (Karnak et al. 2014) and *KRAS*-mutant NSCLC (Parsels et al. 2018a). Mechanistically, in addition to the established functions of WEE1 and PARP in the cell cycle and SSB repair, respectively, replication stress contributes to radiosensitization by WEE1 and PARP inhibition. Specifically, this replication stress involves depletion of nucleotide pools and PARP1-DNA binding (i.e., PARP trapping). Overall, these studies implicate DNA replication stress as an effective therapeutic target for radiosensitization and suggest that targets directly involved in maintaining DNA replication forks stability may be especially efficacious. One such combination is ATR and PARP. Given the direct involvement of ATR in mitigating DNA replication stress and the effects of trapped PARP on DNA replication, the combination of ATR inhibitors and PARP inhibitors as a radiosensitizing strategy is appealing, especially in cancers with elevated replication stress.

Accumulating evidence suggests that the inevitable recurrence of GBM after chemo-RT is largely driven by radioresistant GBM cancer stem-like cells (GSC), which drive resistance to DNA-damaging therapies through constitutive upregulation of ATR and CHK1 kinase (Carruthers et al. 2018). One potential source of replication stress in GSCs is the elevated transcription of "very long genes" by RNA polymerase that may inadvertently collide with late replicating regions of the genome, activating the ATR replication stress response, which in turn promotes cell survival and radioresistance. PARP inhibitor alone is insufficient to radiosensitize this GSC population; however, combining ATR inhibitors and PARP inhibitors induces profound radiosensitization.

Clinical trials are currently underway assessing numerous DDR inhibitor–DDR inhibitor combinations, including combinations of inhibitors targeting ATR-PARP (NCT02723864), WEE1-PARP (NCT02511795), and ATM-PARP (NCT02588105). Unfortunately, no clinical studies are currently evaluating the combination of multiple DDR inhibitors in the setting of RT. A major obstacle is the overlapping toxicity profiles of many DDR inhibitors—especially myelosuppression—that will need to be addressed through optimizing dosing and treatment scheduling of the DDR inhibitor–DDR inhibitor combinations before introducing RT.

5 Sequencing: Mechanistic Considerations

The majority of the clinical trials evaluating DDR inhibitors have administered the drug in a logical sequence relative to the timing of irradiation, that is, by administrating DDR inhibitors *before* the initiation of RT, these agents are able to preemptively neutralize various DNA repair pathways, thereby maximizing the lethality of subsequent DNA-damaging RT. Another important consideration is the optimization of DDR inhibitor-induced anti-tumoral activity. Since most radiosensitizers—with the possible exception of ATR inhibitors—lead to adaptive upregulation of PD-L1 expression, treatment regimens involving RT and most DDR inhibitors will need to consider anti-PD-1/PD-L1 to address immunosuppressive negative feedback mechanisms. While no randomized controlled trials have evaluated the impact of the timing of ICB administration relative to RT, preclinical studies have predominately supported initiating ICB before—or concurrent with— RT (Dovedi et al. 2014; Young et al. 2016). Mechanistically, this is supported by significant upregulation of tumor PD-L1 expression at 24-48 h post-RT (Sato et al. 2017) and elevated PD-1 expression on tumor-infiltrating CD4$^+$ and CD8$^+$ T cells at 24 h post-RT (Dovedi et al. 2014). Delaying the blockade of PD-1/PD-L1 signaling until after the completion of an RT cycle might limit efficacy due to anergy of tumor-reactive CD8$^+$ T cell by that later timepoint.

In the landmark PACIFIC trial in locally advanced NSCLC, patients derived an OS survival benefit from anti-PD-L1 treatment using a trial design in which they received potentially lymphocyte-depleting interventions before anti-PD-L1 therapy (i.e., durvalumab): chemotherapy, conventional fractionated RT, and irradiation of draining lymph nodes where T cells are primed to TAAs of irradiated tumor cells (Antonia et al. 2018). A post hoc analysis showed that patients who received durvalumab within 14 days following completion of chemo-RT demonstrated a greater OS benefit compared to those who received durvalumab later although selection bias can also explain this observation. If positive outcomes were achieved in this setting of potential immunosuppression, one could speculate that the potential benefits might be even more pronounced with *hypofractionated* RT, *concurrent* ICB, and less intensive chemotherapy. Clinical trials with concurrent ICB are in progress in this patient population.

The timing of treatment strategies combining RT with DDR inhibitors and ICB will be critical to optimize patient outcomes. And while preclinical studies suggest starting ICB before—or concurrently with—RT confers improved survival, clinical trials will need to assess this question in a randomized manner.

6   Conclusions

The DDR is a clinically validated target that may be most effective in combination with tumor cell-selective DNA-damaging agents like RT. To improve outcomes with this treatment combination, the development of functionally based predictive biomarker assays will be vital. Genomic biomarkers such as *TP53* mutation status may additionally aid the selection of patients most likely to benefit from RT/drug combinations. Furthermore, there is a prominent immune-modulation component to DDR inhibitor-induced radiosensitization, and it will be critical to optimize anti-tumoral immunity through RT dose, fractionation, treatment modality, DDR inhibitor dose/sequencing, minimizing lymphopenia, and mitigation of negative feedback mechanisms (e.g., PD-L1 expression).

References

Abkevich V et al (2012) Patterns of genomic loss of heterozygosity predict homologous recombination repair defects in epithelial ovarian cancer. Br J Cancer 107(10):1776–1782. https://doi.org/10.1038/bjc.2012.451

Ang KK et al (2010) Human papillomavirus and survival of patients with oropharyngeal cancer. N Engl J Med 363(1):24–35. https://doi.org/10.1056/NEJMoa0912217

Antonia SJ et al (2018) Overall survival with durvalumab after chemoradiotherapy in stage III NSCLC. N Engl J Med 379(24):2342–2350. https://doi.org/10.1056/NEJMoa1809697

Bakkenist CJ, Kastan MB (2003) DNA damage activates ATM through intermolecular autophosphorylation and dimer dissociation. Nature 421(6922):499–506. https://doi.org/10.1038/nature01368

Beck H et al (2012) Cyclin-dependent kinase suppression by WEE1 kinase protects the genome through control of replication initiation and nucleotide consumption. Mol Cell Biol 32(20):4226–4236. https://doi.org/10.1128/MCB.00412-12

Biddlestone-Thorpe L et al (2013) ATM kinase inhibition preferentially sensitizes p53-mutant glioma to ionizing radiation. Clin Cancer Res 19(12):3189–3200. https://doi.org/10.1158/1078-0432.CCR-12-3408

Blackford AN, Jackson SP (2017) ATM, ATR, and DNA-PK: the trinity at the heart of the DNA damage response. Mol Cell 66(6):801–817. https://doi.org/10.1016/j.molcel.2017.05.015

Bridges KA et al (2014) Niraparib (MK-4827), a novel poly(ADP-ribose) polymerase inhibitor, radiosensitizes human lung and breast cancer cells. Oncotarget 5(13):5076–5086. https://doi.org/10.18632/oncotarget.2083

Bryant HE et al (2005) Specific killing of BRCA2-deficient tumours with inhibitors of poly(ADP-ribose) polymerase. Nature 434(7035):913–917. https://doi.org/10.1038/nature03443

Buisson R et al (2015) Distinct but concerted roles of ATR, DNA-PK, and Chk1 in countering replication stress during S phase. Mol Cell 59(6):1011–1024. https://doi.org/10.1016/j.molcel.2015.07.029

Bunting SF et al (2010) 53BP1 inhibits homologous recombination in Brca1-deficient cells by blocking resection of DNA breaks. Cell 141(2):243–254

Cancer Genome Atlas Network (2012) Comprehensive molecular portraits of human breast tumours. Nature 490(7418):61–70. https://doi.org/10.1038/nature11412

Caron M-C et al (2019) Poly(ADP-ribose) polymerase-1 antagonizes DNA resection at double-strand breaks. Nat Commun 10(1):2954. https://doi.org/10.1038/s41467-019-10741-9

Carr M et al (2019) Abstract 2923: DNA-PK inhibitor, M3814, is a potent inducer of inflammatory micronucleation in irradiated p53-deficient cancer cells: implications for combination radio-immunotherapy. Cancer Res.. American Association for Cancer Research 79(13 Supplement):2923. https://doi.org/10.1158/1538-7445.AM2019-2923

Carruthers RD et al (2018) Replication stress drives constitutive activation of the DNA damage response and radioresistance in glioblastoma stem-like cells. Cancer Res 78(17):5060–5071. https://doi.org/10.1158/0008-5472.CAN-18-0569

Ceccaldi R, Rondinelli B, D'Andrea AD (2016a) Repair pathway choices and consequences at the double-strand break. Trends Cell Biol 26(1):52–64. https://doi.org/10.1016/j.tcb.2015.07.009

Ceccaldi R, Sarangi P, D'Andrea AD (2016b) The Fanconi anaemia pathway: new players and new functions. Nat Rev Mol Cell Biol 17(6):337–349. https://doi.org/10.1038/nrm.2016.48

Ciszewski WM et al (2014) DNA-PK inhibition by NU7441 sensitizes breast cancer cells to ionizing radiation and doxorubicin. Breast Cancer Res Treat 143(1):47–55. https://doi.org/10.1007/s10549-013-2785-6

Cuneo KC et al (2016) Wee1 kinase inhibitor AZD1775 radiosensitizes hepatocellular carcinoma regardless of TP53 mutational status through induction of replication stress. Int J Radiat Oncol Biol Phys 95(2):782–790. https://doi.org/10.1016/j.ijrobp.2016.01.028

Cuneo KC et al (2019) Dose escalation trial of the Wee1 inhibitor Adavosertib (AZD1775) in combination with gemcitabine and radiation for patients with locally advanced pancreatic cancer. J Clin Oncol:JCO1900730. https://doi.org/10.1200/JCO.19.00730

DeVita VT Jr, Lawrence TS, Rosenberg SA (2018) In: DeVita SA Jr, Vincent T, Lawrence TS, Rosenberg (eds) Essentials of radiation therapy: from cancer: principles & practice of oncology, 11th edn. Lippincott Williams & Wilkins (LWW), Philadelphia, PA

Dillon MT et al (2017) Radiosensitization by the ATR inhibitor AZD6738 through generation of acentric micronuclei. Mol Cancer Ther 16(1):25–34. https://doi.org/10.1158/1535-7163. MCT-16-0239

Dillon MT et al (2018) PATRIOT: a phase I study to assess the tolerability, safety and biological effects of a specific ataxia telangiectasia and Rad3-related (ATR) inhibitor (AZD6738) as a single agent and in combination with palliative radiation therapy in patients with solid tumours. Clin Transl Radiat Oncol 12:16–20. https://doi.org/10.1016/j.ctro.2018.06.001

Dillon MT et al (2019) ATR inhibition potentiates the radiation-induced inflammatory tumor microenvironment. Clin Cancer Res 25(11):3392–3403. https://doi.org/10.1158/1078-0432. CCR-18-1821

Ding L et al (2018) PARP inhibition elicits STING-dependent antitumor immunity in Brca1-deficient ovarian cancer. Cell Rep 25(11):2972–2980.e5. https://doi.org/10.1016/j.celrep.2018.11.054

Dinkelborg PH, Wang M, Gheorghiu L, Gurski JM, Hong TS, Cyril H, Juric BD, Jimenez RB, Borgmann K, Willers H, (2019) A common Chk1-dependent phenotype of DNA double-strand break suppression in two distinct radioresistant cancer types. Breast Cancer Res Treat 174(3):605–613

Dovedi SJ et al (2014) Acquired resistance to fractionated radiotherapy can be overcome by concurrent PD-L1 blockade. Cancer Res 74(19):5458–5468. https://doi.org/10.1158/0008-5472. CAN-14-1258

Dréan A, Lord CJ, Ashworth A (2016) PARP inhibitor combination therapy. Crit Rev Oncol Hematol 108:73–85. https://doi.org/10.1016/j.critrevonc.2016.10.010

Dunne V et al (2017) Inhibition of ataxia telangiectasia related-3 (ATR) improves therapeutic index in preclinical models of non-small cell lung cancer (NSCLC) radiotherapy. Radiother Oncol 124(3):475–481. https://doi.org/10.1016/j.radonc.2017.06.025

Durant ST et al (2018) The brain-penetrant clinical ATM inhibitor AZD1390 radiosensitizes and improves survival of preclinical brain tumor models. Sci Adv 4(6):eaat1719. https://doi. org/10.1126/sciadv.aat1719

Engelke CG et al (2013) Sensitization of pancreatic cancer to chemoradiation by the Chk1 inhibitor MK8776. Clin Cancer Res 19(16):4412–4421. https://doi.org/10.1158/1078-0432. CCR-12-3748

Farmer H et al (2005) Targeting the DNA repair defect in BRCA mutant cells as a therapeutic strategy. Nature 434(7035):917–921. https://doi.org/10.1038/nature03445

Forment JV et al (2011) Structure-specific DNA endonuclease Mus81/Eme1 generates DNA damage caused by Chk1 inactivation. PLoS One. Edited by M. Muzi-Falconi 6(8):e23517. https://doi.org/10.1371/journal.pone.0023517

Frederick MJ et al (2011) Phosphoproteomic analysis of signaling pathways in head and neck squamous cell carcinoma patient samples. Am J Pathol 178(2):548–571. https://doi. org/10.1016/j.ajpath.2010.10.044

Galluzzi L et al (2017) Immunogenic cell death in cancer and infectious disease. Nat Rev Immunol 17(2):97–111. https://doi.org/10.1038/nri.2016.107

Haahr P et al (2016) Activation of the ATR kinase by the RPA-binding protein ETAA1. Nat Cell Biol 18(11):1196–1207. https://doi.org/10.1038/ncb3422

Halazonetis TD, Gorgoulis VG, Bartek J (2008) An oncogene-induced DNA damage model for cancer development. Science 319(5868):1352–1355. https://doi.org/10.1126/science.1140735

Hamilton DH et al (2014) WEE1 inhibition alleviates resistance to immune attack of tumor cells undergoing epithelial-mesenchymal transition. Cancer Res 74(9):2510–2519. https://doi. org/10.1158/0008-5472.CAN-13-1894

Hammel P et al (2016) Effect of chemoradiotherapy vs chemotherapy on survival in patients with locally advanced pancreatic cancer controlled after 4 months of gemcitabine with or without Erlotinib. JAMA 315(17):1844. https://doi.org/10.1001/jama.2016.4324

Hanzlikova H et al (2018) The importance of poly(ADP-ribose) polymerase as a sensor of Unligated Okazaki fragments during DNA replication. Mol Cell 71(2):319–331.e3. https://doi.org/10.1016/j.molcel.2018.06.004

Harding SM et al (2017) Mitotic progression following DNA damage enables pattern recognition within micronuclei. Nature 548(7668):466–470. https://doi.org/10.1038/nature23470

Hatch EM et al (2013) Catastrophic nuclear envelope collapse in cancer cell micronuclei. Cell 154(1):47–60. https://doi.org/10.1016/j.cell.2013.06.007

Heeke AL et al (2018) Prevalence of homologous recombination-related gene mutations across multiple cancer types. JCO Precis Oncol. NIH Public Access, 2018. https://doi.org/10.1200/PO.17.00286

Huntoon CJ et al (2013) ATR inhibition broadly sensitizes ovarian cancer cells to chemotherapy independent of BRCA status. Cancer Res 73(12):3683–3691. https://doi.org/10.1158/0008-5472.CAN-13-0110

Jagsi R et al (2018) Concurrent veliparib with chest wall and nodal radiotherapy in patients with inflammatory or locoregionally recurrent breast cancer: the TBCRC 024 phase I multicenter study. J Clin Oncol 36(13):1317–1322. https://doi.org/10.1200/JCO.2017.77.2665

Jiao S et al (2017) PARP inhibitor upregulates PD-L1 expression and enhances cancer-associated immunosuppression. Clin Cancer Res 23(14):3711–3720. https://doi.org/10.1158/1078-0432.CCR-16-3215

Kakarougkas A, Jeggo PA (2014) DNA DSB repair pathway choice: an orchestrated handover mechanism. Br J Radiol 87(1035):20130685. https://doi.org/10.1259/bjr.20130685

Karam SD et al (2018) Final report of a phase I trial of olaparib with cetuximab and radiation for heavy smoker patients with locally advanced head and neck cancer. Clin Cancer Res 24(20):4949–4959. https://doi.org/10.1158/1078-0432.CCR-18-0467

Karnak D et al (2014) Combined inhibition of Wee1 and PARP1/2 for radiosensitization in pancreatic cancer. Clin Cancer Res 20(19):5085–5096. https://doi.org/10.1158/1078-0432.CCR-14-1038

Kausar T et al (2015) Sensitization of pancreatic cancers to gemcitabine chemoradiation by WEE1 kinase inhibition depends on homologous recombination repair. Neoplasia (New York, NY) 17(10):757–766. https://doi.org/10.1016/j.neo.2015.09.006

Kotsantis P, Petermann E, Boulton SJ (2018) Mechanisms of oncogene-induced replication stress: jigsaw falling into place. Cancer Discov 8(5):537–555. https://doi.org/10.1158/2159-8290.CD-17-1461

Krajewska M et al (2013) Forced activation of Cdk1 via wee1 inhibition impairs homologous recombination. Oncogene 32(24):3001–3008. https://doi.org/10.1038/onc.2012.296

Krajewska M et al (2015) ATR inhibition preferentially targets homologous recombination-deficient tumor cells. Oncogene 34(26):3474–3481. https://doi.org/10.1038/onc.2014.276

Kumagai A et al (2006) TopBP1 activates the ATR-ATRIP complex. Cell 124(5):943–955. https://doi.org/10.1016/j.cell.2005.12.041

Kwok M et al (2016) ATR inhibition induces synthetic lethality and overcomes chemoresistance in TP53- or ATM-defective chronic lymphocytic leukemia cells. Blood 127(5):582–595. https://doi.org/10.1182/blood-2015-05-644872

Laird JH et al (2018) Talazoparib is a potent Radiosensitizer in small cell lung cancer cell lines and Xenografts. Clin Cancer Res 24(20):5143–5152. https://doi.org/10.1158/1078-0432.CCR-18-0401

Lesueur P et al (2017) Poly-(ADP-ribose)-polymerase inhibitors as radiosensitizers: a systematic review of pre-clinical and clinical human studies. Oncotarget 8(40):69105–69124. https://doi.org/10.18632/oncotarget.19079

Li YH et al (2012) Inhibition of non-homologous end joining repair impairs pancreatic cancer growth and enhances radiation response. PLoS One 7(6):1–10. https://doi.org/10.1371/journal. pone.0039588

Lord CJ, Ashworth A (2017) PARP inhibitors: synthetic lethality in the clinic. Science 355(6330):1152–1158. https://doi.org/10.1126/science.aam7344

Maya-Mendoza A et al (2018) High speed of fork progression induces DNA replication stress and genomic instability. Nature 559(7713):279–284. https://doi.org/10.1038/s41586-018-0261-5

Minn AJ (2015) Interferons and the immunogenic effects of cancer therapy. Trends Immunol 36(11):725–737. https://doi.org/10.1016/j.it.2015.09.007

Morgan MA, Lawrence TS (2015) Molecular pathways: overcoming radiation resistance by targeting DNA damage response pathways. Clin Cancer Res 21(13):2898–2904. https://doi. org/10.1158/1078-0432.CCR-13-3229

Morgan MA et al (2010) Mechanism of radiosensitization by the Chk1/2 inhibitor AZD7762 involves abrogation of the G2 checkpoint and inhibition of homologous recombinational DNA repair. Cancer Res 70(12):4972–4981. https://doi.org/10.1158/0008-5472.CAN-09-3573

Morgan MA et al (2014) Improving the efficacy of chemoradiation with targeted agents. Cancer Discov 4(3):280–291. https://doi.org/10.1158/2159-8290.CD-13-0337

Mouw KW et al (2017) DNA damage and repair biomarkers of immunotherapy response. Cancer Discov 7(7):675–693. https://doi.org/10.1158/2159-8290.CD-17-0226

Nik-Zainal S et al (2016) Landscape of somatic mutations in 560 breast cancer whole-genome sequences. Nature 534(7605):47–54. https://doi.org/10.1038/nature17676

Parsels LA, Karnak D et al (2018a) PARP1 trapping and DNA replication stress enhance Radiosensitization with combined WEE1 and PARP inhibitors. Mol Cancer Res 16(2):222–232. https://doi.org/10.1158/1541-7786.MCR-17-0455

Parsels LA, Parsels JD et al (2018b) The contribution of DNA replication stress marked by high-intensity, pan-nuclear γH2AX staining to chemosensitization by CHK1 and WEE1 inhibitors. Cell Cycle 17(9):1076–1086. https://doi.org/10.1080/15384101.2018.1475827

Patel AG, Sarkaria JN, Kaufmann SH (2011) Nonhomologous end joining drives poly(ADP-ribose) polymerase (PARP) inhibitor lethality in homologous recombination-deficient cells. Proc Natl Acad Sci 108(8):3406–3411. https://doi.org/10.1073/pnas.1013715108

Patel P, Sun L, Robbins Y, Clavijo, Paul E, et al (2019) 'Enhancing direct cytotoxicity and response to immune checkpoint blockade following ionizing radiation with Wee1 kinase inhibition', OncoImmunology. Taylor and Francis Inc., 8(11). https://doi.org/10.1080/21624 02X.2019.1638207

Petermann E, Woodcock M, Helleday T (2010) Chk1 promotes replication fork progression by controlling replication initiation. Proc Natl Acad Sci U S A 107(37):16090–16095. https://doi. org/10.1073/pnas.1005031107

Pilié PG et al (2019) State-of-the-art strategies for targeting the DNA damage response in cancer. Nat Rev Clin Oncol. Springer US 16(2):81–104. https://doi.org/10.1038/s41571-018-0114-z

Pommier Y, OConnor MJ, de Bono J (2016) Laying a trap to kill cancer cells: PARP inhibitors and their mechanisms of action. Sci Transl Med 8(362):362ps17–362ps17. https://doi.org/10.1126/ scitranslmed.aaf9246

Reaper PM et al (2011) Selective killing of ATM- or p53-deficient cancer cells through inhibition of ATR. Nat Chem Biol 7(7):428–430. https://doi.org/10.1038/nchembio.573

Reichert ZR, Wahl DR, Morgan MA (2016) Translation of targeted radiation sensitizers into clinical trials. Semin Radiat Oncol 26(4):261–270. https://doi.org/10.1016/j.semradonc.2016.06.001

Sarcar B et al (2011) Targeting radiation-induced G(2) checkpoint activation with the Wee-1 inhibitor MK-1775 in glioblastoma cell lines. Mol Cancer Ther 10(12):2405–2414. https://doi. org/10.1158/1535-7163.MCT-11-0469

Sato H et al (2017) DNA double-strand break repair pathway regulates PD-L1 expression in cancer cells. Nat Commun 8(1):1751. https://doi.org/10.1038/s41467-017-01883-9

Sen T et al (2019) Targeting DNA damage response promotes antitumor immunity through STING-mediated T-cell activation in small cell lung cancer. Cancer Discov 9(5):646–661. https://doi.org/10.1158/2159-8290.CD-18-1020

Shaheen FS et al (2011) Targeting the DNA double strand break repair machinery in prostate cancer. PLoS One 6(5):1–7. https://doi.org/10.1371/journal.pone.0020311

Shen J et al (2015) ARID1A deficiency impairs the DNA damage checkpoint and sensitizes cells to PARP inhibitors. Cancer Discov 5(7):752–767. https://doi.org/10.1158/2159-8290.CD-14-0849

Shen J et al (2019) PARPi triggers the STING-dependent immune response and enhances the therapeutic efficacy of immune checkpoint blockade independent of BRCAness. Cancer Res 79(2):311–319. https://doi.org/10.1158/0008-5472.CAN-18-1003

Sørensen CS, Syljuåsen RG (2012) Safeguarding genome integrity: the checkpoint kinases ATR, CHK1 and WEE1 restrain CDK activity during normal DNA replication. Nucleic Acids Res 40(2):477–486. https://doi.org/10.1093/nar/gkr697

Sørensen CS et al (2005) The cell-cycle checkpoint kinase Chk1 is required for mammalian homologous recombination repair. Nat Cell Biol 7(2):195–201. https://doi.org/10.1038/ncb1212

Sun L et al (2018) WEE1 kinase inhibition reverses G2/M cell cycle checkpoint activation to sensitize cancer cells to immunotherapy. Onco Targets Ther 7(10):e1488359. https://doi.org/10.1080/2162402X.2018.1488359

Sun Q et al (2019) Therapeutic implications of p53 status on cancer cell fate following exposure to ionizing radiation and the DNA-PK inhibitor M3814. Mol Cancer Res,. p. molcanres.0362.2019. https://doi.org/10.1158/1541-7786.MCR-19-0362

Syljuåsen RG et al (2005) Inhibition of human Chk1 causes increased initiation of DNA replication, phosphorylation of ATR targets, and DNA breakage. Mol Cell Biol 25(9):3553–3562. https://doi.org/10.1128/MCB.25.9.3553-3562.2005

Thompson R, Montano R, Eastman A (2012) The Mre11 nuclease is critical for the sensitivity of cells to Chk1 inhibition. PLoS One. Edited by K. Borgmann 7(8):e44021. https://doi.org/10.1371/journal.pone.0044021

Timme CR et al (2018) The DNA-PK inhibitor VX-984 enhances the radiosensitivity of glioblastoma cells grown *In Vitro* and as orthotopic xenografts. Mol Cancer Ther 17(6):1207–1216. https://doi.org/10.1158/1535-7163.MCT-17-1267

Toledo LI et al (2013) ATR prohibits replication catastrophe by preventing global exhaustion of RPA. Cell 155(5):1088–1103. https://doi.org/10.1016/j.cell.2013.10.043

Tu X et al (2018) ATR inhibition is a promising radiosensitizing strategy for triple-negative breast cancer. Mol Cancer Ther 17(11):2462–2472. https://doi.org/10.1158/1535-7163.MCT-18-0470

Tuli R et al (2019) A phase 1 study of veliparib, a PARP-1/2 inhibitor, with gemcitabine and radiotherapy in locally advanced pancreatic cancer. EBioMedicine 40:375–381. https://doi.org/10.1016/j.ebiom.2018.12.060

Turner N, Tutt A, Ashworth A (2004) Hallmarks of "BRCAness" in sporadic cancers. Nat Rev Cancer 4(10):814–819. https://doi.org/10.1038/nrc1457

Van Triest B et al (2018) A phase Ia/Ib trial of the DNA-PK inhibitor M3814 in combination with radiotherapy (RT) in patients (pts) with advanced solid tumors: dose-escalation results. J Clin Oncol 36(15_suppl):2518. https://doi.org/10.1200/JCO.2018.36.15_suppl.2518

Vendetti FP et al (2015) The orally active and bioavailable ATR kinase inhibitor AZD6738 potentiates the anti-tumor effects of cisplatin to resolve ATM-deficient non-small cell lung cancer in vivo. Oncotarget 6(42):44289–44305. https://doi.org/10.18632/oncotarget.6247

Vendetti FP et al (2018) ATR kinase inhibitor AZD6738 potentiates CD8+ T cell–dependent antitumor activity following radiation. J Clin Investig 128(9):3926–3940. https://doi.org/10.1172/JCI96519

Watkins JA et al (2014) Genomic scars as biomarkers of homologous recombination deficiency and drug response in breast and ovarian cancers. Breast Cancer Res 16(3):211. https://doi.org/10.1186/bcr3670

Weidhaas JB et al (2017) The KRAS-variant and Cetuximab response in head and neck squamous cell cancer: a secondary analysis of a randomized clinical trial. JAMA Oncol. American Medical Association 3(4):483–491. https://doi.org/10.1001/jamaoncol.2016.5478

Willers H, Dahm-Daphi J, Powell SN (2004) Repair of radiation damage to DNA. Br J Cancer 90(7):1297–1301. https://doi.org/10.1038/sj.bjc.6601729

Young KH et al (2016) Optimizing timing of immunotherapy improves control of tumors by hypofractionated radiation therapy. PLoS One. Edited by F. Mattei 11(6):e0157164. https://doi.org/10.1371/journal.pone.0157164

Zeng L et al (2017) Combining Chk1/2 inhibition with cetuximab and radiation enhances in vitro and in vivo cytotoxicity in head and neck squamous cell carcinoma. Mol Cancer Ther 16(4):591–600. https://doi.org/10.1158/1535-7163.MCT-16-0352

Zhang Q et al (2019) Inhibition of ATM increases interferon signaling and sensitizes pancreatic cancer to immune checkpoint blockade therapy. Cancer Res., p. canres.0761.2019. https://doi.org/10.1158/0008-5472.CAN-19-0761

Zhao Y et al (2006) Preclinical evaluation of a potent novel DNA-dependent protein kinase inhibitor NU7441. Cancer Res 66(10):5354–5362. https://doi.org/10.1158/0008-5472.CAN-05-4275

Chapter 10
Targeting Tumor Metabolism to Overcome Radioresistance

Daniel Wahl, Michael Petronek, Rashmi Ramachandran, John Floberg, Bryan G. Allen, and Julie K. Schwarz

Abstract Metabolic reprogramming is a hallmark of cancer. Altered metabolism provides a survival advantage for cancer cells during tumorigenesis by supplying resources needed for uncontrolled growth and increased rates of cell division. As tumors grow beyond the limits of diffusion, altered metabolism provides a selective advantage in the context of nutrient deprivation. Many cancer therapies, including radiation, are known to impact tumor metabolism while the metabolic state of a cancer may contribute to radioresistance. Preclinical and clinical evidence exists to support combinations of radiation therapy with drugs that affect, for example,

D. Wahl
Department of Radiation Oncology, University of Michigan, Ann Arbor, MI, USA

M. Petronek
Department of Radiation Oncology, Free Radical and Radiation Biology Program, University of Iowa, Iowa City, IA, USA

R. Ramachandran
Department of Radiation Oncology, Washington University School of Medicine, Saint Louis, MO, USA

J. Floberg
Department of Human Oncology, University of Wisconsin School of Medicine and Public Health, Milwaukee, WI, USA

B. G. Allen
Department of Radiation Oncology, Free Radical and Radiation Biology Program, Holden Comprehensive Cancer Center, University of Iowa, Carver College of Medicine, Iowa City, IA, USA

J. K. Schwarz (✉)
Department of Radiation Oncology, Washington University School of Medicine, Saint Louis, MO, USA

Alvin J. Siteman Cancer Center, Washington University School of Medicine, Saint Louis, MO, USA

Department of Cell Biology and Physiology, Washington University School of Medicine, Saint Louis, MO, USA
e-mail: jschwarz@wustl.edu

© Springer Nature Switzerland AG 2020
H. Willers, I. Eke (eds.), *Molecular Targeted Radiosensitizers*, Cancer Drug Discovery and Development, https://doi.org/10.1007/978-3-030-49701-9_10

oxidative, glucose, glutamine, one-carbon, nucleotide, or iron metabolism in cancers. Work is ongoing to determine optimal strategies for combining these drugs with conventionally fractionated and hypofractionated radiation schemes. New strategies, including dietary manipulation during the course of radiation therapy, are currently being explored. Targeting tumor metabolism is a rapidly evolving and promising field of oncology and will be reviewed here in more detail.

Keywords Ascorbate · Calorie restriction · Glucose metabolism · Glutaminolysis · Glycolysis · Iron metabolism · Hallmarks of cancer · Ketogenic diet · Metabolic reprogramming · NAD · NADP · Nucleoside analogs · Nucleotide metabolism · One-carbon metabolism · Pentose phosphate pathway · Radioresistance · Ribonucleotide reductase · Thymidylate synthase

1 Introduction

Altered metabolism is a phenomenon that is generalizable across many cancer types, so much so that it has been included as one of the hallmarks of cancer (Hanahan and Weinberg 2011; Pavlova and Thompson 2016). Altered metabolism provides a survival advantage for cancer cells during tumorigenesis by supplying resources needed for uncontrolled growth and increased rates of cell division. As tumors grow beyond the limits of diffusion, altered metabolism provides a selective advantage in the context of nutrient deprivation (DeBerardinis and Chandel 2016). While the individual details of metabolic adaptations may diverge across tumor types, some general themes emerge which provide an opportunity for the rational design of cancer cell-selective, metabolically targeted therapies (Luengo et al. 2017). Drugs that target tumor metabolism can be administered alone, in combination with other drugs as well as in combination with radiation therapy (Floberg and Schwarz 2019). In this chapter, we will review tumor metabolic reprogramming with a focus on established mechanisms of metabolic adaptation that provide the strongest scientific rationale for combination treatment with radiotherapy.

2 Tumor Metabolic Reprogramming

Tumor metabolic alterations are cell lineage dependent and influenced by the local microenvironment (Luengo et al. 2017). Mutations in individual metabolic enzymes, although they do exist, are relatively rare in cancer. More commonly, classical oncogene and tumor suppressor pathways induce tumor metabolic reprogramming via direct effects on gene transcription. For example, the PI3K/AKT/mTOR pathway, which normally transmits signals from growth factor receptors to stimulate glycolytic flux, fatty acid and amino acid biosynthetic pathways needed to support cell growth, is frequently hyperactivated in cancer, and cancers with PI3K/AKT/mTOR pathway activation display increased rates of glucose uptake and glycolysis in addition to a unique set of associated targetable metabolic vulnerabilities (Yuan and Cantley 2008; Dibble and Manning 2013; Saxton and Sabatini 2017; Sabatini 2017; Ilic et al. 2017). Similarly, the *MYC* family of regulator and proto-oncogenes code for transcription factors that stimulate the expression of several genes directly involved in glycolysis, glutaminolysis, fatty acid synthesis, serine, and mitochondrial metabolism, and each of these pathways be targeted by new classes of developing anti-metabolic drugs (Stine et al. 2015).

The tumor suppressor p53 (*TP53*), which was previously thought to execute its tumor suppressive function via effects on DNA repair, cell cycle arrest, apoptosis, and/or senescence, is able to control the expression of many metabolic genes including *GLS2, FDXR, FUCA1, PRKAB1, PANK1,* and *TIGAR* (Li et al. 2012; Kruiswijk et al. 2015; Fischer 2017). Although the precise nature of p53 target gene regulation is cell lineage and context dependent, wild-type p53 is thought to support the increased activity of the pentose phosphate pathway and mitochondrial oxidative phosphorylation at the expense of glycolysis. A key player in this effect is p53-induced expression of *TIGAR*, a fructose bisphosphastase, which removes a phosphate group from fructose-2,6-bisphosphate (F-2,6-BP) an allosteric regulator of glycolysis and gluconeogenesis (Bensaad et al. 2006; Ko et al. 2016; Bartrons et al. 2018). Work is ongoing to determine how the expression of p53 target genes, including metabolic genes, is affected in the setting of tumor-specific *TP53* mutations.

An emerging concept is the identification of oncometabolites or the products of tumor-associated metabolic alterations such as 2-hydroxyglutarate (2-HG) by mutant isocitrate dehydrogenase 1 or 2 (IDH1 or IDH2) in glioma and other cancers (Collins et al. 2017; Ward et al. 2010). High levels of 2-HG suppress the activity of enzymes that require a-ketoglutarate as a cofactor, including the histone demethylases. This enzymatic modification further affects gene transcription via changes in chromatin structure induced by hypermethylation of histones and CpG islands in DNA (Figueroa et al. 2010; Lu et al. 2012; Turcan et al. 2012). Thus, a complicated picture emerges in which cancer-associated mutations have metabolic effects which not only provide selective advantages for survival, growth, and replication in the setting of nutrient deprivation but also promote alterations in gene expression and chromatin structure which can become a source of further adaptation (Turcan et al. 2018). In this way, tumor metabolic alterations become a critical source of plasticity, rapid adaptability, tumor heterogeneity, and evolution essential for tumor progression and resistance to anti-cancer therapies including radiation.

3 Glucose Metabolism in Cancer

Nearly all cancers show increased glucose utilization, commonly referred to as the Warburg effect. This phenomenon has been put to clinical use through [F-18]fluorodeoxy-glucose positron emission tomography (FDG-PET) imaging, and this strategy is currently used to image many cancer types (Warburg 1924; Hanahan and Weinberg 2011; Gambhir 2002). The underlying cause for increased glucose uptake in cancer is a combination of tumor metabolic reprogramming outlined above and tumor microenvironments with scarce oxygen, glucose, and other nutrients, which select for tumor phenotypes that upregulate glucose uptake and glycolysis (Gatenby and Gillies 2004; Graeber et al. 1996; Gatenby and Vincent 2003). The importance of this phenomenon has been demonstrated by the prognostic significance of FDG-PET, both the initial FDG uptake by tumors and the change in FDG uptake throughout treatment, across a broad number of cancers (Berghmans et al. 2008; Haioun et al. 2005; Brun et al. 2002; Kidd et al. 2007; Westerterp et al. 2005; Schwarz et al. 2007). Increased glucose utilization therefore appears to be related to the initial aggressiveness of cancer and a predictor of how well cancer will respond to therapies including chemotherapy and radiation. Glucose utilization by tumors also decreases during the course of cancer therapy, and post-therapy assessments of tumor glucose uptake by FDG-PET imaging are reliable surrogates for long-term survival outcomes after radiation including both local control and overall survival outcomes.

3.1   Glycolysis

Glycolysis is an oxygen-independent metabolic pathway that converts glucose into pyruvate and serves as a principle means of ATP generation for many cancers, even in the presence of oxygen (Warburg 1924; Hanahan and Weinberg 2011). Glycolysis also plays a key role in the regulation of reductive/oxidative (redox) metabolism in cancer cells. For example, cervical cancer cells that demonstrate increased glycolysis also show increased levels of oxidative stress and are susceptible to combination drug strategies targeting glycolysis as well as other redox metabolic pathways (Rashmi et al. 2018). Several potential therapeutic targets within the glycolysis pathway are shown in Fig. 10.1. Furthest upstream, the GLUT family of glucose transporters can be targeted. For example, WZB117 is an inhibitor of GLUT1, and the protease inhibitor ritonavir has off-target inhibitory effects on the GLUT4 transporter. Both have demonstrated anti-neoplastic effects in preclinical models (Shibuya et al. 2015; Liu et al. 2012; McBrayer et al. 2012). Hexokinase, the first enzyme in the glycolysis pathway, is another potential upstream target. Drugs that target hexokinase that have been investigated in the preclinical and clinical settings include 2-deoxyglucose (2-DG) and lonidamine (El Mjiyad et al. 2011; Pelicano et al. 2006). 2-DG has been extensively studied, including a number of preclinical models with promising results, as well as in human glioblastoma patients in combination with radiation therapy (Zhao et al. 2013; Pelicano et al. 2006; Kennedy et al. 2013; Mohanti et al. 1996; Singh et al. 2005). Ultimately however, the clinical efficacy of 2-DG seems to be limited by unacceptable side effects at high doses, and limited efficacy at lower doses (Vander Heiden 2011). Lonidamine has likewise proven toxic for clinical use (Price et al. 1996). Further downstream, bromopyru-

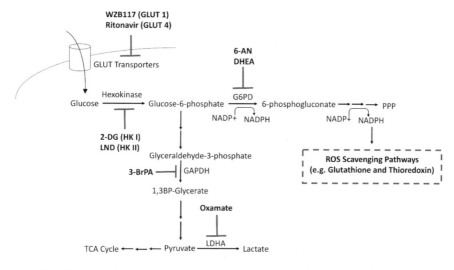

Fig. 10.1 Glycolysis, the pentose phosphate pathway, and potential targets for anti-cancer therapy. Blocking glucose metabolism can inhibit a major energy source for cancer cells as well as a source of NADPH, one of the principal reducing equivalents in cells. Drugs that inhibit various steps in glycolysis and the pentose phosphate pathway (PPP) are shown in bold. Abbreviations: HK, hexokinase; 2-DG, 2-deoxyglucose; LND, lonidamide; G6PD, glucose-6-phosphate dehydrogenase; 6-AN, 6-aminonicotinamide; DHEA, dehydroepiandrosterone; PPP, pentose phosphate pathway; GAPDH, glyceraldehyde 3-phosphate dehydrogenase; 3-BrPA, 3-bromopyruvate; LDHA, lactate dehydrogenase A; TCA cycle, tricarboxylic acid cycle (Adapted and reprinted from Seminars in Radiation Oncology, Vol. 19(1), John M Floberg and Julie K Schwarz, Manipulation of Glucose and Hydroperoxide Metabolism to Improve Radiation Response, pp. 33–41, 2019, with permission from Elsevier)

vate and oxamate have been studied as glycolytic inhibitors. For example, oxamate increases the efficacy of systemic agents such as trastuzumab in preclinical models (Zhao et al. 2011). Bromopyruvate has likewise shown promise in preclinical models, including in abrogating radiation resistance (Gunda et al. 2017). However, progress toward clinical use of these drugs is slow primarily due to normal tissue effects.

3.2   The Pentose Phosphate Pathway

Another glucose metabolic pathway important to cancer cells is the pentose phosphate pathway (PPP). The PPP is one of the principle sources of nicotinamide adenine dinucleotide phosphate (NADPH), which provides electrons for reactive oxygen species (ROS) scavenging pathways, namely the glutathione and thioredoxin pathways (Fig. 10.1). These pathways are in turn critical to managing oxidative stress in cancer cells and help drive progression and treatment resistance (Harris et al. 2015; DeNicola et al. 2011; Diehn et al. 2009). There have been some attempts to target the PPP directly, for example, using 6-aminonicotinamide (6-AN) or dehydroepiandrosterone (DHEA). 6-AN is an inhibitor of glucose-6-phosphate dehydrogenase (G6PD) that is toxic to cancer cells in vitro, but whose use is limited in vivo by toxicity to normal cells (Pelicano et al. 2006). Perhaps the most effective therapeutic strategy targeting redox metabolism is the combined inhibition of glycolysis and the PPP and/or the ROS scavenging pathways that depend upon the PPP for NADPH (Floberg and Schwarz 2019). For example, inhibiting the pentose cycle with DHEA, thioredoxin metabolism with auranofin, and glycolysis with 2-DG is significantly more toxic to breast, prostate, and cervical cancer cells than inhibition of glycolysis alone (Li et al. 2015). Alternatively, targeting both of the principle cellular ROS scavenging pathways, the thioredoxin and glutathione pathways, in addition to glycolysis is toxic to cervical cancer cells, and enhances their sensitivity to radiation, particularly in cells that show high baseline levels of FDG uptake (Rashmi et al. 2018). These results suggest that FDG-PET imaging could be explored as a predictive marker for identifying cancers that would be sensitive to drug strategies that target the combination of glycolysis and redox metabolic pathways.

4   Glutaminolysis

Glutamine is an essential amino acid in the human body (Alberghina and Gaglio 2014). It plays a major role as the precursor for the synthesis of nucleotides, proteins, amino acids, and other biologically important molecules such as GSH glutathione (GSH) and nicotinamide adenine dinucleotide phosphate (NADPH), which help maintain redox balance (Lee et al. 2009). Glutamine is also consumed in greater quantities and at a quicker rate by cancer cells, compared to normal cells (Vaupel et al. 1989). Apart from glucose, proliferating tumor cells depend on glutamine as an important energy resource and as substrates for biosynthetic pathways. Enhanced glycolysis leads to diminished TCA cycle intermediates. Thus, glycolytic tumor cells exhibit an enhanced dependency on exogenous glutamine, which is commonly referred to as glutamine addiction. Glutamine is indispensable to the survival of certain cancer cells, and glutamine deprivation results in cell death. Glutamine is converted to glutamate and an ammonium ion by the enzyme glutaminase (GLS). Glutamate is further converted to alpha-ketoglutarate (α-KG) by glutamate dehydrogenase (GLUD) which then enters the TCA cycle to provide energy and biosynthetic intermediates (glutamine anapleurosis) (Altman et al. 2016). GLS exists in multiple tissue-specific versions, encoded by two genes in mammals, kidney-type glutaminase (GLS1) and liver-type glutaminase (GLS2). GLS1 expression has been reported to show positive correlation with malignancy in cancer cells and growth rate in normal cells (Matre et al. 2016).

CB-839 (Glutaminase Inhibitor Telaglenastat) is a potent, selective, and orally bioavailable non-competitive inhibitor of GLS and an NCI Cancer Therapy Evaluation Program (CTEP)-supported agent that selectively and irreversibly inhibits GLS (Gross et al. 2014; Vogl et al. 2015; Wang et al. 2015). Preclinical data supporting the use of CB-839 in cancer therapy is growing. In a patient-derived TNBC mouse xenograft model, CB-839 (200 mg/kg, p.o.) inhibits tumor growth by 61% relative to vehicle control, and more recent studies have shown that CB-839 is effective in combination with mTOR inhibition in preclinical models of triple-negative and advanced estrogen receptor-positive disease (Demas et al. 2019; Shibata et al. 1988). CB-839 also possesses anti-proliferative properties against acute myeloid leukemia (AML) as a monotherapeutic agent or in conjunction with redox-directed therapies including arsenic trioxide (ATO) or homoharringtonine (HHT). In KRAS mutant non-small cell lung cancer (NSCLC), LKB1 loss and activation of the KEAP/NRF2 pathway are associated with increased sensitivity to CB-839 monotherapy (Galan-Cobo et al. 2019). In addition, CB-839 is active in combination with erlotinib in EGFR-driven NSCLC (Gregory et al. 2019). Several emerging drug strategies pair CB-839 with other metabolically targeted drugs, including transporters and enzymes associated with glycolysis and lipid oxidation (Reis et al. 2019; Reckzeh et al. 2019). Esophageal squamous cell carcinoma cells (ESCC) and ESCC cells with acquired CDK4/6 resistance are sensitive to CB-839 in combination with metformin or phenformin (Jacque et al. 2015; Matre et al. 2016; Momcilovic et al. 2017; Qie et al. 2019). Currently CB-839 is being evaluated in Phase II clinical trials in several drug combinations including cabozantinib, talazoparib, nivolumab, and palbociclib in patients with advanced or metastatic Renal Cell Carcinoma (RCC), melanoma, and NSCLC (NCT02771626, NCT03875313, NCT03965845, NCT03428217). Several Phase I/II trial studies are evaluating CB-839 in combination with panitumumab, irinotecan hydrochloride, azacitidine, capecitabine, and osimertinib in patients with colorectal cancer, myelodysplastic syndrome and NSCLC (NCT03047993, NCT02861300, NCT03831932, NCT03263429).

Given the association between sensitivity to CB-839 and tumor oxidative stress, it is interesting to speculate that CB-839 would synergize with radiation therapy. In the preclinical setting, CB-839 increased radiation therapy sensitivity of glutamine-dependent IDH1 mutant glioma cells, leading to prolonged survival of mice bearing these tumors (Zhang 2018). This phenotype is due to the ability of 2-HG to inhibit branched chain amino acid aminotransferases, which renders IDH mutant cancers entirely dependent on glutaminase for the generation of gluthathione (McBrayer et al. 2018). These preclinical studies have motivated an ongoing phase 1b clinical trial that studies the side effects and best dose of CB-839 in combination with radiation therapy and temozolomide in treating patients with IDH-mutated diffuse or anaplastic astrocytoma (NCT03528642). CB-839 has also been shown to sensitize KRAS mutant NSCLC to radiation treatment in in vitro and in vivo models. (Chakrabarti 2015; Boysen et al. 2019). Research in our laboratory has demonstrated high potency of CB-839 monotherapy and drug combinations for highly glycolytic, radiation-resistant cervical cancer, and work is ongoing to determine the best strategy to combine CB-839 with radiation in cervical cancer preclinical models (Ramachandran and Schwarz, *In Preparation*).

5 Nucleotide Metabolism and the Radiation Response

Combining radiation with nucleotide metabolism inhibitors is a standard of care treatment for many malignancies including gastric, rectal, and pancreatic cancer. The efficacy of these combination therapies hints at the important biologic relationships between nucleotide metabolism and radiation-induced DNA damage. Indeed, an unbiased phosphoproteomic analysis performed 1 h after radiation treatment revealed that of 421 annotated phosphorylation events, with nearly half occurring on proteins related to DNA and nucleic acid metabolism (Matsuoka et al. 2007). The mechanistic and therapeutic links between DNA damage and nucleotide metabolism have been extensively investigated, particularly at the levels of ribonucleotide reductase and thymidylate synthase.

5.1 Ribonucleotide Reductase

Ribonucleotide reductase (RNR) is an oligomeric enzymatic complex that converts nucleotide diphosphates into deoxynucleotide disphosphates, which can eventually be incorporated into DNA. In mammals, RNR functions as an $\alpha_2\beta_2$ hetero-tetramer where the α subunit is encoded by the *RRM1* gene and the β subunit is encoded by both the *RRM2* and the *RRM2B* genes (Kauppi et al. 1996; Nordlund and Reichard 2006). RNR activity varies with the cell cycle and is maximal during S phase when deoxynucleotide need is greatest. This regulation is largely due to increased transcription of *RRM2* during S phase and degradation of the *RRM2* gene-product during mitosis (Nordlund and Reichard 2006). After DNA damage, *RRM2B* is transcriptionally activated in a p53-dependent fashion, leading to an acute increase in RNR activity and the production of deoxynucleotides (Elledge and Davis 1989; Tanaka et al. 2000). The RNR protein also rapidly migrates to sites of DNA damage, which ensures that deoxynucleotides are synthesized in close proximity to where they are needed for DNA repair (Niida et al. 2010).

Inhibition of RNR activity potentiates the effects of radiation. Gemcitabine (2′, 2′-difluorodeoxycytidine) is the most widely used clinical RNR inhibitor. Once inside cells, gemcitabine must be phosphorylated by deoxycytidine kinase to generate its active diphosphate (difluorodeoxycytidine disphosphate, dFdCDP) and triphosphate (difluorodeoxycytidine triphosphate, dFdCTP) forms (Heinemann et al. 1988). The triphosphate metabolite is the dominant mediator of gemcitabine-induced cytotoxicity due to its ability to compete with dCTP for incorporation into DNA (Huang et al. 1991). The diphosphate analog of gemcitabine, which inhibits RNR and depletes deoxynucleotides (especially dATP), is the principal metabolite responsible for radiosensitization (Lawrence et al. 1999). Gemcitabine treatment radiosensitizes multiple cancer models in vitro and in vivo (Shewach et al. 1994; Lawrence et al. 1996; Fehlauer et al. 2006; Pauwels et al. 2005). RNR Inhibition using genetic silencing (Zhao et al. 2019) or agents other than gemcitabine (Kunos et al. 2010) produces similar effects.

Gemcitabine has been combined with radiation to treat many cancers including glioblastoma (Kim et al. 2016), head and neck squamous cell cancers (Popovtzer et al. 2014), and NSCLC (Lee et al. 2005). Concurrent gemcitabine and radiation continue to form the backbone of standard treatments for patients with locally advanced unresectable pancreatic (Loehrer et al. 2011; Cuneo et al. 2019) and bladder cancer (Choudhury et al. 2011). While this combination is well tolerated for bladder and pancreatic cancer, gemcitabine causes unacceptable mucosal toxicity when combined with radiation when it is used to treat patients with head and neck cancer (Popovtzer et al. 2014). These results emphasize the need to fully understand the metabolism of nearby normal tissue in addition to the cancer itself when designing combination therapies. RNR inhibition using triapine has also been extensively studied in vitro and in vivo and is currently being tested in clinical trials in combination with radiation for cervical cancer (NCT02466971).

5.2   Thymidylate Synthase

Thymidylate synthase (TS) catalyzes the reductive methylation of deoxyuridine monophosphate to deoxythymidine monophosphate, which is driven by the conversion of methylene tetrahydrofolate to dihydrofolate (Carreras and Santi 1995). Thus, its activity is critical for the production of deoxythimidine triphosphate and subsequent DNA synthesis. Knockdown of TS radiosensitizes colon cancer cells and is associated with depletion of deoxythymidine triphosphate and deoxyguanosine triphosphate (Flanagan et al. 2012). Enhancement ratios achieved with TS knockdown are substantial (Flanagan et al. 2012).

Pharmacologic inhibition of TS achieves similar results (Flanagan et al. 2012). The most commonly used class of TS inhibitors are the fluoropyrimidines, which include 5-fluorouracil (5-FU) and 5-fluoro-2′deoxyuridine (FdUrd) (Grem 2000). 5-FU can be converted into fluorouracil triphosphate (F-UTP), which directly incorporates into RNA and exerts effects independently of TS. However, the radiosensitizing effects of 5-FU appear related to its ability to inhibit TS and deplete intracellular TTP pools (Flanagan et al. 2012). Indeed, metabolites of 5-FU that can inhibit TS but not be directly incorporated into RNA are potent radiosensitizers in vitro (Flanagan et al. 2012; Bruso et al. 1990).

The combination of 5-FU and radiation is a standard of care for many malignancies, especially those of the gastrointestinal tract. As early as the 1960s, a randomized trial of nearly 200 patients with unresectable cancers of the stomach, pancreas, and large bowel suggested that the addition of 5-FU to radiotherapy provided a several month survival benefit compared to radiation therapy alone (Moertel et al. 1969). The addition of 5-FU also caused a modest increase in radiation-associated toxicity. Similar results were obtained in the last decade for neoadjuvant therapy of rectal cancer. A randomized trial of more than 700 patients from France showed that the addition of 5-FU to preoperative radiotherapy for locally advanced rectal cancer more than doubled the rates of pathologic complete response and halved the rates of local recurrence (Gerard et al. 2006). Toxicity was modestly increased with this regimen and there was no change in overall survival. Similar results were seen in a second large randomized trial for locally advanced rectal cancer conducted at numerous European sites (Bosset et al. 2005). Capecitabine, an orally administered prodrug of 5-FU, confers similar or improved oncologic outcomes compared to infusional 5-FU when combined with radiation for rectal cancer with less hematologic toxicity (Hofheinz et al. 2012). Thus, antifolates combined with radiotherapy remain a part of standard of care treatment for locally advanced rectal cancer (Beets and Beets-Tan 2012). Antifolates continue to be used in combination with radiation for the treatment of anal cancer (Meulendijks et al. 2014; Bartelink et al. 1997), cholangiocarcinoma (Ben-Josef et al. 2015), gastric cancer (Macdonald et al. 2001), and others.

5.3   Nucleoside Analogs

Because of the success of combining radiation with ribonucleotide reductase and thymidylate synthase inhibitors, there is interest in developing other pharmacologic agents that target nucleotide metabolism to be combined with radiation therapy. Iodinated pyrimidine analogs such as IUdR (5-iodo-2′-deoxyuridine) and IPdR (5-iodo-2-pyrimidinone-2′deoxyribose) are, like 5-FU, halogenated compounds related to uridine (Saif et al. 2007). However, these drugs exert their radiosensitizing effects through direct incorporation into DNA rather than by inhibiting TS and depleting dTTP (Saif et al. 2007). While IUdR can only be administered through intravenous (IV) infusion, IPdR is an orally bioavailable prodrug of IUdR that undergoes conversion to the active IUdR in the liver (Kinsella et al. 1998). Once it enters cells, IUdR is phosphorylated by thymidine kinase and eventually converted into its triphosphate form, which competes with dTTP for incorporation into DNA. The magnitude of radiosensitization achieved by IUdR is directly proportional to the amount incorporated into DNA (Lawrence et al. 1990).

   IUdR was developed for clinical use and tested in combination with radiation in clinical trials in the 1980s and 1990s in cancers such as glioblastoma and high-grade sarcoma (Robertson et al. 1995; Kinsella et al. 1988). Unfortunately, the half-life of IUdR after bolus infusion is less than 5 min, which caused the cessation of clinical development due to the need for continuous infusions and difficulties finding effective doses without dose-limiting systemic toxicity (Belanger et al. 1986). These challenges led to the prioritization of the orally bioavailable IPdR for clinical development. A first-in-human phase 0 trial of IPdR in ten patients with advanced malignancies revealed no treatment-related adverse events when drug was administered by itself (Kummar et al. 2013). Phase I studies are ongoing that combine IPdR with radiation for gastrointestinal cancers (NCT02381561) and patients undergoing whole brain radiotherapy for brain metastases (NCT02993146).

   The successful use of nucleotide metabolism inhibitors in combination with radiation indicates that the cancer cell metabolism is sufficiently distinct from normal tissues to allow for a favorable therapeutic window where efficacy can be increased without causing unacceptable normal tissue toxicity. As our understanding of the fundamental metabolic alterations that distinguish cancer cells from normal tissues grows, there is every reason to believe that a similar therapeutic window will exist for such pathways as iron homeostasis, redox balance, and glutamine catabolism. In order to understand how to best combine altered metabolism inhibitors with radiotherapy without affecting normal tissue toxicity, it will be critical to understand both the mechanisms by which radiation interacts with individual metabolic pathways and the level at which normal tissues differ from nearby cancer cells.

6 One-Carbon Metabolism and the Radiation Response

6.1 One-Carbon Metabolism Overview

One-carbon metabolism broadly refers to three interlinking pathways: the folate cycle, the methionine cycle, and the transsulfuration pathway (Fig. 10.2) (Ducker and Rabinowitz 2017). Together, these metabolic pathways are crucial for the biosynthesis of nucleotides and fatty acids, the maintenance of redox balance, and methylation reactions throughout the cell. The backbone carrier of one of the carbon units is the folate molecule, which in mammals is acquired from folic acid. Once folic acid enters cells, it undergoes serial NADPH-driven reductions to tetrahydrofolate (THF). A one-carbon methyl group, which can be derived from serine via the serine hydroxymethyltransferase enzymes or from glycine via the glycine cleavage system, is then added to THF to form 5,10-methylene THF (Schirch and Szebenyi 2005; Pai et al. 2015). Other sources of one-carbon units include glucose, whose carbons enter the cycle through conversion to serine; histidine, whose catabolism generates 5,10-methylene THF directly; and formate, which can combine with THF to generate 10-formyl-THF in an ATP-dependent fashion (Brosnan and Brosnan 2016). 5,10-methylene THF can be further reduced by NADPH through the action of methylene-THF reductase to generate 5-methyl THF.

These three one-carbon carrying folate derivatives (5,10-methylene THF, 10-formyl-THF, and 5-methyl THF) have distinct cellular functions. 5,10-methylene THF is the one-carbon donor used by thymidylate synthase to convert deoxyuridine monophosphate to deoxythymidine monophosphate (Ducker and Rabinowitz 2017). 10-formyl-THF donates two carbons during the de novo formation of purine rings at the GAR transformylase and AICAR transformylase steps (Lane and Fan 2015). Through these reactions, one-carbon metabolism has a clear intersection with nucleotide synthesis, the importance of which likely varies based on how dependent a cell is on de novo purine synthesis compared to salvage pathways. 5-methyl THF is used to re-methylate homocysteine to generate methionine by the cobalamin-dependent enzyme methionine synthase (Banerjee and Matthews 1990). Methionine is then conjugated to adenosine in an ATP-dependent fashion to form S-adenosylmethionine (SAM) by members of the methionine adenosyltransferase

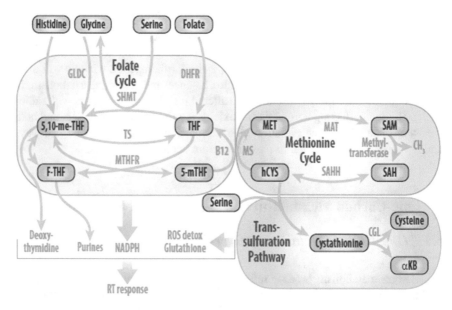

Fig. 10.2 One-carbon metabolic pathways. Dietary folate enters the folate cycle and is converted to tetrahydrofolate (THF) by dihydrofolate reductase (DHFR). THF is converted to 5,10-methylene-THF (5,10-me-THF) by either serine hydroxymethyl transferase (SHMT) or glycine decarboxylase (GLDC). Serine and glycine are derived from numerous sources including glycolytic intermediates. 5,10-me-THF can be used to generate deoxythymidine or converted to either 5-methyl-THF (5-mTHF) or 10-formyl-THF (F-THF), which feed into methionine synthesis or de novo purine synthesis. Methionine synthase (MS) and its cofactor vitamin B12 catalyze the demethylation of 5-mTHF to regenerate THF and convert homocysteine (hCYS) to form methionine (MET). This step links the folate and methionine cycles. Methionine adenosyltransferase (MAT) combines ATP and MET to form S-adenosylmethionine (SAM), which is the major cellular methyl donor. When it loses its methyl group, SAM is converted to S-adenosyl homocysteine (SAH), which is converted back to homocysteine by S-adenosyl homocysteine hydrolase (SAHH)-mediated deadenylation. In the transsulfuration pathway, hCYS condenses with serine to form cystathionine, which can be cleaved by cystathione lyase (CGL) to form cysteine and α-ketobutyrate (αKB). Cysteine is then used to generate glutathione to help maintain cellular redox balance

enzyme family (Quinlan et al. 2017). Because SAM is the major methyl donor in the cell, these series of reactions link one-carbon metabolism to epigenetic methylation reactions, sulfur metabolism and the biosynthesis of polyamines, creatine and lipid head groups (Ducker and Rabinowitz 2017). The one-carbon pathway is also linked to redox balance, as serine and homocysteine can combine to form cystathionine and eventually glutathione (Locasale 2013). In addition to these canonical outputs of nucleotides, methyl groups, and glutathione, the one-carbon pathway was recently discovered to be a major generator of cellular reducing power in the form of NADPH (Fan et al. 2014). In some contexts, the cytosolic and mitochondrial forms of methylene tetrahydrofolate dehydrogenase (MTHFD) can produce NADPH levels comparable to those produced by the pentose phosphate cycle.

6.2   One-Carbon Pathways in Cancer

One-carbon metabolic pathways appear to be especially important in cancer. Numerous cytosolic and mitochondrial enzymes involved in one-carbon metabolism are upregulated at the transcript level in breast, colon, lung, and ovarian cancer compared to normal tissue controls (Mehrmohamadi et al. 2014). Indeed, the mitochondrial enzyme *MTHFD2* is the most consistently overexpressed metabolic transcript across all cancers (Nilsson et al. 2014). *PHGDH*, whose protein product catalyzes the first step in de novo serine synthesis, is recurrently amplified in several cancer types most notably breast cancer and melanoma (Mullarky et al. 2011; Possemato et al. 2011). Inhibition of PHGDH, either through genetic approaches or using small molecules, slows the growth of PHGDH overexpressing cancers in vitro or in mouse models, and thus *PHGDH* is considered a candidate oncogene (Pacold et al. 2016). *SHMT2,* whose protein product catalyzes the entry of serine-derived carbons into the one-carbon cycle in the mitochondria, is also overexpressed in a variety of cancers and appears to be especially important for the growth of B-cell lymphomas (Ducker et al. 2017). The entry of serine into one-carbon metabolism may be especially important for cancers to adapt to hypoxia. In high-grade gliomas, SHMT2 is preferentially expressed in ischemic regions and is important for maintaining viability in hypoxia (Kim et al. 2015). Similar findings are seen in MYC-driven cancers, which rely on SHMT2 to generate NADPH and maintain viability under hypoxia (Ye et al. 2014).

6.3   Pharmacologic Targeting of the One-Carbon Pathway

While one-carbon enzyme inhibitors such as PHGDH, SHMT2, and MAT2a are under development with uncertain efficacy in patients (Locasale 2013), folate metabolism inhibitors have been a mainstay of cancer therapy for more than 70 years (Visentin et al. 2012). Aminopterin was the first anti-folate used clinically in the 1940s and achieved temporary remissions in children with acute lymphoblastic leukemia (Farber and Diamond 1948). This was followed by methotrexate (MTX), which was introduced in the 1950s and remains a standard cancer therapy (Grommes and DeAngelis 2017). Pemetrexed was recently introduced where it is now a standard treatment for mesothelioma and NSCLC (Vogelzang et al. 2003; Cohen et al. 2010).

Both aminopterin and methotrexate are structural analogs of folic acid and achieve their pharmacologic effects by inhibiting DHFR and depleting THF levels, resulting in pleiotropic effects on nucleotide metabolism (Bokkerink et al. 1986) and cellular methylation reactions (Wang and Chiang 2012). In support of this hypothesis, perturbations that slow the consumption of THF (such as the inhibition of histidine catabolism) can limit the efficacy of MTX (Kanarek et al. 2018). MTX may also exert some of its effects by directly inhibiting thymidylate synthase or the folate-requiring reactions of de novo purine synthesis (Allegra et al. 1985a, b). Pemetrexed has a slightly different action mechanism in that it directly inhibits THF-requiring enzymes such as thymidylate synthase, rather than inhibiting DHFR and depleting THF levels (Allegra et al. 1985b). Upregulation of thymidylate synthase is closely associated with the development of resistance to pemetrexed (Zhang et al. 2011).

Efforts have also been made to target one-carbon metabolism through dietary modification. Starving tumor-bearing mice of the two main carbon inputs of the one-carbon pathways (serine and glycine) slows tumor growth and forced cancers to upregulate de novo serine synthesis to maintain glutathione levels in a p53-dependent fashion (Maddocks et al. 2012, 2017). Similar results are seen when methionine is depleted from the diet. Mice fed diets completely lacking in methionine had decreased circulating levels of methionine and its related metabolites (Gao et al. 2019). Administering this diet to mice bearing colorectal tumors slowed tumor growth and depleted key metabolites including dTTP, L-cysteine, and L-homocysteine. These changes in tumor metabolism were associated with increased sensitivity to anti-metabolite chemotherapies. Importantly, methionine restriction is achievable in humans. Restricting methionine levels by 80% in six healthy adults caused perturbations in numerous metabolites related to one-carbon metabolism including glutathione and numerous nucleotide species. Whether this diet will be tolerable in patients with cancer is uncertain, but worthy of further investigation.

6.4   Interactions between One-Carbon Metabolism and the Radiation Response

The mechanisms by which radiation kills cancer cells have numerous points of intersection with one-carbon metabolism including purine synthesis, dTMP synthesis, and redox balance. Pemetrexed radiosensitizes a variety of cancer cell lines of different origins when used in vitro with enhancement ratios between 1.2 and 2.1 (Bischof et al. 2002, 2003). Pemetrexed has also been combined with radiation in cancer patients. While studies in NSCLC showed promising oncologic outcomes with minimal toxicity (Brade et al. 2011, 2016), large field-irradiation administered after pemetrexed caused high rates of fatal pneumonitis in patients with mesothelioma (Allen et al. 2006). As early as the 1960s, methotrexate had been combined with radiation for patients with head and neck squamous cell carcinoma, leading to both increased efficacy of radiation and increased toxicity (Condit et al. 1964). Single arm studies combining radiation and methotrexate to treat patients with leptomeningeal disease have shown promising results (Hitchins et al. 1987; Pan et al. 2016), but this approach is not a standard of care, due in part to the high toxicity rates seen when these agents are combined (Peylan-Ramu et al. 1978). When studied in vitro, methotrexate appears to confer less radiosensitization than pemetrexed

(Kim et al. 2012). These results suggest that thymidylate synthase inhibition (which is direct in the case of pemetrexed and indirect in the case of methotrexate) may be responsible for the radiosensitizing properties of antifolates.

Perturbing one-carbon metabolism by eating a methionine-restricted diet also modulates the effects of radiotherapy. In mice bearing autochthonous sarcomas lacking functional Kras and p53, a methionine-restricted diet had no effect on tumor growth on its own but increased the median time to tumor tripling from approximately 17 days with radiation alone to 27 days with radiation combined with methionine-restricted diet (Gao et al. 2019). This efficacy was associated with perturbations in intratumoral concentrations of metabolites related to nucleotide and antioxidant metabolism. Whether methionine restriction will favorably combine with radiation in patients, or whether it will also potentiate the effects of radiation on normal tissues is not yet known.

7 NAD and NADP Metabolism

Nicotinamide adenine dinucleotide (NAD^+) is a dinucleotide that consists of adenine and nicotinomide moieties whose ribose sugars are linked by phosphates. Nicotinamide adenine dinucleotide phosphate ($NADP^+$) is identical to NAD^+ apart from an additional phosphate group at the $2'$ position of the adenine ribose (Ying 2008). NAD^+ and $NADP^+$ are the oxidized species of these molecules and can also exist in reduced species (NADH and NADPH). These structurally similar redox pairs are regulated separately and control distinct intracellular functions. NAD^+/NADH levels are critical for mitochondrial ATP production and as a substrate for numerous enzymes including the poly ADP-ribose polymerase (PARP) family and the sirtuins. $NADP^+$/NADPH levels, on the other hand, are critical for mediating the reductive biosynthesis of antioxidants, fatty acids, and deoxynucleotides and for the function of the peroxisome (Pollak et al. 2007).

7.1 NAD⁺ Synthesis

NAD^+ can be synthesized through two pathways: de novo NAD^+ synthesis or NAD^+ salvage. In the de novo synthetic pathway, tryptophan is metabolized through the kynurenine pathway to generate quinolinate, which is then joined with activated ribose by quinolinate phosphoribosyl transferase to form nicotinate mononucleotide (NMN). NMN then combines with ATP to form nicotinate adenine dinucleotide, in a reaction catalyzed by the nicotinamide nucleotide adenyltransferase (NMNAT) family of enzymes. Finally, glutamine donates its amide nitrogen to convert the carboxylic acid group of nicotinate to an amide in an ATP-dependent fashion to generate NAD^+. In the salvage pathway, nicotinate or nicotinamide (either from the diet or from NAD^+-consuming enzymes) are re-formed into NAD^+. Nicotinate is joined to activated ribose to form NMN by the action of the enzyme nicotinate phos-phoribosyltransferase (NAPRT). As noted above, NMN must still be linked with adenosine and amidated by glutamine to generate NAD^+. Nicotinamide is joined to activated ribose by a different enzyme (nicotinamide phosphoribosyltransferase (NAMPT)) and then linked with adenosine to form NAD^+ (Bogan and Brenner 2008). Once NAD^+ is synthesized, it can be consumed by numerous NAD^+-dependent enzymes or interconverted with its reduced form (NADH), which does not consume the NAD^+ backbone.

7.2   NAD⁺ and the Radiation Response

NAD^+ is a critical cofactor in the DNA damage response (Lewis et al. 2019). Within seconds of DNA damage, the PARP enzymes are recruited to single-strand break sites where they consume large amounts of NAD^+ to transfer numerous ADP-ribose moieties onto themselves and neighboring nuclear proteins (De Vos et al. 2012). This poly-ADP ribosylation (PARylation) facilitates the recruitment of various members of the DNA repair pathways that have PAR binding domains, which leads to the successful repair of damage (Pleschke et al. 2000). Pharmacologically inhib-iting this signaling axis sensitizes numerous cancer types to ionizing radiation in in vitro and in vivo preclinical models (Speers et al. 2014). This approach is being tested in the clinic where PARP inhibitors are being combined with radiation in numerous diseases including glioblastoma (Lesueur et al. 2019), aggressive breast cancers (Jagsi et al. 2018), and others (Speers et al. 2014; George et al. 2019).

Inhibiting NAD^+ synthesis can also potentiate the radiation response. Tryptophan catabolism inhibitors (and thus de novo NAD^+ synthesis) increase the responsiveness of glioblastoma multiforme (GBM) xenografts to radiation in both flank and intracra-nial models (Kesarwani et al. 2018). Whether these radiosensitizing effects are due to NAD^+ depletion or a reversal of the immunosuppression induced by other trypto-phan products such as kynurenine is not certain. When normal liver is irradiated, the activity of both NMNAT and NAMPT increases, suggesting that NAD^+ salvage may play an important role in mitigating the effects of radiation (Batra and Kislay 2013). Indeed, mice eating a nicotinamide-supplemented diet have reduced DNA damage markers in the liver following radiation (Batra and Kislay 2013). NAMPT is overex-pressed in a variety of cancers (Wang et al. 2011; Cerna et al. 2012) and its inhibition synergizes with radiotherapy in both head and neck squamous cell carcinoma and glioblastoma (Kato et al. 2010; Gujar et al. 2016). NAMPT activity may be espe-cially important in cancers with mutated isocitrate dehydrogenase 1 (IDH1). Mutant IDH1 expression (and accumulation of the oncometabolite 2-hydroxyglutarate) represses the expression of *NAPRT1*, which forces these cells to rely on NAMPT to generate NAD^+. As a result, pharmacological NAMPT inhibitors kill IDH1 mutant glioma cell lines at 1000-fold lower concentrations than they do IDH1 wild-type cell lines (Tateishi et al. 2015). Whether these inhibitors also selectively potentiate radia-tion in IDH1 mutant tumors is not yet known.

7.3 NADP⁺ and the Radiation Response

NADP$^+$ is formed when NAD$^+$ is phosphorylated by the enzyme NAD kinase (Love et al. 2015). Once formed, NADP$^+$ can be reduced by only a handful of enzymes to generate NADPH, the primary carrier of electrons for reductive biosynthesis in the cell. The reducing power carried by NADPH is used by the cell to keep antioxidants in their active (reduced) states, synthesize lipids, and generate deoxyribonucleotides from ribonucleotides. Unlike the NAD$^+$/NADH pool, which predominantly exists in its oxidized form under physiologic conditions, the vast majority of the NADP$^+$/NADPH pool exits in its reduced form (NADPH), which underlies the importance of the biosynthetic reactions driven by NADPH (Ying 2008).

As discussed earlier, the oxidation of glucose-derived carbons through the pentose phosphate cycle is an important method to keep the NADPH pool reduced. In the last few years, alternative NADPH producers have been found to play important roles in maintaining redox balance in the cell. These include the methylene tetrahydrofolate dehydrogenase enzymes (discussed above in the one-carbon metabolism section), malic enzymes, isocitrate dehydrogenase (IDH) enzymes, and nicotinamide nucleotide transhydrogenase (NNT).

There are three IDH enzymes in mammalian cells. IDH1 is expressed in the cytosol and couples the reversible oxidation of isocitrate to the reduction of NADP$^+$ to generate 2-oxoglutarate and NADPH. IDH1 is a dominant producer of NADPH in glioblastoma and has important interactions with the radiation response (Calvert et al. 2017; Wahl et al. 2017). IDH1 expression is induced by radiation both in GBM and other cancers and its inhibition radiosensitizes GBM models in vitro and in vivo by depleting NADPH and NADPH-dependent metabolites such as reduced glutathione and deoxynucleotides (Wahl et al. 2017; Lee et al. 2004). Pharmacologic IDH1 inhibitors have now been described (Jakob et al. 2018). Whether such compounds will have clinical utility is uncertain, however the lack of significant phenotype in mice with whole body IDH1 knockout suggests that there may be a therapeutic window for this strategy (Itsumi et al. 2015). IDH2, which catalyzes the same reaction in the mitochondria also protects cancers from radiation (Lee et al. 2007), though whether this enzyme is differentially important in cancerous and non-cancerous tissues is not known. IDH3 exists in the mitochondria and is an integral part of the TCA cycle by virtue of its dependence on NAD$^+$ rather than NADP$^+$. While the enzymatic activity of IDH3 is important for some cancers, it is not known to have a role in antioxidant maintenance or the radiation response (May et al. 2019).

Malic enzyme (ME) catalyzes the reversible oxidation of malate to pyruvate, which is coupled to NAD(P)$^+$ conversion to NAD(P)H and the release of carbon dioxide. There are three malic enzyme isoforms: ME1, which is cytosolic and NADP$^+$ dependent; ME2, which is mitochondrial and prefers NAD$^+$; and ME3, which is mitochondrial and prefers NADP$^+$ (Pongratz et al. 2007). ME1 appears to be especially important for maintaining NADPH levels in *KRAS* mutated pancreatic cancers (Son et al. 2013). In these cancers, the mutant *KRAS* shunts glutamine-derived carbons into cytosolic malate, which is metabolized by ME1 to generate large amounts of NADPH. ME1 Inhibition, or numerous other members of this metabolic pathway, slows PDAC growth and perturbs redox balance (Son et al. 2013). This aberrant metabolic re-wiring and dependence on ME1 may exist in other *KRAS* mutated cancers as well. ME1 may also help control the response of cancer to radiotherapy. Increased ME1expression, or the related enzyme GOT1, is associated with poor response to radiotherapy in NSCLC patients (Chakrabarti 2015). Whether ME1 knockdown or its related enzymes promotes the radiation response in vitro or in vivo is not known.

Like the other NADPH-producing enzymes, nicotinamide nucleotide transhydrogenase (NNT) may play a role in mediating redox balance in cancer cells (Li et al. 2018; Chortis et al. 2018). NNT is a mitochondrial enzyme that transfers reducing equivalents from NADH to NADPH and thus may partially couple the bioenergetics and biosynthetic redox pools, but little is known about its role in the radiotherapy response (Ronchi et al. 2016). Thus, most NADPH-producing enzymes can play important roles in maintaining the redox balance of cancer cells depending on the origin tissue or the governing oncogenes present. Because both normal tissues and cancers must use NADPH-dependent molecules to survive the radiation response, a key issue in exploiting this pathway is selectivity. In order to overcome radiation resistance in cancers without causing excessive normal tissue toxicity, a key goal will be to inhibit those NADPH-producing pathways that are especially important to the malignancy in question.

8   Iron Metabolism in Cancer

8.1   *Role of Intracellular Labile Iron in Radiosensitivity*

Iron metabolism is an integral and often overlooked part of cellular function. Within a cell, there are complex metabolic networks geared towards maintaining stable intracellular iron levels. At the center of this network is the labile iron pool (LIP) (Petronek et al. 2019). Unchelated iron (Fe^{2+}) may participate in reactions that cause significant cell damage through its ability to react with oxygen and participate in Fenton chemistry (Wardman and Candeias 1996; Hursting and Kari 1999). Dysregulation of the iron metabolic network is linked to a myriad of diseases including numerous cancers, Alzheimer's disease, Parkinson's disease, iron-deficient anemia, chronic kidney disease, and Friedreich Ataxia (Torti and Torti 2011; Li and Reichmann 2016; Dev and Babitt 2017).

Iron is considered redox active because it can serve as either an electron donor (Fe^{2+} to Fe^{3+}) or an electron acceptor (Fe^{3+} to Fe^{2+}). Due to its redox activity, iron is involved in many different cellular reactions (Miller et al. 1990). The three major classes of iron containing proteins are iron-sulfur containing proteins, heme-containing proteins, and iron enzymes that do not contain heme or iron-sulfur clusters (Kaplan and Ward 2013). However, due to its reactive nature, labile iron is readily able to contribute to intracellular oxidative stress when not stored properly or utilized in proteins. The LIP contains unbound chelatable iron that makes up a small portion of the total iron of the cell ($\leq 2\%$). The LIP is made up of primarily ferrous (Fe^{2+}) iron ($\geq 95\%$) (Breuer et al. 2008; Kruszewski 2003). Despite the LIP making up such a small portion of the total iron content, it is extremely well regulated due to the damage it can cause to a cell. The LIP contributes to the oxidative stress of the cell through the generation of ROS via reactions with molecular oxygen and Fenton chemistry (see Eqs. 1–3) (Wardman and Candeias 1996; Qian and Buettner 1999; Kruszewski 2003; Silva and Faustino 2015). Because of its strong contribution as a catalyst for ROS generation, the LIP concentration acts as a strong trigger for intracellular iron metabolism.

$$Fe^{3+} + O_2^- \rightarrow Fe^{2+} + O_2 \tag{1}$$

$$Fe^{2+} + H_2O_2 \rightarrow Fe^{3+} + OH^- + HO^. \tag{2}$$

$$Net\,reaction: O_2^- + H_2O_2 \xrightarrow{Fe} O_2 + OH^- + HO^. \tag{3}$$

In the realm of radiation biology, low-linear energy transfer (LET) radiations induce cellular damage primarily through the generation of ROS through the indirect action of therapeutic radiation (Radiobiology for the Radiologist 2012; Azzam et al. 2012; Kawamura et al. 2018). In the modeling of indirect action, the radiolysis of water accounts for approximately two-third of radiation-induced damage through the generation of the hydroxyl radical (Radiobiology for the Radiologist 2012). A lesser noted consequence of indirect action is iron labilization. By generating a large flux of reactive free radical species, natural by-products include the labilization of iron due to the thermodynamic favorability of such reactions, described in detail by Petronek et al. (Petronek et al. 2019). The role that the LIP plays in cell death following radiation exposure has been demonstrated in keratinocytes and fibroblasts following exposure to ultraviolet—A (UV-A) radiation (Reelfs et al. 2004; Zhong et al. 2004). Following irradiation, both keratinocytes and fibroblasts experienced an increase in the LIP resulting in the onset of necrosis. The onset of necrosis following exposure to UV-A radiation was blunted by treatment with the iron chelators, Desferal and Hemin. Supporting the notion that increased LIP may be a key contributor to radiation-induced cell death, there appeared to be an inverse relationship between the radiation dose required to induce cell death and the labilization of iron (Zhong et al. 2004). In a Fredrich's Ataxia (FRDA) fibroblast model, it was shown that FRDA phenotypic fibroblasts were prone to an increased mitochondrial LIP. The increased mitochondrial LIP was central to FRDA-associated sensitivity to UV-A radiation as iron chelation was able to significantly reduce their radiosensitivity (Reelfs et al. 2019). While the true effect of LIP modulation has yet to be illuminated, a well-characterized example of the impact the LIP can have on radiosensitization is the use of pharmacological ascorbate (ascorbate plasma concentrations ≥ 10 mM).

8.2 Pharmacologic Ascorbate Works as a Radiosensitizer through Labile Iron

Ascorbic acid (AscH$_2$), colloquially known as vitamin C, is a ketolactone with ionizable hydroxyl groups at the 2nd and 3rd positions. At a physiologic pH of 7.4, the most prevalent form is the ascorbate monoanion (AscH$^-$) as the hydroxyl groups have pK$_a$s at 4.2 and 11.6 (Du et al. 2012). Ascorbate may act as a reducing agent capable of undergoing a reversible Michaelis oxidation to dehydroascorbic acid (DHA) (Eqs. 4 and 5) with a radical intermediate (ascorbate radical; Asc$^{\bullet-}$) (Du et al. 2012; Bielski 1982). The ascorbate radical is considered an unreactive radical species due to its rapid dismutation to DHA (Bielski 1982).

$$AscH_2 \leftrightarrow Asc^- + 2H^+ \tag{4}$$

$$2Asc^- + H^+ \leftrightarrow AscH^- + DHA \tag{5}$$

Ascorbate may undergo pH-dependent autoxidation via the formation of the ascorbate dianion (AscH^{2-}) (see Eq. 6) (Bielski 1982; Du et al. 2012).

$$AscH^{2-} + O_2 \rightarrow Asc^- + O_2^- \tag{6}$$

$$k \approx 3 \times 10^{-1} M^{-1} s^{-1}$$

Therefore, ascorbate may be oxidized to produce superoxide without the aid of catalytic metals. However, this reaction occurs very slowly and is not likely to occur significantly at physiological pH due to the limited amount of the AscH^{2-} present.

Ascorbate oxidation occurs more readily in the presence of catalytic metals (Buettner and Jurkiewicz 1996; Frei and Lawson 2008). Ascorbate can act as a one-electron reducing agent converting ferric (Fe^{3+}) to ferrous (Fe^{2+}) iron resulting in the production of an ascorbate radical (see Eq. 7). In the presence of oxygen, ferrous iron is able to generate superoxide (see Eq. 8). The superoxide radical is then dismuted by superoxide dismutase (SOD) to produce H$_2$O$_2$ and O$_2$ (Eq. 9).

$$AscH^- + Fe^{3+} \rightarrow Fe^{2+} + Asc^- \tag{7}$$

$$Fe^{2+} + O_2 \rightarrow Fe^{3+} + O_2^- \tag{8}$$

$$2O_2^- + 2H^+ \xrightarrow{SOD} H_2O_2 + O_2 \tag{9}$$

H$_2$O$_2$ is a by-product of the high doses of ascorbate delivered throughout treatment and is the central determinant of the cytotoxic effects of ascorbate. When ascorbate exists in millimolar levels, the autoxidation of ascorbate (Eq. 9) produces considerable amounts of H$_2$O$_2$ without the aid of catalytic metals. An ascorbate concentration of 20 mM will consist of $\approx$ 1 μM Asc^{2-} (pH = 7.4) and may result in a flux of H_2O_2 at a rate of approximately 10 nM s^{-1} (Du et al. 2012).

Due to its ability to act as a reducing agent, ascorbate can effectively labilize iron in cancerous cells. By increasing the labile iron pool, there is more iron available to participate in oxidation reactions with ascorbate, O_2, and H_2O_2 to produce toxic ROS. Moser et al. showed that combining ascorbate with ionizing radiation had an additive effect in increasing labile iron pools in MIA PaCa-2 tumor homogenates (Moser et al. 2013). Schoenfeld, et al. went on to show that ascorbate selectively increases the labile iron pool in non-small cell lung cancer and glioblastoma cells in vitro relative to normal cells, sensitizing the neoplastic cells to chemoradiation therapy (Schoenfeld et al. 2017). In vitro knockdown of TfR and overexpression of ferritin rescued cells from the cytotoxic effects of ascorbate evidence that the ascorbate driven increase in labile iron is central to its sensitizing effects (Schoenfeld et al. 2017).

8.3 Clinical Relevance of Pharmacological Ascorbate

In the 1970s, the potential utility of supraphysiological doses of ascorbate (pharmacological ascorbate; achieving mM plasma ascorbate concentrations) given intravenously was established in multiple trials showing safety and efficacy in the treatment of various terminal patients (Cameron and Pauling 1976, 1978; Cameron et al. 1975; Cameron and Campbell 1974). However, two randomized, double-blind clinical trials with high dose oral ascorbate failed to show a clinical benefit relative to placebo (Creagan et al. 1979). This caused a significant reduction in interest in using pharmacologic ascorbate as an anti-cancer agent.

It was later discovered that oral ascorbate administration does not achieve mM plasma ascorbate concentrations necessary to provide anti-cancer effects. In the plasma, the steady-state concentration of ascorbate is $\approx$ 80 μM following an oral dose of 200 mg. As oral doses exceed 200 mg, plasma saturation occurs at approximately 1000 mg with a plasma concentration of $\approx$ 220 μM (Levine et al. 1996; Graumlich et al. 1997). However, an intravenous ascorbate dose of 50 g is able to achieve plasma concentrations of 13.4 mM (Padayatty et al. 2004). A pilot clinical trial using pharmacological ascorbate delivered intravenously showed that a 10 g dose was able to achieve an average plasma concentration of 1.1 mM (Riordan et al. 2004). Therefore, it was determined that best way to effectively deliver pharmacological doses of ascorbate is intravenously.

Since determining an efficacious delivery approach, there has been a resurgence of interest in evaluating the potential anti-cancer capabilities of pharmacological ascorbate. In 2004, Riordan, et al. found pharmacological ascorbate be safe and tolerable in renal cell carcinoma, colorectal cancer, pancreatic cancer, non-Hodgkin's lymphoma, and breast cancer (Riordan et al. 2004). Riordan, et al. then performed a pilot study of intravenous, pharmacological ascorbate in 24, terminally ill cancer patients. All patients in the study were vitamin C deficient prior to beginning the trial and following the infusion of pharmacological ascorbate the mean plasma concentrations reached 1.1 mM. The most common adverse events that this study reported included minor nausea, edema, xerostomia, and dry skin. One patient experienced the development of a kidney stone 13 days into treatment but had a history of renal calculi (Riordan et al. 2004). In 2008, a phase I clinical trial including both solid tumor and hematologic malignancies demonstrated no significant toxicity but also failed to show any anti-cancer responses and concluded that although pharmacological ascorbate may be well tolerated in patients, the promise of ascorbate as an anti-cancer therapy may lie in its use with other cytotoxic therapeutic agents (Hoffer et al. 2008). In 2012, Monti et al. completed a phase I clinical trial combining pharmacological ascorbate with gemcitabine and erlotinib for patients with stage IV pancreatic ductal carcinoma. Over the course of 8 weeks, 14 patients received ascorbate 3 times per week in combination with gemcitabine and erlotinib with 9 of the 14 patients completing the trial. In the patients who completed the trial, seven had stable disease while two showed progression according to the RESIST criteria. The study reported 15 non-serious adverse events and eight serious adverse events, which the investigators believed were attributed to erlotinib and gemcitabine (Monti et al. 2012). In 2014, a phase I clinical trial of 14 stage IV pancreas cancer patients combined pharmacological ascorbate with gemcitabine to assess safety and efficacy. This dose-escalation study gave two infusions of pharmacological ascorbate (15–125 g intravenous; ≥ 20 mM plasma concentration) per week during 4-week chemotherapy cycles. Patients received ascorbate infusions until experiencing a grade 3 dose-limiting toxicity or disease progression (as defined by RESIST criteria). Nine of the 14 subjects enrolled were able to complete at least two treatment cycles. The most common side effects noted were dry mouth, nausea, and diarrhea and no dose-limiting toxicities were observed. At the time of publication (August 2014), the average overall survival was 15 ± 2 months and average time to progression was 26 ± 7 weeks. In this setting, pharmacological ascorbate showed a drastic enhancement of treatment with gemcitabine where historical overall survival was 6 months and the historical average time to progression of 9 weeks (Welsh et al. 2013). Also, in 2014, a phase 1 clinical trial in ovarian cancer showed that pharmacological ascorbate enhanced chemosensitivity in murine models and protected against carboplatin and paclitaxel chemotherapy-associated toxicity in human subjects (Ma et al. 2014). A recent phase 1 clinical trial of newly diagnosed glioblastoma (GBM) patients assessed the potential efficacy of ascorbate with radiation. Eleven patients received pharmacological ascorbate concurrently with radiation and temozolomide chemotherapy followed by adjuvant ascorbate and temozolomide. Throughout the study, the only adverse events attributable to pharmacological ascorbate were dry mouth and chills. The median progression-free survival was 9.4 months and the median overall survival was 18 months (Allen et al. 2019). Patients receiving temozolomide and radiation alone who lacked methylation of the O^6-methylguanine-DNA methyltransferase (MGMT) promoter region had significantly reduced survival (median OS = 12.7 vs. 21.7 months) (Stupp et al. 2005). In eight patients treated with pharmacological ascorbate with temozolomide and radiation lacking MGMT promoter methylation, the median progression-free survival was 10 months and median overall survival was 23 months (Allen et al. 2019). A phase 1 clinical trial in locally advanced pancreas cancer combining pharmacological ascorbate with therapeutic ionizing radiation and gemcitabine chemotherapy demonstrated a significant improvement in progression-free overall survival from 4.6 months to 13.7 months relative to patients receiving radiation and chemotherapy alone (Alexander et al. 2018). Furthermore, pharmacological ascorbate protected against radiation and chemotherapy-induced intestinal damage (Alexander et al. 2018). These results support the hypothesis that by working through the labilization of iron, pharmacological ascorbate has the potential to enhance current standard clinical practices, including radiation therapy.

9 Dietary Strategies

9.1 Diet and Cancer

It is estimated that approximately one-third of all cancer-related deaths worldwide are related to diet (Doll and Peto 1981). The large differences in cancer incidence rates among the various world populations suggest that lifestyle and diet contribute to the development of many common cancers. The hypothesis that diet can influence both cancer risk and response to cancer therapy is supported by both descriptive and epidemiologic research (Koriech 1994). The relationships among the processes of metabolism, aging, and cancer have created a re-emergence of interest in dietary modifications as an approach to enhance cancer therapy. Recent results of laboratory and clinical trial research encourage further exploration into the association between cancer and patient diet (Koriech 1994).

Many cancer therapies exploit fundamental metabolic differences between cancer cells and normal cells. Relative to normal cells, cancer cells have increased glucose uptake, increased frequency of mutations in mitochondrial and nuclear DNA encoding for electron transport chain complexes, and increased levels of the ROS including hydrogen peroxide (H_2O_2) and superoxide ($O_2^{\cdot-}$) (Polyak et al. 1998; Fliss et al. 2000; Spitz et al. 2000; Nishikawa et al. 2001; Liu et al. 2001; Petros et al. 2005; Zhou et al. 2007; Kroemer and Pouyssegur 2008; Aykin-Burns et al. 2009; Schoenfeld et al. 2017). Fluorodeoxyglucose positron emission tomography (FDG-PET) as a part of cancer imaging is based upon increased cancer glucose demand related to the surrounding normal tissues (Rigo et al. 1996). It has long been proposed that cancer cells have increased glucose demand because they have defective mitochondrial respiration requiring increased glycolysis as a compensatory mechanism for energy production (Warburg 1956). Defective mitochondrial respiration can result in pro-tumorigenic mitochondrial ROS production (Ishikawa et al. 2008). In addition to increased glycolysis, cancer cells also have an increased pentose phosphate pathway activity to produce the reducing agent, nicotinamide adenine dinucleotide phosphate (NADPH). NADPH is a necessary cofactor for the reduction of H_2O_2 and organic peroxides via glutathione/glutathione peroxidase and thioredoxin/thioredoxin peroxidase pathways (Buettner 2011) to reduce cellular oxidative stress. Previous studies showed that glucose deprivation selectively increases cancer cell oxidative stress relative to normal cells and that treatment with a $O_2^{\cdot-}$ or H_2O_2 scavengers restores the oxidative stress levels in the cell (Ahmad et al. 2005; Aykin-Burns et al. 2009).

Since cancer cells depend upon glucose metabolism for both energy production and the generation of NADPH to mitigate the increased ROS from defective mitochondrial metabolism, it is reasonable to propose that approaches which decrease cancer cell glucose availability would selectively sensitize cancer cells to ROS inducing anti-cancer approaches. Anthracyclines, platinum-containing complexes, DNA-alkylating agents, epipodophyllotoxins, and camptothecins are chemotherapy agents that induce oxidative stress (Conklin 2004). Therapeutic radiation can damage cells either by direct or indirect action. In direct action, ionizing radiation interacts directly with DNA, creating structural damage that may result in cell damage or cell death (Radiobiology for the Radiologist 2012). In indirect action, therapeutic radiation ionizes water and other organic molecules forming free radicals including the hydroxyl radical (HO•) and alkoxy radical (RO$_2$•) (Radiobiology for the Radiologist 2012). These free radicals are highly reactive and can damage cellular proteins, DNA, and lipids resulting in cell damage or death.

9.2   Ketogenic Diets

Ketogenic diets are high in fat (90% of calorie intake), low in protein (8%) and carbohydrate (2%) content (Allen et al. 2014). Because of the minimal carbohydrate and protein calorie intake, fat metabolism serves as the main energy source for the body. Fatty acid oxidation produces ketone bodies which can then be converted to acetyl-CoA and enter the citric acid cycle producing adenosine triphosphate (ATP). Since the early twentieth century, ketogenic diets have been used to successfully treat childhood epilepsy (Wheless 2004). A recent clinical study in treatment-intractable epilepsy randomized children to consuming a ketogenic diet or continued standard of care (control) found that the diet group experienced significantly fewer seizures than the control group (Neal et al. 2008).

Ketogenic diets have recently been studied as a complementary approach to enhance cancer therapy in both animal models and early phase clinical trials. In the 1980s, colon cancer mouse xenografts fed a ketogenic diet had decreased tumor size and reduced weight loss (Tisdale et al. 1987). Additional animal studies identified that high fat diets decreased tumor growth and improved survival in models of malignant glioma (Seyfried et al. 2003; Maurer et al. 2011), colon (Beck and Tisdale 1989), stomach (Otto et al. 2008), and prostate cancers (Freedland et al. 2008; Mavropoulos et al. 2009). Ketogenic diets enhanced radiation effectiveness improving overall survival in non-small cell lung cancer (Allen et al. 2013), pancreas cancer (Zahra et al. 2017), malignant glioma (Abdelwahab et al. 2012) animal models. In addition, ketogenic diets enhanced radiation and chemotherapy effectiveness in an NSCLC mouse model (Abdelwahab et al. 2012).

Early clinical examples of consuming a ketogenic diet to enhance cancer therapy include a case report of two pediatric patients with advanced stage malignant astrocytoma. They consumed a 60% medium chain triglyceride oil-based diet, demonstrating reduced tumor FDG-PET uptake compared to pre-diet imaging (Nebeling et al. 1995). A case report of a 65-year-old female diagnosed with a GBM tumor consumed a ketogenic diet while receiving standard radiation and temozolomide therapy for 2 months; no detectable tumor was found on FDG-PET or MR imaging (Zuccoli et al. 2010). A randomized controlled trial in women with ovarian or endometrial cancer found that ketogenic diets reduced fatigue associated with cancer therapy (Cohen et al. 2018). A pilot study of ketogenic diets in 20 subjects with recurrent GBM found ketogenic diets to be feasible and safe but without clinical activity when used as a single agent (Rieger et al. 2014). Some ongoing and active clinical trials combining a ketogenic diet include: a phase 2 trial in children with malignant or recurrent/refractory brain tumors (NCT03328858), phase 1 trial refractory/end stage GBM (NCT01865162), phase 2 trial in GBM (NCT02302235), phase 1 trial combining a ketogenic diet with letrozole in estrogen receptor-positive breast cancer (NCT03962647), and a trial combining a ketogenic diet and palliative chemotherapy in stage IV breast cancer (NCT03535701). However, some patients have difficulty tolerating a ketogenic diet in combination with standard cancer therapy. Phase 1 clinical trial patients who combined a ketogenic diet with radiation and chemotherapy in locally advanced lung and pancreas cancer had difficulty complying with the diet and had poor tolerance (Zahra et al. 2017). Observed toxicities included grade 4 hyperuricemia and grade 3 nausea, dehydration, and hypokalemia (Zahra et al. 2017). A clinical trial combining a ketogenic diet with radiation and chemotherapy in GBM found that ketogenic diets may exacerbate nausea and gastric distress (Schwartz et al. 2018).

Many preclinical studies have demonstrated the effectiveness of ketogenic diets when combined with radiation and chemotherapy in improving cancer outcomes. Early clinical studies with a ketogenic diet alone or in combination with traditional cancer therapies are promising. However, some cancer patients are not able to tolerate a ketogenic diet in combination with radiation therapy and/or chemotherapy due to the gastrointestinal side effects and risk of hyperuricemia. Careful patient selection is necessary when considering a ketogenic diet trial as an anti-cancer therapy.

9.3 Calorie Restriction

Reducing calorie intake by 20–40% without limiting essential vitamins and nutrients has been demonstrated to increase life span across a variety of species (Champ et al. 2013). The process of calorie restriction can be achieved either via intermittent fasting or by overall dietary reduction (Hursting and Kari 1999; Hursting et al. 2003). Calorie restriction slows degenerative pathologies including cataract formation, cardiomyopathy, nephropathy, and cancer initiation (Hursting and Kari 1999). Several animal studies have demonstrated that calorie restriction protects against spontaneous and chemically induced cancers (Weindruch et al. 1988; Hursting et al. 1993; Silverstone and Tannenbaum 1951). Similarly, humans with anorexia nervosa have a much lower risk of developing cancer than the general population (Mellemkjaer et al. 2001; Michels and Ekbom 2004). Alternatively, obesity is associated with higher risks of developing cancer as well as cancer-associated mortality (Calle et al. 2003; Hite et al. 2011). Because of the strong correlation between the processes governing aging, obesity, and cancer; calorie restriction has recently re-emerged as a possible dietary modification to enhance traditional cancer therapy (Hursting and Kari 1999; Campisi 2013).

As far back as the early 1900s, it was shown that animals fed a calorie restricted diet had slower tumor growth rates and metastasis relative to mice fed ad libitum (Hursting et al. 2003; Rous 1914; Campisi 2013). More recent animal studies identified that calorie restriction increases survival times after cancer initiation (Berrigan et al. 2002; Cheney et al. 1983). Likewise, patients who have undergone gastric bypass surgery frequently reduce their calorie intake by >50% and have significantly reduced lower cancer incidence rates relative to obese control patients (Dias et al. 2006; Adams et al. 2009).

The mechanisms responsible for calorie restriction's anti-cancer properties resemble those of ketogenic diets. Both calorie restriction and ketogenic diets decrease the secretion of proliferation promoting hormones including growth hormone, insulin, and insulin-like growth factor I (IGF-1) (Baserga 1992; Parr 1996; Dunn et al. 1997). IGF-1 modulates cell proliferation by binding to insulin-like growth factor receptors (IGF-1R) which in turn activate the PI3K/AKT pathway promoting cell growth and inhibiting apoptosis (Resnicoff et al. 1994; Champ et al. 2013). Calorie restriction reduces serum IGF-1, insulin, and IGF-1R expression in breast cancer animal models (Ruggeri et al. 1989). Therapeutic radiation increases IGF-1R expression on tumor cells likely as a survival mechanism following radiation-induced DNA damage (Cosaceanu et al. 2007). Inhibition of IGF-1R leads to enhanced radiation sensitivity, inhibited proliferation, and induced apoptosis in breast cancer cell lines (Wen et al. 2001). Fasting mice for 72 h showed a 70% reduction in circulating IGF-1 (Lee et al. 2010). Calorie restriction also decreases insulin receptor and phosphatidylinositol-3-kinase expression resulting in enhanced radiation sensitivity and reduced tumor growth in both in vivo and in vitro models (Price and Youmell 1996; Cataldi et al. 2001; Kandel et al. 2002; Gupta et al. 2003; Soderlund et al. 2005). These data suggest that the combination of radiation with calorie restriction or ketogenic diets enhance tumor cell killing.

Calorie restriction is currently being assessed as an adjuvant to radiation and chemotherapy in variety of clinical trials. Current active and ongoing clinical trials include a caloric restriction diet prior to surgery in patients with endometrial, prostate, or breast cancer (NCT02983279); calorie restricted ketogenic diet as a treatment in malignant tumors (NCT03160599); caloric restriction and exercise for the protection from anthracycline toxicities in breast cancer (NCT03131024); and the effect of caloric restriction on post-operative complications in sarcoma patients treated with neoadjuvant radiation therapy (NCT02792270). However, methods of measuring adherence to calorie restriction diets is difficult relying predominantly on food journals, interviews, and questionnaires (Heilbronn et al. 2006). In addition, caloric restriction may not be suitable for all cancer patients as possible complications include weight loss, impaired wound healing, and impaired immune function (Reed et al. 1996; Fontana et al. 2010).

In conclusion, the data supporting an association between dietary modification and the influence on cancer incidence, treatment, and survival is strong. Both ketogenic diets and caloric restriction downregulate several molecular pathways involved in cancer cell progression and survival. The exciting clinical trials utilizing ketogenic diets and caloric restriction may change the treatment paradigm for a variety of malignancies.

10 Conclusion

Metabolic reprogramming is a hallmark of cancer, and many cancer therapies, including radiation, are known to impact tumor metabolism. A strong preclinical rationale exists to combine drugs that increase intracellular oxidative stress and/or interfere with nucleotide metabolism with primary radiation therapy. Preclinical and clinical evidence support the combined use of a number of metabolically targeted agents with radiation therapy. Work is ongoing to determine the optimized strategy for combining these drugs with conventionally fractionated and hypofractionated schemes. New strategies, including dietary manipulation during the course of radiation therapy, are currently being explored.

References

Abdelwahab MG, Fenton KE, Preul MC, Rho JM, Lynch A, Stafford P, Scheck AC (2012) The ketogenic diet is an effective adjuvant to radiation therapy for the treatment of malignant glioma. PLoS One 7(5):e36197. https://doi.org/10.1371/journal.pone.0036197

Adams TD, Stroup AM, Gress RE, Adams KF, Calle EE, Smith SC, Halverson RC, Simper SC, Hopkins PN, Hunt SC (2009) Cancer incidence and mortality after gastric bypass surgery. Obesity (Silver Spring) 17(4):796–802. https://doi.org/10.1038/oby.2008.610

Ahmad IM, Aykin-Burns N, Sim JE, Walsh SA, Higashikubo R, Buettner GR, Venkataraman S, Mackey MA, Flanagan SW, Oberley LW, Spitz DR (2005) Mitochondrial O2*- and H2O2 mediate glucose deprivation-induced stress in human cancer cells. J Biol Chem 280(6):4254–4263. https://doi.org/10.1074/jbc.M411662200

Alberghina L, Gaglio D (2014) Redox control of glutamine utilization in cancer. Cell Death Dis 5:e1561. https://doi.org/10.1038/cddis.2014.513

Alexander MS, Wilkes JG, Schroeder SR, Buettner GR, Wagner BA, Du J, Gibson-Corley K, O'Leary BR, Spitz DR, Buatti JM, Berg DJ, Bodeker KL, Vollstedt S, Brown HA, Allen BG, Cullen JJ (2018) Pharmacologic ascorbate reduces radiation-induced normal tissue toxicity and enhances tumor radiosensitization in pancreatic cancer. Cancer Res 78(24):6838–6851. https://doi.org/10.1158/0008-5472.CAN-18-1680

Allegra CJ, Chabner BA, Drake JC, Lutz R, Rodbard D, Jolivet J (1985a) Enhanced inhibition of thymidylate synthase by methotrexate polyglutamates. J Biol Chem 260(17):9720–9726

Allegra CJ, Drake JC, Jolivet J, Chabner BA (1985b) Inhibition of phosphoribosylaminoimidazolecarboxamide transformylase by methotrexate and dihydrofolic acid polyglutamates. Proc Natl Acad Sci U S A 82(15):4881–4885. https://doi.org/10.1073/pnas.82.15.4881

Allen AM, Czerminska M, Janne PA, Sugarbaker DJ, Bueno R, Harris JR, Court L, Baldini EH (2006) Fatal pneumonitis associated with intensity-modulated radiation therapy for mesothelioma. Int J Radiat Oncol Biol Phys 65(3):640–645. https://doi.org/10.1016/j.ijrobp.2006.03.012

Allen BG, Bhatia SK, Anderson CM, Eichenberger-Gilmore JM, Sibenaller ZA, Mapuskar KA, Schoenfeld JD, Buatti JM, Spitz DR, Fath MA (2014) Ketogenic diets as an adjuvant cancer therapy: history and potential mechanism. Redox Biol 2:963–970. https://doi.org/10.1016/j.redox.2014.08.002

Allen BG, Bhatia SK, Buatti JM, Brandt KE, Lindholm KE, Button AM, Szweda LI, Smith BJ, Spitz DR, Fath MA (2013) Ketogenic diets enhance oxidative stress and radio-chemotherapy responses in lung cancer xenografts. Clin Cancer Res 19(14):3905–3913. https://doi.org/10.1158/1078-0432.CCR-12-0287

Allen BG, Bodeker KL, Smith MC, Monga V, Sandhu S, Hohl RJ, Carlisle TL, Brown HA, Hollenbeck NJ, Vollstedt S, Greenlee JDW, Howard MA, Mapuskar KA, Seyedin SN, Caster JM, Jones KA, Cullen JJ, Berg DJ, Wagner BA, Buettner GR, TenNapel MJ, Smith BJ, Spitz DR, Buatti JM (2019) First-in-human phase 1 clinical trial of pharmacological ascorbate combined with radiation and temozolomide for newly diagnosed glioblastoma. Clin Cancer Res. https://doi.org/10.1158/1078-0432.CCR-19-0594

Altman BJ, Stine ZE, Dang CV (2016) From Krebs to clinic: glutamine metabolism to cancer therapy. Nat Rev Cancer 16(10):619–634. https://doi.org/10.1038/nrc.2016.71

Aykin-Burns N, Ahmad IM, Zhu Y, Oberley LW, Spitz DR (2009) Increased levels of superoxide and H2O2 mediate the differential susceptibility of cancer cells versus normal cells to glucose deprivation. Biochem J 418(1):29–37. https://doi.org/10.1042/BJ20081258

Azzam EI, Jay-Gerin JP, Pain D (2012) Ionizing radiation-induced metabolic oxidative stress and prolonged cell injury. Cancer Lett 327(1–2):48–60. https://doi.org/10.1016/j.canlet.2011.12.012

Banerjee RV, Matthews RG (1990) Cobalamin-dependent methionine synthase. FASEB J 4(5):1450–1459. https://doi.org/10.1096/fasebj.4.5.2407589

Bartelink H, Roelofsen F, Eschwege F, Rougier P, Bosset JF, Gonzalez DG, Peiffert D, van Glabbeke M, Pierart M (1997) Concomitant radiotherapy and chemotherapy is superior to radiotherapy alone in the treatment of locally advanced anal cancer: results of a phase III randomized trial of the European Organization for Research and Treatment of Cancer Radiotherapy and Gastrointestinal Cooperative Groups. J Clin Oncol Off J Am Soc Clin Oncol 15(5):2040–2049. https://doi.org/10.1200/jco.1997.15.5.2040

Bartrons R, Simon-Molas H, Rodriguez-Garcia A, Castano E, Navarro-Sabate A, Manzano A, Martinez-Outschoorn UE (2018) Fructose 2,6-Bisphosphate in cancer cell metabolism. Front Oncol 8:331. https://doi.org/10.3389/fonc.2018.00331

Baserga R (1992) The double life of the IGF-1 receptor. Receptor 2(4):261–266

Batra V, Kislay B (2013) Mitigation of gamma-radiation induced abasic sites in genomic DNA by dietary nicotinamide supplementation: metabolic up-regulation of NAD(+) biosynthesis. Mutat Res 749(1–2):28–38. https://doi.org/10.1016/j.mrfmmm.2013.07.001

Beck SA, Tisdale MJ (1989) Nitrogen excretion in cancer cachexia and its modification by a high fat diet in mice. Cancer Res 49(14):3800–3804

Beets GL, Beets-Tan RG (2012) Capecitabine in the treatment of rectal cancer. Lancet Oncol 13(6):560–561. https://doi.org/10.1016/s1470-2045(12)70170-5

Belanger K, Klecker RW Jr, Rowland J, Kinsella TJ, Collins JM (1986) Incorporation of iododeoxyuridine into DNA of granulocytes in patients. Cancer Res 46(12 Pt 1):6509–6512

Ben-Josef E, Guthrie KA, El-Khoueiry AB, Corless CL, Zalupski MM, Lowy AM, Thomas CR Jr, Alberts SR, Dawson LA, Micetich KC, Thomas MB, Siegel AB, Blanke CD (2015) SWOG S0809: a phase II intergroup trial of adjuvant capecitabine and gemcitabine followed by radiotherapy and concurrent capecitabine in extrahepatic cholangiocarcinoma and gallbladder carcinoma. J Clin Oncol Off J Am Soc Clin Oncol 33(24):2617–2622. https://doi.org/10.1200/JCO.2014.60.2219

Bensaad K, Tsuruta A, Selak MA, Vidal MN, Nakano K, Bartrons R, Gottlieb E, Vousden KH (2006) TIGAR, a p53-inducible regulator of glycolysis and apoptosis. Cell 126(1):107–120. https://doi.org/10.1016/j.cell.2006.05.036

Berghmans T, Dusart M, Paesmans M, Hossein-Foucher C, Buvat I, Castaigne C, Scherpereel A, Mascaux C, Moreau M, Roelandts M, Alard S, Meert AP, Patz EF, Lafitte JJ, Sculier JP, Project ELCWPftILCS (2008) Primary tumor standardized uptake value (SUVmax) measured on fluorodeoxyglucose positron emission tomography (FDG-PET) is of prognostic value for survival in non-small cell lung cancer (NSCLC): a systematic review and meta-analysis (MA) by the European Lung Cancer Working Party for the IASLC Lung Cancer Staging Project. J Thorac Oncol 3(1):6–12. https://doi.org/10.1097/JTO.0b013e31815e6d6b

Berrigan D, Perkins SN, Haines DC, Hursting SD (2002) Adult-onset calorie restriction and fasting delay spontaneous tumorigenesis in p53-deficient mice. Carcinogenesis 23(5):817–822. https://doi.org/10.1093/carcin/23.5.817

Bielski BHJ (1982) Chemistry of ascorbic acid radicals. In: Ascorbic acid: chemistry, metabolism, and uses, vol 200.. Advances in Chemistry, vol 200. American Chemical Society, pp 81–100. https://doi.org/10.1021/ba-1982-0200.ch004

Bischof M, Huber P, Stoffregen C, Wannenmacher M, Weber KJ (2003) Radiosensitization by pemetrexed of human colon carcinoma cells in different cell cycle phases. Int J Radiat Oncol Biol Phys 57(1):289–292. https://doi.org/10.1016/s0360-3016(03)00595-9

Bischof M, Weber KJ, Blatter J, Wannenmacher M, Latz D (2002) Interaction of pemetrexed disodium (ALIMTA, multitargeted antifolate) and irradiation in vitro. Int J Radiat Oncol Biol Phys 52(5):1381–1388. https://doi.org/10.1016/s0360-3016(01)02794-8

Bogan KL, Brenner C (2008) Nicotinic acid, nicotinamide, and nicotinamide riboside: a molecular evaluation of NAD+ precursor vitamins in human nutrition. Annu Rev Nutr 28:115–130. https://doi.org/10.1146/annurev.nutr.28.061807.155443

Bokkerink JP, De Abreu RA, Bakker MA, Hulscher TW, Van Baal JM, De Vaan GA (1986) Dose-related effects of methotrexate on purine and pyrimidine nucleotides and on cell-kinetic parameters in MOLT-4 malignant human T-lymphoblasts. Biochem Pharmacol 35(20):3557–3564. https://doi.org/10.1016/0006-2952(86)90626-x

Bosset J-F, Calais G, Mineur L, Maingon P, Radosevic-Jelic L, Daban A, Bardet E, Beny A, Briffaux A, Collette L (2005) Enhanced tumorocidal effect of chemotherapy with preoperative radiotherapy for rectal cancer: preliminary results—EORTC 22921. J Clin Oncol 23(24):5620–5627. https://doi.org/10.1200/JCO.2005.02.113

Boysen G, Jamshidi-Parsian A, Davis MA, Siegel ER, Simecka CM, Kore RA, Dings RPM, Griffin RJ (2019) Glutaminase inhibitor CB-839 increases radiation sensitivity of lung tumor cells and human lung tumor xenografts in mice. Int J Radiat Biol 95(4):436–442. https://doi.org/10.1080/09553002.2018.1558299

Brade A, Bezjak A, MacRae R, Laurie S, Sun A, Cho J, Leighl N, Pearson S, Southwood B, Wang L, McGill S, Iscoe N, Shepherd FA (2011) Phase I trial of radiation with concurrent and consolidation pemetrexed and cisplatin in patients with unresectable stage IIIA/B non-small-cell lung cancer. Int J Radiat Oncol Biol Phys 79(5):1395–1401. https://doi.org/10.1016/j.ijrobp.2010.01.014

Brade A, MacRae R, Laurie SA, Bezjak A, Burkes R, Chu Q, Goffin JR, Cho J, Hope A, Sun A, Leighl N, Capobianco S, Feld R, Mahalingam E, Hossain A, Iscoe N, Shepherd FA (2016) Phase II study of concurrent pemetrexed, cisplatin, and radiation therapy for stage IIIA/B unresectable non-small cell lung cancer. Clin Lung Cancer 17(2):133–141. https://doi.org/10.1016/j.cllc.2015.12.008

Breuer W, Shvartsman M, Cabantchik ZI (2008) Intracellular labile iron. Int J Biochem Cell Biol 40(3):350–354. https://doi.org/10.1016/j.biocel.2007.03.010

Brosnan ME, Brosnan JT (2016) Formate: the neglected member of one-carbon metabolism. Annu Rev Nutr 36:369–388. https://doi.org/10.1146/annurev-nutr-071715-050738

Brun E, Kjellén E, Tennvall J, Ohlsson T, Sandell A, Perfekt R, Wennerberg J, Strand SE (2002) FDG PET studies during treatment: prediction of therapy outcome in head and neck squamous cell carcinoma. Head Neck 24(2):127–135

Bruso CE, Shewach DS, Lawrence TS (1990) Fluorodeoxyuridine-induced radiosensitization and inhibition of DNA double strand break repair in human colon cancer cells. Int J Radiat Oncol Biol Phys 19(6):1411–1417. https://doi.org/10.1016/0360-3016(90)90352-k

Buettner GR (2011) Superoxide dismutase in redox biology: the roles of superoxide and hydrogen peroxide. Anti Cancer Agents Med Chem 11(4):341–346

Buettner GR, Jurkiewicz BA (1996) Catalytic metals, ascorbate and free radicals: combinations to avoid. Radiat Res 145(5):532–541

Calle EE, Rodriguez C, Walker-Thurmond K, Thun MJ (2003) Overweight, obesity, and mortality from cancer in a prospectively studied cohort of U.S. adults. N Engl J Med 348(17):1625–1638. https://doi.org/10.1056/NEJMoa021423

Calvert AE, Chalastanis A, Wu Y, Hurley LA, Kouri FM, Bi Y, Kachman M, May JL, Bartom E, Hua Y, Mishra RK, Schiltz GE, Dubrovskyi O, Mazar AP, Peter ME, Zheng H, James CD, Burant CF, Chandel NS, Davuluri RV, Horbinski C, Stegh AH (2017) Cancer-associated IDH1 promotes growth and resistance to targeted therapies in the absence of mutation. Cell Rep 19(9):1858–1873. https://doi.org/10.1016/j.celrep.2017.05.014

Cameron E, Campbell A (1974) The orthomolecular treatment of cancer. II. Clinical trial of high-dose ascorbic acid supplements in advanced human cancer. Chem Biol Interact 9(4):285–315. https://doi.org/10.1016/0009-2797(74)90019-2

Cameron E, Campbell A, Jack T (1975) The orthomolecular treatment of cancer. III. Reticulum cell sarcoma: double complete regression induced by high-dose ascorbic acid therapy. Chem Biol Interact 11(5):387–393. https://doi.org/10.1016/0009-2797(75)90007-1

Cameron E, Pauling L (1976) Supplemental ascorbate in the supportive treatment of cancer: prolongation of survival times in terminal human cancer. Proc Natl Acad Sci U S A 73(10):3685–3689. https://doi.org/10.1073/pnas.73.10.3685

Cameron E, Pauling L (1978) Supplemental ascorbate in the supportive treatment of cancer: reevaluation of prolongation of survival times in terminal human cancer. Proc Natl Acad Sci U S A 75(9):4538–4542. https://doi.org/10.1073/pnas.75.9.4538

Campisi J (2013) Aging, cellular senescence, and cancer. Annu Rev Physiol 75:685–705. https://doi.org/10.1146/annurev-physiol-030212-183653

Carreras CW, Santi DV (1995) The catalytic mechanism and structure of thymidylate synthase. Annu Rev Biochem 64:721–762. https://doi.org/10.1146/annurev.bi.64.070195.003445

Cataldi A, Zauli G, Di Pietro R, Castorina S, Rana R (2001) Involvement of the pathway phosphatidylinositol-3-kinase/AKT-1 in the establishment of the survival response to ionizing radiation. Cell Signal 13(5):369–375. https://doi.org/10.1016/s0898-6568(01)00147-4

Cerna D, Li H, Flaherty S, Takebe N, Coleman CN, Yoo SS (2012) Inhibition of nicotinamide phosphoribosyltransferase (NAMPT) activity by small molecule GMX1778 regulates reactive oxygen species (ROS)-mediated cytotoxicity in a p53- and nicotinic acid phosphoribosyltransferase1 (NAPRT1)-dependent manner. J Biol Chem 287(26):22408–22417. https://doi.org/10.1074/jbc.M112.357301

Chakrabarti G (2015) Mutant KRAS associated malic enzyme 1 expression is a predictive marker for radiation therapy response in non-small cell lung cancer. Radiat Oncol 10(1):145. https://doi.org/10.1186/s13014-015-0457-x

Champ CE, Baserga R, Mishra MV, Jin L, Sotgia F, Lisanti MP, Pestell RG, Dicker AP, Simone NL (2013) Nutrient restriction and radiation therapy for cancer treatment: when less is more. Oncologist 18(1):97–103. https://doi.org/10.1634/theoncologist.2012-0164

Cheney KE, Liu RK, Smith GS, Meredith PJ, Mickey MR, Walford RL (1983) The effect of dietary restriction of varying duration on survival, tumor patterns, immune function, and body temperature in B10C3F1 female mice. J Gerontol 38(4):420–430. https://doi.org/10.1093/geronj/38.4.420

Chortis V, Taylor AE, Doig CL, Walsh MD, Meimaridou E, Jenkinson C, Rodriguez-Blanco G, Ronchi CL, Jafri A, Metherell LA, Hebenstreit D, Dunn WB, Arlt W, Foster PA (2018) Nicotinamide nucleotide transhydrogenase as a novel treatment target in adrenocortical carcinoma. Endocrinology 159(8):2836–2849. https://doi.org/10.1210/en.2018-00014

Choudhury A, Swindell R, Logue JP, Elliott PA, Livsey JE, Wise M, Symonds P, Wylie JP, Ramani V, Sangar V, Lyons J, Bottomley I, McCaul D, Clarke NW, Kiltie AE, Cowan RA (2011) Phase II study of conformal hypofractionated radiotherapy with concurrent gemcitabine in muscle-invasive bladder cancer. J Clin Oncol Off J Am Soc Clin Oncol 29(6):733–738. https://doi.org/10.1200/jco.2010.31.5721

Cohen CW, Fontaine KR, Arend RC, Soleymani T, Gower BA (2018) Favorable effects of a ketogenic diet on physical function, perceived energy, and food cravings in women with ovarian or endometrial cancer: a randomized, controlled trial. Nutrients 10(9). https://doi.org/10.3390/nu10091187

Cohen MH, Cortazar P, Justice R, Pazdur R (2010) Approval summary: pemetrexed maintenance therapy of advanced/metastatic nonsquamous, non-small cell lung cancer (NSCLC). Oncologist 15(12):1352–1358. https://doi.org/10.1634/theoncologist.2010-0224

Collins RRJ, Patel K, Putnam WC, Kapur P, Rakheja D (2017) Oncometabolites: a new paradigm for oncology, metabolism, and the clinical laboratory. Clin Chem 63(12):1812–1820. https://doi.org/10.1373/clinchem.2016.267666

Condit PT, Ridings GR, Coin JW, Williams GR, Mitchell D Jr, Boles GW (1964) Methotrexate and radiation in the treatment of patients with cancer. Cancer Res 24:1524–1533

Conklin KA (2004) Chemotherapy-associated oxidative stress: impact on chemotherapeutic effectiveness. Integr Cancer Ther 3(4):294–300. https://doi.org/10.1177/1534735404270335

Cosaceanu D, Budiu RA, Carapancea M, Castro J, Lewensohn R, Dricu A (2007) Ionizing radiation activates IGF-1R triggering a cytoprotective signaling by interfering with Ku-DNA binding and by modulating Ku86 expression via a p38 kinase-dependent mechanism. Oncogene 26(17):2423–2434. https://doi.org/10.1038/sj.onc.1210037

Creagan ET, Moertel CG, O'Fallon JR, Schutt AJ, O'Connell MJ, Rubin J, Frytak S (1979) Failure of high-dose vitamin C (ascorbic acid) therapy to benefit patients with advanced cancer. A controlled trial. N Engl J Med 301(13):687–690. https://doi.org/10.1056/NEJM197909273011303

Cuneo KC, Morgan MA, Sahai V, Schipper MJ, Parsels LA, Parsels JD, Devasia T, Al-Hawaray M, Cho CS, Nathan H, Maybaum J, Zalupski MM, Lawrence TS (2019) Dose escalation trial of the Wee1 inhibitor Adavosertib (AZD1775) in combination with gemcitabine and radiation for patients with locally advanced pancreatic cancer. J Clin Oncol:Jco1900730. https://doi.org/10.1200/jco.19.00730

De Vos M, Schreiber V, Dantzer F (2012) The diverse roles and clinical relevance of PARPs in DNA damage repair: current state of the art. Biochem Pharmacol 84(2):137–146. https://doi.org/10.1016/j.bcp.2012.03.018

DeBerardinis RJ, Chandel NS (2016) Fundamentals of cancer metabolism. Sci Adv 2(5):e1600200. https://doi.org/10.1126/sciadv.1600200

Demas DM, Demo S, Fallah Y, Clarke R, Nephew KP, Althouse S, Sandusky G, He W, Shajahan-Haq AN (2019) Glutamine metabolism drives growth in advanced hormone receptor positive breast cancer. Front Oncol 9:686. https://doi.org/10.3389/fonc.2019.00686

DeNicola GM, Karreth FA, Humpton TJ, Gopinathan A, Wei C, Frese K, Mangal D, Yu KH, Yeo CJ, Calhoun ES, Scrimieri F, Winter JM, Hruban RH, Iacobuzio-Donahue C, Kern SE, Blair IA, Tuveson DA (2011) Oncogene-induced Nrf2 transcription promotes ROS detoxification and tumorigenesis. Nature 475(7354):106–109. https://doi.org/10.1038/nature10189

Dev S, Babitt JL (2017) Overview of iron metabolism in health and disease. Hemodial Int 21(Suppl 1):S6–S20. https://doi.org/10.1111/hdi.12542

Dias MC, Ribeiro AG, Scabim VM, Faintuch J, Zilberstein B, Gama-Rodrigues JJ (2006) Dietary intake of female bariatric patients after anti-obesity gastroplasty. Clinics (Sao Paulo) 61(2):93–98. https://doi.org/10.1590/s1807-59322006000200002

Dibble CC, Manning BD (2013) Signal integration by mTORC1 coordinates nutrient input with biosynthetic output. Nat Cell Biol 15(6):555–564. https://doi.org/10.1038/ncb2763

Diehn M, Cho RW, Lobo NA, Kalisky T, Dorie MJ, Kulp AN, Qian D, Lam JS, Ailles LE, Wong M, Joshua B, Kaplan MJ, Wapnir I, Dirbas FM, Somlo G, Garberoglio C, Paz B, Shen J, Lau SK, Quake SR, Brown JM, Weissman IL, Clarke MF (2009) Association of reactive oxygen species levels and radioresistance in cancer stem cells. Nature 458(7239):780–783. https://doi.org/10.1038/nature07733

Doll R, Peto R (1981) The causes of cancer: quantitative estimates of avoidable risks of cancer in the United States today. J Natl Cancer Inst 66(6):1191–1308

Du J, Cullen JJ, Buettner GR (2012) Ascorbic acid: chemistry, biology and the treatment of cancer. Biochim Biophys Acta 1826(2):443–457. https://doi.org/10.1016/j.bbcan.2012.06.003

Ducker GS, Ghergurovich JM, Mainolfi N, Suri V, Jeong SK, Hsin-Jung Li S, Friedman A, Manfredi MG, Gitai Z, Kim H, Rabinowitz JD (2017) Human SHMT inhibitors reveal defective glycine import as a targetable metabolic vulnerability of diffuse large B-cell lymphoma. Proc Natl Acad Sci 114(43):11404–11409. https://doi.org/10.1073/pnas.1706617114

Ducker GS, Rabinowitz JD (2017) One-carbon metabolism in health and disease. Cell Metab 25(1):27–42. https://doi.org/10.1016/j.cmet.2016.08.009

Dunn SE, Kari FW, French J, Leininger JR, Travlos G, Wilson R, Barrett JC (1997) Dietary restriction reduces insulin-like growth factor I levels, which modulates apoptosis, cell proliferation, and tumor progression in p53-deficient mice. Cancer Res 57(21):4667–4672

El Mjiyad N, Caro-Maldonado A, Ramirez-Peinado S, Munoz-Pinedo C (2011) Sugar-free approaches to cancer cell killing. Oncogene 30(3):253–264. https://doi.org/10.1038/onc.2010.466

Elledge SJ, Davis RW (1989) DNA damage induction of ribonucleotide reductase. Mol Cell Biol 9(11):4932–4940. https://doi.org/10.1128/mcb.9.11.4932

Fan J, Ye J, Kamphorst JJ, Shlomi T, Thompson CB, Rabinowitz JD (2014) Quantitative flux analysis reveals folate-dependent NADPH production. Nature 510(7504):298–302. https://doi.org/10.1038/nature13236

Farber S, Diamond LK (1948) Temporary remissions in acute leukemia in children produced by folic acid antagonist, 4-aminopteroyl-glutamic acid. N Engl J Med 238(23):787–793. https://doi.org/10.1056/nejm194806032382301

Fehlauer F, Muench M, Smid EJ, Slotman B, Richter E, Van der Valk P, Sminia P (2006) Combined modality therapy of gemcitabine and irradiation on human glioma spheroids derived from cell lines and biopsy tissue. Oncol Rep 15(1):97–105

Figueroa ME, Abdel-Wahab O, Lu C, Ward PS, Patel J, Shih A, Li Y, Bhagwat N, Vasanthakumar A, Fernandez HF, Tallman MS, Sun Z, Wolniak K, Peeters JK, Liu W, Choe SE, Fantin VR, Paietta E, Lowenberg B, Licht JD, Godley LA, Delwel R, Valk PJ, Thompson CB, Levine RL, Melnick A (2010) Leukemic IDH1 and IDH2 mutations result in a hypermethylation phenotype, disrupt TET2 function, and impair hematopoietic differentiation. Cancer Cell 18(6):553–567. https://doi.org/10.1016/j.ccr.2010.11.015

Fischer M (2017) Census and evaluation of p53 target genes. Oncogene 36(28):3943–3956. https://doi.org/10.1038/onc.2016.502

Flanagan SA, Cooper KS, Mannava S, Nikiforov MA, Shewach DS (2012) Short hairpin RNA suppression of thymidylate synthase produces DNA mismatches and results in excellent radiosensitization. Int J Radiat Oncol Biol Phys 84(5):e613–e620. https://doi.org/10.1016/j.ijrobp.2012.06.050

Fliss MS, Usadel H, Caballero OL, Wu L, Buta MR, Eleff SM, Jen J, Sidransky D (2000) Facile detection of mitochondrial DNA mutations in tumors and bodily fluids. Science 287(5460):2017–2019. https://doi.org/10.1126/science.287.5460.2017

Floberg JM, Schwarz JK (2019) Manipulation of glucose and hydroperoxide metabolism to improve radiation response. Semin Radiat Oncol 29(1):33–41. https://doi.org/10.1016/j.semradonc.2018.10.007

Fontana L, Partridge L, Longo VD (2010) Extending healthy life span—from yeast to humans. Science 328(5976):321–326. https://doi.org/10.1126/science.1172539

Freedland SJ, Mavropoulos J, Wang A, Darshan M, Demark-Wahnefried W, Aronson WJ, Cohen P, Hwang D, Peterson B, Fields T, Pizzo SV, Isaacs WB (2008) Carbohydrate restriction, prostate cancer growth, and the insulin-like growth factor axis. Prostate 68(1):11–19. https://doi.org/10.1002/pros.20683

Frei B, Lawson S (2008) Vitamin C and cancer revisited. Proc Natl Acad Sci U S A 105(32):11037–11038. https://doi.org/10.1073/pnas.0806433105

Galan-Cobo A, Sitthideatphaiboon P, Qu X, Poteete A, Pisegna MA, Tong P, Chen PH, Boroughs LK, Rodriguez MLM, Zhang W, Parlati F, Wang J, Gandhi V, Skoulidis F, DeBerardinis RJ, Minna JD, Heymach JV (2019) LKB1 and KEAP1/NRF2 pathways cooperatively promote metabolic reprogramming with enhanced glutamine dependence in KRAS-mutant lung adenocarcinoma. Cancer Res 79(13):3251–3267. https://doi.org/10.1158/0008-5472.CAN-18-3527

Gambhir SS (2002) Molecular imaging of cancer with positron emission tomography. Nat Rev Cancer 2(9):683–693. https://doi.org/10.1038/nrc882

Gao X, Sanderson SM, Dai Z, Reid MA, Cooper DE, Lu M, Richie JP Jr, Ciccarella A, Calcagnotto A, Mikhael PG, Mentch SJ, Liu J, Ables G, Kirsch DG, Hsu DS, Nichenametla SN, Locasale JW (2019) Dietary methionine influences therapy in mouse cancer models and alters human metabolism. Nature 572(7769):397–401. https://doi.org/10.1038/s41586-019-1437-3

Gatenby RA, Gillies RJ (2004) Why do cancers have high aerobic glycolysis? Nat Rev Cancer 4(11):891–899. https://doi.org/10.1038/nrc1478

Gatenby RA, Vincent TL (2003) An evolutionary model of carcinogenesis. Cancer Res 63(19):6212–6220

George TJ, Yothers G, Hong TS, Russell MM, You YN, Parker W, Jacobs SA, Lucas PC, Gollub MJ, Hall WA, Kachnic LA, Vijayvergia N, Wolmark N (2019) NRG-GI002: a phase II clinical trial platform using total neoadjuvant therapy (TNT) in locally advanced rectal cancer (LARC)—first experimental arm (EA) initial results. J Clin Oncol 37(15_suppl):3505–3505. https://doi.org/10.1200/JCO.2019.37.15_suppl.3505

Gerard JP, Conroy T, Bonnetain F, Bouche O, Chapet O, Closon-Dejardin MT, Untereiner M, Leduc B, Francois E, Maurel J, Seitz JF, Buecher B, Mackiewicz R, Ducreux M, Bedenne L (2006) Preoperative radiotherapy with or without concurrent fluorouracil and leucovorin in T3-4 rectal cancers: results of FFCD 9203. J Clin Oncol Off J Am Soc Clin Oncol 24(28):4620–4625. https://doi.org/10.1200/jco.2006.06.7629

Graeber TG, Osmanian C, Jacks T, Housman DE, Koch CJ, Lowe SW, Giaccia AJ (1996) Hypoxia-mediated selection of cells with diminished apoptotic potential in solid tumours. Nature 379(6560):88–91. https://doi.org/10.1038/379088a0

Graumlich JF, Ludden TM, Conry-Cantilena C, Cantilena LR Jr, Wang Y, Levine M (1997) Pharmacokinetic model of ascorbic acid in healthy male volunteers during depletion and repletion. Pharm Res 14(9):1133–1139. https://doi.org/10.1023/a:1012186203165

Gregory MA, Nemkov T, Park HJ, Zaberezhnyy V, Gehrke S, Adane B, Jordan CT, Hansen KC, D'Alessandro A, DeGregori J (2019) Targeting glutamine metabolism and redox state for Leukemia therapy. Clin Cancer Res 25(13):4079–4090. https://doi.org/10.1158/1078-0432.CCR-18-3223

Grem JL (2000) 5-Fluorouracil: forty-plus and still ticking. A review of its preclinical and clinical development. Investig New Drugs 18(4):299–313. https://doi.org/10.1023/a:1006416410198

Grommes C, DeAngelis LM (2017) Primary CNS lymphoma. J Clin Oncol 35(21):2410–2418. https://doi.org/10.1200/JCO.2017.72.7602

Gross MI, Demo SD, Dennison JB, Chen L, Chernov-Rogan T, Goyal B, Janes JR, Laidig GJ, Lewis ER, Li J, Mackinnon AL, Parlati F, Rodriguez ML, Shwonek PJ, Sjogren EB, Stanton TF, Wang T, Yang J, Zhao F, Bennett MK (2014) Antitumor activity of the glutaminase inhibitor CB-839 in triple-negative breast cancer. Mol Cancer Ther 13(4):890–901. https://doi.org/10.1158/1535-7163.MCT-13-0870

Gujar AD, Le S, Mao DD, Dadey DYA, Turski A, Sasaki Y, Aum D, Luo J, Dahiya S, Yuan L, Rich KM, Milbrandt J, Hallahan DE, Yano H, Tran DD, Kim AH (2016) An NAD$^+$-dependent transcriptional program governs self-renewal and radiation resistance in glioblastoma. Proc Natl Acad Sci 113(51):E8247–E8256. https://doi.org/10.1073/pnas.1610921114

Gunda V, Souchek J, Abrego J, Shukla SK, Goode GD, Vernucci E, Dasgupta A, Chaika NV, King RJ, Li S, Wang S, Yu F, Bessho T, Lin C, Singh PK (2017) MUC1-mediated metabolic alterations regulate response to radiotherapy in pancreatic cancer. Clin Cancer Res 23(19):5881–5891. https://doi.org/10.1158/1078-0432.CCR-17-1151

Gupta AK, Cerniglia GJ, Mick R, Ahmed MS, Bakanauskas VJ, Muschel RJ, McKenna WG (2003) Radiation sensitization of human cancer cells in vivo by inhibiting the activity of PI3K using LY294002. Int J Radiat Oncol Biol Phys 56(3):846–853. https://doi.org/10.1016/s0360-3016(03)00214-1

Haioun C, Itti E, Rahmouni A, Brice P, Rain JD, Belhadj K, Gaulard P, Garderet L, Lepage E, Reyes F, Meignan M (2005) [18F]fluoro-2-deoxy-D-glucose positron emission tomography (FDG-PET) in aggressive lymphoma: an early prognostic tool for predicting patient outcome. Blood 106(4):1376–1381. https://doi.org/10.1182/blood-2005-01-0272

Hanahan D, Weinberg RA (2011) Hallmarks of cancer: the next generation. Cell 144(5):646–674. https://doi.org/10.1016/j.cell.2011.02.013

Harris IS, Treloar AE, Inoue S, Sasaki M, Gorrini C, Lee KC, Yung KY, Brenner D, Knobbe-Thomsen CB, Cox MA, Elia A, Berger T, Cescon DW, Adeoye A, Brustle A, Molyneux SD, Mason JM, Li WY, Yamamoto K, Wakeham A, Berman HK, Khokha R, Done SJ, Kavanagh TJ, Lam CW, Mak TW (2015) Glutathione and thioredoxin antioxidant pathways synergize to drive cancer initiation and progression. Cancer Cell 27(2):211–222. https://doi.org/10.1016/j.ccell.2014.11.019

Heilbronn LK, de Jonge L, Frisard MI, DeLany JP, Larson-Meyer DE, Rood J, Nguyen T, Martin CK, Volaufova J, Most MM, Greenway FL, Smith SR, Deutsch WA, Williamson DA, Ravussin E, Pennington CT (2006) Effect of 6-month calorie restriction on biomarkers of longevity, metabolic adaptation, and oxidative stress in overweight individuals: a randomized controlled trial. JAMA 295(13):1539–1548. https://doi.org/10.1001/jama.295.13.1539

Heinemann V, Hertel LW, Grindey GB, Plunkett W (1988) Comparison of the cellular pharmacokinetics and toxicity of 2′,2′-difluorodeoxycytidine and 1-beta-D-arabinofuranosylcytosine. Cancer Res 48(14):4024–4031

Hitchins RN, Bell DR, Woods RL, Levi JA (1987) A prospective randomized trial of single-agent versus combination chemotherapy in meningeal carcinomatosis. J Clin Oncol 5(10):1655–1662. https://doi.org/10.1200/JCO.1987.5.10.1655

Hite AH, Berkowitz VG, Berkowitz K (2011) Low-carbohydrate diet review: shifting the paradigm. Nutr Clin Pract 26(3):300–308. https://doi.org/10.1177/0884533611405791

Hoffer LJ, Levine M, Assouline S, Melnychuk D, Padayatty SJ, Rosadiuk K, Rousseau C, Robitaille L, Miller WH Jr (2008) Phase I clinical trial of i.v. ascorbic acid in advanced malignancy. Ann Oncol 19(11):1969–1974. https://doi.org/10.1093/annonc/mdn377

Hofheinz RD, Wenz F, Post S, Matzdorff A, Laechelt S, Hartmann JT, Muller L, Link H, Moehler M, Kettner E, Fritz E, Hieber U, Lindemann HW, Grunewald M, Kremers S, Constantin C, Hipp M, Hartung G, Gencer D, Kienle P, Burkholder I, Hochhaus A (2012) Chemoradiotherapy with capecitabine versus fluorouracil for locally advanced rectal cancer: a randomised, multicentre, non-inferiority, phase 3 trial. Lancet Oncol 13(6):579–588. https://doi.org/10.1016/s1470-2045(12)70116-x

Huang P, Chubb S, Hertel LW, Grindey GB, Plunkett W (1991) Action of 2′,2′-difluorodeoxycytidine on DNA synthesis. Cancer Res 51(22):6110–6117

Hursting SD, Kari FW (1999) The anti-carcinogenic effects of dietary restriction: mechanisms and future directions. Mutat Res 443(1–2):235–249. https://doi.org/10.1016/s1383-5742(99)00021-6

Hursting SD, Lavigne JA, Berrigan D, Perkins SN, Barrett JC (2003) Calorie restriction, aging, and cancer prevention: mechanisms of action and applicability to humans. Annu Rev Med 54:131–152. https://doi.org/10.1146/annurev.med.54.101601.152156

Hursting SD, Switzer BR, French JE, Kari FW (1993) The growth hormone: insulin-like growth factor 1 axis is a mediator of diet restriction-induced inhibition of mononuclear cell leukemia in Fischer rats. Cancer Res 53(12):2750–2757

Ilic N, Birsoy K, Aguirre AJ, Kory N, Pacold ME, Singh S, Moody SE, DeAngelo JD, Spardy NA, Freinkman E, Weir BA, Tsherniak A, Cowley GS, Root DE, Asara JM, Vazquez F, Widlund HR, Sabatini DM, Hahn WC (2017) PIK3CA mutant tumors depend on oxoglutarate dehydrogenase. Proc Natl Acad Sci U S A 114(17):E3434–E3443. https://doi.org/10.1073/pnas.1617922114

Ishikawa K, Takenaga K, Akimoto M, Koshikawa N, Yamaguchi A, Imanishi H, Nakada K, Honma Y, Hayashi J (2008) ROS-generating mitochondrial DNA mutations can regulate tumor cell metastasis. Science 320(5876):661–664. https://doi.org/10.1126/science.1156906

Itsumi M, Inoue S, Elia AJ, Murakami K, Sasaki M, Lind EF, Brenner D, Harris IS, Chio II, Afzal S, Cairns RA, Cescon DW, Elford AR, Ye J, Lang PA, Li WY, Wakeham A, Duncan GS, Haight J, You-Ten A, Snow B, Yamamoto K, Ohashi PS, Mak TW (2015) Idh1 protects murine hepatocytes from endotoxin-induced oxidative stress by regulating the intracellular NADP(+)/NADPH ratio. Cell Death Differ 22(11):1837–1845. https://doi.org/10.1038/cdd.2015.38

Jacque N, Ronchetti AM, Larrue C, Meunier G, Birsen R, Willems L, Saland E, Decroocq J, Maciel TT, Lambert M, Poulain L, Hospital MA, Sujobert P, Joseph L, Chapuis N, Lacombe C, Moura IC, Demo S, Sarry JE, Recher C, Mayeux P, Tamburini J, Bouscary D (2015) Targeting glutaminolysis has antileukemic activity in acute myeloid leukemia and synergizes with BCL-2 inhibition. Blood 126(11):1346–1356. https://doi.org/10.1182/blood-2015-01-621870

Jagsi R, Griffith KA, Bellon JR, Woodward WA, Horton JK, Ho A, Feng FY, Speers C, Overmoyer B, Sabel M, Schott AF, Pierce L (2018) Concurrent veliparib with chest wall and nodal radiotherapy in patients with inflammatory or locoregionally recurrent breast cancer: the TBCRC 024 phase I multicenter study. J Clin Oncol Off J Am Soc Clin Oncol 36(13):1317–1322. https://doi.org/10.1200/jco.2017.77.2665

Jakob CG, Upadhyay AK, Donner PL, Nicholl E, Addo SN, Qiu W, Ling C, Gopalakrishnan SM, Torrent M, Cepa SP, Shanley J, Shoemaker AR, Sun CC, Vasudevan A, Woller KR, Shotwell JB, Shaw B, Bian Z, Hutti JE (2018) Novel modes of inhibition of wild-type Isocitrate dehydrogenase 1 (IDH1): direct covalent modification of His315. J Med Chem 61(15):6647–6657. https://doi.org/10.1021/acs.jmedchem.8b00305

Kanarek N, Keys HR, Cantor JR, Lewis CA, Chan SH, Kunchok T, Abu-Remaileh M, Freinkman E, Schweitzer LD, Sabatini DM (2018) Histidine catabolism is a major determinant of methotrexate sensitivity. Nature 559(7715):632–636. https://doi.org/10.1038/s41586-018-0316-7

Kandel ES, Skeen J, Majewski N, Di Cristofano A, Pandolfi PP, Feliciano CS, Gartel A, Hay N (2002) Activation of Akt/protein kinase B overcomes a G(2)/m cell cycle checkpoint induced by DNA damage. Mol Cell Biol 22(22):7831–7841. https://doi.org/10.1128/mcb.22.22.7831-7841.2002

Kaplan J, Ward DM (2013) The essential nature of iron usage and regulation. Curr Biol 23(15):R642–R646. https://doi.org/10.1016/j.cub.2013.05.033

Kato H, Ito E, Shi W, Alajez NM, Yue S, Lee C, Chan N, Bhogal N, Coackley CL, Vines D, Green D, Waldron J, Gullane P, Bristow R, Liu FF (2010) Efficacy of combining GMX1777 with radiation therapy for human head and neck carcinoma. Clin Cancer Res 16(3):898–911. https://doi.org/10.1158/1078-0432.ccr-09-1945

Kauppi B, Nielsen BB, Ramaswamy S, Kjøller Larsen I, Thelander M, Thelander L, Eklund H (1996) The three-dimensional structure of mammalian ribonucleotide reductase protein R2 reveals a more-accessible iron-radical site than Escherichia coli R2. J Mol Biol 262(5):706–720. https://doi.org/10.1006/jmbi.1996.0546

Kawamura K, Qi F, Kobayashi J (2018) Potential relationship between the biological effects of low-dose irradiation and mitochondrial ROS production. J Radiat Res 59(suppl_2):ii91–ii97. https://doi.org/10.1093/jrr/rrx091

Kennedy CR, Tilkens SB, Guan H, Garner JA, Or PM, Chan AM (2013) Differential sensitivities of glioblastoma cell lines towards metabolic and signaling pathway inhibitions. Cancer Lett 336(2):299–306. https://doi.org/10.1016/j.canlet.2013.03.020

Kesarwani P, Prabhu A, Kant S, Kumar P, Graham SF, Buelow KL, Wilson GD, Miller CR, Chinnaiyan P (2018) Tryptophan metabolism contributes to radiation-induced immune checkpoint reactivation in glioblastoma. Clin Cancer Res 24(15):3632–3643. https://doi.org/10.1158/1078-0432.ccr-18-0041

Kidd EA, Siegel BA, Dehdashti F, Grigsby PW (2007) The standardized uptake value for F-18 fluorodeoxyglucose is a sensitive predictive biomarker for cervical cancer treatment response and survival. Cancer 110(8):1738–1744. https://doi.org/10.1002/cncr.22974

Kim A, Lee JE, Jang WS, Lee SJ, Park S, Kang HJ, Lee SS (2012) A combination of methotrexate and irradiation promotes cell death in NK/T-cell lymphoma cells via down-regulation of NF-kappaB signaling. Leuk Res 36(3):350–357. https://doi.org/10.1016/j.leukres.2011.07.027

Kim D, Fiske BP, Birsoy K, Freinkman E, Kami K, Possemato RL, Chudnovsky Y, Pacold ME, Chen WW, Cantor JR, Shelton LM, Gui DY, Kwon M, Ramkissoon SH, Ligon KL, Kang SW, Snuderl M, Vander Heiden MG, Sabatini DM (2015) SHMT2 drives glioma cell survival in ischaemia but imposes a dependence on glycine clearance. Nature 520(7547):363–367. https://doi.org/10.1038/nature14363

Kim MM, Camelo-Piragua S, Schipper M, Tao Y, Normolle D, Junck L, Mammoser A, Betz BL, Cao Y, Kim CJ, Heth J, Sagher O, Lawrence TS, Tsien CI (2016) Gemcitabine plus radiation therapy for high-grade glioma: long-term results of a phase 1 dose-escalation study. Int J Radiat Oncol Biol Phys 94(2):305–311. https://doi.org/10.1016/j.ijrobp.2015.10.032

Kinsella TJ, Collins J, Rowland J, Klecker R Jr, Wright D, Katz D, Steinberg SM, Glastein E (1988) Pharmacology and phase I/II study of continuous intravenous infusions of iododeoxyuridine and hyperfractionated radiotherapy in patients with glioblastoma multiforme. J Clin Oncol Off J Am Soc Clin Oncol 6(5):871–879. https://doi.org/10.1200/jco.1988.6.5.871

Kinsella TJ, Kunugi KA, Vielhuber KA, Potter DM, Fitzsimmons ME, Collins JM (1998) Preclinical evaluation of 5-iodo-2-pyrimidinone-2′-deoxyribose as a prodrug for 5-iodo-2′-deoxyuridine-mediated radiosensitization in mouse and human tissues. Clin Cancer Res 4(1):99–109

Ko YH, Domingo-Vidal M, Roche M, Lin Z, Whitaker-Menezes D, Seifert E, Capparelli C, Tuluc M, Birbe RC, Tassone P, Curry JM, Navarro-Sabate A, Manzano A, Bartrons R, Caro J, Martinez-Outschoorn U (2016) TP53-inducible glycolysis and apoptosis regulator (TIGAR) metabolically reprograms carcinoma and stromal cells in breast cancer. J Biol Chem 291(51):26291–26303. https://doi.org/10.1074/jbc.M116.740209

Koriech OM (1994) Diet and cancer. J Family Community Med 1(1):2–11

Kroemer G, Pouyssegur J (2008) Tumor cell metabolism: cancer's Achilles' heel. Cancer Cell 13(6):472–482. https://doi.org/10.1016/j.ccr.2008.05.005

Kruiswijk F, Labuschagne CF, Vousden KH (2015) p53 in survival, death and metabolic health: a lifeguard with a licence to kill. Nat Rev Mol Cell Biol 16(7):393–405. https://doi.org/10.1038/nrm4007

Kruszewski M (2003) Labile iron pool: the main determinant of cellular response to oxidative stress. Mutat Res 531(1–2):81–92. https://doi.org/10.1016/j.mrfmmm.2003.08.004

Kummar S, Anderson L, Hill K, Majerova E, Allen D, Horneffer Y, Ivy SP, Rubinstein L, Harris P, Doroshow JH, Collins JM (2013) First-in-human phase 0 trial of oral 5-iodo-2-pyrimidinone-2′-deoxyribose in patients with advanced malignancies. Clin Cancer Res 19(7):1852–1857. https://doi.org/10.1158/1078-0432.ccr-12-3118

Kunos CA, Radivoyevitch T, Pink J, Chiu SM, Stefan T, Jacobberger J, Kinsella TJ (2010) Ribonucleotide reductase inhibition enhances chemoradiosensitivity of human cervical cancers. Radiat Res 174(5):574–581. https://doi.org/10.1667/RR2273.1

Lane AN, Fan TWM (2015) Regulation of mammalian nucleotide metabolism and biosynthesis. Nucleic Acids Res 43(4):2466–2485. https://doi.org/10.1093/nar/gkv047

Lawrence TS, Chang EY, Hahn TM, Hertel LW, Shewach DS (1996) Radiosensitization of pancreatic cancer cells by 2′,2′-difluoro-2′-deoxycytidine. Int J Radiat Oncol Biol Phys 34(4):867–872. https://doi.org/10.1016/0360-3016(95)02134-5

Lawrence TS, Davis MA, Maybaum J, Stetson PL, Ensminger WD (1990) The dependence of halogenated pyrimidine incorporation and radiosensitization on the duration of drug exposure. Int J Radiat Oncol Biol Phys 18(6):1393–1398. https://doi.org/10.1016/0360-3016(90)90313-9

Lawrence TS, Eisbruch A, McGinn CJ, Fields MT, Shewach DS (1999) Radiosensitization by gemcitabine. Oncology (Williston Park) 13(10 Suppl 5):55–60

Lee C, Safdie FM, Raffaghello L, Wei M, Madia F, Parrella E, Hwang D, Cohen P, Bianchi G, Longo VD (2010) Reduced levels of IGF-I mediate differential protection of normal and cancer cells in response to fasting and improve chemotherapeutic index. Cancer Res 70(4):1564–1572. https://doi.org/10.1158/0008-5472.CAN-09-3228

Lee DH, Han JY, Cho KH, Pyo HR, Kim HY, Yoon SJ, Lee JS (2005) Phase II study of induction chemotherapy with gemcitabine and vinorelbine followed by concurrent chemoradiotherapy with oral etoposide and cisplatin in patients with inoperable stage III non-small-cell lung cancer. Int J Radiat Oncol Biol Phys 63(4):1037–1044. https://doi.org/10.1016/j.ijrobp.2005.04.034

Lee EW, Lee MS, Camus S, Ghim J, Yang MR, Oh W, Ha NC, Lane DP, Song J (2009) Differential regulation of p53 and p21 by MKRN1 E3 ligase controls cell cycle arrest and apoptosis. EMBO J 28(14):2100–2113. https://doi.org/10.1038/emboj.2009.164

Lee JH, Kim SY, Kil IS, Park JW (2007) Regulation of ionizing radiation-induced apoptosis by mitochondrial NADP+-dependent isocitrate dehydrogenase. J Biol Chem 282(18):13385–13394. https://doi.org/10.1074/jbc.M700303200

Lee SH, Jo SH, Lee SM, Koh HJ, Song H, Park JW, Lee WH, Huh TL (2004) Role of NADP+-dependent isocitrate dehydrogenase (NADP+-ICDH) on cellular defence against oxidative injury by gamma-rays. Int J Radiat Biol 80(9):635–642. https://doi.org/10.1080/09553000400007680

Lesueur P, Lequesne J, Grellard J-M, Dugué A, Coquan E, Brachet P-E, Geffrelot J, Kao W, Emery E, Berro DH, Castera L, Goardon N, Lacroix J, Lange M, Capel A, Leconte A, Andre B, Léger A, Lelaidier A, Clarisse B, Stefan D (2019) Phase I/IIa study of concomitant radiotherapy with olaparib and temozolomide in unresectable or partially resectable glioblastoma: OLA-TMZ-RTE-01 trial protocol. BMC Cancer 19(1):198. https://doi.org/10.1186/s12885-019-5413-y

Levine M, Conry-Cantilena C, Wang Y, Welch RW, Washko PW, Dhariwal KR, Park JB, Lazarev A, Graumlich JF, King J, Cantilena LR (1996) Vitamin C pharmacokinetics in healthy volunteers: evidence for a recommended dietary allowance. Proc Natl Acad Sci U S A 93(8):3704–3709. https://doi.org/10.1073/pnas.93.8.3704

Lewis JE, Singh N, Holmila RJ, Sumer BD, Williams NS, Furdui CM, Kemp ML, Boothman DA (2019) Targeting NAD(+) metabolism to enhance radiation therapy responses. Semin Radiat Oncol 29(1):6–15. https://doi.org/10.1016/j.semradonc.2018.10.009

Li K, Reichmann H (2016) Role of iron in neurodegenerative diseases. J Neural Transm (Vienna) 123(4):389–399. https://doi.org/10.1007/s00702-016-1508-7

Li L, Fath MA, Scarbrough PM, Watson WH, Spitz DR (2015) Combined inhibition of glycolysis, the pentose cycle, and thioredoxin metabolism selectively increases cytotoxicity and oxidative stress in human breast and prostate cancer. Redox Biol 4:127–135. https://doi.org/10.1016/j.redox.2014.12.001

Li S, Zhuang Z, Wu T, Lin J-C, Liu Z-X, Zhou L-F, Dai T, Lu L, Ju H-Q (2018) Nicotinamide nucleotide transhydrogenase-mediated redox homeostasis promotes tumor growth and metastasis in gastric cancer. Redox Biol 18:246–255. https://doi.org/10.1016/j.redox.2018.07.017

Li T, Kon N, Jiang L, Tan M, Ludwig T, Zhao Y, Baer R, Gu W (2012) Tumor suppression in the absence of p53-mediated cell-cycle arrest, apoptosis, and senescence. Cell 149(6):1269–1283. https://doi.org/10.1016/j.cell.2012.04.026

Liu VW, Shi HH, Cheung AN, Chiu PM, Leung TW, Nagley P, Wong LC, Ngan HY (2001) High incidence of somatic mitochondrial DNA mutations in human ovarian carcinomas. Cancer Res 61(16):5998–6001

Liu Y, Cao Y, Zhang W, Bergmeier S, Qian Y, Akbar H, Colvin R, Ding J, Tong L, Wu S, Hines J, Chen X (2012) A small-molecule inhibitor of glucose transporter 1 downregulates glycolysis, induces cell-cycle arrest, and inhibits cancer cell growth in vitro and in vivo. Mol Cancer Ther 11(8):1672–1682. https://doi.org/10.1158/1535-7163.MCT-12-0131

Locasale JW (2013) Serine, glycine and one-carbon units: cancer metabolism in full circle. Nat Rev Cancer 13(8):572–583. https://doi.org/10.1038/nrc3557

Loehrer PJ, Feng Y, Cardenes H, Wagner L, Brell JM, Cella D, Flynn P, Ramanathan RK, Crane CH, Alberts SR, Benson AB (2011) Gemcitabine alone versus gemcitabine plus radiotherapy in patients with locally advanced pancreatic cancer: an eastern cooperative oncology group trial. J Clin Oncol 29(31):4105–4112. https://doi.org/10.1200/JCO.2011.34.8904

Love NR, Pollak N, Dölle C, Niere M, Chen Y, Oliveri P, Amaya E, Patel S, Ziegler M (2015) NAD kinase controls animal NADP biosynthesis and is modulated via evolutionarily divergent calmodulin-dependent mechanisms. Proc Natl Acad Sci 112(5):1386–1391. https://doi.org/10.1073/pnas.1417290112

Lu C, Ward PS, Kapoor GS, Rohle D, Turcan S, Abdel-Wahab O, Edwards CR, Khanin R, Figueroa ME, Melnick A, Wellen KE, O'Rourke DM, Berger SL, Chan TA, Levine RL, Mellinghoff IK, Thompson CB (2012) IDH mutation impairs histone demethylation and results in a block to cell differentiation. Nature 483(7390):474–478. https://doi.org/10.1038/nature10860

Luengo A, Gui DY, Vander Heiden MG (2017) Targeting metabolism for cancer therapy. Cell Chem Biol 24(9):1161–1180. https://doi.org/10.1016/j.chembiol.2017.08.028

Ma Y, Chapman J, Levine M, Polireddy K, Drisko J, Chen Q (2014) High-dose parenteral ascorbate enhanced chemosensitivity of ovarian cancer and reduced toxicity of chemotherapy. Sci Transl Med 6(222):222ra218. https://doi.org/10.1126/scitranslmed.3007154

Macdonald JS, Smalley SR, Benedetti J, Hundahl SA, Estes NC, Stemmermann GN, Haller DG, Ajani JA, Gunderson LL, Jessup JM, Martenson JA (2001) Chemoradiotherapy after surgery compared with surgery alone for adenocarcinoma of the stomach or gastroesophageal junction. N Engl J Med 345(10):725–730. https://doi.org/10.1056/NEJMoa010187

Maddocks ODK, Athineos D, Cheung EC, Lee P, Zhang T, van den Broek NJF, Mackay GM, Labuschagne CF, Gay D, Kruiswijk F, Blagih J, Vincent DF, Campbell KJ, Ceteci F, Sansom OJ, Blyth K, Vousden KH (2017) Modulating the therapeutic response of tumours to dietary serine and glycine starvation. Nature 544:372. https://doi.org/10.1038/nature22056. https://www.nature.com/articles/nature22056#supplementary-information

Maddocks ODK, Berkers CR, Mason SM, Zheng L, Blyth K, Gottlieb E, Vousden KH (2012) Serine starvation induces stress and p53-dependent metabolic remodelling in cancer cells. Nature 493:542. https://doi.org/10.1038/nature11743. https://www.nature.com/articles/nature11743#supplementary-information

Matre P, Velez J, Jacamo R, Qi Y, Su X, Cai T, Chan SM, Lodi A, Sweeney SR, Ma H, Davis RE, Baran N, Haferlach T, Su X, Flores ER, Gonzalez D, Konoplev S, Samudio I, DiNardo C, Majeti R, Schimmer AD, Li W, Wang T, Tiziani S, Konopleva M (2016) Inhibiting glutaminase in acute myeloid leukemia: metabolic dependency of selected AML subtypes. Oncotarget 7(48):79722–79735. https://doi.org/10.18632/oncotarget.12944

Matsuoka S, Ballif BA, Smogorzewska A, McDonald ER, Hurov KE, Luo J, Bakalarski CE, Zhao Z, Solimini N, Lerenthal Y, Shiloh Y, Gygi SP, Elledge SJ (2007) ATM and ATR substrate analysis reveals extensive protein networks responsive to DNA damage. Science (New York, NY) 316(5828):1160–1166. https://doi.org/10.1126/science.1140321

Maurer GD, Brucker DP, Bahr O, Harter PN, Hattingen E, Walenta S, Mueller-Klieser W, Steinbach JP, Rieger J (2011) Differential utilization of ketone bodies by neurons and glioma cell lines: a rationale for ketogenic diet as experimental glioma therapy. BMC Cancer 11:315. https://doi.org/10.1186/1471-2407-11-315

Mavropoulos JC, Buschemeyer WC 3rd, Tewari AK, Rokhfeld D, Pollak M, Zhao Y, Febbo PG, Cohen P, Hwang D, Devi G, Demark-Wahnefried W, Westman EC, Peterson BL, Pizzo SV, Freedland SJ (2009) The effects of varying dietary carbohydrate and fat content on survival in a murine LNCaP prostate cancer xenograft model. Cancer Prev Res (Phila) 2(6):557–565. https://doi.org/10.1158/1940-6207.CAPR-08-0188

May JL, Kouri FM, Hurley LA, Liu J, Tommasini-Ghelfi S, Ji Y, Gao P, Calvert AE, Lee A, Chandel NS, Davuluri RV, Horbinski CM, Locasale JW, Stegh AH (2019) IDH3alpha regulates one-carbon metabolism in glioblastoma. Sci Adv 5(1):eaat0456. https://doi.org/10.1126/sciadv.aat0456

McBrayer SK, Cheng JC, Singhal S, Krett NL, Rosen ST, Shanmugam M (2012) Multiple myeloma exhibits novel dependence on GLUT4, GLUT8, and GLUT11: implications for glucose transporter-directed therapy. Blood 119(20):4686–4697. https://doi.org/10.1182/blood-2011-09-377846

McBrayer SK, Mayers JR, DiNatale GJ, Shi DD, Khanal J, Chakraborty AA, Sarosiek KA, Briggs KJ, Robbins AK, Sewastianik T, Shareef SJ, Olenchock BA, Parker SJ, Tateishi K, Spinelli JB, Islam M, Haigis MC, Looper RE, Ligon KL, Bernstein BE, Carrasco RD, Cahill DP, Asara JM, Metallo CM, Yennawar NH, Vander Heiden MG, Kaelin WG Jr (2018) Transaminase inhibition by 2-hydroxyglutarate impairs glutamate biosynthesis and redox homeostasis in glioma. Cell 175(1):101–116. e125. https://doi.org/10.1016/j.cell.2018.08.038

Mehrmohamadi M, Liu X, Shestov AA, Locasale JW (2014) Characterization of the usage of the serine metabolic network in human cancer. Cell Rep 9(4):1507–1519. https://doi.org/10.1016/j.celrep.2014.10.026

Mellemkjaer L, Emborg C, Gridley G, Munk-Jorgensen P, Johansen C, Tjonneland A, Kjaer SK, Olsen JH (2001) Anorexia nervosa and cancer risk. Cancer Causes Control 12(2):173–177

Meulendijks D, Dewit L, Tomasoa NB, van Tinteren H, Beijnen JH, Schellens JHM, Cats A (2014) Chemoradiotherapy with capecitabine for locally advanced anal carcinoma: an alternative treatment option. Br J Cancer 111(9):1726–1733. https://doi.org/10.1038/bjc.2014.467

Michels KB, Ekbom A (2004) Caloric restriction and incidence of breast cancer. JAMA 291(10):1226–1230. https://doi.org/10.1001/jama.291.10.1226

Miller DM, Buettner GR, Aust SD (1990) Transition metals as catalysts of "autoxidation" reactions. Free Radic Biol Med 8(1):95–108. https://doi.org/10.1016/0891-5849(90)90148-c

Moertel C, Reitemeier R, Childs D, Colby M, Holbrook M (1969) Combined 5-fluorouracil and supervoltage radiation therapy of locally unresectable gastrointestinal cancer. Lancet 294(7626):865–867. https://doi.org/10.1016/S0140-6736(69)92326-5

Mohanti BK, Rath GK, Anantha N, Kannan V, Das BS, Chandramouli BA, Banerjee AK, Das S, Jena A, Ravichandran R, Sahi UP, Kumar R, Kapoor N, Kalia VK, Dwarakanath BS, Jain V (1996) Improving cancer radiotherapy with 2-deoxy-D-glucose: phase I/II clinical trials on human cerebral gliomas. Int J Radiat Oncol Biol Phys 35(1):103–111

Momcilovic M, Bailey ST, Lee JT, Fishbein MC, Magyar C, Braas D, Graeber T, Jackson NJ, Czernin J, Emberley E, Gross M, Janes J, Mackinnon A, Pan A, Rodriguez M, Works M, Zhang W, Parlati F, Demo S, Garon E, Krysan K, Walser TC, Dubinett SM, Sadeghi S, Christofk HR, Shackelford DB (2017) Targeted inhibition of EGFR and glutaminase induces metabolic crisis in EGFR mutant lung cancer. Cell Rep 18(3):601–610. https://doi.org/10.1016/j.celrep.2016.12.061

Monti DA, Mitchell E, Bazzan AJ, Littman S, Zabrecky G, Yeo CJ, Pillai MV, Newberg AB, Deshmukh S, Levine M (2012) Phase I evaluation of intravenous ascorbic acid in combination with gemcitabine and erlotinib in patients with metastatic pancreatic cancer. PLoS One 7(1):e29794. https://doi.org/10.1371/journal.pone.0029794

Moser JC, Rawal M, Wagner BA, Du J, Cullen JJ, Buettner GR (2013) Pharmacological ascorbate and ionizing radiation (IR) increase labile iron in pancreatic cancer. Redox Biol 2:22–27. https://doi.org/10.1016/j.redox.2013.11.005

Mullarky E, Mattaini KR, Vander Heiden MG, Cantley LC, Locasale JW (2011) PHGDH amplification and altered glucose metabolism in human melanoma. Pigment Cell Melanoma Res 24(6):1112–1115. https://doi.org/10.1111/j.1755-148X.2011.00919.x

Neal EG, Chaffe H, Schwartz RH, Lawson MS, Edwards N, Fitzsimmons G, Whitney A, Cross JH (2008) The ketogenic diet for the treatment of childhood epilepsy: a randomised controlled trial. Lancet Neurol 7(6):500–506. https://doi.org/10.1016/S1474-4422(08)70092-9

Nebeling LC, Miraldi F, Shurin SB, Lerner E (1995) Effects of a ketogenic diet on tumor metabolism and nutritional status in pediatric oncology patients: two case reports. J Am Coll Nutr 14(2):202–208. https://doi.org/10.1080/07315724.1995.10718495

Niida H, Katsuno Y, Sengoku M, Shimada M, Yukawa M, Ikura M, Ikura T, Kohno K, Shima H, Suzuki H, Tashiro S, Nakanishi M (2010) Essential role of Tip60-dependent recruitment of ribonucleotide reductase at DNA damage sites in DNA repair during G1 phase. Genes Dev 24(4):333–338. https://doi.org/10.1101/gad.1863810

Nilsson R, Jain M, Madhusudhan N, Sheppard NG, Strittmatter L, Kampf C, Huang J, Asplund A, Mootha VK (2014) Metabolic enzyme expression highlights a key role for MTHFD2 and the mitochondrial folate pathway in cancer. Nat Commun 5(1):3128. https://doi.org/10.1038/ncomms4128

Nishikawa M, Nishiguchi S, Shiomi S, Tamori A, Koh N, Takeda T, Kubo S, Hirohashi K, Kinoshita H, Sato E, Inoue M (2001) Somatic mutation of mitochondrial DNA in cancerous and noncancerous liver tissue in individuals with hepatocellular carcinoma. Cancer Res 61(5):1843–1845

Nordlund P, Reichard P (2006) Ribonucleotide reductases. Annu Rev Biochem 75(1):681–706. https://doi.org/10.1146/annurev.biochem.75.103004.142443

Otto C, Kaemmerer U, Illert B, Muehling B, Pfetzer N, Wittig R, Voelker HU, Thiede A, Coy JF (2008) Growth of human gastric cancer cells in nude mice is delayed by a ketogenic diet supplemented with omega-3 fatty acids and medium-chain triglycerides. BMC Cancer 8:122. https://doi.org/10.1186/1471-2407-8-122

Pacold ME, Brimacombe KR, Chan SH, Rohde JM, Lewis CA, Swier LJ, Possemato R, Chen WW, Sullivan LB, Fiske BP, Cho S, Freinkman E, Birsoy K, Abu-Remaileh M, Shaul YD, Liu CM, Zhou M, Koh MJ, Chung H, Davidson SM, Luengo A, Wang AQ, Xu X, Yasgar A, Liu L, Rai G, Westover KD, Vander Heiden MG, Shen M, Gray NS, Boxer MB, Sabatini DM (2016) A PHGDH inhibitor reveals coordination of serine synthesis and one-carbon unit fate. Nat Chem Biol 12(6):452–458. https://doi.org/10.1038/nchembio.2070

Padayatty SJ, Sun H, Wang Y, Riordan HD, Hewitt SM, Katz A, Wesley RA, Levine M (2004) Vitamin C pharmacokinetics: implications for oral and intravenous use. Ann Intern Med 140(7):533–537. https://doi.org/10.7326/0003-4819-140-7-200404060-00010

Pai YJ, Leung KY, Savery D, Hutchin T, Prunty H, Heales S, Brosnan ME, Brosnan JT, Copp AJ, Greene ND (2015) Glycine decarboxylase deficiency causes neural tube defects and features of non-ketotic hyperglycinemia in mice. Nat Commun 6:6388. https://doi.org/10.1038/ncomms7388

Pan Z, Yang G, He H, Zhao G, Yuan T, Li Y, Shi W, Gao P, Dong L, Li Y (2016) Concurrent radiotherapy and intrathecal methotrexate for treating leptomeningeal metastasis from solid tumors with adverse prognostic factors: a prospective and single-arm study. Int J Cancer 139(8):1864–1872. https://doi.org/10.1002/ijc.30214

Parr T (1996) Insulin exposure controls the rate of mammalian aging. Mech Ageing Dev 88(1–2):75–82. https://doi.org/10.1016/0047-6374(96)01723-x

Pauwels B, Korst AEC, Lardon F, Vermorken JB (2005) Combined modality therapy of gemcitabine and radiation. Oncologist 10(1):34–51. https://doi.org/10.1634/theoncologist.10-1-34

Pavlova NN, Thompson CB (2016) The emerging hallmarks of cancer metabolism. Cell Metab 23(1):27–47. https://doi.org/10.1016/j.cmet.2015.12.006

Pelicano H, Martin DS, Xu RH, Huang P (2006) Glycolysis inhibition for anticancer treatment. Oncogene 25(34):4633–4646. https://doi.org/10.1038/sj.onc.1209597

Petronek MS, Spitz DR, Buettner GR, Allen BG (2019) Linking cancer metabolic dysfunction and genetic instability through the lens of iron metabolism. Cancers (Basel) 11(8). https://doi.org/10.3390/cancers11081077

Petros JA, Baumann AK, Ruiz-Pesini E, Amin MB, Sun CQ, Hall J, Lim S, Issa MM, Flanders WD, Hosseini SH, Marshall FF, Wallace DC (2005) mtDNA mutations increase tumorigenicity in prostate cancer. Proc Natl Acad Sci U S A 102(3):719–724. https://doi.org/10.1073/pnas.0408894102

Peylan-Ramu N, Poplack DG, Pizzo PA, Adornato BT, Di Chiro G (1978) Abnormal CT scans of the brain in asymptomatic children with acute lymphocytic leukemia after prophylactic treatment of the central nervous system with radiation and intrathecal chemotherapy. N Engl J Med 298(15):815–818. https://doi.org/10.1056/nejm197804132981504

Pleschke JM, Kleczkowska HE, Strohm M, Althaus FR (2000) Poly(ADP-ribose) binds to specific domains in DNA damage checkpoint proteins. J Biol Chem 275(52):40974–40980. https://doi.org/10.1074/jbc.M006520200

Pollak N, Dolle C, Ziegler M (2007) The power to reduce: pyridine nucleotides--small molecules with a multitude of functions. Biochem J 402(2):205–218. https://doi.org/10.1042/BJ20061638

Polyak K, Li Y, Zhu H, Lengauer C, Willson JK, Markowitz SD, Trush MA, Kinzler KW, Vogelstein B (1998) Somatic mutations of the mitochondrial genome in human colorectal tumours. Nat Genet 20(3):291–293. https://doi.org/10.1038/3108

Pongratz RL, Kibbey RG, Shulman GI, Cline GW (2007) Cytosolic and mitochondrial malic enzyme isoforms differentially control insulin secretion. J Biol Chem 282(1):200–207. https://doi.org/10.1074/jbc.M602954200

Popovtzer A, Normolle D, Worden FP, Prince ME, Chepeha DB, Wolf GT, Bradford CR, Lawrence TS, Eisbruch A (2014) Phase I trial of radiotherapy concurrent with twice-weekly gemcitabine for head and neck cancer: translation from preclinical investigations aiming to improve the therapeutic ratio. Transl Oncol 7(4):479–483. https://doi.org/10.1016/j.tranon.2014.04.016

Possemato R, Marks KM, Shaul YD, Pacold ME, Kim D, Birsoy K, Sethumadhavan S, Woo H-K, Jang HG, Jha AK, Chen WW, Barrett FG, Stransky N, Tsun Z-Y, Cowley GS, Barretina J, Kalaany NY, Hsu PP, Ottina K, Chan AM, Yuan B, Garraway LA, Root DE, Mino-Kenudson M, Brachtel EF, Driggers EM, Sabatini DM (2011) Functional genomics reveal that the serine synthesis pathway is essential in breast cancer. Nature 476(7360):346–350. https://doi.org/10.1038/nature10350

Price BD, Youmell MB (1996) The phosphatidylinositol 3-kinase inhibitor wortmannin sensitizes murine fibroblasts and human tumor cells to radiation and blocks induction of p53 following DNA damage. Cancer Res 56(2):246–250

Price GS, Page RL, Riviere JE, Cline JM, Thrall DE (1996) Pharmacokinetics and toxicity of oral and intravenous lonidamine in dogs. Cancer Chemother Pharmacol 38(2):129–135

Qian SY, Buettner GR (1999) Iron and dioxygen chemistry is an important route to initiation of biological free radical oxidations: an electron paramagnetic resonance spin trapping study. Free Radic Biol Med 26(11–12):1447–1456. https://doi.org/10.1016/s0891-5849(99)00002-7

Qie S, Yoshida A, Parnham S, Oleinik N, Beeson GC, Beeson CC, Ogretmen B, Bass AJ, Wong KK, Rustgi AK, Diehl JA (2019) Targeting glutamine-addiction and overcoming CDK4/6 inhibitor resistance in human esophageal squamous cell carcinoma. Nat Commun 10(1):1296. https://doi.org/10.1038/s41467-019-09179-w

Quinlan CL, Kaiser SE, Bolaños B, Nowlin D, Grantner R, Karlicek-Bryant S, Feng JL, Jenkinson S, Freeman-Cook K, Dann SG, Wang X, Wells PA, Fantin VR, Stewart AE, Grant SK (2017) Targeting S-adenosylmethionine biosynthesis with a novel allosteric inhibitor of Mat2A. Nat Chem Biol 13:785. https://doi.org/10.1038/nchembio.2384. https://www.nature.com/articles/nchembio.2384#supplementary-information

Lippincott Williams & Wilkins (2012) Radiobiology for the radiologist, 7th edn. Lippincott Williams & Wilkins. Wolters Kluwer, Philadelphia, PA

Rashmi R, Huang X, Floberg JM, Elhammali AE, McCormick ML, Patti GJ, Spitz DR, Schwarz JK (2018) Radioresistant cervical cancers are sensitive to inhibition of glycolysis and redox metabolism. Cancer Res 78(6):1392–1403. https://doi.org/10.1158/0008-5472.CAN-17-2367

Reckzeh ES, Karageorgis G, Schwalfenberg M, Ceballos J, Nowacki J, Stroet MCM, Binici A, Knauer L, Brand S, Choidas A, Strohmann C, Ziegler S, Waldmann H (2019) Inhibition of glucose transporters and glutaminase synergistically impairs tumor cell growth. Cell Chem Biol 26(9):1214–1228. e1225. https://doi.org/10.1016/j.chembiol.2019.06.005

Reed MJ, Penn PE, Li Y, Birnbaum R, Vernon RB, Johnson TS, Pendergrass WR, Sage EH, Abrass IB, Wolf NS (1996) Enhanced cell proliferation and biosynthesis mediate improved wound repair in refed, caloric-restricted mice. Mech Ageing Dev 89(1):21–43. https://doi.org/10.1016/0047-6374(96)01737-x

Reelfs O, Abbate V, Cilibrizzi A, Pook MA, Hider RC, Pourzand C (2019) The role of mitochondrial labile iron in Friedreich's ataxia skin fibroblasts sensitivity to ultraviolet A. Metallomics 11(3):656–665. https://doi.org/10.1039/c8mt00257f

Reelfs O, Tyrrell RM, Pourzand C (2004) Ultraviolet a radiation-induced immediate iron release is a key modulator of the activation of NF-kappaB in human skin fibroblasts. J Invest Dermatol 122(6):1440–1447. https://doi.org/10.1111/j.0022-202X.2004.22620.x

Reis LMD, Adamoski D, Ornitz Oliveira Souza R, Rodrigues Ascencao CF, Sousa de Oliveira KR, Correa-da-Silva F, Malta de Sa Patroni F, Meira Dias M, Consonni SR, Mendes de Moraes-Vieira PM, Silber AM, SMG D (2019) Dual inhibition of glutaminase and carnitine palmitoyltransferase decreases growth and migration of glutaminase inhibition-resistant triple-negative breast cancer cells. J Biol Chem 294(24):9342–9357. https://doi.org/10.1074/jbc.RA119.008180

Resnicoff M, Coppola D, Sell C, Rubin R, Ferrone S, Baserga R (1994) Growth inhibition of human melanoma cells in nude mice by antisense strategies to the type 1 insulin-like growth factor receptor. Cancer Res 54(18):4848–4850

Rieger J, Bahr O, Maurer GD, Hattingen E, Franz K, Brucker D, Walenta S, Kammerer U, Coy JF, Weller M, Steinbach JP (2014) ERGO: a pilot study of ketogenic diet in recurrent glioblastoma. Int J Oncol 44(6):1843–1852. https://doi.org/10.3892/ijo.2014.2382

Rigo P, Paulus P, Kaschten BJ, Hustinx R, Bury T, Jerusalem G, Benoit T, Foidart-Willems J (1996) Oncological applications of positron emission tomography with fluorine-18 fluorode-oxyglucose. Eur J Nucl Med 23(12):1641–1674. https://doi.org/10.1007/bf01249629

Riordan HD, Riordan NH, Jackson JA, Casciari JJ, Hunninghake R, Gonzalez MJ, Mora EM, Miranda-Massari JR, Rosario N, Rivera A (2004) Intravenous vitamin C as a chemotherapy agent: a report on clinical cases. P R Health Sci J 23(2):115–118

Robertson JM, Sondak VK, Weiss SA, Sussman JJ, Chang AE, Lawrence TS (1995) Preoperative radiation therapy and iododeoxyuridine for large retroperitoneal sarcomas. Int J Radiat Oncol Biol Phys 31(1):87–92. https://doi.org/10.1016/0360-3016(94)00341-h

Ronchi JA, Francisco A, Passos LAC, Figueira TR, Castilho RF (2016) The contribution of nicotinamide nucleotide transhydrogenase to peroxide detoxification is dependent on the respiratory state and counterbalanced by other sources of NADPH in liver mitochondria. J Biol Chem 291(38):20173–20187. https://doi.org/10.1074/jbc.M116.730473

Rous P (1914) The influence of diet on transplanted and spontaneous mouse tumors. J Exp Med 20(5):433–451. https://doi.org/10.1084/jem.20.5.433

Ruggeri BA, Klurfeld DM, Kritchevsky D, Furlanetto RW (1989) Caloric restriction and 7,12-dimethylbenz(a)anthracene-induced mammary tumor growth in rats: alterations in circulating insulin, insulin-like growth factors I and II, and epidermal growth factor. Cancer Res 49(15):4130–4134

Sabatini DM (2017) Twenty-five years of mTOR: uncovering the link from nutrients to growth. Proc Natl Acad Sci U S A 114(45):11818–11825. https://doi.org/10.1073/pnas.1716173114

Saif MW, Berk G, Cheng YC, Kinsella TJ (2007) IPdR: a novel oral radiosensitizer. Expert Opin Investig Drugs 16(9):1415–1424. https://doi.org/10.1517/13543784.16.9.1415

Saxton RA, Sabatini DM (2017) mTOR Signaling in growth, metabolism, and disease. Cell 168(6):960–976. https://doi.org/10.1016/j.cell.2017.02.004

Schirch V, Szebenyi DM (2005) Serine hydroxymethyltransferase revisited. Curr Opin Chem Biol 9(5):482–487. https://doi.org/10.1016/j.cbpa.2005.08.017

Schoenfeld JD, Sibenaller ZA, Mapuskar KA, Wagner BA, Cramer-Morales KL, Furqan M, Sandhu S, Carlisle TL, Smith MC, Abu Hejleh T, Berg DJ, Zhang J, Keech J, Parekh KR, Bhatia S, Monga V, Bodeker KL, Ahmann L, Vollstedt S, Brown H, Shanahan Kauffman EP, Schall ME, Hohl RJ, Clamon GH, Greenlee JD, Howard MA, Schultz MK, Smith BJ, Riley DP, Domann FE, Cullen JJ, Buettner GR, Buatti JM, Spitz DR, Allen BG (2017) O2(−) and H2O2-mediated disruption of Fe metabolism causes the differential susceptibility of NSCLC and GBM cancer cells to pharmacological ascorbate. Cancer Cell 31(4):487–500. e488. https://doi.org/10.1016/j.ccell.2017.02.018

Schwartz KA, Noel M, Nikolai M, Chang HT (2018) Investigating the ketogenic diet as treatment for primary aggressive brain cancer: challenges and lessons learned. Front Nutr 5:11. https://doi.org/10.3389/fnut.2018.00011

Schwarz JK, Siegel BA, Dehdashti F, Grigsby PW (2007) Association of posttherapy positron emission tomography with tumor response and survival in cervical carcinoma. JAMA 298(19):2289–2295. https://doi.org/10.1001/jama.298.19.2289

Seyfried TN, Sanderson TM, El-Abbadi MM, McGowan R, Mukherjee P (2003) Role of glucose and ketone bodies in the metabolic control of experimental brain cancer. Br J Cancer 89(7):1375–1382. https://doi.org/10.1038/sj.bjc.6601269

Shewach DS, Hahn TM, Chang E, Hertel LW, Lawrence TS (1994) Metabolism of 2′,2′-difluoro-2′-deoxycytidine and radiation sensitization of human colon carcinoma cells. Cancer Res 54(12):3218–3223

Shibata S, Satake N, Hester RK, Kurahashi K, Ito M (1988) The mode of vasoinhibitory action of a pyridazione derivative (MCI-154), a new cardiotonic agent, on contractile responses induced by alpha-adrenoceptor agonists and 45Ca influx in isolated vascular smooth muscles. Eur J Pharmacol 145(2):113–121. https://doi.org/10.1016/0014-2999(88)90222-1

Shibuya K, Okada M, Suzuki S, Seino M, Seino S, Takeda H, Kitanaka C (2015) Targeting the facilitative glucose transporter GLUT1 inhibits the self-renewal and tumor-initiating capacity of cancer stem cells. Oncotarget 6(2):651–661. https://doi.org/10.18632/oncotarget.2892

Silva B, Faustino P (2015) An overview of molecular basis of iron metabolism regulation and the associated pathologies. Biochim Biophys Acta 1852(7):1347–1359. https://doi.org/10.1016/j.bbadis.2015.03.011

Silverstone H, Tannenbaum A (1951) Proportion of dietary protein and the formation of spontaneous hepatomas in the mouse. Cancer Res 11(6):442–446

Singh D, Banerji AK, Dwarakanath BS, Tripathi RP, Gupta JP, Mathew TL, Ravindranath T, Jain V (2005) Optimizing cancer radiotherapy with 2-deoxy-d-glucose dose escalation studies in patients with glioblastoma multiforme. Strahlenther Onkol 181(8):507–514. https://doi.org/10.1007/s00066-005-1320-z

Soderlund K, Perez-Tenorio G, Stal O (2005) Activation of the phosphatidylinositol 3-kinase/Akt pathway prevents radiation-induced apoptosis in breast cancer cells. Int J Oncol 26(1):25–32

Son J, Lyssiotis CA, Ying H, Wang X, Hua S, Ligorio M, Perera RM, Ferrone CR, Mullarky E, Shyh-Chang N, Kang Y, Fleming JB, Bardeesy N, Asara JM, Haigis MC, DePinho RA, Cantley LC, Kimmelman AC (2013) Glutamine supports pancreatic cancer growth through a KRAS-regulated metabolic pathway. Nature 496(7443):101–105. https://doi.org/10.1038/nature12040

Speers C, Feng FY, Pierce LJ (2014) PARP-1 inhibitors and radiotherapy sensitivity: future prospects for therapy? Breast Cancer Management 3(3):281–296. https://doi.org/10.2217/bmt.14.6

Spitz DR, Sim JE, Ridnour LA, Galoforo SS, Lee YJ (2000) Glucose deprivation-induced oxidative stress in human tumor cells. A fundamental defect in metabolism? Ann N Y Acad Sci 899:349–362. https://doi.org/10.1111/j.1749-6632.2000.tb06199.x

Stine ZE, Walton ZE, Altman BJ, Hsieh AL, Dang CV (2015) MYC, metabolism, and cancer. Cancer Discov 5(10):1024–1039. https://doi.org/10.1158/2159-8290.CD-15-0507

Stupp R, Mason WP, van den Bent MJ, Weller M, Fisher B, Taphoorn MJ, Belanger K, Brandes AA, Marosi C, Bogdahn U, Curschmann J, Janzer RC, Ludwin SK, Gorlia T, Allgeier A, Lacombe D, Cairncross JG, Eisenhauer E, Mirimanoff RO, European Organisation for R, Treatment of Cancer Brain T, Radiotherapy G, National Cancer Institute of Canada Clinical Trials G (2005) Radiotherapy plus concomitant and adjuvant temozolomide for glioblastoma. N Engl J Med 352(10):987–996. https://doi.org/10.1056/NEJMoa043330

Tanaka H, Arakawa H, Yamaguchi T, Shiraishi K, Fukuda S, Matsui K, Takei Y, Nakamura Y (2000) A ribonucleotide reductase gene involved in a p53-dependent cell-cycle checkpoint for DNA damage. Nature 404(6773):42–49. https://doi.org/10.1038/35003506

Tateishi K, Wakimoto H, Iafrate AJ, Tanaka S, Loebel F, Lelic N, Wiederschain D, Bedel O, Deng G, Zhang B, He T, Shi X, Gerszten RE, Zhang Y, Yeh J-RJ, Curry WT, Zhao D, Sundaram S, Nigim F, Koerner MVA, Ho Q, Fisher DE, Roider EM, Kemeny LV, Samuels Y, Flaherty KT, Batchelor TT, Chi AS, Cahill DP (2015) Extreme vulnerability of IDH1 mutant cancers to NAD+ depletion. Cancer Cell 28(6):773–784. https://doi.org/10.1016/j.ccell.2015.11.006

Tisdale MJ, Brennan RA, Fearon KC (1987) Reduction of weight loss and tumour size in a cachexia model by a high fat diet. Br J Cancer 56(1):39–43. https://doi.org/10.1038/bjc.1987.149

Torti SV, Torti FM (2011) Ironing out cancer. Cancer Res 71(5):1511–1514. https://doi.org/10.1158/0008-5472.CAN-10-3614

Turcan S, Makarov V, Taranda J, Wang Y, Fabius AWM, Wu W, Zheng Y, El-Amine N, Haddock S, Nanjangud G, LeKaye HC, Brennan C, Cross J, Huse JT, Kelleher NL, Osten P, Thompson CB, Chan TA (2018) Mutant-IDH1-dependent chromatin state reprogramming, reversibility, and persistence. Nat Genet 50(1):62–72. https://doi.org/10.1038/s41588-017-0001-z

Turcan S, Rohle D, Goenka A, Walsh LA, Fang F, Yilmaz E, Campos C, Fabius AW, Lu C, Ward PS, Thompson CB, Kaufman A, Guryanova O, Levine R, Heguy A, Viale A, Morris LG, Huse JT, Mellinghoff IK, Chan TA (2012) IDH1 mutation is sufficient to establish the glioma hypermethylator phenotype. Nature 483(7390):479–483. https://doi.org/10.1038/nature10866

Vander Heiden MG (2011) Targeting cancer metabolism: a therapeutic window opens. Nat Rev Drug Discov 10(9):671–684. https://doi.org/10.1038/nrd3504

Vaupel P, Kallinowski F, Okunieff P (1989) Blood flow, oxygen and nutrient supply, and metabolic microenvironment of human tumors: a review. Cancer Res 49(23):6449–6465

Visentin M, Zhao R, Goldman ID (2012) The antifolates. Hematol Oncol Clin North Am 26(3):629–6ix. https://doi.org/10.1016/j.hoc.2012.02.002

Vogelzang NJ, Rusthoven JJ, Symanowski J, Denham C, Kaukel E, Ruffie P, Gatzemeier U, Boyer M, Emri S, Manegold C, Niyikiza C, Paoletti P (2003) Phase III study of pemetrexed in combination with cisplatin versus cisplatin alone in patients with malignant pleural mesothelioma. J Clin Oncol Off J Am Soc Clin Oncol 21(14):2636–2644. https://doi.org/10.1200/jco.2003.11.136

Vogl DTYA, Stewart K, Orford KW, Bennett M, Siegel D, Berdeja JG (2015) Phase 1 study of CB-839, a first-in-class, glutaminase inhibitor in patients with multiple myeloma and lymphoma. Blood 126(23):3059

Wahl DR, Dresser J, Wilder-Romans K, Parsels JD, Zhao SG, Davis M, Zhao L, Kachman M, Wernisch S, Burant CF, Morgan MA, Feng FY, Speers C, Lyssiotis CA, Lawrence TS (2017) Glioblastoma therapy can be augmented by targeting IDH1-mediated NADPH biosynthesis. Cancer Res 77(4):960–970. https://doi.org/10.1158/0008-5472.can-16-2008

Wang B, Hasan MK, Alvarado E, Yuan H, Wu H, Chen WY (2011) NAMPT overexpression in prostate cancer and its contribution to tumor cell survival and stress response. Oncogene 30(8):907–921. https://doi.org/10.1038/onc.2010.468

Wang ES, Frankfurt O, Orford KW, Bennett M, Flinn IW, Maris M, Konopleva M (2015) Phase 1 study of CB-839, a first-in-class, orally administered small molecule inhibitor of glutaminase in patients with relapsed/refractory leukemia. Blood 126(23):2566

Wang Y-C, Chiang E-PI (2012) Low-dose methotrexate inhibits methionine S-adenosyltransferase in vitro and in vivo. Mol Med 18(1):423–432. https://doi.org/10.2119/molmed.2011.00048

Warburg O (1924) Uber den Stoffwechsel der Carcinomzelle. 12. https://doi.org/10.1007/BF01504608

Warburg O (1956) On the origin of cancer cells. Science 123(3191):309–314. https://doi.org/10.1126/science.123.3191.309

Ward PS, Patel J, Wise DR, Abdel-Wahab O, Bennett BD, Coller HA, Cross JR, Fantin VR, Hedvat CV, Perl AE, Rabinowitz JD, Carroll M, Su SM, Sharp KA, Levine RL, Thompson CB (2010) The common feature of leukemia-associated IDH1 and IDH2 mutations is a neomorphic enzyme activity converting alpha-ketoglutarate to 2-hydroxyglutarate. Cancer Cell 17(3):225–234. https://doi.org/10.1016/j.ccr.2010.01.020

Wardman P, Candeias LP (1996) Fenton chemistry: an introduction. Radiat Res 145(5):523–531

Weindruch R, Naylor PH, Goldstein AL, Walford RL (1988) Influences of aging and dietary restriction on serum thymosin alpha 1 levels in mice. J Gerontol 43(2):B40–B42. https://doi.org/10.1093/geronj/43.2.b40

Welsh JL, Wagner BA, van't Erve TJ, Zehr PS, Berg DJ, Halfdanarson TR, Yee NS, Bodeker KL, Du J, Roberts LJ 2nd, Drisko J, Levine M, Buettner GR, Cullen JJ (2013) Pharmacological ascorbate with gemcitabine for the control of metastatic and node-positive pancreatic cancer (PACMAN): results from a phase I clinical trial. Cancer Chemother Pharmacol 71(3):765–775. https://doi.org/10.1007/s00280-013-2070-8

Wen B, Deutsch E, Marangoni E, Frascona V, Maggiorella L, Abdulkarim B, Chavaudra N, Bourhis J (2001) Tyrphostin AG 1024 modulates radiosensitivity in human breast cancer cells. Br J Cancer 85(12):2017–2021. https://doi.org/10.1054/bjoc.2001.2171

Westerterp M, van Westreenen HL, Reitsma JB, Hoekstra OS, Stoker J, Fockens P, Jager PL, Van Eck-Smit BL, Plukker JT, van Lanschot JJ, Sloof GW (2005) Esophageal cancer: CT, endoscopic US, and FDG PET for assessment of response to neoadjuvant therapy—systematic review. Radiology 236(3):841–851. https://doi.org/10.1148/radiol.2363041042

Wheless JW (2004) History and origin of the ketogenic diet. In: Stafstrom CE, Rho JM (eds) Epilepsy and the ketogenic diet. Humana Press, Totowa, NJ, pp 31–50

Ye J, Fan J, Venneti S, Wan Y-W, Pawel BR, Zhang J, Finley LWS, Lu C, Lindsten T, Cross JR, Qing G, Liu Z, Simon MC, Rabinowitz JD, Thompson CB (2014) Serine catabolism regulates mitochondrial redox control during hypoxia. Cancer Discov 4(12):1406–1417. https://doi.org/10.1158/2159-8290.cd-14-0250

Ying W (2008) NAD+/NADH and NADP+/NADPH in cellular functions and cell death: regulation and biological consequences. Antioxid Redox Signal 10(2):179–206. https://doi.org/10.1089/ars.2007.1672

Yuan TL, Cantley LC (2008) PI3K pathway alterations in cancer: variations on a theme. Oncogene 27(41):5497–5510. https://doi.org/10.1038/onc.2008.245

Zahra A, Fath MA, Opat E, Mapuskar KA, Bhatia SK, Ma DC, Rodman SN III, Snyders TP, Chenard CA, Eichenberger-Gilmore JM, Bodeker KL, Ahmann L, Smith BJ, Vollstedt SA, Brown HA, Hejleh TA, Clamon GH, Berg DJ, Szweda LI, Spitz DR, Buatti JM, Allen BG (2017) Consuming a ketogenic diet while receiving radiation and chemotherapy for locally advanced lung cancer and pancreatic cancer: the University of Iowa experience of two phase 1 clinical trials. Radiat Res 187(6):743–754. https://doi.org/10.1667/RR14668.1

Zhang D, Ochi N, Takigawa N, Tanimoto Y, Chen Y, Ichihara E, Hotta K, Tabata M, Tanimoto M, Kiura K (2011) Establishment of pemetrexed-resistant non-small cell lung cancer cell lines. Cancer Lett 309(2):228–235. https://doi.org/10.1016/j.canlet.2011.06.006

Zhang Q (2018) It takes two to tango: IDH mutation and glutaminase inhibition in glioma. Sci Transl Med 10(460):344. https://doi.org/10.1126/scitranslmed.aav0344

Zhao H, Zheng GH, Li GC, Xin L, Wang YS, Chen Y, Zheng XM (2019) Long noncoding RNA LINC00958 regulates cell sensitivity to radiotherapy through RRM2 by binding to microRNA-5095 in cervical cancer. J Cell Physiol 234(12):23349–23359. https://doi.org/10.1002/jcp.28902

Zhao Y, Butler EB, Tan M (2013) Targeting cellular metabolism to improve cancer therapeutics. Cell Death Dis 4:e532. https://doi.org/10.1038/cddis.2013.60

Zhao Y, Liu H, Liu Z, Ding Y, Ledoux SP, Wilson GL, Voellmy R, Lin Y, Lin W, Nahta R, Liu B, Fodstad O, Chen J, Wu Y, Price JE, Tan M (2011) Overcoming trastuzumab resistance in breast cancer by targeting dysregulated glucose metabolism. Cancer Res 71(13):4585–4597. https://doi.org/10.1158/0008-5472.CAN-11-0127

Zhong JL, Yiakouvaki A, Holley P, Tyrrell RM, Pourzand C (2004) Susceptibility of skin cells to UVA-induced necrotic cell death reflects the intracellular level of labile iron. J Invest Dermatol 123(4):771–780. https://doi.org/10.1111/j.0022-202X.2004.23419.x

Zhou S, Kachhap S, Sun W, Wu G, Chuang A, Poeta L, Grumbine L, Mithani SK, Chatterjee A, Koch W, Westra WH, Maitra A, Glazer C, Carducci M, Sidransky D, McFate T, Verma A, Califano JA (2007) Frequency and phenotypic implications of mitochondrial DNA mutations in human squamous cell cancers of the head and neck. Proc Natl Acad Sci U S A 104(18):7540–7545. https://doi.org/10.1073/pnas.0610818104

Zuccoli G, Marcello N, Pisanello A, Servadei F, Vaccaro S, Mukherjee P, Seyfried TN (2010) Metabolic management of glioblastoma multiforme using standard therapy together with a restricted ketogenic diet: case report. Nutr Metab (Lond) 7:33. https://doi.org/10.1186/1743-7075-7-33

Chapter 11
Targeting Tumor Hypoxia

Michael Skwarski, Elizabeth Bowler ⓘ**, Joseph D. Wilson** ⓘ**,**
Geoff S. Higgins ⓘ**, and Ester M. Hammond** ⓘ

Abstract Hypoxia (oxygen levels below 1–2%) is a common finding in solid tumors. The development of tumor hypoxia can be viewed as an imbalance between oxygen supply and demand. Tumor hypoxia significantly impacts tumor radiosensitivity and subsequently leads to poor clinical outcomes in patients treated with radiation therapy. The presence of molecular oxygen supports the production of lethal DNA damage in irradiated cells; therefore, the radiation dose required under severely hypoxic conditions to achieve a certain biological effect is generally 2- to 3-fold higher than the dose needed under normoxic conditions (i.e., oxygen enhancement ratio (OER) = 2–3). Several therapeutic approaches have been historically used and are emerging to target tumor hypoxia in order to improve radiation therapy outcomes. These include hyperbaric oxygen, correction of anemia, combination of radiation with carbogen and nicotinamide (ARCON), oxygen mimetics such as nimorazole, hypoxia-activated prodrugs, vascular normalization strategies (reviewed in Chap. 12), and emerging therapies to target tumor oxidative phosphorylation. Even though tumor hypoxia has long been established as a negative factor for radiation therapy outcomes in the clinic, we still lack robust, widely available, and adequately validated biomarkers for assessing tumor hypoxia in patients. This has not only significantly impeded the investigation of the efficacy of hypoxia modifiers, but it has also resulted in an inability to accurately select patients who are likely to benefit from such treatment. It is likely that only when hypoxia biomarkers are widely available will hypoxia modification enter the era of personalized medicine and improve outcomes.

Keywords Anemia · ARCON · Atovaquone · Hyperbaric oxygen · Hypoxia, acute · Hypoxia, chronic · Hypoxia-inducible factors · Oxidative phosphorylation · Oxygen consumption rate · Oxygen enhancement ratio · Oxygen mimetics · Radioresistance · Tissue oxygenation · Tumor metabolism · Tumor microenvironment · Vascular normalization

M. Skwarski · E. Bowler · J. D. Wilson · G. S. Higgins · E. M. Hammond (✉)
Department of Oncology, Oxford Institute for Radiation Oncology, University of Oxford, Oxford, UK
e-mail: ester.hammond@oncology.ox.ac.uk

© Springer Nature Switzerland AG 2020
H. Willers, I. Eke (eds.), *Molecular Targeted Radiosensitizers*, Cancer Drug Discovery and Development, https://doi.org/10.1007/978-3-030-49701-9_11

1 Introduction

Oxygen is vital for all living cells and plays a primordial role in key cellular activities. Central to our evolution into large and complex multicellular organisms has been the development of an intricate vascular system to ensure the adequate supply of oxygen to support cellular function (Pittman 2011). At the ends of the branching vascular network, capillaries provide the blood–tissue interface for oxygen delivery. In terms of distance, the diffusion limit for oxygen in tissue is in the region of 100–200 µM (Thomlinson and Gray 1955); therefore, cells must be within this proximity of a functional vessel to ensure adequate oxygenation. Given the limit of oxygen diffusion, tissue oxygenation is not binary, but rather exists in continuous gradients. Interestingly, the permission of low and near sub-physiological levels of oxygen are important for certain normal tissue functions, such as fetal development, tissue healing, and liver zonation (Dunwoodie 2009). However, the presence of such low levels of oxygen in healthy tissue is highly restricted and tightly regulated for specific purposes only.

When discussing tissue oxygenation, it is firstly important to define the units used and the relevant nomenclature. Several units are used to report oxygen levels and include the international system pressure unit the Pascal (Pa) beside millimeter of mercury (mmHg) (1 kPa = 7.5 mmHg) and the percentage of oxygen (1 kPa = 1%), both commonly used in medicine. The term "normoxia" refers to the atmospheric oxygen level of 21% (160 mmHg). "Tissue normoxia," also referred to as "physioxia," varies depending on tissue type and is significantly lower than atmospheric normoxia (Hammond et al. 2014). For example, in outer layers of skin the oxygen levels are in region of 1% (8 mmHg) (Wang et al. 2003), whilst in lung tissue they are 6% (42 mmHg) (Le et al. 2006) and 10% (72 mmHg) in the kidney (Müller et al. 1998). It is important to note that these values are significantly lower than the majority of in vitro experiments aimed to replicate tissue normoxia, which are conducted using 95% air and 5% carbon dioxide, and thus performed at around 20% oxygen (150 mmHg). The term "hypoxia" should be reserved for oxygen levels below that of the normoxia range for the tissue in question (Carreau et al. 2011), and generally refers to levels below 1–2% (7.5–15 mmHg).

In contrast to normal tissues, hypoxia is a common finding in solid tumors. The development of tumor hypoxia can be viewed as an imbalance between oxygen supply and demand. Rapid proliferation and high metabolic rates result in high oxygen consumption, which quickly surpasses supply. The subsequent hypoxic microenvironment results in the upregulation of angiogenic factors and thus turns on the "angiogenic switch" stimulating tumor neovascularization (Semenza 2012), a phenomenon first described over a century ago (Goldmann 1908). However, despite an abundance of new vessels, the resulting microvasculature is invariably highly dysregulated and "chaotic" (Jain 2014). In particular, the vessels are tortuous, friable, and leaky. The highly abnormal endothelium results in non-laminar flow and further leakiness predisposes to thrombosis and edema, which further impedes perfusion (Hashizume et al. 2000; Dvorak et al. 1999). Overall, the tumor vasculature is sub-functional and unable to match the oxygen demand of tumors and therefore, hypoxic regions arise.

The paradox that increased tumor angiogenesis can result in decreased perfusion is well established (Yang et al. 2017). In fact, frequently used anti-angiogenesis therapies, such as anti-vascular endothelial growth factor (VEGF) agents including bevacizumab, aim to exploit this phenomenon. These drugs improve tumor perfusion by inhibiting uncontrolled angiogenesis, enabling more regulated vessel development and leading to "vascular normalization" (Jain 2014). When combined with chemotherapy, as is often the case, this results in improved drug delivery to tumors.

Traditionally, tumor hypoxia is classified as either chronic or acute. Chronic hypoxia occurs in tumor regions located beyond the diffusion capacity of oxygen and is fairly stable. In contrast, acute hypoxia, also referred to as transient or cycling hypoxia, refers to regions of dynamic changes in oxygenation with the potential for reoxygenation (Brown 1979; Michiels et al. 2016). Transient hypoxia is commonly observed in tumors with in vivo studies demonstrating that up to 20% of the tumor volume may be affected (Bennewith and Durand 2004), with cycle lengths ranging from seconds to days. It is postulated that high frequency hypoxia cycling arises from alterations in vessel perfusion and red cell flux, whereas remodeling of vasculature is responsible for low frequency cycling occurring over a matter of days (Dewhirst 2009). Clinically, in patients with head and neck tumors, for example, significant change in the location of hypoxic regions has been observed using hypoxia imaging a short number of days apart (Nehmeh et al. 2008). Interestingly, chronic and acute hypoxia result in differing cancer cellular signaling responses, thus further highlighting them as distinct pathophysiological entities.

Overall, due to the complex spatiotemporal distribution of tumor hypoxia, accurate characterization of hypoxia within tumors is challenging with results from sample-based measurement potentially not representative of the tumor as a whole. Nevertheless, the presence of measurable hypoxia is an almost universal feature of tumors. Certain tumor types have consistently been shown to contain higher levels of hypoxia than others (Horsman et al. 2012). For example, polarographic oxygen electrode measurements in patients with non-small cell lung carcinoma (NSCLC) have shown median oxygen levels ranging from 14 to 17 mmHg (Le et al. 2006; Falk et al. 1992), whilst in head and neck squamous cell carcinoma (HNSCC) the average level was 9 mmHg (Falk et al. 1992; Nordsmark et al. 2005) and only in the region of 2 mmHg in prostate cancer (Movsas et al. 2000, 2002), therefore highlighting an additional layer of complexity in the study of tumor hypoxia.

2   The Cellular Response to Hypoxia: Hypoxia-Inducible Factors

Central to the cellular response to hypoxia are the hypoxia-inducible factors (HIFs)—the principal oxygen sensing machinery. The HIF family of transcription factors includes the well-studied HIF1 and HIF2, as well as HIF3. Each of these factors consists of an oxygen-sensitive and tightly regulated HIF-α subunit (HIF1-α, HIF2-α, or HIF3-α, respectively), which forms a heterodimer with a constitutively expressed HIF1-β subunit (also known as ARNT) (Wang et al. 1995). The HIF-α subunit contains two highly preserved proline residues (HP402/P564 for HIF1-α and P405/P531 for HIF2-α), which are hydroxylated in the presence of oxygen by prolyl hydroxylase domain-containing proteins (PHDs). This in turn permits binding to the von Hippel-Lindau (VHL) tumor suppressor protein, leading to HIF-α ubiquitination and its targeting for degradation (Ohh et al. 2000; Jaakkola et al. 2001). Under hypoxic conditions, HIF-α is stabilized through decreased hydroxylation, allowing binding with HIF1-β and translocation to the nucleus where it recognizes and binds to hypoxia-responsive elements (HREs), resulting in the transcription of a multitude of target genes (Liu et al. 2012). An additional layer of HIF regulation occurs at the level of recruitment of coactivators. Further oxygen-dependent hydroxylation of HIF1-α, and to a lesser extent HIF2-α, occurs on the C-terminal transactivation domain on aspartate reside 803 by factor-inhibiting HIF1 (FIH) (Lando et al. 2002; McNeill et al. 2002), which results in the inability of HIF1 to transactivate certain target genes (Dayan et al. 2006). The oxygen tension required to inactivate FIH is lower than that of the PHDs (Koivunen et al. 2004), thus enabling a graded transcriptional response dependent upon the severity of hypoxia.

HIF1-α and HIF2-α have differing expression profiles in tissues and tumors, with expression of HIF1-α ubiquitous whereas HIF2-α far more restricted (Wiesener et al. 2003). Together with the difference in their target genes, this provides a differential HIF-responsive transcriptome dependent on tissue and tumor type. Further still, in chronic hypoxia, HIF1-α levels rapidly increase and are stabilized within hours but within days decrease to much lower expression levels (Ginouvès et al. 2008). HIF1 has been shown to upregulate PHDs, which appear to retain enough activity to hydroxylate HIF1-α even under lower oxygen tensions, resulting in its reinstated degradation (Ginouvès et al. 2008; Berra et al. 2003). In contrast, cycling hypoxia results in an enhanced activity and stabilization of HIF1-α, at much greater levels than witnessed in chronic hypoxia (Dewhirst et al. 2008). The sophisticated regulation of HIF signaling points to its importance in regulating wide-ranging aspects of cellular function, with an ever-growing number of HIF target genes identified (Dengler et al. 2014; Choudhry and Harris 2018). Perhaps therefore unsurprisingly, hypoxia-related HIF signaling contributes significantly to tumorigenesis by directly contributing to the majority of the hallmarks of cancer, with its effects ranging from stimulation of invasion and metastasis, to promotion of sustained proliferation and immune system evasion (Petrova et al. 2018; LaGory and Giaccia 2016; Rankin et al. 2016). Overall, through such means, tumor hypoxia results in an aggressive tumor phenotype.

3   Tumor Hypoxia as a Barrier to Radiation Therapy

There is overwhelming evidence that tumor hypoxia significantly impedes tumor radiation sensitivity and subsequently leads to poor clinical outcomes in patients treated with radiation therapy. Nearly three quarters of a century ago the seminal work of Thomlinson and Gray demonstrated that the cellular response to ionizing radiation is highly dependent upon the presence of oxygen (Gray et al. 1953; Wright and Howard-Flanders 1957; Palcic et al. 1982). In the majority of cell types studied, the ratio of radiation dose required under severely hypoxic or anoxic conditions versus normoxic conditions to achieve the same biological effect, termed the oxygen enhancement ratio (OER), is typically 2.5–3.5 for ionizing radiation such as X-rays or γ-rays which are characterized by low linear energy transfer (LET). The most pronounced change in radiosensitivity occurs as oxygen levels increase from 0 to 30 mmHg (0–4%), with further increases in oxygenation having little additional effect. As a significant proportion of tumor oxygen readings fall within this range, with normal tissue readings normally above this range, this highlights the everyday clinical challenge of treating tumors successfully without causing excessive surrounding normal tissue toxicity.

In order to understand how oxygen potentiates cellular radiosensitivity, it is first important to briefly consider how ionizing radiation results in cellular damage. Radiation results in damage through its effects on DNA, with DNA double-strand breaks being the principle cytotoxic lesions. The effects on DNA can be viewed as either direct or indirect. Direct damage results from ionization of the DNA without the involvement of intermediate steps, and is the principal way by which high LET radiation, such as neutrons and α particles, exert their effect (Hall and Giaccia 2011). By contrast, megavoltage (MV) photons do not produce chemical and biological damage by themselves, but rather predominantly as a result of indirect ionization when they are absorbed in the material through which they pass and their energy is transferred to produce fast-moving charged particles that in turn elicit DNA damage (Hall and Giaccia 2011). At the energies used by most clinical linear accelerators, the MV photons predominantly interact with "free" electrons of the absorbing material with some of the photon energy transferred to the electron in the form of kinetic energy and the scattered photon traveling further into the material interacting with more "free" electrons (Compton Effect) (Steel 2002). This ultimately leads to a large number of fast electrons, which can ionize other atoms in the irradiated material. As cells are 80% comprised of water, it is important to consider the radiochemistry of water. Following exposure to ionizing radiation, water becomes ionized as shown:

$$\text{Photon} \searrow$$
$$H_2O \longrightarrow H_2O^+ + e^-$$

H_2O^+ is an ion radical and rapidly interacts with another water molecule to form the highly reactive hydroxyl radical (OH•) as follows:

$$H_2O^+ + H_2O \rightarrow H_3O^+ + OH^•$$

Such free radicals interact with the DNA molecule and cause damage. The mechanisms responsible for oxygen increasing cellular radiosensitivity can now be explained as outlined by the Oxygen Fixation Hypothesis first described in the 1950s (Alper and Howard-Flanders 1956). Following irradiation, DNA damage can be restored through reactions with free radical scavengers such as sulfydryl-containing compounds (Held et al. 1984; Hutchinson 1961). However, in the presence of molecular oxygen, DNA damage can be "fixed" by the DNA radical reacting with oxygen to form RO2•, which is significantly less amenable to scavenger restoration (Chapman 1979).

4 Tumor Hypoxia and Poor Radiotherapy Clinical Outcomes

Given the multitude of tumor adaptations to hypoxia contributing to many cancer hallmarks, it is not surprising that the presence of tumor hypoxia has been repeatedly shown to be a negative prognostic factor and to be associated with resistance to therapy regardless of treatment modality used (Le et al. 2006; Walsh et al. 2014; Scharping et al. 2017; Doktorova et al. 2015). However, given that oxygen is a direct "facilitator" of radiation-induced DNA damage, it is perhaps unsurprising that the impact of hypoxia on radiation therapy outcomes is most profound. The effect of hypoxia on radiation therapy outcomes has been most studied in patients with HNSCC. In a large analysis of data from numerous HNSCC radiation therapy studies, Nordsmark et al. demonstrated that pre-treatment hypoxia directly measured using oxygen electrodes was a highly significant prognostic factor for overall survival after radiotherapy alone, or in combination with surgery, chemotherapy, or a radiosensitizer (Nordsmark et al. 2005). Multivariate analysis in this study found that pre-treatment proportion of pO_2 values ≤ 2.5 mmHg ($HP_{2.5}$) was independently prognostic for poor survival using a hypoxia threshold of $HP_{2.5} < 20\%$ (median value). Furthermore, the negative impact of hypoxia on radiation therapy efficacy can be deduced from the large study of 918 patients with HNSCC randomized to receive CHART versus conventional radiation (Dische et al. 1997). Although this study failed to show improved locoregional tumor control (LRC) or overall survival (OS) with CHART, a retrospective subgroup analysis of pre-treatment tissue from nearly 200 patients demonstrated that expression of endogenous markers of hypoxia for the HIF-1 and HIF-2 pathway was strongly associated with post-radiation failure. This led the authors to postulate that hypoxic tumors were resistant to the potential benefit of CHART due to insufficient time for tumor reoxygenation to occur during treatment (Koukourakis et al. 2006).

In other tumor types, hypoxia has also been shown to predict poor radiation therapy outcomes (Rischin et al. 2006; Eschmann et al. 2005; Milosevic et al. 2012). For example, in patients with NSCLC, higher baseline levels of hypoxia, as determined by multiple hypoxia PET imaging parameters, was predictive of lower rates of local control following radical radiotherapy (Eschmann et al. 2005). In another study in patients with localized prostate cancer receiving radical radiotherapy, direct measurement of tumor oxygenation revealed that the presence of hypoxia, using a HP_{10} cut-off of 63% (median value), was associated with local recurrence within the gland and early biochemical failure (Milosevic et al. 2012).

5 Measuring Tumor Hypoxia in the Clinical Setting

Key to determining the impact of hypoxia on therapy outcomes has been our developing ability to accurately measure tumor hypoxia in patient samples. Over the last few decades, a wide range of methods have been used to study tumor hypoxia in patients, each with specific advantages as well as limitations. The various methods will be summarized here and have been reviewed (Hammond et al. 2014; O'Connor et al. 2019; Lee et al. 2014).

Direct measurements of tumor oxygenation using glass electrodes began in the 1960s with many early studies demonstrating the relationship between tumor oxygen level and radiation response, especially in cervical cancer and HNSCC (Kolstad 1968; Gatenby et al. 1988). However, our understanding of tumor oxygenation increased exponentially in the early 1990s with the introduction of the commercially available Eppendorf pO_2 histograph, also referred to as the polarographic electrode (Vaupel et al. 2007). This technique, which is able to measure oxygen tensions as low as 1–2 mmHg, demonstrated the significant intra- and inter-tumor variability in oxygenation and a large number of clinical studies quickly utilized this technique to demonstrate the correlation between hypoxia and poor clinical outcomes, as previously described. There were numerous limitations of electrode-based methods for studying tumor oxygenation. Determining oxygen tensions was limited to only accessible tumors and the invasive nature of the procedure, which requires the insertion of the probe along multiple tracks in order to collect sufficient readings, was understandably viewed as somewhat unattractive by patients and clinicians. Furthermore, due to the complex spatiotemporal heterogeneity of hypoxia within tumors, this method was subject to sampling error. Therefore, although this technique is regarded by many as the gold standard for evaluating hypoxia, it has been universally discontinued.

More recently, the most widely adopted approach for preclinical and clinical assessment of hypoxia has become the use of exogenously administered nitroimidazole-based agents. Such electron-deficient nitroaromatic compounds are selectively reduced by intracellular nitroreductase enzymes under hypoxic conditions to form reactive products, which bind irreversibly to nucleophilic molecules within the cell. Different nitroreductase enzymes in the cytoplasm, mitochondria, and microsomes are capable of the reductive metabolism of nitroheterocycles and include

NADPH-cytochrome P450 reductase, cytochrome b5 reductase, xanthine oxidase, aldehyde dehydrogenase, and DT-diaphorase (Kedderis and Miwa 1988). The reduction of nitroimidazoles is accomplished by tissue nitroreductases that are plentiful and which do not represent a rate-limiting factor (Prekeges et al. 1991), thus enabling repeated evaluation of hypoxia by such agents without reaching enzyme saturation. Importantly, bioreduction and intracellular retention of nitroimidazole compounds is inversely proportional to oxygen levels and requires intact nitroreductase enzymes. As a result, it detects only viable hypoxic cells and does not accumulate in regions of tumor necrosis. Typically, such agents have minimal protein binding, permitting efficient transport from blood into tissues (Kizaka-Kondoh and Konse-Nagasawa 2009) and as they are not actively metabolized, their diffusion distance is significantly greater than that of molecular oxygen (Dische 1985), and therefore can still reach poorly perfused areas typical of hypoxic regions. Also of importance is that in vitro experiments have demonstrated that nitroimidazoles are retained over the same oxygen range at which the OER is observed, with sharply increasing retention below oxygen tensions of 10 mmHg (Kizaka-Kondoh and Konse-Nagasawa 2009), therefore highlighting them as clinically relevant markers for the study of tumor hypoxia in radiation oncology. The stability of nitroimidazole adducts in viable hypoxic tissues permits immunohistochemical quantification to be carried out after the administration of nitroimidazole-based agents. Such agents have been widely used to study tumor hypoxia and include EF5 (Lord et al. 1993) and pimonidazole hydrochloride (Raleigh et al. 1999). The degree of immunodetection of such agents has been shown to correlate well with polarographic electrode readings predominantly in preclinical studies (Raleigh et al. 1999). However, as with direct measurements, sampling-specific tumor regions may be unrepresentative of hypoxia throughout the tumor. In addition, obtaining tissue for this purpose is an invasive procedure, which has associated practical limitations.

Nitroimidazoles also provide an exciting and clinically attractive opportunity for the noninvasive evaluation of tumor hypoxia by using PET-CT imaging with radiolabeled nitroimidazole-based tracers (Chapman 1979). [^{18}F]-fluoromisonidazole (FMISO) is the prototypical and most widely used radiotracer for this purpose. In vitro experiments have demonstrated that the under anoxic conditions, [^{3}H]-FMISO binding was approximately 25-fold greater than normoxic controls with binding reduced to 40% at oxygen pressures of 4 mm Hg (Martin et al. 1992), thus demonstrating FMISO as a marker of severe and clinically relevant hypoxia. Relevant to measuring hypoxia in tumors, in vivo data demonstrates no correlation between regional blood flow and FMISO retention with numerous studies concluding that FMISO uptake is independent of blood flow (Martin et al. 1992). In vivo, agreement between FMISO and pimonidazole immunohistochemistry has been observed (Dubois et al. 2004); however, such studies are lacking in patients. In the clinical setting, numerous studies have demonstrated the ability of FMISO to identify heterogeneously distributed hypoxic tissue within human tumors (Rajendran and Krohn 2005).

The partition coefficient describes the lipophilic/hydrophilic nature of molecules and is commonly evaluated as the distribution coefficient between octanol and water. As FMISO partitions nearly equally between octanol and water, once distribution equilibrium is achieved, all tissues should have the same concentration of tracer as blood. Only regions of hypoxia or organs involved in excretion or metabolism will have uptake levels greater than blood. The advantage is that the concentration ratio for normoxic tissue to blood will be very close to one and will be completely independent of blood flow. However, because of such partitioning characteristics of FMISO, whole body clearance is relatively slow, resulting in limited image contrast and requiring imaging following a relatively long period of time after injection of tracer (Rajendran and Krohn 2015). These limitations have led to the development of newer tracers such as [^{18}F]-fluoroazomycin arabinoside (FAZA), which have higher normal tissue clearance kinetics with improved hypoxia-to-normoxia contrast (Fleming et al. 2015).

Clinical imaging protocols for using FMISO PET-CT in the study of tumor hypoxia are fairly well established (McGowan et al. 2019; Koh et al. 1992), with increasing validation and high reproducibility of FMISO demonstrated in NSCLC (Grkovski et al. 2016) and HNSCC (Okamoto et al. 2013). This imaging technique enables the assessment of hypoxia heterogeneity within tumors and for multiple measurements per individual patient. However, the limitations are that it is prohibitively expensive for use in large studies, is associated with logistical challenges in terms of tracer supply and subjects patients to not insignificant radiation exposure. Oxygen-enhanced MRI (OE-MRI) imaging potentially enables the quantification of tumor hypoxia without exposing patients to additional ionizing radiation. Although it has yet to be widely used in clinical studies, OE-MRI might be associated with fewer logistical hurdles than nitroimidazole PET imaging (O'Connor et al. 2019).

As our understanding of the complex tumor response to hypoxia continues to improve, methods used for the assessment of hypoxia have shifted to measuring endogenous markers of this response. The majority of such markers are known to be direct transcription targets of HIF-1 as the detection of HIF-1 itself is challenging due to its instability and rapid degradation.

In terms of tumor tissue hypoxia analysis, immunohistochemistry for carbonic anhydrase IX (CAIX) has been commonly performed. CAIX is a transmembrane metalloenzyme that belongs to the family of α-carbonic anhydrases, which catalyze the reversible hydration of carbon dioxide to bicarbonate ions and protons, thereby regulating the cellular and extracellular pH (Pastorek et al. 1994). Sixteen human CA isoforms have been identified, but it is CAIX that is most strongly induced by hypoxia in a broad range of cell types. Expression of CAIX is tightly regulated by HIF-1-dependent HRE and subsequently, levels are highly responsive to hypoxia (Wykoff et al. 2000). High expression of CAIX has consistently been reported in human tumors and shown to predict poor clinical outcomes (Giatromanolaki et al. 2001; Kaluz et al. 2009). CAIX expression as detected by immunohistochemistry has been shown to grossly co-localize with that of HIF-1 as well as pimonidazole staining (Olive et al. 2001; Gillies et al. 2011) and has also been shown to correlate with direct pO_2 measurements (Le et al. 2006).

When considering such endogenous markers of hypoxia, it is important to appreciate that their expression level may be influenced by numerous factors other than oxygen level, such as other cellular signaling pathways (Hughes et al. 2018). In addition, the level of oxygenation and thus severity of hypoxia required to induce HIF signaling (and increase associated response proteins such as CAIX) differs to that required for the retention of exogenous nitroimidazoles. On detailed inspection of tumor tissue staining, binding of pimonidazole is more restricted to severely hypoxic and peri-necrotic regions as compared to HIF-1 expression (Sobhanifar et al. 2005). In addition, HIF1 expression and its response proteins can also be found in regions of cycling hypoxia, which are not necessarily positive for nitroimidazole retention at the time of measurement. In recognition of the complex tumor response to hypoxia, gene expression profiling is becoming more commonly used to evaluate the transcriptional response to hypoxia with numerous hypoxic metagene signatures now identified and increasingly well validated (Buffa et al. 2010; Winter et al. 2007). Importantly, the clinical utility of these gene expression signatures is enhanced by the fact that they can be derived from routine, formalin-fixed tumor samples. For a comprehensive review, see Harris et al. (Harris et al. 2015).

In addition to tumor tissue-based measurements, endogenous markers of hypoxia also provide the opportunity for identifying circulating hypoxic biomarkers, which may ultimately function as a plasma hypoxia signature. One of the most well-studied circulating markers to this effect is VEGF. Numerous studies have demonstrated the correlation between plasma VEGF levels and direct tumor oxygen measurements (Dunst et al. 2001), with higher levels predicting poor treatment response and outcomes in numerous tumor types (Ostheimer et al. 2014).

Another circulating hypoxia marker which has been studied extensively is osteopontin. This multifunctioning glycoprotein is recognized to play an important role in signaling pathways involved in many aspects of cancer progression including promoting proliferation, angiogenesis, and metastasis (Zhao et al. 2018). Osteopontin is upregulated under hypoxic conditions by AKT activation and stimulation of the ras-activated enhancer (RAE) in the OPN promoter (Zhu et al. 2005). Circulating osteopontin levels have been demonstrated to correlate inversely with polarographic electrode oxygen measurements and function as a prognostic and predictive biomarker with regard to radiotherapy outcomes in NSCLC (Ostheimer et al. 2014; Le et al. 2006) and HNSCC (Nordsmark et al. 2007; Petrik et al. 2006; Overgaard et al. 2005; Le et al. 2003). In NSCLC, a recent meta-analysis has demonstrated that osteopontin as measured by both IHC and as a circulating marker, is highly predictive of overall survival (Wang et al. 2015).

A different class of hypoxia-related circulating biomarkers are microRNAs (miRNAs). These approximately 21 nucleotide non-coding RNAs are key post-transcriptional regulators of gene expression (Krol et al. 2010). In the cellular response to hypoxia, and directly targeted by HIF-1α, miR-210 has emerged as the "master hypoxiaMIR" (Dang and Myers 2015). Shown to correlate with other measures of tumor hypoxia, both tissue and circulating miR-210 have been reported to be diagnostic, predictive, and prognostic hypoxia-related biomarkers in a number of tumor types (Chakraborty and Das 2016; Madhavan et al. 2016; Jiang et al. 2018; Świtlik et al. 2019).

6 Historical Hypoxia Modification Strategies with Radiation Therapy

Over the last half-century, numerous strategies have been investigated in an attempt to overcome the detrimental effect of tumor hypoxia on radiation therapy outcomes.

6.1 Increasing Tumor Oxygenation

Early approaches to address tumor hypoxia focused on increasing tumor oxygen delivery. One such method involved patients breathing 100% oxygen under hyperbaric conditions (HBO). A meta-analysis of HBO in patients with HNSCC treated with radiotherapy demonstrated a small but significant improvement in locoregional control (Overgaard 2011). A comprehensive Cochrane review of 19 clinical trials which delivered HBO concluded that HBO improved local control rates in cervix and HNSCC, but these benefits were small and may have only arisen in the context of unconventional fractionation schedules. In addition, HBO was associated with significant adverse effects, including oxygen toxic seizures and severe tissue radiation injury (Bennett et al. 2005). Given the modest benefit observed, practical inconvenience of treatment delivery and safety concerns, HBO was not adopted into clinical practice.

6.2 Correction of Anemia

Additional methods aimed at increasing tumor oxygenation have focused on administering blood transfusions to increase hemoglobin levels. Anemia is a very common finding in patients presenting for radiotherapy with 40 to 64% of patients being anemic prior to treatment with anemia shown to be associated with worse LRC and survival in numerous tumor types (Harrison et al. 2002; Lee et al. 1998). However, although the etiology of anemia in patients can be multifactorial, it often reflects patients with higher disease burden and therefore those who are more likely to have poor clinical outcomes. Numerous studies, mainly in HNSCC and carcinoma of the cervix, have investigated correcting anemia with blood transfusions during radiation treatment with overall mixed results observed (Varlotto and Stevenson 2005). An alternative method explored for correcting anemia during radiotherapy in HNSCC has been erythropoietin injections. However, unfortunately a significant detrimental impact on survival was observed with this approach (Henke et al. 2006), postulated to be attributable to promoting tumor cell proliferation through stimulation of tumor erythropoietin receptors (Henke et al. 2003).

6.3   ARCON

Other studies have aimed to improve oxygen delivery to tumors during radiation therapy by reversing acute hypoxia by combining the vasodilator nicotinamide with inhaled carbogen (95% oxygen and 5% carbon dioxide). This approach has been used as part of the Accelerated Radiation, Carbogen, and Nicotinamide (ARCON) regime and has demonstrated promising LRC rates and toxicity in large phase II studies in patients with HNSCC (Kaanders et al. 2002) and bladder cancer (Hoskin et al. 2009). Subsequently, in a phase III trial in laryngeal cancer, ARCON was well tolerated and resulted in improved LRC rates, with the poor regional control seen in more hypoxic tumors specifically addressed by this approach (Janssens et al. 2012). Furthermore, in bladder cancer the phase III BCON trial demonstrated improvement in LRC and OS using this treatment (Hoskin et al. 2010). However, due to the not insignificant practical challenges involved in delivering this regime, it has not been widely adopted.

6.4   Oxygen Mimetics

An alternative approach to address hypoxia-mediated radioresistance has been to combine drugs which function as "oxygen mimetics" by promoting the fixation of free radical damage following radiotherapy. These agents belong to the nitroimidazole class of agents, which undergo bioreduction and intracellular trapping under hypoxic conditions, as previously described. Misonidazole was the first of such agents to be shown to result in radiosensitization in vitro (Asquith et al. 1974) and subsequently a number of clinical studies were conducted in many different tumor types combining this agent with radiotherapy (Mäntylä et al. 1982; Bleehen et al. 1981; Overgaard et al. 1989a, b; Papavasiliou et al. 1983). With a few exceptions, generally the results did not demonstrate significant improvements in radiotherapy outcomes and this was associated with high toxicity, in particular with regard to peripheral neuropathy, preventing dose escalation to levels thought to be required to produce tumor radiosensitization (Melgaard et al. 1988). Subsequently, other nitroimidazoles were developed with more favorable toxicity profiles, of which the 5-nitroimidazole nimorazole has been the most widely studied in combination with radiotherapy. In the large randomized phase III Danish Head and Neck Cancer (DAHANCA) study, nimorazole significantly improved LRC in carcinoma of the supraglottic larynx and pharynx (Overgaard et al. 1998). This study, and others in different tumor sites in the head and neck with the addition of cytotoxic chemotherapy, demonstrated acceptable toxicity (Bentzen et al. 2015; Metwally et al. 2014). Despite such promising results, nimorazole is only routinely used in Denmark, with the lack of demonstrated improvement in OS limiting its uptake elsewhere. The results of the randomized nimorazole with radiation versus radiation alone UK phase III study in HNSCC (NIMRAD) are currently awaited (Thomson et al. 2014).

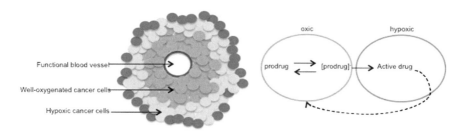

Fig. 11.1 Schematic representation of tumor hypoxia and the mechanism of action of hypoxia-activated prodrugs. As described regions of hypoxia occur at distances of 100–200 μM from functional blood vessels due to the metabolism of oxygen by the tumor cells. Hypoxia-activated prodrugs, which traditionally release a cytotoxin but more recently are molecularly targeted inhibitors, are inactive in oxic conditions but in response to hypoxia become reduced to release the active agent. In some cases, the active agent not only kills the hypoxic cells but also enters the surrounding oxic cells through a bystander mechanism

6.5 Hypoxia-Activated Cytotoxic Prodrugs

Hypoxia-activated prodrugs have also been explored in an effort to target hypoxic cells directly and have been reviewed recently (Mistry et al. 2017). Such agents also become preferentially activated and reduced in low oxygen tensions but this time to form highly cytotoxic species (Fig. 11.1). The most well-known molecule in this class is tirapazamine, which has been shown preclinically to be significantly more cytotoxic under hypoxic conditions (Zeman et al. 1986). Unfortunately, randomized phase III studies using tirapazamine in combination with chemoradiation in carcinoma of the cervix (DiSilvestro et al. 2014) and HNSCC (Rischin et al. 2010) have failed to demonstrate improvement in outcomes. More recently, molecularly targeted hypoxia-activated prodrugs have been described which, instead of being reduced to release a cytotoxin, release an inhibitor of a molecular target (reviewed in (Mistry et al. 2017)). It should be noted that patient stratification is likely to be absolutely essential to this approach as mechanism of action for these agents requires hypoxia, i.e., they cannot and should not work in non-hypoxic tumors.

6.6 Vascular "Normalization"

Intracellular signal transduction pathways are known to play an important role in determining tumor response to radiation with the well-studied EGFR/Ras/PI3K/AKT pathway shown to be of particular importance. Preclinical experiments have demonstrated that inhibitors of EGFR, Ras, PI3K, and AKT produce marked "normalization" of tumor microvasculature with increased perfusion and alleviation of tumor hypoxia (Qayum et al. 2009; Cerniglia et al. 2009). Furthermore, in xenograft models it was observed that PI3K inhibition resulted in significant tumor growth delay after radiation because of vascular remodeling, which was independent and synergistic to increasing intrinsic radiosensitivity (Fokas et al. 2012). Excitingly, recently the specific PI3K inhibitor buparlisib has been shown to result in a reduction in tumor hypoxia as measured by FMISO PET in patients with advanced NSCLC and to be well tolerated in combination with palliative thoracic radiation (McGowan et al. 2019) although no assessment of radiation response was possible in this study.

Novel strategies to normalize tumor angiogenesis and microenvironment to improve hypoxia and radiation outcomes are comprehensively described in Chap. 12.

6.7 Summary of Past Approaches

Over the last three decades, a truly wide range of different approaches has been employed to tackle hypoxia-mediated radioresistance and a meta-analysis of such treatments in HNSCC has demonstrated improvement in LRC and OS, thus providing level 1a evidence for hypoxia modification with radiation. However, due to inconsistency of results observed over the years with any outcome improvements only modest at best, no such treatment is widely used. Concerns regarding toxicity and challenges in practical delivery have further curbed enthusiasm. It is now well recognized that one of the major reasons why hypoxia modification has failed to show significant changes in radiation therapy outcomes is that there has been a complete lack of selecting patients for treatment based on tumor hypoxia and therefore likely to benefit most from such intervention. The reasons for this are largely due to the fact that there is currently no agreement as to which measure of hypoxia should be used for this purpose with many current techniques lacking sufficient validation. We should also consider our selection of in vivo models for testing of hypoxia modifying therapies. The tendency is to choose cell line/tumor models with levels of hypoxia, which are perhaps non-realistic of human tumors. Undeniably, novel and more efficacious hypoxia modification treatments are also required and more recently attention has focused on modulation of tumor metabolism, as will be discussed below.

7 Oxidative Phosphorylation as an Emerging Target to Tackle Tumor Hypoxia

In contrast to previous methods largely aimed at increasing oxygen delivery to tumors, an alternative and exciting novel strategy to tackle tumor hypoxia is to reduce the tumor oxygen consumption rate (OCR), thus addressing the other side of the oxygen supply and demand equation. More specifically, there is growing interest in reducing tumor OCR through inhibition of oxidative phosphorylation (OXPHOS).

7.1 Overview of Cellular Respiration

Cellular respiration describes a series of well-characterized metabolic reactions by which cells convert available nutrients into biochemical energy in the form of adenosine triphosphate (ATP). The most readily available source of cellular energy is glucose and molecular oxygen plays a key role in its conversion to ATP. The first step in cellular respiration in most organisms is glycolysis, also referred to as the Embden-Meyerhof-Parnas pathway. This oxygen-independent pathway constitutes a ten-step multienzyme process occurring in the cytosol and converts one molecule of glucose into two molecules of pyruvate whilst producing two reduced nicotinamide adenine dinuceotide (NADH) and two ATP molecules (net yield). The fate of pyruvate and cellular respiration hereon is highly dependent on the presence of molecular oxygen (Lunt and Vander Heiden 2011). In the absence of oxygen, pyruvate is reduced to lactate by lactate dehydrogenase (LDH). This results in the regeneration of NAD^+ through NADH oxidation and as NAD^+ is required during glycolysis for ATP production, this enables ongoing cellular energy production under anaerobic conditions. Lactate may be converted back to pyruvate by LDH and used for aerobic respiration if oxygenation has increased, or it diffuses into the circulation and can be converted back into glucose by the liver in the Cori cycle.

In contrast, in the presence of oxygen, pyruvate generated during glycolysis enters the mitochondrial matrix, where it undergoes oxidative decarboxylation by a series of enzymes which make up the pyruvate dehydrogenase complex (PDH) and is converted into *acetyl coenzyme A (acetyl CoA)*. Acetyl CoA enters the citric acid cycle, also known as the Krebs or tricarboxylic acid cycle, by combining with oxaloacetate to form citrate, which is systematically converted back to oxaloacetate and then combines with acetyl CoA, and so the cycle repeats. Each full cycle produces one guanosine triphosphate (GTP), one reduced flavin adenine dinucleotide ($FADH_2$) and three NADH molecules. $FADH_2$ and NADH move to the inner mitochondrial membrane and facilitate ATP production during the process of OXPHOS (Lunt and Vander Heiden 2011).

The *electron transport chain (ETC)* uses NADH and $FADH_2$ produced by the Krebs cycle and NADH from glycolysis to produce ATP. Electrons from NADH and $FADH_2$ are released and transferred systematically through protein complexes located in the inner mitochondrial membrane, thus forming the ETC. These inner membrane protein complexes include four enzyme complexes, complex I, complex II, complex III, and complex IV, and two coenzymes, ubiquinone (also known as co-enzyme Q) and cytochrome c. As electrons are passed from one electron carrier to another, it results in their reduction and then oxidation, which releases enough energy to pump hydrogen ions across the inner membrane into the space between in the inner and outer mitochondrial membranes. The accumulation of protons in this intermembrane space creates a steep electrochemical gradient across the inner membrane. As protons traverse the protein pore complex *ATP synthase* embedded in the inner membrane back into the mitochondrial matrix, the shaft of the complex rotates and catalyzes the production of ATP by attaching a phosphate to ADP. In total, for every glucose molecule that enters aerobic respiration, a net yield of 36 ATPs is produced. Once the electrons have passed through the ETC, they are combined with molecular oxygen and hydrogen ions to form water molecules. Therefore, oxygen can be viewed as the terminal electron acceptor and electron flow through the ETC ceases without oxygen. The ETC couples the transfer of electrons from donor molecules to oxygen with ATP production, thus representing the process known as OXPHOS (Kühlbrandt 2015).

7.2 Altered Metabolism in Cancer and the Impact of Tumor Hypoxia

A well-established hallmark of cancer is highly abnormal energy metabolism (Jones and Thompson 2009; Hanahan and Weinberg 2011). First observed by Otto Warburg in 1920s (Koppenol et al. 2011), cancer cells reprogram energy metabolism to predominantly rely on glycolysis, even in the presence of normal oxygenation. This phenomenon of "aerobic glycolysis" is characterized by marked increase in glucose uptake by cancer cells, largely by upregulation of glucose transporters such as *transporter 1* (GLUT1) (Jones and Thompson 2009). Although relying on glycolysis for energy metabolism may seem counterintuitive due to lower yields of ATP per molecule of glucose molecule compared with OXPHOS, the sheer abundance of glucose due to increased uptake results in far greater ATP production and at a faster rate.

Pro-proliferative signal transduction pathways are known to function as glycolytic drivers with increased PI3K/AKT/mTOR signaling and overexpression of RAS and c-myc known to be of key importance (Jones and Thompson 2009; DeBerardinis et al. 2008). For example, AKT has been shown to be perhaps the most important as it appears to be sufficient to drive glycolysis independently (Elstrom et al. 2004), whilst c-myc increases transcription of GLUT1, as well as multiple key enzymes involved in glycolysis (Osthus et al. 2000; Dang et al. 1997).

Tumor hypoxia also plays an important role in fueling glycolysis, primarily through HIF-1 signaling. For example, HIF-1 upregulates GLUT1 as well as virtually all of the glycolytic enzymes, with key examples being HK, PGI, and LDH (Dang and Semenza 1999; Semenza 2010). In addition, HIF-1 also increases expression of PDH kinase 1 which inhibits PDH complex activity, thus preventing the irreversible conversion of pyruvate into acetyl CoA and entry into the citric acid cycle (Kim et al. 2006), and therefore functions as an important switch between glycolysis and OXPHOS respiration. Within the mitochondria itself, HIF-1 tightly regulates the expression of different isoforms of subunit COX4 and the function of ETC complex IV of the electron transport chain, thus impacting on ATP production and oxygen consumption (Fukuda et al. 2007). More recently, it is increasingly recognized that HIF-1 also regulates the expression of a wide range of miRNAs which fine tune metabolic pathways, as outlined in a comprehensive review (Orang et al. 2019).

In terms of OXPHOS activity in cancer, downregulation has been demonstrated in several tumor types and attributed to mitochondrial DNA (mtDNA) mutations, or reduced mtDNA content, given that mtDNA codes for many of the subunits of OXPHOS protein complexes I to V (Yu 2011). Such downregulation of OXPHOS has been demonstrated to correlate with poor clinical outcomes in many cancers and shown to be associated with invasive and metastatic tumor phenotypes (Gaude and Frezza 2016).

7.3 Emergence of the Importance of OXPHOS in Cancer

Because of the observation that glycolysis is upregulated and OXPHOS is down-regulated in tumors, it has become a long-held belief that OXPHOS is largely redundant in cancer and thus has been largely forgotten. However, more recently it has been demonstrated that in a number of tumor types mitochondrial metabolism is not downregulated, including pancreatic and endometrial cancer as well as in lymphoma and high OXPHOS subtype melanoma (Moreno-Sánchez et al. 2007; Weinberg and Chandel 2015). In addition, it has increasingly become recognized that OXPHOS is indeed active in cancer cells and does in fact contribute, although to a varying degree, to cellular energy production (Zu and Guppy 2004). Such is the higher yield of ATP production with OXPHOS compared with glycolysis, that it has been shown that when OXPHOS activity is reduced as low as 6%, it still contributes to 50% of the cell's energy requirements (Mookerjee et al. 2017). In a meta-analysis of normal cell types and cancer cell lines, the average contribution of OXPHOS to ATP production was 80% in normal cells and 83% in cancer cells (Zu and Guppy 2004). Despite the often severely hypoxic conditions within tumors, the level of oxygen, the key determinant of the oxygen consumption rate (OCR) (Moreno-Sánchez et al. 2009; Vaupel and Mayer 2012), is generally above that which would impair mitochondrial respiration as the K_{mO2} of COX is as low as 0.1–0.8 µM in different biological systems (Moreno-Sánchez et al. 2007).

The previous explanation that decreased OXPHOS in cancer is attributable to significantly decreased or mutated mitochondrial (mt) DNA is controversial. In fact, many types of cancer have increased mtDNA content relative to normal tissue (Reznik et al. 2016; Yu 2011). With regard to mtDNA mutations, analysis of paired tumor and normal tissue samples has revealed deleterious somatic tumor-specific mtDNA mutations in the majority of rectal and colon adenocarcinomas (Larman et al. 2012). Furthermore, such mutations were identified in all mtDNA genes many of which were predicted to impair OXPHOS. Interestingly, it has been shown that cancer cells with these mutations in OXPHOS-related genes such as complex I subunits, have much higher sensitivity to complex I inhibitors (Birsoy et al. 2014), indicating these mutations play an important role in cancer cell function.

Further still, in vitro experiments using ethidium bromide to deplete mitochondrial DNA have demonstrated that reduction of mitochondrial respiration dramatically changes the behavior of cancer cells and decreases tumorigenic potential (Cavalli et al. 1997). This is supported by a number of different cancer cell in vivo models, which have demonstrated that depletion of mitochondrial respiratory complexes results in delayed tumor formation following transplantation and an inability of cancer cells to metastasize (Tan et al. 2015). Interestingly, when tumors did eventually form and disseminate, they showed marked reactivation of OXPHOS due to acquisition of host mitochondrial DNA. There is also growing evidence that reliance on OXPHOS, and in fact impaired glycolysis, is a key feature of cancer stem cells and quiescent cancer cells resistant to standard therapies and responsible for repopulation of tumors after treatment (Viale et al. 2015).

Perhaps one important role of OXPHOS in carcinogenesis is the production of reactive oxygen species (ROS). High levels of ROS production has long been recognized to be a classical feature of tumors (Szatrowski and Nathan 1991) with many early studies focused on the DNA damaging effects of ROS, which is believed to be tumorigenic by promoting genomic instability (Ames et al. 1993). However, more recently a paradigm shift has occurred in our understanding of ROS with a more nuanced view of the importance of ROS as signaling pathway molecules, promoting tumorigenesis by regulation of cellular proliferation, metabolic alterations, and angiogenesis (Sullivan and Chandel 2014).

Therefore, after decades of disregard, OXPHOS has re-emerged as a functioning and important part of cancer cellular function. As OXPHOS consumes significant quantities of oxygen, inhibition of this process is a novel approach to reduce tumor oxygen consumption and therefore tackle tumor hypoxia.

7.4 OCR Inhibition to Alleviate Tumor Hypoxia

Over the last few years, there has been growing interest in using OXPHOS inhibitors to reduce tumor OCR. Such an approach would permit unconsumed oxygen to diffuse into adjacent low oxygen regions and therefore alleviate tumor hypoxia. Indeed, 3D multicellular spheroid studies have demonstrated that OCR reduction alleviates central hypoxic regions by increasing the availability of free oxygen (Secomb et al. 1995; Grimes et al. 2014). In support of this approach, mathematical modeling suggests that only a 30% decrease in OCR would abolish severe hypoxia (Grimes et al. 2014) and that reduction in OCR is likely to be a more effective strategy to reduce hypoxia than previous methods aimed at increasing oxygen supply (Secomb et al. 1995).

Inhibition of OXPHOS has been shown to reduce OCR in many different cancer cell types, indicating potential wide applicability (Ashton et al. 2016). Also this approach is thought less susceptible to poor tumor perfusion as such inhibitors would initially target OXPHOS in well-perfused and non-hypoxic regions, which would then result in oxygen rapidly diffusing to adjacent regions of chronic hypoxia, thus targeting "hard to reach" tumor regions indirectly (Ashton et al. 2018).

A number of FDA-approved drugs are known to inhibit OXPHOS through off-target effects and have gained attention as potentially clinically useful OCR inhibitors (Ashton et al. 2018). In particular, the anti-diabetic medication metformin has been most studied in this context. This biguanide is the most widely prescribed medication for treatment of type II diabetes mellitus and exerts its glucose-lowering effect through inhibition of hepatic gluconeogenesis (Hunter et al. 2018). The potential of metformin as an anti-cancer agent first came to light when large epidemiological and retrospective studies demonstrated that diabetic patients taking metformin had significantly lower incidence of cancer and better clinical outcomes following treatment, including in the context of radiotherapy, than patients with diabetes taking alternative medication (Cao et al. 2017; Koritzinsky 2015; Pernicova and Korbonits 2014). The observed benefits of metformin have been attributed to a number of its effects, including systemically lowered insulin/insulin-like growth factor-1 (IGF-1) as well as potential inhibition of mammalian target of rapamycin (mTOR), activation of AMP-activated kinase (AMPK), and reduction in ROS (Belfiore et al. 2009; Algire et al. 2012; Dowling et al. 2007). The mechanism by which metformin reduces OCR is through inhibition of complex I of the ETC (Owen et al. 2000). Preclinical data has shown that metformin reduces OCR in numerous cancer cell lines leading to alleviation of hypoxia in spheroids as well as in xenograft models with corresponding improvement in radiation response (Ashton et al. 2016; Zannella et al. 2013; De Bruycker et al. 2019).

However, unfortunately despite such promise, clinically achievable concentrations of metformin are significantly lower than those required in preclinical models to result in meaningful OCR reduction, and thus unlikely to be a good anti-hypoxia agent. Furthermore, in a number of cell types, metformin was shown to be ineffective at inhibiting OCR, suggesting potential limited applicability (Ashton et al. 2016). A recent clinical study in breast cancer has demonstrated that metformin does alter tumor metabolism, switching it to a glycolytic phenotype (Lord et al. 2018), suggesting sufficient tumor metabolism modulatory activity in patients; however, no hypoxia measures were utilized. A recent randomized study of concurrent chemoradiation therapy with or without metformin in locally advanced NSCLC failed to demonstrate improvement in outcomes (Tsakiridis et al. 2019). Recently, Lord et al. reported that treatment of breast cancer patients with metformin, which inhibits OXPHOS through complex I rather than complex III inhibition, resulted in a shift in tumor metabolism from OXPHOS to glycolysis (Lord et al. 2018), therefore supporting that metabolic reprograming is achievable using OXPHOS inhibitors in the clinical setting. As glycolysis has long been associated with tumor progression and metastasis (Heiden and DeBerardinis 2017), some may voice concern that this approach may be detrimental in terms of disease progression. However, retrospective studies have unanimously demonstrated superior outcomes for cancer patients receiving metformin compared to diabetic patients taking alternative medication, with such improvements independent of diabetic control (Cao et al. 2017;

Koritzinsky 2015; Pernicova and Korbonits 2014; Belfiore et al. 2009; Algire et al. 2012; Dowling et al. 2007). A number of clinical studies are currently underway to investigate the effect of metformin on tumor hypoxia with no reported results as of yet.

Numerous other FDA-approved drugs, as well as new experimental agents, have been shown to inhibit OXPHOS preclinically but several have significant toxicity and unfavorable pharmacokinetics, and are thus unattractive candidates (Wang et al. 2003; Ashton et al. 2016). In one early phase study of the novel complex I inhibitor BAY87–2243, the trial was terminated early due to unexpected toxicity (Kirkpatrick and Powis 2017), demonstrating the importance of carefully assessing the safety of such agents, especially when combined with chemotherapy or radiation.

Another complex I inhibitor papaverine has also been shown to reduce hypoxia and improve tumor radiation response preclinically (Benej et al. 2018). Parpaverine is an FDA-approved compound conventionally used to treat arterial spasm; this is independent of its ability to inhibit complex I, but instead by inhibiting phosphodies-terase 10A (PDE10A). An attractive property of parpaverine is that pre-treatment of just 45 min resulted in a significant reduction in tumor hypoxia, and subsequent radiosensitization. This relatively short pre-treatment time adds to the potential of parpaverine being translated to a clinical setting. Papaverine is undergoing phase I testing in combination with stereotactic ablative body radiotherapy (SABR) in NSCLC but unfortunately, once again, no hypoxia readouts have been included in the study design.

Overall, preclinical data is highly encouraging for developing OXPHOS inhibi-tors in order to reduce OCR and thus tumor hypoxia. However, the translation of such agents into the clinical setting has proven challenging with no clinical evidence to date of alleviation of tumor hypoxia. Any agent being developed for this purpose must not only have strong preclinical data to support its effect on OCR and hypoxia, but do so at clinically relevant concentrations and with favorable toxicity profile.

7.5 Atovaquone as a Novel Tumor Hypoxia Modifier and Radiosensitizer

The recent discovery that the commonly prescribed and well-tolerated antimalarial drug atovaquone meets criteria of affecting OCR/hypoxia at clinically relevant con-centrations and acceptable toxicity is of great promise. Atovaquone is an FDA-approved drug in widespread clinical use for over 20 years. It is currently used as a single agent for the treatment of the *Pneumocystis* pneumonia caused by the oppor-tunistic fungus *Pneumocystis jirovecii*, and in combination with proguanil for the prophylaxis and treatment of malaria caused by the protozoa *Plasmodium falciparum*.

Atovaquone (2-[trans-4-(4′-chlorophenyl) cyclohexyl]-3-hydroxy-1,4-naphtho-quinone, 566C80) is a ubiquinone (co-enzyme Q10) analogue which emerged in 1991 as the leading compound with efficacy against malaria and opportunistic infections such as *Pneumocystis* pneumonia in immunosuppressed patients with favorable pharmacokinetic properties (Hudson et al. 1991). Following required improvements in synthesis methodology, atovaquone became a commonly used antimicrobial in patients from the mid-1990s. Today, in combination with proguanil, atovaquone accounts for over 70% of malarial prophylaxis prescriptions in the USA (LaRocque et al. 2012).

The mechanism of action of atovaquone against *Plasmodium falciparum* is mediated through inhibition of mitochondrial complex III (Fry and Pudney 1992; Srivastava et al. 1997), whereas the mechanism responsible for atovaquone's activity against *Pneumocystis* species still remains unknown. Complex III, also known as cytochrome bc_1 complex or co-enzyme Q cytochrome c reductase, is a multi-subunit transmembrane protein located in the inner mitochondrial membrane which couples the electron transfer from ubiquinol, the reduced form of ubiquinone or co-enzyme Q, to cytochrome *c,* resulting in the movement of four protons across the lipid bilayer and thereby contributing significantly to ATP production. Atovaquone binds to the catalytic Q_o site through hydrogen bonding to the Rieske iron-sulfur proteins which form the most important catalytic subunit of complex III required for transfer of electrons from ubiquinol during the ETC (Birth et al. 2014; Mather et al. 2005). By disrupting mitochondrial respiration in this way, atovaquone significantly prevents energy production in parasites. In addition, atovaquone also acts by blocking essential pyrimidine biosynthesis, which has been shown to be the predominant metabolic function of complex III in *Plasmodium falciparum* (Painter et al. 2007).

Atovaquone causes very few side effects and has an excellent safety profile. Adverse events which have potentially been attributed to atovaquone are generally very mild and most commonly include rash, fever, vomiting, diarrhea, abdominal pain, and headache (MEPRON (atovaquone) Suspension–GSKSource, Anon. n.d.-a; Wellvone 750 mg/5 ml oral suspension—Summary of Product Characteristics (SmPC)—(emc), Anon. n.d.-b). Encouragingly, an overdose of atovaquone with 31,500 mg resulted in no observed toxicity (Cheung 1999).

Using a Seahorse XF analyzer, Ashton et al. (Ashton et al. 2016) conducted a high-throughput screen of 1697 FDA-approved drugs to assess their effect on OCR in FaDu hypopharyngeal cancer cells. Subsequently, it was demonstrated that 10 µM atovaquone dramatically reduced OCR by approximately 80–90% in A549 NSCLC, H1299 NSCLC, H460 NSCLC, HCT116 colorectal cancer, DLD-1 colorectal cancer, MCF7 breast cancer, and T24 bladder cancer cells. A lesser but still impressive reduction of 58% in OCR was seen in PSN-1 pancreatic cancer cells. Furthermore, the effect on OCR was dose-dependent with smaller but still significant decreases in OCR observed at 2 µM (Ashton et al. 2016). Atovaquone was then demonstrated to completely alleviate hypoxia in 3D spheroids of FaDu, H1299, and HCT116 3D cells, again at clinically achievable concentrations. Combination of atovaquone treatment and radiation in FaDu spheroids resulted in increased growth delay following irradiation. In vivo experiments provided further support for atovaquone as a tumor hypoxia modifier and radiosensitizer. Using FaDu and HT116 mice xenograft models, 7 days of atovaquone treatment was shown to eradicate tumor hypoxia as detected by tumor EF5 staining, with mean mice plasma levels comparable to those seen in patients. There was no effect on tumor growth in FaDu xenografts with atovaquone treatment alone, but marked tumor growth delay was observed when combined with radiation (Ashton et al. 2016).

Mechanistic experiments in FaDu cells demonstrated that, as per its antimicrobial mode of action, atovaquone specifically inhibits mitochondrial complex III. With regard to radiosensitization, colony formation assays performed under different oxygen conditions revealed that atovaquone did not alter radiosensitivity, indicating that atovaquone is not an intrinsic radiosensitizer (Ashton et al. 2016).

Overall, this data provides compelling evidence that atovaquone decreases OCR through mitochondrial complex III inhibition, which results in a reduction in tumor hypoxia and in turn results in tumor radiosensitization. Given that hypoxia is predominantly a tumor-specific phenomenon, it is hypothesized that atovaquone would preferentially sensitize tumors and not normal tissues to radiation and thus improve the therapeutic index for radiation therapy.

A number of recent studies have also demonstrated that atovaquone inhibits cancer cell proliferation. For example, atovaquone has been shown to inhibit proliferation and induce apoptosis in renal cell carcinoma cells through a mechanism dependent upon mitochondrial complex III inhibition and increased ROS production (Chen et al. 2018). This group also showed that in vitro and in vivo atovaquone increased the efficacy of 5-fluorouracil (5-FU) and interferon-α (IFN-α) in this tumor type. Further still, in hepatocellular carcinoma (HCC) cells, atovaquone significantly inhibited proliferation through S phase cell cycle arrest with both intrinsic and extrinsic apoptotic pathway induction associated with upregulation of p53 and p21. Further investigation revealed that atovaquone induced double-stranded DNA breaks, leading to sustained activation of ataxia-telangiectasia mutated (ATM) kinase and its downstream molecules such as cell cycle checkpoint kinase-2 (CHK2) and H2AX. Subsequent in vivo experiments demonstrated that atovaquone-inhibited tumor growth and prolonged survival of tumor-bearing mice (Gao et al. 2018). However, in this study atovaquone did not have any significant effect on tumor growth. Furthermore, as previously described Ashton et al. did not observe any direct antiproliferative effect of atovaquone in numerous cancer cell types or tumor growth delay in xenograft models (Ashton et al. 2016), thus suggesting that perhaps the antiproliferative effects of atovaquone are dependent on cell type, as well as specific experimental conditions.

Lastly, atovaquone has also recently been shown to have direct activity against cancer stem-like cells (CSCs). In MCF7 breast cancer cells, atovaquone inhibits oxygen consumption and induces glycolysis as well as oxidative stress. Given that MCF7-derived CSCs are highly dependent on mitochondrial respiration, atovaquone inhibits CSC proliferation with an IC-50 of just 1 μM. Furthermore, in certain CSC populations, atovaquone induces apoptosis (Fiorillo et al. 2016).

Overall, there is therefore growing evidence that in addition to hypoxia modification and thus its potential as a radiosensitizer, atovaquone may be a multifunctioning anti-cancer agent. Atovaquone is extremely well tolerated, which is of key importance especially for combining it with toxic therapies such as radiation and chemotherapy where the therapeutic window is often already very narrow. The finding that atovaquone is so well tolerated is somewhat surprising given that OXPHOS is an integral part of normal cellular function and the main source of energy production. Perhaps the answer lies in the fact that atovaquone has been shown not to alter the metabolic state of normal cells. For example, in normal human fibroblasts no alteration in metabolic function were observed following atovaquone treatment (Fiorillo et al. 2016). This apparent cancer-specific inhibition of OXPHOS adds further impetus for developing this agent as an anti-cancer treatment.

8   Summary

Tumor hypoxia is arguably the best validated target in oncology due to its multifarious role in tumorigenesis and the profound resistance to radiation therapy it confers. In no other tumor type is the need for improving tumor radiosensitivity more evident than in locally advanced NSCLC where exceptionally poor outcomes following chemoradiation are unfortunately part of everyday clinical practice. Therefore, the development of novel hypoxia modifiers to improve radiation efficacy represents an unmet and urgent clinical need for this patient population. An exciting new strategy to tackle tumor hypoxia is reprogramming cellular metabolism through inhibition of OXPHOS to reduce tumor OCR. The commonly prescribed antimicrobial drug atovaquone has emerged as the most promising agent for this purpose. However, despite decades of clinical research combining promising hypoxia modifiers with radiotherapy, no such agent has been adopted into widespread clinical use. The reasons for this are clear and multifactorial. Although improvement in outcomes has been observed, it has been modest at best and often with concerns regarding toxicity or practical deliverability (Overgaard 2011). However, perhaps of greater importance is that there has been an almost complete absence of proof-of-principle studies to confirm the ability of such agents to reduce tumor hypoxia in patients. The barrier to conducting such studies has undeniably been a lack of robust, widely available and adequately validated biomarkers for the clinical evaluating tumor hypoxia. This has not only significantly impeded the investigation of the efficacy of hypoxia modifiers, but it has also resulted in an inability to accurately select patients who are likely to benefit most from such treatment. It is likely that only when hypoxia biomarkers are widely available will hypoxia modification enter the well-established era of personalized medicine and significant improvements in outcomes be realized.

Acknowledgments MS gratefully acknowledges the support of the Howat Foundation. JDW is grateful for support from the Royal College of Radiologists, and Oriel College, Oxford.

References

Algire C, Moiseeva O, Deschênes-Simard X, Amrein L, Petruccelli L, Birman E, Viollet B, Ferbeyre G, Pollak MN (2012) Metformin reduces endogenous reactive oxygen species and associated DNA damage. Cancer Prev Res (Phila) 5(4):536–543. https://doi.org/10.1158/1940-6207. CAPR-11-0536

Alper T, Howard-Flanders P (1956) Role of oxygen in modifying the radiosensitivity of E. coli B. Nature 178(4540):978–979

Ames BN, Shigenaga MK, Hagen TM (1993) Oxidants, antioxidants, and the degenerative diseases of aging. Proc Natl Acad Sci U S A 90(17):7915–7922

Anon. (n.d.-a) MEPRON (atovaquone) Suspension-GSKSource

Anon. (n.d.-b) Wellvone 750mg/5ml oral suspension - Summary of Product Characteristics (SmPC)—(emc)

Ashton TM, Fokas E, Kunz-Schughart LA, Folkes LK, Anbalagan S, Huether M, Kelly CJ, Pirovano G, Buffa FM, Hammond EM, Stratford M, Muschel RJ, Higgins GS, McKenna WG (2016) The anti-malarial atovaquone increases radiosensitivity by alleviating tumour hypoxia. Nat Commun 7. https://doi.org/10.1038/ncomms12308

Ashton TM, McKenna WG, Kunz-Schughart LA, Higgins GS (2018) Oxidative phosphorylation as an emerging target in cancer therapy. Clin Cancer Res 24(11):2482–2490. https://doi.org/10.1158/1078-0432.CCR-17-3070

Asquith JC, Watts ME, Patel K, Smithen CE, Adams GE (1974) Electron affinic sensitization. V. Radiosensitization of hypoxic bacteria and mammalian cells in vitro by some nitroimidazoles and nitropyrazoles. Radiat Res 60(1):108–118

Belfiore A, Frasca F, Pandini G, Sciacca L, Vigneri R (2009) Insulin receptor isoforms and insulin receptor/insulin-like growth factor receptor hybrids in physiology and disease. Endocr Rev 30(6):586–623. https://doi.org/10.1210/er.2008-0047

Benej M, Hong X, Vibhute S, Scott S, Wu J, Graves E, Le Q-T, Koong AC, Giaccia AJ, Yu B, Chen C-S, Papandreou I, Denko NC (2018) Papaverine and its derivatives radiosensitize solid tumors by inhibiting mitochondrial metabolism. Proc Natl Acad Sci U S A 115(42):10756–10761. https://doi.org/10.1073/pnas.1808945115

Bennett M, Feldmeier J, Smee R, Milross C (2005) Hyperbaric oxygenation for tumour sensitisation to radiotherapy. Cochrane Database Syst Rev 4:CD005007. https://doi.org/10.1002/14651858. CD005007.pub2

Bennewith KL, Durand RE (2004) Quantifying transient hypoxia in human tumor xenografts by flow cytometry. Cancer Res 64(17):6183–6189. https://doi.org/10.1158/0008-5472. CAN-04-0289

Bentzen J, Toustrup K, Eriksen JG, Primdahl H, Andersen LJ, Overgaard J (2015) Locally advanced head and neck cancer treated with accelerated radiotherapy, the hypoxic modifier nimorazole and weekly cisplatin. Results from the DAHANCA 18 phase II study. Acta Oncol 54(7):1001–1007. https://doi.org/10.3109/0284186X.2014.992547

Berra E, Benizri E, Ginouvès A, Volmat V, Roux D, Pouysségur J (2003) HIF prolyl-hydroxylase 2 is the key oxygen sensor setting low steady-state levels of HIF-1α in normoxia. EMBO J 22(16):4082–4090. https://doi.org/10.1093/emboj/cdg392

Birsoy K, Possemato R, Lorbeer FK, Bayraktar EC, Thiru P, Yucel B, Wang T, Chen WW, Clish CB, Sabatini DM (2014) Metabolic determinants of cancer cell sensitivity to glucose limitation and biguanides. Nature 508(7494):108–112. https://doi.org/10.1038/nature13110

Birth D, Kao W-C, Hunte C (2014) Structural analysis of atovaquone-inhibited cytochrome bc_1 complex reveals the molecular basis of antimalarial drug action. Nat Commun 5:4029. https://doi.org/10.1038/ncomms5029

Bleehen NM, Wiltshire CR, Plowman PN, Watson JV, Gleave JR, Holmes AE, Lewin WS, Treip CS, Hawkins TD (1981) A randomized study of misonidazole and radiotherapy for grade 3 and 4 cerebral astrocytoma. Br J Cancer 43(4):436–442

Brown JM (1979) Evidence for acutely hypoxic cells in mouse tumours, and a possible mechanism of reoxygenation. Br J Radiol 52(620):650–656. https://doi.org/10.1259/0007-1285-52-620-650

Buffa FM, Harris AL, West CM, Miller CJ (2010) Large meta-analysis of multiple cancers reveals a common, compact and highly prognostic hypoxia metagene. Br J Cancer 102(2):428–435. https://doi.org/10.1038/sj.bjc.6605450

Cao X, Wu Y, Wang J, Liu K, Wang X (2017) The effect of metformin on mortality among diabetic cancer patients: a systematic review and meta-analysis. JNCI Cancer Spectr 1(1). https://doi.org/10.1093/jncics/pkx007

Carreau A, Hafny-Rahbi BE, Matejuk A, Grillon C, Kieda C (2011) Why is the partial oxygen pressure of human tissues a crucial parameter? Small molecules and hypoxia. J Cell Mol Med 15(6):1239–1253. https://doi.org/10.1111/j.1582-4934.2011.01258.x

Cavalli LR, Varella-Garcia M, Liang BC (1997) Diminished tumorigenic phenotype after depletion of mitochondrial DNA. Cell Growth Differ 8(11):1189–1198

Cerniglia GJ, Pore N, Tsai JH, Schultz S, Mick R, Choe R, Xing X, Durduran T, Yodh AG, Evans SM, Koch CJ, Hahn SM, Quon H, Sehgal CM, Lee WMF, Maity A (2009) Epidermal growth factor receptor inhibition modulates the microenvironment by vascular normalization to improve chemotherapy and radiotherapy efficacy. PLoS One 4(8):e6539. https://doi.org/10.1371/journal.pone.0006539

Chakraborty C, Das S (2016) Profiling cell-free and circulating miRNA: a clinical diagnostic tool for different cancers. Tumour Biol 37(5):5705–5714. https://doi.org/10.1007/s13277-016-4907-3

Chapman JD (1979) Hypoxic sensitizers--implications for radiation therapy. N Engl J Med 301(26):1429–1432. https://doi.org/10.1056/NEJM197912273012606

Chen D, Sun X, Zhang X, Cao J (2018) Targeting mitochondria by anthelmintic drug atovaquone sensitizes renal cell carcinoma to chemotherapy and immunotherapy. J Biochem Mol Toxicol 32(9):e22195. https://doi.org/10.1002/jbt.22195

Cheung TW (1999) Overdose of atovaquone in a patient with AIDS. AIDS 13(14):1984–1985

Choudhry H, Harris AL (2018) Advances in hypoxia-inducible factor biology. Cell Metab 27(2):281–298. https://doi.org/10.1016/j.cmet.2017.10.005

Dang CV, Lewis BC, Dolde C, Dang G, Shim H (1997) Oncogenes in tumor metabolism, tumorigenesis, and apoptosis. J Bioenerg Biomembr 29(4):345–354

Dang CV, Semenza GL (1999) Oncogenic alterations of metabolism. Trends Biochem Sci 24(2):68–72. https://doi.org/10.1016/S0968-0004(98)01344-9

Dang K, Myers KA (2015) The role of hypoxia-induced miR-210 in cancer progression. Int J Mol Sci 16(3):6353–6372. https://doi.org/10.3390/ijms16036353

Dayan F, Roux D, Brahimi-Horn MC, Pouyssegur J, Mazure NM (2006) The oxygen sensor factor-inhibiting hypoxia-inducible factor-1 controls expression of distinct genes through the bifunctional transcriptional character of hypoxia-inducible factor-1alpha. Cancer Res 66(7):3688–3698. https://doi.org/10.1158/0008-5472.CAN-05-4564

De Bruycker S, Vangestel C, Van den Wyngaert T, Pauwels P, Wyffels L, Staelens S, Stroobants S (2019) 18F-Flortanidazole hypoxia PET holds promise as a prognostic and predictive imaging biomarker in a lung cancer xenograft model treated with metformin and radiotherapy. J Nucl Med 60(1):34–40. https://doi.org/10.2967/jnumed.118.212225

DeBerardinis RJ, Lum JJ, Hatzivassiliou G, Thompson CB (2008) The biology of cancer: metabolic reprogramming fuels cell growth and proliferation. Cell Metab 7(1):11–20. https://doi.org/10.1016/j.cmet.2007.10.002

Dengler VL, Galbraith M, Espinosa JM (2014) Transcriptional regulation by hypoxia inducible factors. Crit Rev Biochem Mol Biol 49(1):1–15. https://doi.org/10.3109/10409238.2013.838205

Dewhirst MW (2009) Relationships between cycling hypoxia, HIF-1, angiogenesis and oxidative stress. Radiat Res 172(6):653–665. https://doi.org/10.1667/RR1926.1

Dewhirst MW, Cao Y, Moeller B (2008) Cycling hypoxia and free radicals regulate angiogenesis and radiotherapy response. Nat Rev Cancer 8(6):425–437. https://doi.org/10.1038/nrc2397

Dische S (1985) Chemical sensitizers for hypoxic cells: a decade of experience in clinical radiotherapy. Radiother Oncol 3(2):97–115

Dische S, Saunders M, Barrett A, Harvey A, Gibson D, Parmar M (1997) A randomised multicentre trial of CHART versus conventional radiotherapy in head and neck cancer. Radiother Oncol 44(2):123–136

DiSilvestro PA, Ali S, Craighead PS, Lucci JA, Lee Y-C, Cohn DE, Spirtos NM, Tewari KS, Muller C, Gajewski WH, Steinhoff MM, Monk BJ (2014) Phase III randomized trial of weekly cisplatin and irradiation versus cisplatin and tirapazamine and irradiation in stages IB2, IIA, IIB, IIIB, and IVA cervical carcinoma limited to the pelvis: a Gynecologic Oncology Group study. J Clin Oncol 32(5):458–464. https://doi.org/10.1200/JCO.2013.51.4265

Doktorova H, Hrabeta J, Khalil MA, Eckschlager T (2015) Hypoxia-induced chemoresistance in cancer cells: the role of not only HIF-1. Biomed Papers 159(2):166–177. https://doi.org/10.5507/bp.2015.025

Dowling RJO, Zakikhani M, Fantus IG, Pollak M, Sonenberg N (2007) Metformin inhibits mammalian target of rapamycin-dependent translation initiation in breast cancer cells. Cancer Res 67(22):10804–10812. https://doi.org/10.1158/0008-5472.CAN-07-2310

Dubois L, Landuyt W, Haustermans K, Dupont P, Bormans G, Vermaelen P, Flamen P, Verbeken E, Mortelmans L (2004) Evaluation of hypoxia in an experimental rat tumour model by [(18) F]fluoromisonidazole PET and immunohistochemistry. Br J Cancer 91(11):1947–1954. https://doi.org/10.1038/sj.bjc.6602219

Dunst J, Stadler P, Becker A, Kuhnt T, Lautenschläger C, Molls M, Haensgen G (2001) Tumor hypoxia and systemic levels of vascular endothelial growth factor (VEGF) in head and neck cancers. Strahlenther Onkol 177(9):469–473

Dunwoodie SL (2009) The role of hypoxia in development of the mammalian embryo. Dev Cell 17(6):755–773. https://doi.org/10.1016/j.devcel.2009.11.008

Dvorak HF, Nagy JA, Feng D, Brown LF, Dvorak AM (1999) Vascular permeability factor/vascular endothelial growth factor and the significance of microvascular hyperpermeability in angiogenesis. Curr Top Microbiol Immunol 237:97–132

Elstrom RL, Bauer DE, Buzzai M, Karnauskas R, Harris MH, Plas DR, Zhuang H, Cinalli RM, Alavi A, Rudin CM, Thompson CB (2004) Akt stimulates aerobic glycolysis in cancer cells. Cancer Res 64(11):3892–3899. https://doi.org/10.1158/0008-5472.CAN-03-2904

Eschmann S-M, Paulsen F, Reimold M, Dittmann H, Welz S, Reischl G, Machulla H-J, Bares R (2005) Prognostic impact of hypoxia imaging with 18F-misonidazole PET in non-small cell lung cancer and head and neck cancer before radiotherapy. J Nucl Med 46(2):253–260

Falk SJ, Ward R, Bleehen NM (1992) The influence of carbogen breathing on tumour tissue oxygenation in man evaluated by computerised pO2 histography. Br J Cancer 66(5):919–924

Fiorillo M, Lamb R, Tanowitz HB, Mutti L, Krstic-Demonacos M, Cappello AR, Martinez-Outschoorn UE, Sotgia F, Lisanti MP (2016) Repurposing atovaquone: targeting mitochondrial complex III and OXPHOS to eradicate cancer stem cells. Oncotarget 7(23):34084–34099. https://doi.org/10.18632/oncotarget.9122

Fleming IN, Manavaki R, Blower PJ, West C, Williams KJ, Harris AL, Domarkas J, Lord S, Baldry C, Gilbert FJ (2015) Imaging tumour hypoxia with positron emission tomography. Br J Cancer 112(2):238–250. https://doi.org/10.1038/bjc.2014.610

Fokas E, Im JH, Hill S, Yameen S, Stratford M, Beech J, Hackl W, Maira S-M, Bernhard EJ, McKenna WG, Muschel RJ (2012) Dual inhibition of the PI3K/mTOR pathway increases tumor radiosensitivity by normalizing tumor vasculature. Cancer Res 72(1):239–248. https://doi.org/10.1158/0008-5472.CAN-11-2263

Fry M, Pudney M (1992) Site of action of the antimalarial hydroxynaphthoquinone, 2-[trans-4-(4'-chlorophenyl) cyclohexyl]-3-hydroxy-1,4-naphthoquinone (566C80). Biochem Pharmacol 43(7):1545–1553

Fukuda R, Zhang H, Kim J-w, Shimoda L, Dang CV, Semenza GL (2007) HIF-1 regulates cytochrome oxidase subunits to optimize efficiency of respiration in hypoxic cells. Cell 129(1):111–122. https://doi.org/10.1016/j.cell.2007.01.047

Gao X, Liu X, Shan W, Liu Q, Wang C, Zheng J, Yao H, Tang R, Zheng J (2018) Anti-malarial atovaquone exhibits anti-tumor effects by inducing DNA damage in hepatocellular carcinoma. Am J Cancer Res 8(9):1697–1711

Gatenby RA, Kessler HB, Rosenblum JS, Coia LR, Moldofsky PJ, Hartz WH, Broder GJ (1988) Oxygen distribution in squamous cell carcinoma metastases and its relationship to outcome of radiation therapy. Int J Radiat Oncol Biol Phys 14(5):831–838. https://doi.org/10.1016/0360-3016(88)90002-8

Gaude E, Frezza C (2016) Tissue-specific and convergent metabolic transformation of cancer correlates with metastatic potential and patient survival. Nat Commun 7:13041. https://doi.org/10.1038/ncomms13041

Giatromanolaki A, Koukourakis MI, Sivridis E, Pastorek J, Wykoff CC, Gatter KC, Harris AL (2001) Expression of hypoxia-inducible carbonic anhydrase-9 relates to angiogenic pathways and independently to poor outcome in non-small cell lung cancer. Cancer Res 61(21):7992–7998

Gillies RM, Robinson SP, McPhail LD, Carter ND, Murray JF (2011) Immunohistochemical assessment of intrinsic and extrinsic markers of hypoxia in reproductive tissue: differential expression of HIF1α and HIF2α in rat oviduct and endometrium. J Mol Hist 42(4):341–354. https://doi.org/10.1007/s10735-011-9338-2

Ginouvès A, Ilc K, Macías N, Pouysségur J, Berra E (2008) PHDs overactivation during chronic hypoxia "desensitizes" HIFalpha and protects cells from necrosis. Proc Natl Acad Sci U S A 105(12):4745–4750. https://doi.org/10.1073/pnas.0705680105

Goldmann E (1908) The growth of malignant disease in man and the lower animals, with special reference to the vascular system. Proc R Soc Med 1(Surg Sect):1–13

Gray LH, Conger AD, Ebert M, Hornsey S, Scott OCA (1953) The concentration of oxygen dissolved in tissues at the time of irradiation as a factor in radiotherapy. Br J Radiol 26(312):638–648. https://doi.org/10.1259/0007-1285-26-312-638

Grimes DR, Kelly C, Bloch K, Partridge M (2014) A method for estimating the oxygen consumption rate in multicellular tumour spheroids. J R Soc Interface 11(92):20131124. https://doi.org/10.1098/rsif.2013.1124

Grkovski M, Schwartz J, Rimner A, Schöder H, Carlin SD, Zanzonico PB, Humm JL, Nehmeh SA (2016) Reproducibility of 18F-fluoromisonidazole intratumour distribution in non-small cell lung cancer. EJNMMI Res 6. https://doi.org/10.1186/s13550-016-0210-y

Hall E, Giaccia A (2011) Radiobiology for the radiologist, 7th edn. Lippincottt Williams & Wilkins, Philadelphia, PA

Hammond EM, Asselin MC, Forster D, O'Connor JP, Senra JM, Williams KJ (2014) The meaning, measurement and modification of hypoxia in the laboratory and the clinic. Clin Oncol (R Coll Radiol) 26(5):277–288. https://doi.org/10.1016/j.clon.2014.02.002

Hanahan D, Weinberg RA (2011) Hallmarks of cancer: the next generation. Cell 144(5):646–674. https://doi.org/10.1016/j.cell.2011.02.013

Harris BHL, Barberis A, West CML, Buffa FM (2015) Gene expression signatures as biomarkers of tumour hypoxia. Clin Oncol (R Coll Radiol) 27(10):547–560. https://doi.org/10.1016/j.clon.2015.07.004

Harrison LB, Chadha M, Hill RJ, Hu K, Shasha D (2002) Impact of tumor hypoxia and anemia on radiation therapy outcomes. Oncologist 7(6):492–508

Hashizume H, Baluk P, Morikawa S, McLean JW, Thurston G, Roberge S, Jain RK, McDonald DM (2000) Openings between defective endothelial cells explain tumor vessel leakiness. Am J Pathol 156(4):1363–1380

Heiden MGV, DeBerardinis RJ (2017) Understanding the intersections between metabolism and cancer biology. Cell 168(4):657–669. https://doi.org/10.1016/j.cell.2016.12.039

Held KD, Harrop HA, Michael BD (1984) Effects of oxygen and sulphydryl-containing compounds on irradiated transforming DNA. II. Glutathione, cysteine and cysteamine. Int J Radiat Biol Relat Stud Phys Chem Med 45(6):615–626

Henke M, Laszig R, Rübe C, Schäfer U, Haase K-D, Schilcher B, Mose S, Beer KT, Burger U, Dougherty C, Frommhold H (2003) Erythropoietin to treat head and neck cancer patients with anaemia undergoing radiotherapy: randomised, double-blind, placebo-controlled trial. Lancet 362(9392):1255–1260. https://doi.org/10.1016/S0140-6736(03)14567-9

Henke M, Mattern D, Pepe M, Bézay C, Weissenberger C, Werner M, Pajonk F (2006) Do erythropoietin receptors on cancer cells explain unexpected clinical findings? J Clin Oncol 24(29):4708–4713. https://doi.org/10.1200/JCO.2006.06.2737

Horsman MR, Mortensen LS, Petersen JB, Busk M, Overgaard J (2012) Imaging hypoxia to improve radiotherapy outcome. Nat Rev Clin Oncol 9(12):674–687. https://doi.org/10.1038/nrclinonc.2012.171

Hoskin P, Rojas A, Saunders M (2009) Accelerated radiotherapy, carbogen, and nicotinamide (ARCON) in the treatment of advanced bladder cancer: mature results of a phase II non-randomized study. Int J Radiat Oncol Biol Phys 73(5):1425–1431. https://doi.org/10.1016/j.ijrobp.2008.06.1950

Hoskin PJ, Rojas AM, Bentzen SM, Saunders MI (2010) Radiotherapy with concurrent car-bogen and nicotinamide in bladder carcinoma. J Clin Oncol. https://doi.org/10.1200/JCO.2010.28.4950

Hudson AT, Dickins M, Ginger CD, Gutteridge WE, Holdich T, Hutchinson DB, Pudney M, Randall AW, Latter VS (1991) 566C80: a potent broad spectrum anti-infective agent with activity against malaria and opportunistic infections in AIDS patients. Drugs Exp Clin Res 17(9):427–435

Hughes VS, Wiggins JM, Siemann DW (2018) Tumor oxygenation and cancer therapy—then and now. Br J Radiol 92(1093):20170955. https://doi.org/10.1259/bjr.20170955

Hunter RW, Hughey CC, Lantier L, Sundelin EI, Peggie M, Zeqiraj E, Sicheri F, Jessen N, Wasserman DH, Sakamoto K (2018) Metformin reduces liver glucose production by inhi-bition of fructose-1-6-bisphosphatase. Nat Med 24(9):1395. https://doi.org/10.1038/s41591-018-0159-7

Hutchinson F (1961) Sulfhydryl groups and the oxygen effect on irradiated dilute solutions of enzymes and nucleic acids. Radiat Res 14:721–731

Jaakkola P, Mole DR, Tian YM, Wilson MI, Gielbert J, Gaskell SJ, von Kriegsheim A, Hebestreit HF, Mukherji M, Schofield CJ, Maxwell PH, Pugh CW, Ratcliffe PJ (2001) Targeting of HIF-alpha to the von Hippel-Lindau ubiquitylation complex by O2-regulated prolyl hydroxylation. Science 292(5516):468–472. https://doi.org/10.1126/science.1059796

Jain RK (2014) Antiangiogenesis strategies revisited: from starving tumors to alleviating hypoxia. Cancer Cell 26(5):605–622. https://doi.org/10.1016/j.ccell.2014.10.006

Janssens GO, Rademakers SE, Terhaard CH, Doornaert PA, Bijl HP, van den Ende P, Chin A, Marres HA, de Bree R, van der Kogel AJ, Hoogsteen IJ, Bussink J, Span PN, Kaanders JH (2012) Accelerated radiotherapy with carbogen and nicotinamide for laryngeal cancer: results of a phase III randomized trial. J Clin Oncol 30(15):1777–1783. https://doi.org/10.1200/JCO.2011.35.9315

Jiang M, Li X, Quan X, Li X, Zhou B (2018, 2018) Clinically correlated MicroRNAs in the diag-nosis of non-small cell lung cancer: a systematic review and meta-analysis. Biomed Res Int. https://doi.org/10.1155/2018/5930951

Jones RG, Thompson CB (2009) Tumor suppressors and cell metabolism: a recipe for cancer growth. Genes Dev 23(5):537–548. https://doi.org/10.1101/gad.1756509

Kaanders JHAM, Pop LAM, Marres HAM, Bruaset I, van den Hoogen FJA, Merkx MAW, van der Kogel AJ (2002) ARCON: experience in 215 patients with advanced head-and-neck cancer. Int J Radiat Oncol Biol Phys 52(3):769–778

Kaluz S, Kaluzová M, Liao S-Y, Lerman M, Stanbridge EJ (2009) Transcriptional control of the tumor- and hypoxia-marker carbonic anhydrase 9: a one transcription factor (HIF-1) show? Biochim Biophys Acta 1795(2):162–172. https://doi.org/10.1016/j.bbcan.2009.01.001

Kedderis GL, Miwa GT (1988) The metabolic activation of nitroheterocyclic therapeutic agents. Drug Metab Rev 19(1):33–62. https://doi.org/10.3109/03602538809049618

Kim J-w, Tchernyshyov I, Semenza GL, Dang CV (2006) HIF-1-mediated expression of pyruvate dehydrogenase kinase: a metabolic switch required for cellular adaptation to hypoxia. Cell Metab 3(3):177–185. https://doi.org/10.1016/j.cmet.2006.02.002

Kirkpatrick DL, Powis G (2017) Clinically evaluated cancer drugs inhibiting redox signaling. Antioxid Redox Signal 26(6):262–273. https://doi.org/10.1089/ars.2016.6633

Kizaka-Kondoh S, Konse-Nagasawa H (2009) Significance of nitroimidazole compounds and hypoxia-inducible factor-1 for imaging tumor hypoxia. Cancer Sci 100(8):1366–1373. https://doi.org/10.1111/j.1349-7006.2009.01195.x

Koh WJ, Rasey JS, Evans ML, Grierson JR, Lewellen TK, Graham MM, Krohn KA, Griffin TW (1992) Imaging of hypoxia in human tumors with [F-18]fluoromisonidazole. Int J Radiat Oncol Biol Phys 22(1):199–212

Koivunen P, Hirsilä M, Günzler V, Kivirikko KI, Myllyharju J (2004) Catalytic properties of the asparaginyl hydroxylase (FIH) in the oxygen sensing pathway are distinct from those of its prolyl 4-hydroxylases. J Biol Chem 279(11):9899–9904. https://doi.org/10.1074/jbc.M312254200

Kolstad P (1968) Intercapillary distance, oxygen tension and local recurrence in cervix cancer. Scand J Clin Lab Invest Suppl 106:145–157

Koppenol WH, Bounds PL, Dang CV (2011) Otto Warburg's contributions to current concepts of cancer metabolism. Nat Rev Cancer 11(5):325–337. https://doi.org/10.1038/nrc3038

Koritzinsky M (2015) Metformin: a novel biological modifier of tumor response to radiation therapy. Int J Radiat Oncol Biol Phys 93(2):454–464. https://doi.org/10.1016/j.ijrobp.2015.06.003

Koukourakis MI, Bentzen SM, Giatromanolaki A, Wilson GD, Daley FM, Saunders MI, Dische S, Sivridis E, Harris AL (2006) Endogenous markers of two separate hypoxia response pathways (hypoxia inducible factor 2 alpha and carbonic anhydrase 9) are associated with radiotherapy failure in head and neck cancer patients recruited in the CHART randomized trial. J Clin Oncol 24(5):727–735. https://doi.org/10.1200/JCO.2005.02.7474

Krol J, Loedige I, Filipowicz W (2010) The widespread regulation of microRNA biogenesis, function and decay. Nat Rev Genet 11(9):597–610. https://doi.org/10.1038/nrg2843

Kühlbrandt W (2015) Structure and function of mitochondrial membrane protein complexes. BMC Biol 13(1):89. https://doi.org/10.1186/s12915-015-0201-x

LaGory EL, Giaccia AJ (2016) The ever expanding role of HIF in tumour and stromal biology. Nat Cell Biol 18(4):356–365. https://doi.org/10.1038/ncb3330

Lando D, Peet DJ, Gorman JJ, Whelan DA, Whitelaw ML, Bruick RK (2002) FIH-1 is an asparaginyl hydroxylase enzyme that regulates the transcriptional activity of hypoxia-inducible factor. Genes Dev 16(12):1466–1471. https://doi.org/10.1101/gad.991402

Larman TC, DePalma SR, Hadjipanayis AG, Cancer Genome Atlas Research N, Protopopov A, Zhang J, Gabriel SB, Chin L, Seidman CE, Kucherlapati R, Seidman JG (2012) Spectrum of somatic mitochondrial mutations in five cancers. Proc Natl Acad Sci U S A 109(35):14087–14091. https://doi.org/10.1073/pnas.1211502109

LaRocque RC, Rao SR, Lee J, Ansdell V, Yates JA, Schwartz BS, Knouse M, Cahill J, Hagmann S, Vinetz J, Connor BA, Goad JA, Oladele A, Alvarez S, Stauffer W, Walker P, Kozarsky P, Franco-Paredes C, Dismukes R, Rosen J, Hynes NA, Jacquerioz F, McLellan S, Hale D, Sofarelli T, Schoenfeld D, Marano N, Brunette G, Jentes ES, Yanni E, Sotir MJ, Ryan ET, Global TravEpiNet C (2012) Global TravEpiNet: a national consortium of clinics providing care to international travelers—analysis of demographic characteristics, travel destinations, and pretravel healthcare of high-risk US international travelers, 2009–2011. Clin Infect Dis 54(4):455–462. https://doi.org/10.1093/cid/cir839

Le Q-T, Chen E, Salim A, Cao H, Kong CS, Whyte R, Donington J, Cannon W, Wakelee H, Tibshirani R, Mitchell JD, Richardson D, O'Byrne KJ, Koong AC, Giaccia AJ (2006) An evaluation of tumor oxygenation and gene expression in patients with early stage non–small cell lung cancers. Clin Cancer Res 12(5):1507–1514. https://doi.org/10.1158/1078-0432.CCR-05-2049

Le Q-T, Sutphin PD, Raychaudhuri S, Yu SCT, Terris DJ, Lin HS, Lum B, Pinto HA, Koong AC, Giaccia AJ (2003) Identification of osteopontin as a prognostic plasma marker for head and neck squamous cell carcinomas. Clin Cancer Res 9(1):59–67

Lee CT, Boss MK, Dewhirst MW (2014) Imaging tumor hypoxia to advance radiation oncology. Antioxid Redox Signal 21(2):313–337. https://doi.org/10.1089/ars.2013.5759

Lee WR, Berkey B, Marcial V, Fu KK, Cooper JS, Vikram B, Coia LR, Rotman M, Ortiz H (1998) Anemia is associated with decreased survival and increased locoregional failure in patients with locally advanced head and neck carcinoma: a secondary analysis of RTOG 85-27. Int J Radiat Oncol Biol Phys 42(5):1069–1075

Liu W, Shen S-M, Zhao X-Y, Chen G-Q (2012) Targeted genes and interacting proteins of hypoxia inducible factor-1. Int J Biochem Mol Biol 3(2):165–178

Lord EM, Harwell L, Koch CJ (1993) Detection of hypoxic cells by monoclonal antibody recognizing 2-nitroimidazole adducts. Cancer Res 53(23):5721–5726

Lord SR, Cheng W-C, Liu D, Gaude E, Haider S, Metcalf T, Patel N, Teoh EJ, Gleeson F, Bradley K, Wigfield S, Zois C, McGowan DR, Ah-See M-L, Thompson AM, Sharma A, Bidaut L, Pollak M, Roy PG, Karpe F, James T, English R, Adams RF, Campo L, Ayers L, Snell C, Roxanis I, Frezza C, Fenwick JD, Buffa FM, Harris AL (2018) Integrated pharmacodynamic analysis identifies two metabolic adaption pathways to metformin in breast cancer. Cell Metab 28(5):679–688.e674. https://doi.org/10.1016/j.cmet.2018.08.021

Lunt SY, Vander Heiden MG (2011) Aerobic glycolysis: meeting the metabolic requirements of cell proliferation. Annu Rev Cell Dev Biol 27(1):441–464. https://doi.org/10.1146/annurev-cellbio-092910-154237

Madhavan D, Peng C, Wallwiener M, Zucknick M, Nees J, Schott S, Rudolph A, Riethdorf S, Trumpp A, Pantel K, Sohn C, Chang-Claude J, Schneeweiss A, Burwinkel B (2016) Circulating miRNAs with prognostic value in metastatic breast cancer and for early detection of metastasis. Carcinogenesis 37(5):461–470. https://doi.org/10.1093/carcin/bgw008

Mäntylä MJ, Nordman EM, Ruotsalainen PJ, Kylmämaa TT (1982) Misonidazole and radiotherapy in lung cancer: a randomized double-blind trial. Int J Radiat Oncol Biol Phys 8(10):1719–1720. https://doi.org/10.1016/0360-3016(82)90292-9

Martin GV, Caldwell JH, Graham MM, Grierson JR, Kroll K, Cowan MJ, Lewellen TK, Rasey JS, Casciari JJ, Krohn KA (1992) Noninvasive detection of hypoxic myocardium using fluorine-18-fluoromisonidazole and positron emission tomography. J Nucl Med 33(12):2202–2208

Mather MW, Darrouzet E, Valkova-Valchanova M, Cooley JW, McIntosh MT, Daldal F, Vaidya AB (2005) Uncovering the molecular mode of action of the antimalarial drug atovaquone using a bacterial system. J Biol Chem 280(29):27458–27465. https://doi.org/10.1074/jbc.M502319200

McGowan DR, Skwarski M, Bradley KM, Campo L, Fenwick JD, Gleeson FV, Green M, Horne A, Maughan TS, McCole MG, Mohammed S, Muschel RJ, Ng SM, Panakis N, Prevo R, Strauss VY, Stuart R, Tacconi EMC, Vallis KA, McKenna WG, Macpherson RE, Higgins GS (2019) Buparlisib with thoracic radiotherapy and its effect on tumour hypoxia: a phase I study in patients with advanced non-small cell lung carcinoma. Eur J Cancer 113:87–95. https://doi.org/10.1016/j.ejca.2019.03.015

McNeill LA, Hewitson KS, Claridge TD, Seibel JF, Horsfall LE, Schofield CJ (2002) Hypoxia-inducible factor asparaginyl hydroxylase (FIH-1) catalyses hydroxylation at the beta-carbon of asparagine-803. Biochem J 367(Pt 3):571–575. https://doi.org/10.1042/BJ20021162

Melgaard B, Køhler O, Sand Hansen H, Overgaard J, Munck-Hansen J, Paulson OB (1988) Misonidazole neuropathy. A prospective study. J Neuro-Oncol 6(3):227–230

Metwally MAH, Frederiksen KD, Overgaard J (2014) Compliance and toxicity of the hypoxic radiosensitizer nimorazole in the treatment of patients with head and neck squamous cell carcinoma (HNSCC). Acta Oncol 53(5):654–661. https://doi.org/10.3109/0284186X.2013.864050

Michiels C, Tellier C, Feron O (2016) Cycling hypoxia: a key feature of the tumor microenvironment. Biochimica et Biophysica Acta (BBA)—Reviews on Cancer 1866(1):76–86. https://doi.org/10.1016/j.bbcan.2016.06.004

Milosevic M, Warde P, Menard C, Chung P, Toi A, Ishkanian A, McLean M, Pintilie M, Sykes J, Gospodarowicz M, Catton C, Hill RP, Bristow R (2012) Tumor hypoxia predicts biochemical failure following radiotherapy for clinically localized prostate cancer. Clin Cancer Res 18(7):2108–2114. https://doi.org/10.1158/1078-0432.CCR-11-2711

Mistry IN, Thomas M, Calder EDD, Conway SJ, Hammond EM (2017) Clinical advances of hypoxia-activated prodrugs in combination with radiation therapy. Int J Radiat Oncol Biol Phys 98(5):1183–1196. https://doi.org/10.1016/j.ijrobp.2017.03.024

Mookerjee SA, Gerencser AA, Nicholls DG, Brand MD (2017) Quantifying intracellular rates of glycolytic and oxidative ATP production and consumption using extracellular flux measurements. J Biol Chem 292(17):7189–7207. https://doi.org/10.1074/jbc.M116.774471

Moreno-Sánchez R, Rodríguez-Enríquez S, Marín-Hernández A, Saavedra E (2007) Energy metabolism in tumor cells. FEBS J 274(6):1393–1418. https://doi.org/10.1111/j.1742-4658.2007.05686.x

Moreno-Sánchez R, Rodríguez-Enríquez S, Saavedra E, Marín-Hernández A, Gallardo-Pérez JC (2009) The bioenergetics of cancer: is glycolysis the main ATP supplier in all tumor cells? Biofactors 35(2):209–225. https://doi.org/10.1002/biof.31

Movsas B, Chapman JD, Greenberg RE, Hanlon AL, Horwitz EM, Pinover WH, Stobbe C, Hanks GE (2000) Increasing levels of hypoxia in prostate carcinoma correlate significantly with increasing clinical stage and patient age: an Eppendorf pO(2) study. Cancer 89(9):2018–2024

Movsas B, Chapman JD, Hanlon AL, Horwitz EM, Greenberg RE, Stobbe C, Hanks GE, Pollack A (2002) Hypoxic prostate/muscle pO2 ratio predicts for biochemical failure in patients with prostate cancer: preliminary findings. Urology 60(4):634–639

Müller M, Padberg W, Schindler E, Sticher J, Osmer C, Friemann S, Hempelmann G (1998) Renocortical tissue oxygen pressure measurements in patients undergoing living donor kidney transplantation. Anesth Analg 87(2):474–476. https://doi.org/10.1097/00000539-199808000-00045

Nehmeh SA, Lee NY, Schröder H, Squire O, Zanzonico PB, Erdi YE, Greco C, Mageras G, Pham HS, Larson SM, Ling CC, Humm JL (2008) Reproducibility of intratumor distribution of 18F-fluoromisonidazole in head and neck cancer. Int J Radiat Oncol Biol Phys 70(1):235–242. https://doi.org/10.1016/j.ijrobp.2007.08.036

Nordsmark M, Bentzen SM, Rudat V, Brizel D, Lartigau E, Stadler P, Becker A, Adam M, Molls M, Dunst J, Terris DJ, Overgaard J (2005) Prognostic value of tumor oxygenation in 397 head and neck tumors after primary radiation therapy. An international multi-center study. Radiother Oncol 77(1):18–24. https://doi.org/10.1016/j.radonc.2005.06.038

Nordsmark M, Eriksen JG, Gebski V, Alsner J, Horsman MR, Overgaard J (2007) Differential risk assessments from five hypoxia specific assays: the basis for biologically adapted individualized radiotherapy in advanced head and neck cancer patients. Radiother Oncol 83(3):389–397. https://doi.org/10.1016/j.radonc.2007.04.021

O'Connor JPB, Robinson SP, Waterton JC (2019) Imaging tumour hypoxia with oxygen-enhanced MRI and BOLD MRI. Br J Radiol 92(1095):20180642. https://doi.org/10.1259/bjr.20180642

Ohh M, Park CW, Ivan M, Hoffman MA, Kim TY, Huang LE, Pavletich N, Chau V, Kaelin WG (2000) Ubiquitination of hypoxia-inducible factor requires direct binding to the beta-domain of the von Hippel-Lindau protein. Nat Cell Biol 2(7):423–427. https://doi.org/10.1038/35017054

Okamoto S, Shiga T, Yasuda K, Ito YM, Magota K, Kasai K, Kuge Y, Shirato H, Tamaki N (2013) High reproducibility of tumor hypoxia evaluated by 18F-fluoromisonidazole PET for head and neck cancer. J Nucl Med 54(2):201–207. https://doi.org/10.2967/jnumed.112.109330

Olive PL, Aquino-Parsons C, MacPhail SH, Liao SY, Raleigh JA, Lerman MI, Stanbridge EJ (2001) Carbonic anhydrase 9 as an endogenous marker for hypoxic cells in cervical cancer. Cancer Res 61(24):8924–8929

Orang AV, Petersen J, McKinnon RA, Michael MZ (2019) Micromanaging aerobic respiration and glycolysis in cancer cells. Mol Metab 23:98–126. https://doi.org/10.1016/j.molmet.2019.01.014

Ostheimer C, Bache M, Güttler A, Kotzsch M, Vordermark D (2014) A pilot study on potential plasma hypoxia markers in the radiotherapy of non-small cell lung cancer. Strahlenther Onkol 190(3):276. https://doi.org/10.1007/s00066-013-0484-1

Osthus RC, Shim H, Kim S, Li Q, Reddy R, Mukherjee M, Xu Y, Wonsey D, Lee LA, Dang CV (2000) Deregulation of glucose transporter 1 and glycolytic gene expression by c-Myc. J Biol Chem 275(29):21797–21800. https://doi.org/10.1074/jbc.C000023200

Overgaard J (2011) Hypoxic modification of radiotherapy in squamous cell carcinoma of the head and neck—a systematic review and meta-analysis. Radiother Oncol 100(1):22–32. https://doi.org/10.1016/j.radonc.2011.03.004

Overgaard J, Bentzen SM, Kolstad P, Kjoerstad K, Davy M, Bertelsen K, Mäntyla M, Frankendal B, Skryten A, Löftquist I (1989a) Misonidazole combined with radiotherapy in the treatment of carcinoma of the uterine cervix. Int J Radiat Oncol Biol Phys 16(4):1069–1072

Overgaard J, Eriksen JG, Nordsmark M, Alsner J, Horsman MR, Danish H, Neck Cancer Study G (2005) Plasma osteopontin, hypoxia, and response to the hypoxia sensitiser nimorazole in radiotherapy of head and neck cancer: results from the DAHANCA 5 randomised double-blind placebo-controlled trial. Lancet Oncol 6(10):757–764. https://doi.org/10.1016/S1470-2045(05)70292-8

Overgaard J, Hansen HS, Andersen AP, Hjelm-Hansen M, Jørgensen K, Sandberg E, Berthelsen A, Hammer R, Pedersen M (1989b) Misonidazole combined with split-course radiotherapy in the treatment of invasive carcinoma of larynx and pharynx: report from the DAHANCA 2 study. Int J Radiat Oncol Biol Phys 16(4):1065–1068

Overgaard J, Hansen HS, Overgaard M, Bastholt L, Berthelsen A, Specht L, Lindeløv B, Jørgensen K (1998) A randomized double-blind phase III study of nimorazole as a hypoxic radiosensitizer of primary radiotherapy in supraglottic larynx and pharynx carcinoma. Results of the Danish Head and Neck Cancer Study (DAHANCA) protocol 5-85. Radiother Oncol 46(2):135–146

Owen MR, Doran E, Halestrap AP (2000) Evidence that metformin exerts its anti-diabetic effects through inhibition of complex 1 of the mitochondrial respiratory chain. Biochem J 348(Pt 3):607–614

Painter HJ, Morrisey JM, Mather MW, Vaidya AB (2007) Specific role of mitochondrial electron transport in blood-stage Plasmodium falciparum. Nature 446(7131):88–91. https://doi.org/10.1038/nature05572

Palcic B, Brosing JW, Skarsgard LD (1982) Survival measurements at low doses: oxygen enhancement ratio. Br J Cancer 46(6):980–984

Papavasiliou C, Yiogarakis D, Davillas N, Seretakis L, Pappas J, Licourinas M, Theodorou C, Stathopoulos P, Katsoyianni C, Thanos A (1983) Treatment of bladder carcinoma with irradiation combined with misonidazole. Int J Radiat Oncol Biol Phys 9(11):1631–1633

Pastorek J, Pastoreková S, Callebaut I, Mornon JP, Zelník V, Opavský R, Zat'ovicová M, Liao S, Portetelle D, Stanbridge EJ (1994) Cloning and characterization of MN, a human tumor-associated protein with a domain homologous to carbonic anhydrase and a putative helix-loop-helix DNA binding segment. Oncogene 9(10):2877–2888

Pernicova I, Korbonits M (2014) Metformin—mode of action and clinical implications for diabetes and cancer. Nat Rev Endocrinol 10(3):143–156. https://doi.org/10.1038/nrendo.2013.256

Petrik D, Lavori PW, Cao H, Zhu Y, Wong P, Christofferson E, Kaplan MJ, Pinto HA, Sutphin P, Koong AC, Giaccia AJ, Le Q-T (2006) Plasma osteopontin is an independent prognostic marker for head and neck cancers. J Clin Oncol 24(33):5291–5297. https://doi.org/10.1200/JCO.2006.06.8627

Petrova V, Annicchiarico-Petruzzelli M, Melino G, Amelio I (2018) The hypoxic tumour microenvironment. Oncogenesis 7(1). https://doi.org/10.1038/s41389-017-0011-9

Pittman RN (2011) Regulation of tissue oxygenation. Integrated systems physiology: from molecule to function to disease. Morgan & Claypool Life Sciences, San Rafael, CA

Prekeges JL, Rasey JS, Grunbaum Z, Krohn KH (1991) Reduction of fluoromisonidazole, a new imaging agent for hypoxia. Biochem Pharmacol 42(12):2387–2395

Qayum N, Muschel RJ, Im JH, Balathasan L, Koch CJ, Patel S, McKenna WG, Bernhard EJ (2009) Tumor vascular changes mediated by inhibition of oncogenic signaling. Cancer Res 69(15):6347–6354. https://doi.org/10.1158/0008-5472.CAN-09-0657

Rajendran JG, Krohn KA (2005) Imaging hypoxia and angiogenesis in tumors. Radiol Clin N Am 43(1):169–187

Rajendran JG, Krohn KA (2015) F18 Fluoromisonidazole for imaging tumor hypoxia: imaging the microenvironment for personalized cancer therapy. Semin Nucl Med 45(2):151–162. https://doi.org/10.1053/j.semnuclmed.2014.10.006

Raleigh JA, Chou SC, Arteel GE, Horsman MR (1999) Comparisons among pimonidazole binding, oxygen electrode measurements, and radiation response in C3H mouse tumors. Radiat Res 151(5):580–589

Rankin EB, Nam J-M, Giaccia AJ (2016) Hypoxia: signaling in the metastatic cascade. Trends Cancer 2(6):295–304. https://doi.org/10.1016/j.trecan.2016.05.006

Reznik E, Miller ML, Şenbabaoğlu Y, Riaz N, Sarungbam J, Tickoo SK, Al-Ahmadie HA, Lee W, Seshan VE, Hakimi AA, Sander C (2016) Mitochondrial DNA copy number variation across human cancers. elife 5. https://doi.org/10.7554/eLife.10769

Rischin D, Hicks RJ, Fisher R, Binns D, Corry J, Porceddu S, Peters LJ (2006) Prognostic significance of [18F]-Misonidazole positron emission tomography–detected tumor hypoxia in patients with advanced head and neck cancer randomly assigned to chemoradiation with or without tirapazamine: a substudy of Trans-Tasman Radiation Oncology Group Study 98.02. J Clin Oncol 24(13):2098–2104. https://doi.org/10.1200/JCO.2005.05.2878

Rischin D, Peters LJ, O'Sullivan B, Giralt J, Fisher R, Yuen K, Trotti A, Bernier J, Bourhis J, Ringash J, Henke M, Kenny L (2010) Tirapazamine, cisplatin, and radiation versus cisplatin and radiation for advanced squamous cell carcinoma of the head and neck (TROG 02.02, HeadSTART): a phase III trial of the Trans-Tasman Radiation Oncology Group. J Clin Oncol 28(18):2989–2995. https://doi.org/10.1200/JCO.2009.27.4449

Scharping NE, Menk AV, Whetstone RD, Zeng X, Delgoffe GM (2017) Efficacy of PD-1 blockade is potentiated by metformin-induced reduction of tumor hypoxia. Cancer Immunol Res 5(1):9–16. https://doi.org/10.1158/2326-6066.CIR-16-0103

Secomb TW, Hsu R, Ong ET, Gross JF, Dewhirst MW (1995) Analysis of the effects of oxygen supply and demand on hypoxic fraction in tumors. Acta Oncol 34(3):313–316

Semenza GL (2010) HIF-1: upstream and downstream of cancer metabolism. Curr Opin Genet Dev 20(1):51–56. https://doi.org/10.1016/j.gde.2009.10.009

Semenza GL (2012) Hypoxia-inducible factors: mediators of cancer progression and targets for cancer therapy. Trends Pharmacol Sci 33(4):207–214. https://doi.org/10.1016/j.tips.2012.01.005

Sobhanifar S, Aquino-Parsons C, Stanbridge EJ, Olive P (2005) Reduced expression of hypoxia-inducible factor-1α in perinecrotic regions of solid Tumors. Cancer Res 65(16):7259–7266. https://doi.org/10.1158/0008-5472.CAN-04-4480

Srivastava IK, Rottenberg H, Vaidya AB (1997) Atovaquone, a broad spectrum antiparasitic drug, collapses mitochondrial membrane potential in a malarial parasite. J Biol Chem 272(7):3961–3966. https://doi.org/10.1074/jbc.272.7.3961

Steel G (2002) Basic clinical radiobiology, 3rd edn. Oxford University Press, London

Sullivan LB, Chandel NS (2014) Mitochondrial reactive oxygen species and cancer. Cancer Metab 2. https://doi.org/10.1186/2049-3002-2-17

Świtlik WZ, Karbownik MS, Suwalski M, Kozak J, Szemraj J (2019) Serum miR-210-3p as a potential noninvasive biomarker of lung adenocarcinoma: a preliminary study. Genet Test Mol Biomarkers 23(5):353–358. https://doi.org/10.1089/gtmb.2018.0275

Szatrowski TP, Nathan CF (1991) Production of large amounts of hydrogen peroxide by human tumor cells. Cancer Res 51(3):794–798

Tan AS, Baty JW, Dong L-F, Bezawork-Geleta A, Endaya B, Goodwin J, Bajzikova M, Kovarova J, Peterka M, Yan B, Pesdar EA, Sobol M, Filimonenko A, Stuart S, Vondrusova M, Kluckova K, Sachaphibulkij K, Rohlena J, Hozak P, Truksa J, Eccles D, Haupt LM, Griffiths LR, Neuzil J, Berridge MV (2015) Mitochondrial genome acquisition restores respiratory function and tumorigenic potential of cancer cells without mitochondrial DNA. Cell Metab 21(1):81–94. https://doi.org/10.1016/j.cmet.2014.12.003

Thomlinson RH, Gray LH (1955) The histological structure of some human lung cancers and the possible implications for radiotherapy. Br J Cancer 9(4):539–549

Thomson D, Yang H, Baines H, Miles E, Bolton S, West C, Slevin N (2014) NIMRAD—a phase III trial to investigate the use of nimorazole hypoxia modification with intensity-modulated radiotherapy in head and neck cancer. Clin Oncol (R Coll Radiol) 26(6):344–347. https://doi.org/10.1016/j.clon.2014.03.003

Tsakiridis T, Hu C, Skinner HD, Santana-Davila R, Lu B, Erasmus JJ, Doemer A, Videtic GMM, Coster J, Yang X, Lee R, Werner-Wasik M, Schaner PE, McCormack SE, Esparaz B, McGarry R, Bazan JG, Struve T, Bradley JD (2019) Initial reporting of NRG-LU001 (NCT02186847), randomized phase II trial of concurrent chemoradiotherapy (CRT) +/− metformin in locally advanced non-small cell lung cancer (NSCLC). J Clin Oncol 37(15_suppl):8502–8502. https://doi.org/10.1200/JCO.2019.37.15_suppl.8502

Varlotto J, Stevenson MA (2005) Anemia, tumor hypoxemia, and the cancer patient. Int J Radiat Oncol Biol Phys 63(1):25–36. https://doi.org/10.1016/j.ijrobp.2005.04.049

Vaupel P, Höckel M, Mayer A (2007) Detection and characterization of tumor hypoxia using pO2 histography. Antioxid Redox Signal 9(8):1221–1236. https://doi.org/10.1089/ars.2007.1628

Vaupel P, Mayer A (2012) Availability, not respiratory capacity governs oxygen consumption of solid tumors. Int J Biochem Cell Biol 44(9):1477–1481. https://doi.org/10.1016/j.biocel.2012.05.019

Viale A, Corti D, Draetta GF (2015) Tumors and mitochondrial respiration: a neglected connection. Cancer Res 75(18):3687–3691. https://doi.org/10.1158/0008-5472.CAN-15-0491

Walsh JC, Lebedev A, Aten E, Madsen K, Marciano L, Kolb HC (2014) The clinical importance of assessing tumor hypoxia: relationship of tumor hypoxia to prognosis and therapeutic opportunities. Antioxid Redox Signal 21(10):1516–1554. https://doi.org/10.1089/ars.2013.5378

Wang GL, Jiang BH, Rue EA, Semenza GL (1995) Hypoxia-inducible factor 1 is a basic-helix-loop-helix-PAS heterodimer regulated by cellular O2 tension. Proc Natl Acad Sci U S A 92(12):5510–5514

Wang W, Winlove CP, Michel CC (2003) Oxygen partial pressure in outer layers of skin of human finger nail folds. J Physiol 549(Pt 3):855–863. https://doi.org/10.1113/jphysiol.2002.037994

Wang Y, Yang J, Liu H, Bi J-R, Liu Y, Chen Y-Y, Cao J-Y, Lu Y-J (2015) The association between osteopontin and survival in non-small-cell lung cancer patients: a meta-analysis of 13 cohorts. Onco Targets Ther 8:3513–3521. https://doi.org/10.2147/OTT.S94082

Weinberg SE, Chandel NS (2015) Targeting mitochondria metabolism for cancer therapy. Nat Chem Biol 11(1):9–15. https://doi.org/10.1038/nchembio.1712

Wiesener MS, Jürgensen JS, Rosenberger C, Scholze CK, Hörstrup JH, Warnecke C, Mandriota S, Bechmann I, Frei UA, Pugh CW, Ratcliffe PJ, Bachmann S, Maxwell PH, Eckardt K-U (2003) Widespread hypoxia-inducible expression of HIF-2alpha in distinct cell populations of different organs. FASEB J 17(2):271–273. https://doi.org/10.1096/fj.02-0445fje

Winter SC, Buffa FM, Silva P, Miller C, Valentine HR, Turley H, Shah KA, Cox GJ, Corbridge RJ, Homer JJ, Musgrove B, Slevin N, Sloan P, Price P, West CML, Harris AL (2007) Relation of a hypoxia metagene derived from head and neck cancer to prognosis of multiple cancers. Cancer Res 67(7):3441–3449. https://doi.org/10.1158/0008-5472.CAN-06-3322

Wright EA, Howard-Flanders P (1957) The influence of oxygen on the radiosensitivity of mammalian tissues. Acta Radiol 48(1):26–32

Wykoff CC, Beasley NJP, Watson PH, Turner KJ, Pastorek J, Sibtain A, Wilson GD, Turley H, Talks KL, Maxwell PH, Pugh CW, Ratcliffe PJ, Harris AL (2000) Hypoxia-inducible expression of tumor-associated carbonic anhydrases. Cancer Res 60(24):7075–7083

Yang W-H, Xu J, Mu J-B, Xie J (2017) Revision of the concept of anti-angiogenesis and its applications in tumor treatment. Chronic Dis Transl Med 3(1):33–40. https://doi.org/10.1016/j.cdtm.2017.01.002

Yu M (2011) Generation, function and diagnostic value of mitochondrial DNA copy number alterations in human cancers. Life Sci 89(3–4):65–71. https://doi.org/10.1016/j.lfs.2011.05.010

Zannella VE, Dal Pra A, Muaddi H, McKee TD, Stapleton S, Sykes J, Glicksman R, Chaib S, Zamiara P, Milosevic M, Wouters BG, Bristow RG, Koritzinsky M (2013) Reprogramming metabolism with metformin improves tumor oxygenation and radiotherapy response. Clin Cancer Res 19(24):6741–6750. https://doi.org/10.1158/1078-0432.CCR-13-1787

Zeman EM, Brown JM, Lemmon MJ, Hirst VK, Lee WW (1986) SR-4233: a new bioreductive agent with high selective toxicity for hypoxic mammalian cells. Int J Radiat Oncol Biol Phys 12(7):1239–1242. https://doi.org/10.1016/0360-3016(86)90267-1

Zhao H, Chen Q, Alam A, Cui J, Suen KC, Soo AP, Eguchi S, Gu J, Ma D (2018) The role of osteopontin in the progression of solid organ tumour. Cell Death Dis 9(3). https://doi.org/10.1038/s41419-018-0391-6

Zhu Y, Denhardt DT, Cao H, Sutphin PD, Koong AC, Giaccia AJ, Le Q-T (2005) Hypoxia upregulates osteopontin expression in NIH-3T3 cells via a Ras-activated enhancer. Oncogene 24(43):6555–6563. https://doi.org/10.1038/sj.onc.1208800

Zu XL, Guppy M (2004) Cancer metabolism: facts, fantasy, and fiction. Biochem Biophys Res Commun 313(3):459–465. https://doi.org/10.1016/j.bbrc.2003.11.136

Chapter 12
Normalizing the Tumor Microenvironment for Radiosensitization

John D. Martin and Rakesh K. Jain

Abstract Radiation is used in various cancer treatment regimens. However, hypoxia—a hallmark of the tumor microenvironment (TME)—drives disease progression and limits response to radiation, chemo-, immuno-, and targeted therapies. Hypoxia is a prognostic biomarker of worse outcome in most types of solid tumors. Combinations of radiation therapy and molecular targeted radiosensitizers are limited by hypoxia through multiple mechanisms. Thus, targeting the tumor microenvironment to ameliorate hypoxia is a promising strategy for cancer treatment broadly and radiosensitization specifically. Key processes that cause hypoxia are dysregulated angiogenesis and desmoplasia, which induce formation of tumor vessels that are abnormal in structure and function thereby reducing vessels' efficiency in delivering oxygen, other nutrients, immune cells, and drugs. Judiciously inhibiting angiogenesis and desmoplasia normalizes the tumor microenvironment towards alleviating hypoxia and reversing treatment resistance. By increasing oxygen, drug, and anti-tumor immune-cell accumulation and distribution within tumors and their metastases, TME normalization could be a beneficial component of radiation regimens for many patients. We describe opportunities to combine molecular targeted and other radiosensitizers to improve outcomes in cancer patients. We also outline challenges to the preclinical development and clinical translation of these combinations.

Keywords Angiogenesis · Anti-angiogenic therapeutics · Biomarkers · Chemotherapy · Desmoplasia · Immune checkpoint blockade · Immunotherapy · Mechanotherapeutics · Nanoradiosensitizers · Preclinical models · Radioresistance · Stromal normalization · Tumor hypoxia · Tumor microenvironment · Vascular normalization

J. D. Martin
NanoCarrier Co. Ltd., Kashiwa, Chiba, Japan
e-mail: martin@nanocarrier.co.jp

R. K. Jain (✉)
Edwin L. Steele Laboratories, Department of Radiation Oncology, Massachusetts General Hospital and Harvard Medical School, Boston, MA, USA
e-mail: jain@steele.mgh.harvard.edu

© Springer Nature Switzerland AG 2020
H. Willers, I. Eke (eds.), *Molecular Targeted Radiosensitizers*, Cancer Drug Discovery and Development, https://doi.org/10.1007/978-3-030-49701-9_12

1 Introduction

Radiation therapy (RT) is widely used to treat cancer, but its use can be expanded because it can prime tumors to be sensitive to other therapies and also its efficacy can be improved by radiosensitizers (Bristow et al. 2018; Sharabi et al. 2015). Our hypothesis is that tumor progression and treatment resistance are fueled by sub-physiological oxygen concentration—hypoxia—within tumors (Martin et al. 2019b). Furthermore, we propose that RT should be employed to reduce hypoxia towards sensitizing tumors to other therapies. In addition, alleviation of hypoxia can effectively sensitize a tumor for RT alone as well as with other treatments.

The tumor microenvironment (TME)—the non-cancerous components of solid tumors (Fig. 12.1)—is co-opted by cancer cells to promote hypoxia. The abnormal growth (angiogenesis) and structure of vessels (Goel et al. 2011; Carmeliet and Jain 2011a), fibrosis (desmoplasia) (Jain et al. 2014), and immune cells (inflammation) (Datta et al. 2019; Munn and Jain 2019; Mazzone and Bergers 2019) causes tumor blood vessels to inefficiently deliver blood and oxygen to tumor tissue. Accordingly, biomarkers of these processes along with hypoxia are prognostic biomarkers of worse outcome across most cancer types (Martin et al. 2019b). Thus, strategies that normalize the TME towards reversing hypoxia have succeeded in certain cancer types in combination with other therapies and are currently being integrated more

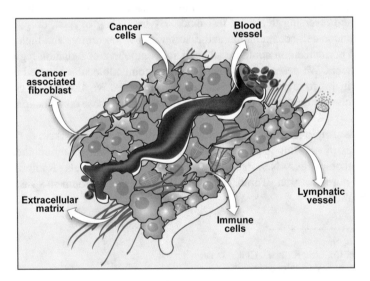

Fig. 12.1 Solid tumors are made up of malignant cancer cells and stroma produced abnormally through dysregulated angiogenesis, desmoplasia, and inflammation. Cancer cells enlist nonmalignant stromal cells, including fibroblasts, immune cells, and blood and lymphatic vascular cells and the extracellular matrix. The result is a pathological molecular, metabolic, and physical microenvironment that promotes tumor progression while resisting therapy and host immune response. From Martin et al. (2019b) with permission

broadly (Jain 2001, 2005, 2008; Carmeliet and Jain 2011b; Goel et al. 2011; Vasudev and Reynolds 2014; Martin et al. 2016, 2019b; Viallard and Larrivée 2017).

Vascular normalization using anti-angiogenic therapies (AAT), cancer-associated fibroblast (CAF)/extracellular matrix (ECM) normalization through CAF reprogramming using mechanotherapeutics (Sheridan 2019) and immunotherapeutics particularly immune checkpoint blockade (ICB) alone or in combination can normalize the TME towards alleviating hypoxia (Martin et al. 2019b). Here, we will describe these strategies in the context of serving as radiosensitizers. In addition, we will explore how RT can prime tumors for other therapies. After discussing considerations for various combinations of these therapies, we will provide an overview of some challenges involved in the translation of preclinical studies investigating various drug combinations to clinical practice.

2 Hypoxia Is a Critical Biomarker of Treatment Resistance and Response

Cancer cells rely on nutrients delivered by nearby vessels to grow and proliferate. However, cancer cells induce these vessels to become inefficient, and the vessels quickly become leaky and collapsed (Hagendoorn et al. 2006). Specifically, cancer cells stimulate angiogenesis to produce immature vessels (Goel et al. 2011) and generate forces that produce solid stress and stimulate CAFs to produce ECM that stores the stress (Jain et al. 2014). The neovasculature in tumors does not fully mature and the result is vessel hyperpermeability and abnormal morphology (Jain 2003). The solid stress compresses vessels. Permeability and compression vary with the tumor type, stage, and location within a single lesion and between lesions in the same patient (Martin et al. 2019b; Yuan et al. 1994; Netti et al. 2000).

While healthy cells require nutrients to grow, cancer cells benefit from inefficient vasculature. Low oxygen concentrations—hypoxia—grant cancer cells a survival advantage by exerting a selection pressure for malignant cells and helping them avoid immune surveillance. Additionally, hypoxia promotes resistance to radiation, chemotherapy, and immunotherapy. Indeed, oxygen is a validated prognostic biomarker and an emerging potential biomarker of response (Martin et al. 2019b).

2.1 Hypoxia Promotes Disease Progression

Hypoxia exerts a selection pressure that enables the most malignant cancer cells to survive despite the apoptotic cues of hypoxia (Wilson and Hay 2011; Carmeliet et al. 1998). Furthermore, hypoxia inhibits tumor-suppressive genes, which enables cancer cells to expand (Thienpont et al. 2016). Additionally, hypoxia promotes more aggressive invasive phenotypes of cancer cells. Specifically, hypoxia influences cancer stem cell (Semenza 2016) and epithelial-to-mesenchymal transition (Philip et al. 2013) phenotypes. Finally, hypoxia facilitates portions of the metastatic cascade, which enables cancer cells to spread throughout the body. For example, hypoxia stimulates production of pro-migratory and ECM-degrading signals that enable cancer cells to move through the tumor, intravasate into vessels and circulate throughout the host (Estrella et al. 2013; Schito and Semenza 2016).

2.2 Hypoxia Promotes Treatment Resistance

Hypoxia promotes treatment resistance to radiation, chemotherapy, and immunotherapy. Besides affecting cancer cells, hypoxia also affects stromal cells in the TME, which ultimately results in immunosuppression and resistance to immunotherapy.

2.2.1 Radiation

Ionizing radiation damages mitochondria thereby promoting reactive oxygen species (ROS) production, which causes DNA damage leading to cell death. However, RT causes less DNA damage in hypoxic tumors (Rockwell et al. 2009). One mechanism involves hypoxia-mediated stabilization of hypoxia-inducible factor 1 (HIF1) thereby inducing glycolysis and accumulation of NADPH, which then scavenges ROS (Meijer et al. 2012). Glycolysis also induces the accumulation of lactate, which upregulates HIF1 to complete a cycle of hypoxia-mediated RT resistance (Lee et al. 2015).

2.2.2 Chemotherapy

Just like oxygen, intravenously administered chemotherapy relies on immature, inefficient tumor blood vessels to reach cancer cells. Thus, the characteristics of vessels that result in hypoxia also result in limited delivery of small-molecule chemotherapy. Indeed, even the delivery of larger nanomedicines, whose transport is also limited by slow diffusion in the extravascular space, is correlated with perfusion in mice (Stapleton et al. 2013). Because the delivery of drugs to a tumor lesion is correlated with the lesion's response to treatment in patients (Lee et al. 2017; Ramanathan et al. 2017), the presence of hypoxia is related to resistance to chemotherapy. Additionally, most—but not all—chemotherapies are less potent in hypoxia. Similarly, weak-base chemotherapies are neutralized by acidity, which is a feature of a hypoxic TME (Martin et al. 2019b).

2.2.3 Immunotherapy

ICB has generated exciting improvements in the survival of a subset of patients. However, ICB is estimated to benefit currently <13% of patients with cancer (Haslam and Prasad 2019) and a substantial fraction of patients will develop immune-related adverse events (Postow et al. 2018). Hypoxia in the TME is a major cause of resistance to ICB through various mechanisms (Martin et al. 2020, Martin et al. 2019b; Fukumura et al. 2018; Datta et al. 2019; Munn and Jain 2019).

Hypoxia induces the expression of chemokines that recruit regulatory T (T_{reg}) cells (Facciabene et al. 2011). These cells support tumor growth by promoting the immune system to tolerate the presence of cancer cells (Facciabene et al. 2011; Togashi et al. 2019). Hypoxia also promotes expression of VEGF, which impairs the immune system's recognition of cancer cells, because VEGF inhibits the maturation of dendritic cells (DCs) (Veglia and Gabrilovich 2017). As a result, DCs cannot effectively present cancer cell antigens to train the immune system to attack cancer cells. Even if DCs can train the immune system, angiogenic signaling impairs leukocytes from binding to the vessel wall and transporting into the extravascular space (Fukumura et al. 2018, 1995). Indeed, T cells move slower in tissues with hypoxia (Rytelewski et al. 2019; Hatfield et al. 2015). Even if T cells can transport into the tumor parenchyma to attack cancer cells, hypoxia limits their function. Hypoxia recruits immunosuppressive cells such as T_{reg} that impair the ability of antitumor T cells to recognize and kill cancer cells (Maenhout et al. 2014; Facciabene et al. 2011). Hypoxia and hypoxia-induced signaling upregulates immune checkpoints on T cells and their ligands on cancer and stromal cells thereby halting the function of T cells (Voron et al. 2015; Palazon et al. 2017; Wallin et al. 2016; Noman et al. 2014, 2015). Similarly, acidity reduces the cytotoxic activity of T cells (Calcinotto et al. 2012). Like drugs and oxygen, some immune cells use blood vessels to traffic to tumors. In hypoxic tumor regions, perfusion is limited, which impairs immune-cell infiltration. Indeed, perfusion is associated with response to ICB in mice (Zheng et al. 2018).

2.3 Hypoxia as a Prognostic Biomarker

Consistent with the mechanistic studies identifying hypoxia as a cause of disease progression and treatment resistance, there are numerous clinical studies validating hypoxia as an independent prognostic biomarker of poor outcome (Martin et al. 2016, 2019b; Wilson and Hay 2011). Paradoxically, oxygen is delivered by blood vessels and researchers have long observed that high vascularization is necessary for tumor growth (Goel et al. 2011). Indeed, microvascular density (MVD) in areas of intense vascularization (Weidner et al. 1992) is an independent, prognostic biomarker of worse response that also has been validated broadly (Martin et al. 2019b). These findings present a paradox because high vascularity is required for tumor growth but the lack of oxygen, which is carried in the blood, also predicts more tumor progression.

3 Components of the TME Cause Hypoxia

Low oxygen predicts worse outcome for patients, but even though vessels carry oxygen, high vascularity also predicts worse outcome (Martin et al. 2019b). To resolve this paradox, in 2001 we postulated that the judicious use of angiogenesis inhibitors, which block the formation of new vessels through angiogenesis could improve vascular function and thus improve oxygenation (Jain 2001, 2005). Here, we will describe how the various components of TME (Fig. 12.1) cause vascular abnormalities in tumors thereby diminishing blood flow and oxygen delivery to tumors.

3.1 Vascular Abnormalities

3.1.1 Structure

The phenotype of endothelial cells (ECs), which make up the vessel wall, is abnormal in tumors. In healthy vessels, ECs are polarized with blood flow and connected tightly to each other. In tumors, they are misaligned with blood flow, loosely connected and sometimes protruding into the vessel lumen or extravascular space (Carmeliet and Jain 2011a; Mazzone et al. 2009). Like normal ECs, tumor ECs also have vesiculo-vacuolar organelles, which provide a trans-EC connection between the lumen and extravascular space that is enhanced by VEGF (Hashizume et al. 2000; Goel et al. 2011; Feng et al. 1996). The cells around vessels—known as pericytes—structurally support vessels and fill gaps between ECs (Carmeliet and Jain 2011a). Although they support EC quiescence, they detach from ECs during angiogenesis (Morikawa et al. 2002). These tumor pericytes are less contractile thereby losing their ability to influence vessel function (Greenberg et al. 2008). In healthy vessels, the vascular basement membrane (BM) holds ECs and pericytes together. In tumors, the BM is discontinuous with holes and thicker regions (Baluk et al. 2003). Thus, the components of tumor vessels have irregular phenotypes (Jain 2003; Carmeliet and Jain 2011a; Goel et al. 2011).

The pathological angiogenic signaling and the abnormal phenotype of vessels results in a heterogeneous collection of vessels within tumors (Arvanitis et al. 2020). Even single vessels, which typically branch according to an orderly hierarchy of arteries, arterioles, capillaries, venules, and veins in normal organs lack these phenotypes and can vary substantially across their length (Less et al. 1991, 1997; Baish et al. 2011). Tumor vessels can feature a large, dilated diameter, and be tortuous rather than being straight (Chauhan et al. 2011; Sevick and Jain 1989a). Other vessels can be collapsed shut and buckled (Griffon-Etienne et al. 1999; Padera et al. 2004; Stylianopoulos et al. 2012). They can be saccular and their branching is irregular (Less et al. 1991). As a result, there are regions of high vessel density and regions of low vessel density. Sometimes, tumor tissue volumes as large as cubic millimeters lack vessels, while in normal tissues there are vessels within at least 100–200 micrometers of each other (Baish et al. 2011).

3.1.2 Function

As tumor vessels undergo angiogenesis and ECs detach from each other and pericytes, vessels become leaky (Carmeliet and Jain 2011a). Vesiculo-vacuolar organelles might also contribute to leakiness (Hashizume et al. 2000; Feng et al. 1996). As fluid leaks from vessels, the pressure difference across the vessel wall is reduced and fluid transport into tumors is slowed (Netti et al. 1996; Chauhan et al. 2011). Additionally, vessel leakiness reduces intravascular blood flow by allowing plasma to leak thereby increasing the red blood cell density within vessels causing blood viscosity to increase (Sevick and Jain 1989b). Also, plasma leaking from vessels into the extravascular space reduces the pressure in vessels upstream thereby reducing the intravascular pressure gradient, which is the driving force of intravascular blood flow (Stylianopoulos et al. 2018). The abnormal phenotype of ECs and pericytes limits their ability to control flow, which is transient in tumors and sometimes reverses direction. Additionally, some tumor vessels that collapsed under elevated solid stress lack blood flow (Chauhan et al. 2013). Non-collapsed, yet compressed vessels have reduced flow rate because shorter vessel diameters impair flow (Stylianopoulos et al. 2018; Less et al. 1997). In various regions within tumors, there is no flow because a local or upstream vessel is collapsed (Less et al. 1991; Stylianopoulos et al. 2012; Chauhan et al. 2013). Thus, abnormal vascular morphology leads to spatial and temporal variations in blood flow (Jain 1988; Sun et al. 2007).

3.2 Causes of Vascular Abnormalities

3.2.1 Angiogenesis

One century ago, researchers observed that the vascular system is associated with tumor growth (Goldman 1907). In the 1940s, more insights into the vasculature of tumors using transparent window techniques were developed (Algire and Chalkley 1945; Ide et al. 1939; Jain et al. 2002, 1997). In 1968, researchers proposed that tumors produce an "angiogenic" substance that stimulates neovascularization (Greenblatt and Philippe 1968). Shortly thereafter in 1971, Folkman put forth the hypothesis that blocking angiogenesis reduces tumor growth and metastasis (Folkman 1971). In 1978, it was observed that tissues acquire angiogenic capacity during neoplastic transformation—and, thus, the concept that anti-angiogenesis could be used to prevent cancer was put forward (Gullino 1978). Decades later, bevacizumab received the first approval as an anti-angiogenic agent (AAT) for treatment of cancer. It is an antibody specific to vascular endothelial growth factor (VEGF) and initially demonstrated increased survival in metastatic colorectal cancer patients with standard chemotherapy (Hurwitz et al. 2004). Now, more than a dozen AAT are approved for various types of cancer in combination with various treatments, including five with ICB (Martin et al. 2019b).

Angiogenesis is regulated by the relative amounts pro- and anti-angiogenic factors (Jain 2005). In normal physiology, this balance is in equilibrium spatially and temporally "angiogenic switch" is "off" except when needed "on" (e.g., during embryonic development, wound healing, formation of the corpus luteum). During tumor initiation and progression, this balance is tipped, and blood vessels form haphazardly to support a growing tumor mass. During "sprouting" angiogenesis, BM and other ECM are digested; ECs divest of pericytes and migrate and proliferate forming a sprout; a lumen forms through canalization; branches form through confluence and anastomoses of sprouts enabling perfusion; and finally, the newly formed vessels invest in BM and pericytes (Carmeliet and Jain 2011a). While in tumors vessels remain immature, typically vessels then differentiate into arterioles, capillaries, and venules (Carmeliet and Jain 2011a; Jain 2003; Jain and Carmeliet 2001; Jain et al. 1997).

Besides sprouting (angiogenesis), there are at least five mechanisms of vascularization of tumors: co-option (Seano and Jain 2020; Voutouri et al. 2019), intussusception (Patan et al. 1996), vasculogenesis (Carmeliet and Jain 2011a; Duda et al. 2006), mimicry (Chang et al. 2000), and cancer cell to EC transdifferentiation (Goel et al. 2011). In co-option, tumor cells migrate and proliferate surrounding vessels forming "perivascular" cuffs. These cuffs expand past the diffusion limit of oxygen and other nutrients. Furthermore, they can collapse vessels as the generate solid stress (Voutouri et al. 2019). In intussusception, a vessel enlarges in response to angiogenic factors from cancer cells, and a tissue column grows in the expanded vessel lumen to separate the lumen into a vessel branch point (Dvorak 2002; Patan et al. 1996, 2001a, b). In tumor vasculogenesis, endothelial precursor cells (EPCs)—transporting from bone marrow niches into the peripheral blood circulation—can also promote neovascularization (Duda et al. 2006; Isner 2002; Rafii et al. 2002). EPCs of non-bone marrow origin can be recruited from adjacent tissues and/or circulation (Ergun et al. 2008; Aicher et al. 2007). In mimicry, the luminal surface of vessels may be lined by cancer cells (Chang et al. 2000). Finally, trans-differentiated cancer cells (Sajithlal et al. 2010) or cancer stem-like cells (Ricci-Vitiani et al. 2010; Soda et al. 2011; Wang et al. 2010; Carmeliet and Jain 2011a) could make up a fraction of ECs in tumor vessels. Thus, "vasculogenesis" is used to describe neovascularization induced by cancer stem cell integration into the vasculature (Kozin et al. 2012). Discerning the relative amounts of these processes could lead to better drugs to ameliorate pathological angiogenesis (Kozin et al. 2011).

3.2.2 Desmoplasia

Another component of the TME are CAFs and the ECM components they produce and maintain thereby providing physical structure to tumors. Through fibroblasts, cancer cells stimulate desmoplasia, which is the growth of fibrotic tissue and ECM. Depending on the tumor type and its stage of differentiation, neoplastic cells may be dispersed in the ECM as individual cells (e.g., lymphomas, melanomas) or as clumps or nests (e.g., carcinomas). In a poorly differentiated carcinoma, the cancer cells may be loosely packed in clumps, whereas in a well-differentiated carcinoma, the cells may be connected with intercellular junctions and tightly packed in a nest enveloped by a BM. Host cells such as fibroblasts may proliferate and migrate from the adjacent connective tissue or from primary tumor to the metastatic site (Duda et al. 2010).

Similar to angiogenesis, desmoplasia is dysregulated in tumors. Cancer cells co-opt fibroblasts through signaling proteins (e.g., transforming growth factor β or TGF-β), transcriptional factors, interleukins, matrix metalloproteinases, and ROS (Sahai et al. 2020). In parallel, hypoxia can induce fibroblasts to produce and maintain ECM through connective tissue growth factor (CTGF), TGF-β, and Sonic hedgehog signaling (Eguchi et al. 2013; Spivak-Kroizman et al. 2013). Once activated, CAFs excessively differentiate, contract, proliferate, and generate ECM components. Like cancer cells, CAFs generate physical forces that are stored in and transmitted by the dense ECM, thereby elevating solid stress levels and leading to compression of blood and lymphatic vessels (Stylianopoulos et al. 2018, 2012). As a result, desmoplasia contributes to elevated interstitial pressure (IFP) in tumors by reducing fluid drainage through collapsed lymphatics (Stylianopoulos et al. 2012) and trapping fluid in extravascular space (Netti et al. 2000). Thus, therapies that reduce solid stress also reduce IFP and therefore have been referred to as mechanotherapeutics (Sheridan 2019), even though these agents also affect other components of TME such as immune cells and ECs (Regan et al. 2019).

By contributing to elevated solid stress and IFP, desmoplasia exacerbates reduced blood flow in tumors. This contributes to hypoxia-induced disease progression. Additionally, solid stress directly promotes disease progression by making cancer cells more invasive (Tse et al. 2012) and the surrounding normal tissue more malignant (Fernández-Sánchez et al. 2015). Desmoplasia also directly promotes angiogenesis and immunosuppression, as certain CAF populations produce angiogenic molecules (Fukumura et al. 1998) and inflammatory cytokines (Öhlund et al. 2017; Costa et al. 2018).

4 TME Normalization Alleviates Hypoxia and Overcomes Resistance

4.1 Vascular Normalization

Microvascular density (MVD) in vascularized areas within tumors (Weidner et al. 1992) and hypoxia (Martin et al. 2016; Wilson and Hay 2011) are two independent biomarkers predictive of worse patient outcome consistent across most cancer types (Martin et al. 2019b). In 2001, we postulated that the judicious use of AAT could increase vascular function and reduce hypoxia (Jain 2001). Afterwards, data from clinical trials have demonstrated that vascular normalization does occur with judicious use of AAT (Carmeliet and Jain 2011b; Goel et al. 2011; Jain 2013, 2014).

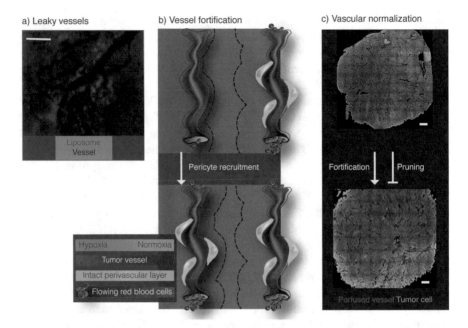

Fig. 12.2 Angiogenesis results in hyperpermeable tumor vessels. (**a**) Intravital microscopy image of murine tumor vessels (black; negative contrast). 24 h post-injection, 90-nm liposomes (bright red) extravasated from and accumulated around leaky tumor vessels (black). The liposomes' extravasation is heterogeneous. Scale bar, 100 µm. (**b**) Schematics of perfusion and hypoxia before and after normalization. In the top image, the schematic depicts untreated tumor vessels, with one vessel having limited flow (few red blood cells) and the other vessel well-perfused (many red blood cells). The tissue around the perfused vessel is normoxic (pink), while the tissue farther from the vessels is hypoxic (purple). The region of normoxia surrounding each vessel is denoted by a black dashed line. Vessel fortification occurs when pericytes are recruited and basement membrane is repaired to produce an intact perivascular layer (green), which leads to increased blood flow that results in normoxia in the surrounding tissue. (**c**) Normalization results in homogenous perfusion throughout tumors. In untreated tumors (green, top panel), perfused vessels are heterogeneous and of limited density (red). Fortifying—not pruning—vascular normalization produces a homogenous distribution of perfused vessels (bottom). Scale bars, 500 µm. From Martin et al. (2019b) with permission

Furthermore, patients with increased tumor vessel function and reduced hypoxia after AAT have better outcomes (Jain 2013, 2014; Martin et al. 2016, 2019b). These clinical results are consistent with the notion that alleviation of hypoxia post-AAT reduces disease progression and treatment resistance. Hypoxia should be investigated to validate whether it is a predictive biomarker of response.

Passive vessel normalization results in pruning of immature vessels (their leakiness shown in Fig. 12.2a), so that the remaining vessels are mature. The vessels are on average more efficient, but the density of the vessels might not be enough to effectively supply the entire tumor volume. Active vessel normalization results in the fortification of immature vessels with perivascular cells, which makes them more mature (Fig. 12.2b). The vessels are on average more efficient and the density of vessels is more likely to be sufficient to supply the entire tumor volume (Fig. 12.2c). Data from clinical trials demonstrate that vascular normalization occurs after judicious administration of AAT (Carmeliet and Jain 2011b; Goel et al. 2011; Jain 2013, 2014; Martin et al. 2019b). There is also clinical evidence that active rather than passive normalization is associated with improved patient response to chemotherapy (Tolaney et al. 2015).

4.2   Hypoxia as a Potential Biomarker of Response to Vascular Normalization

Data from hypothesis-generating clinical trials indicates that patients with tumors that after AAT have increased tumor vessel function (e.g., perfusion, vessel maturity) and alleviated hypoxia derive the most benefit (Jain 2013, 2014; Martin et al. 2016, 2019b). Specifically, in recurrent glioblastoma (GBM) patients, as in mice (Kamoun et al. 2009), cediranib, an oral pan-VEGFR tyrosine kinase inhibitor (TKI), normalizes tumor vessel structure and reduces leakiness (Batchelor et al. 2007). Indeed, progression-free survival (PFS) and overall survival (OS) increased with the relative amount of normalization as quantified by a set of biomarkers characterizing vessel structure and function (Sorensen et al. 2009). This correlation was confirmed subsequently, as cediranib-increased perfusion and oxygenation correlates with survival of GBM patients (Batchelor et al. 2013; Emblem et al. 2013; Sorensen et al. 2012). In breast cancer (BC) patients, similar correlations of normalization with outcome have been observed with nintedanib (Quintela-Fandino et al. 2016), eribulin (Ueda et al. 2016), and bevacizumab (Garcia-Foncillas et al. 2012; Ueda et al. 2014, 2016, 2017). Along these lines, non-small cell lung cancer (NSCLC) patients with increased perfusion after bevacizumab treatment had improved OS (Heist et al. 2015). These potential predictive physiological biomarkers of response to normalizing therapy must now be verified prospectively.

4.3   Stromal Normalization

Stromal or CAF/ECM normalization is a complementary strategy to vessel normalization and is best embodied by the reprogramming of CAFs to a quiescent phenotype (Chauhan et al. 2013, 2019; Sherman et al. 2014; Chen et al. 2019a). While vessel normalization can enhance the function of many tumor vessels, it cannot affect collapsed vessels (Fig. 12.3a). Reprogramming of CAFs normalizes their function thereby limiting their ability to produce and maintain ECM (Sherman et al. 2014; Chauhan et al. 2013, 2019; Chen et al. 2019a). As a result, ECM levels in tumors are reduced. Reprogramming is favored because killing CAFs and/or

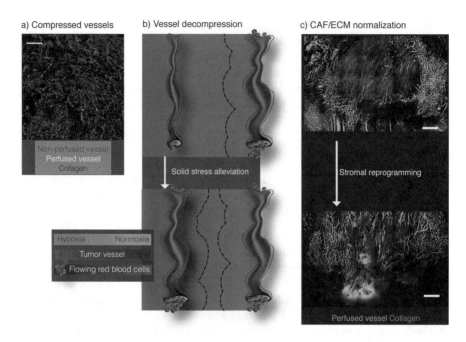

Fig. 12.3 Desmoplasia results in compressed tumor vessels. (**a**) Histological image of murine tumor vessels. Most vessels are non-perfused (red) in this collagen-rich (blue) tumor, and there is a lack of blood flow (yellow). Scale bar, 100 μm. (**b**) Vessel decompression occurs after solid stress is alleviated. The decompressed blood vessel is re-perfused and normoxia around the vessel is restored. (**c**) In untreated tumors (top panel), collagen (blue) and other components of desmoplasia promote vessel compression, such that large regions lack perfused vessels (green). CAF/ECM normalization (bottom) reduces collagen and re-perfuses compressed vessels. Scale bars, 500 μm. From Martin et al. (2019b) with permission

digesting ECM directly could result in tumor progression and immunosuppression (Martin et al. 2019b). By normalizing CAFs and ECM, the fluid and solid stress are reduced towards normal levels (Stylianopoulos et al. 2012, 2013, 2018). Thus, therapies that induce stromal normalization through CAF reprogramming have been referred to as mechanotherapeutics (Sheridan 2019), even though they might have other additional direct effects on stromal cells including immune cells. After CAF reprogramming, vessels are decompressed (Fig. 12.3b) and perfusion is increased (Fig. 12.3c). Furthermore, the transport of oxygen and drugs is increased.

4.4   Combined Vascular and Stromal Normalization

Reprogramming the ECs, pericytes, and/or CAFs participating in creating dysfunctional vessels can normalize vascular function, thereby reducing hypoxia and treatment resistance (Martin et al. 2019b; Mpekris et al. 2020). Nonetheless, combining AAT with mechanotherapies will depend on the context. First, the existing character of the vessels matters. In tumors with hyperpermeable, hypoperfused vessels, the combination will be most effective (Stylianopoulos and Jain 2013). Second, early clinical data supports the notion that often mechanotherapeutics might best precede AAT because more vessels with open lumen pre-AAT might increase outcomes to subsequent AAT and cytotoxic therapy (Tolaney et al. 2015). Also supporting this rationale, vascular destruction caused by AAT leads to hypoxia and resistance (Jain 2013, 2014). By increasing the density of perfused vessels before AAT, mechanotherapeutics could reduce the impact of vessel pruning by AAT. Thus, we hypothesize that maximizing decompressed MVD before AAT will improve outcomes. Some clinical data supports this hypothesis. In GBM patients, angiotensin system inhibitors (ASIs) that can decompress vessels and have other effects on tumors (Regan et al. 2019), increased the amount of perfused vessels (Emblem et al. 2016) and retrospective studies indicate that ASIs alone and in combination with other therapies increases survival of patients (Levin et al. 2017; Martin et al. 2020; Pinter and Jain 2017). AAT preceding mechanotherapeutics is necessary in some cases because AAT can induce CAF activation and ECM deposition, so administering mechanotherapies after AAT could reduce this AAT-induced treatment resistance (Rahbari et al. 2016; Chen et al. 2014, 2015).

4.5 TME Normalization for Immunotherapy

TME normalization has the potential to improve immunotherapy (Fukumura et al. 2018; Martin et al. 2020; Munn and Jain 2019; Mpekris et al. 2020; Arvanitis et al. 2020). As immunotherapy can be radiosensitizing (Sharabi et al. 2015) and RT can prime tumors for immunotherapy, for example, through the abscopal effect (Rodríguez-Ruiz et al. 2018), understanding how TME normalization and immunotherapy interact is necessary to develop radiosensitizing strategies. The cancer-immunity cycle must be perpetuated for immunotherapy to be effective (Fig. 12.4 outer ring). The TME defines the "set-point" of response and resistance to immunotherapies including ICB (Chen and Mellman 2017). We propose that TME normalization can help to overcome resistance at each of the set-points (Fig. 12.4 inner ring) (Martin et al. 2020). These set-points are classified into three main TME phenotypes.

4.5.1 Cancer-Immune TME Phenotypes

The immune-desert phenotype is the phenotype most resistant to immunotherapies (Tumeh et al. 2014). It is characterized by a lack of the following: antitumor immune cells, antigens, and/or their presentation, response to antigen presentation and T cell priming (Fig. 12.4 light orange). TME-normalizing strategies could promote progression through the cycle (Fig. 12.4 blue) towards the immune-excluded

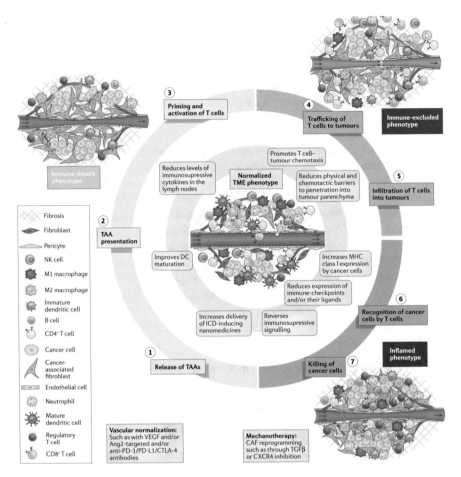

Fig. 12.4 Cancer-immune TME phenotypes define the set-points that predict sensitivity to immunotherapy (Chen and Mellman 2017) while TME normalization perpetuates the cancer-immunity cycle (Martin et al. 2020). TME normalization (blue inner circle) pushes the cycle through the various set-points. In the immune-desert phenotype (yellow), the TME with sparse immune cells is immunosuppressed. The immune system allows malignant cell expansion because often it does not recognize antigens, tolerates the antigens if it does recognize them, and/or eventually fails to prime cytotoxic T cells. Hypoxia affects these steps in the cycle. In the immune-excluded phenotype (purple), the stroma restricts immune-cell infiltration such that immune cells are retained in the tumor periphery and/or stroma. The TME characteristics that distinguish immune-exclusion also reduce the delivery of various radiosensitizers and/or oxygen. In the inflamed phenotype (red), there are proinflammatory cytokines that stimulate the relatively large amounts of immune cells migrating through the parenchyma. However, inhibitory factors often induced by hypoxia reduce antitumor immunity. The structure and function of vessels may be normalized by inhibiting angiogenic factors and/or immune checkpoints. Meanwhile, normalization of CAFs and/or the ECM could decompress vessels collapsed by solid stress. These two strategies work independently or as a combination to improve perfusion, oxygen delivery, and drug distribution. Strategies that cause excessive vessel, CAF and/or ECM depletion could induce disease progression. Immune checkpoint blockade therapies such as anti-programmed cell death protein 1 (PD-1) or programmed cell death 1 ligand 1 (PD-L1) antibodies induce blood vessel maturation in some tumor types

phenotype (Fig. 12.4 purple) because angiogenesis and hypoxia promote the immune-desert phenotype. Specifically, VEGF promotes immunological ignorance by reducing DC maturation thereby interfering with antigen presentation (Veglia and Gabrilovich 2017). Hypoxia also promotes immune tolerance by inducing the expression of chemokines that recruit pro-tumor T_{reg} cells (Facciabene et al. 2011; Togashi et al. 2019).

The immune-excluded phenotype (Fig. 12.4 purple) features immune cells in the tumor periphery and/or stroma but not parenchyma (Chen and Mellman 2017). The infiltration and migration of these immune cells is impaired by abnormal vessels and excessive fibrosis. Increased levels of TGFβ, ECM, and CAFs characterizes immune-exclusion (Mariathasan et al. 2018; Chen et al. 2019a; Chauhan et al. 2019). This phenotype can be more sensitive to ICB than immune-deserts (Fig. 12.4 red) because of the presence of T cells (Mariathasan et al. 2018; Tumeh et al. 2014). Signaling that causes desmoplasia, solid stress, and vessel compression also limits immune cells' cancer cell killing. CAF secretion of chemokines like TGFβ and stromal cell-derived factor 1α (SDF-1α) hamper cytotoxic T lymphocytes (CTLs) as they infiltrate the tumor parenchyma (Chen et al. 2019a; Chauhan et al. 2019; Mariathasan et al. 2018). Also, TGFβ promotes T_{reg} phenotypes in naïve T cells (Togashi et al. 2019). Furthermore, desmoplasia physically impedes CTL migration (Salmon et al. 2012). Angiogenesis also causes immune-exclusion, as its signaling reduces the amount of adhesion factors on vessel walls thereby limiting CTL adhesion and ultimately transport into tumors (Fukumura et al. 2018, 1995; Schmittnaegel et al. 2017). Thus, abnormal angiogenesis and desmoplasia cause hypoxia, and both the signaling and the physiological consequences of these processes directly limit the distribution of CTLs. Indeed, T cell migration is reduced in hypoxic tumor regions (Rytelewski et al. 2019; Hatfield et al. 2015).

The inflamed phenotype (Fig. 12.4 red) feature T cells in the parenchyma and proinflammatory cytokines, which is evidence of an earlier antitumor immune response (Chen and Mellman 2017). In other words, there is a large number of T cells that have T cell receptors (TCRs) against tumor-associated antigens, so inflamed tumors are relatively sensitive to ICI (Mariathasan et al. 2018). Still, this phenotype also has suppressed immune cells that could be reprogrammed towards antitumor immunity through TME normalization. Specifically, VEGF signaling recruits pro-tumor immune cells, such as T_{reg} cells, myeloid-derived suppressor cells

---

Fig. 12.4 (continued) thereby protecting them from excessive pruning by anti-angiogenic agents, which affect immature vessels. Blocking TME-normalizing signaling pathways such as those activated by VEGF, angiopoietin-2, CXCL12/CXCR4, and TGFβ can also alleviate immunosuppression through additional mechanisms. Thus, combination of these therapies that inhibit some of these pathways with radiosensitizers and immunotherapies could have synergy. In conclusion, TME normalization strategies tailored to TME immune phenotype of a tumor could enhance response rates and duration of responses to radiosensitizing immunotherapies. CTLA-4, cytotoxic T-lymphocyte protein 4; MHC, major histocompatibility complex; TME, tumor microenvironment; PD-1, programmed cell death protein 1; PD-L1, programmed cell death 1 ligand 1; TAA, tumor-associated antigen; TME, tumor microenvironment. From Martin et al. (2020) with permission

(MDSCs), and M2-like tumor-associated macrophages (TAMs) (Maenhout et al. 2014). Similarly, hypoxia and CAFs facilitate recruitment of T_{reg} cells (Facciabene et al. 2011; Costa et al. 2018). Another feature of the inflamed phenotype is the expression of immune checkpoints, which reduce the immune-cell activity. Indeed, VEGF causes the upregulation of various immune checkpoints on T cells (Voron et al. 2015; Palazon et al. 2017; Wallin et al. 2016). Additionally, hypoxia through HIF-1α does the same on MDSCs, TAMs, DCs, and cancer cells (Noman et al. 2014, 2015). Finally, acidity (Calcinotto et al. 2012), CAFs (Costa et al. 2018), and collagen density (Kuczek et al. 2019) might impair the cytotoxic activity of CTLs in the parenchyma.

Thus, VEGF and abnormal angiogenesis have a role in promoting the cancer-immunity phenotypes. Meanwhile, immune cells can promote pathological angiogenesis (Mazzone and Bergers 2019; Huang et al. 2018; Tian et al. 2017; Zheng et al. 2018) thereby completing a circularity of abnormal vasculature and pro-tumor immunosuppression. To break from this cycle, we propose normalizing the TME to alleviate hypoxia (Martin et al. 2016, 2019b) and in turn increase immune-cell density and antitumor function (Jain 2014; Martin et al. 2019b; Munn and Jain 2019). This approach is particularly promising because many patients have primary tumors and metastases featuring heterogeneous cancer-immunity phenotypes (Baine et al. 2015; Müller et al. 2016; Lee et al. 2017; Ramanathan et al. 2017).

4.5.2 TME Normalization through Inhibition of Immunosuppressive Signaling Pathways

Increasing tumor perfusion and oxygenation facilitates progression through and perpetuates the cancer-immunity cycle (Fig. 12.4 inner ring) (Zheng et al. 2018). Besides TME-normalizing effects, blocking vascular "abnormalizing" pathways such as VEGF and ANG-2 as well as other pathways such as TGFβ and SDF-1α/ CXCR4 promote antitumor immunity by interfering with immunosuppressive signaling in tumors (Martin et al. 2020; Fukumura et al. 2018; Munn and Jain 2019). Indeed, murine studies demonstrate that vascular normalization can enhance the antitumor efficacy of ICB (Allen et al. 2017; Schmittnaegel et al. 2017; Shigeta et al. 2019), whole cancer cell vaccines (Huang et al. 2012) and adoptive cell therapy (ACT) (Shrimali et al. 2010). These findings mirror the success of AAT with ICB in patients. Indeed, phase III trials showed that combining the anti-VEGF antibody bevacizumab with the ICB atezolizumab and the chemotherapy paclitaxel in patients with metastatic non-squamous NSCLC (Socinski et al. 2018) and the small-molecule VEGFR1–3 inhibitor axitinib with either ICB of avelumab (Motzer et al. 2019) or pembrolizumab (Rini et al. 2019) in patients with advanced-stage RCC. In addition, ICBs can induce immune cells to cause vascular normalization in certain preclinical models (Shigeta et al. 2019; Tian et al. 2017; Zheng et al. 2018). Thus, clinical evidence supports the preclinical observations that combining vascular normalization and ICB might cause a beneficial cycle of efficient vasculature alleviating hypoxia towards simultaneously increasing the antitumor efficacy of AAT and ICB (Shigeta et al. 2019; Munn and Jain 2019; Huang et al. 2018; Martin et al. 2020, Martin et al. 2019b).

Like AAT, mechanotherapeutics, which modify the mechanics of tumor tissue and often directly affect immune cells, are in clinical trials with ICB. Mechanotherapeutics that interfere with TGFβ signaling in CAFs such as angiotensin receptor blockers (ARBs) like losartan (Chauhan et al. 2013, 2019; Diop-Frimpong et al. 2011; Pinter and Jain 2017) could increase the efficacy of immunotherapies through various mechanisms besides alleviating stresses in the TME (Chakravarthy et al. 2018). Among the multiple roles of TGFβ signaling in cancer, it is immunosuppressive (Chakravarthy et al. 2018; Mariathasan et al. 2018; Tauriello et al. 2018). Specifically, TGFβ promotes immune evasion in murine metastases (Tauriello et al. 2018) and excludes T cells from the tumor parenchyma, thereby associating with poor responses to ICB in patients (Mariathasan et al. 2018). Relatedly, TGFβ signaling inhibition increases the amount of adhesion molecules (such as ICAM-1 or VCAM-1) on tumor blood vessels so that leukocytes may better bind tumor vessels and penetrate into tumors (Munn and Jain 2019). In addition, TGFβ signaling inhibition promotes abscopal effects induced by RT (Vanpouille-Box et al. 2015).

Clinical data supports the notion that ARBs may increase efficacy of immunotherapeutics. In patients with pancreatic ductal adenocarcinoma (PDAC), there was more gene expression associated with T cell activation with losartan treatment (Liu et al. 2017). Retrospective analyses largely indicate patients fare better when taking ARBs long-term versus those without long-term ARB use (Martin et al. 2020; Pinter and Jain 2017). These various mechanisms support the ongoing clinical trial in patients with locally advanced PDAC receiving losartan in combination with nivolumab, FOLFIRINOX, and stereotactic body RT (NCT03563248).

4.6 Immunotherapy-Induced Vascular Normalization

While vessel normalization increases immunotherapy efficacy through multiple mechanisms (Fukumura et al. 2018; Martin et al. 2020; Munn and Jain 2019; Arvanitis et al. 2020), ICB activates immune cells, which then normalize vessels (Munn and Jain 2019). In tumor prevention studies, CD4+ rather than CD8+ T cells normalized vessels in an IFN-γ dependent manner (Tian et al. 2017). In one therapeutic setting, CD8+ T cells normalized vessels in an IFN-γ dependent manner (Zheng et al. 2018), while in another setting CD4+ T cells did (Shigeta et al. 2019).

Besides differences in the immune cells that normalize vessels, there is also variability between studies and tumor types of the type of normalization that occurs. Several studies in relatively desmoplastic tumor models such as breast, pancreatic and colorectal cancers have found that AAT and ICB therapies passively normalized vessels, with enhanced vessel maturity after pruning (Allen et al. 2017; Schmittnaegel et al. 2017; Zheng et al. 2018). In hepatocellular carcinoma, which is more vascularized and sensitive to AAT monotherapy (Jayson et al. 2016), AAT (both high and low doses) and ICB combinations fortified vessels resulting in active normalization that avoids pruning (Shigeta et al. 2019).

5 Opportunities for Molecular Targeted Radiosensitizers in Combination Therapy Regimens

Although RT is a local treatment, patients with few metastases in spatially restricted sites may have these oligometastases directly treated by RT, which may prolong OS. This oligometastasis hypothesis puts forth a strategy that might expand the fraction of patients who can benefit from RT with or without radiosensitizers (Bristow et al. 2018; Ko et al. 2018; Pitroda et al. 2019). Nonetheless, even in this setting the TME likely impairs efficacy of RT. Thus, we propose that radiosensitizers could benefit patients with oligometastases thereby increasing the fraction of patients with localized cancer cured by RT (Bristow et al. 2018). In patients with widespread disease, systemically administered radiosensitizers could also induce antitumor efficacy against non-irradiated lesions. First, these systemically administered radiosensitizers will directly act on non-irradiated lesions. Second, these systemic radiosensitizers can make these distant lesions more amenable to abscopal effects induced by RT treatment against the accessible lesion by enabling antitumor immune cells to efficiently infiltrate distant lesions. Third, these systemic radiosensitizers can magnify the generation of abscopal effects by sensitizing the accessible lesion to RT, thereby facilitating immunogenic cell death (ICD) and presentation of tumor antigens to cytotoxic T lymphocytes. Thus, here we will describe combination strategies for RT enhancement by nanomedicine-, TME normalization-, chemotherapy-, and/or immunotherapy-based radiosensitizers.

5.1 Combination with Passively Targeted Systemically or Locally Administered Nano-Radiosensitizers

The most common radiosensitizers are high atomic number metals. When high atomic number metals are irradiated, the metal atoms undergo inner shell ionization, and electrons are emitted. These electrons can directly damage cancer cells or do so indirectly by producing ROS (Liu et al. 2018). Nanomedicines containing these RT-sensitizing materials could enhance the efficacy of RT while enabling a lower dose of irradiation (Liu et al. 2018). Alternatively, nanomedicines encapsulating chemotherapies and/or TME-normalizing drugs may also be used as radiosensitizers (Martin et al. 2020). These nanomedicine-based radiosensitizers can be administered systemically to passively accumulate in tumors through the enhanced permeability and retention effect (Jain and Stylianopoulos 2010; Gerlowski and Jain 1986; Chauhan et al. 2011; Martin et al. 2020; Matsumura and Maeda 1986). They may also be administered through an intratumoral injection in superficially located tumors, where they are retained more than locally administered small molecules (Liu et al. 2018). The approval by the European Medicines Agency (EMA) of intratumoral injections of NBTXR3 hafnium oxide nanoparticles, which enhance the RT abscopal effect in locally advanced soft-tissue sarcomas validates this strategy (Bonvalot et al. 2019). Furthermore, the finding that the efficacy of RT combined with immunotherapy is inversely correlated to the RT dose to healthy immune cells indicates the importance of using radiosensitizers to maximize the dose of RT administered to tumors and limit that to healthy tissue (Jin et al. 2017).

Nano-based chemotherapy can act as a more efficient radio sensitizer than small-molecule chemotherapy for several reasons (Martin et al. 2020). First, systemically administered nanomedicines often have less or altered toxicity compared to small molecules (Chauhan and Jain 2013). Second, nano-based chemotherapy can act similarly to metronomic chemotherapy in normalizing the TME (Mpekris et al. 2017; Panagi et al. 2020). One potential reason is that the constant presence of chemotherapy in the circulation with frequently administered metronomic small-molecule chemotherapy or long-circulating nanomedicine reduces the proliferation of endothelial cells leading to an anti-angiogenic effect. Similarly, it alleviates solid stress by eliminating proliferating cancer cells thereby decompressing vessels. Thus, in some cases, nano-based chemotherapy can act as an anti-angiogenic therapy, a mechanotherapeutic and a cytotoxic chemotherapy that induces immunogenic cell death (ICD).

TME-normalizing strategies often rely on drugs that are repurposed from other diseases to act as mechanotherapeutics in cancer, where they can reprogram CAFs to a quiescent phenotype thereby alleviating stresses, decompressing vessels, restoring perfusion, and reducing hypoxia. Apart from effects on tissue mechanics, these drugs might directly polarize immune cells towards antitumor immunity (Regan et al. 2019). These small-molecule drugs can benefit from nanoformulation because the nanoformulation reduces the normal systemic effects of these drugs while increasing their accrual in the tumor (Martin et al. 2020). For example, ARBs typically used to treat hypertension, when encapsulated in a nanoformulation, did not reduce blood pressure but had increased TME-normalizing effects (Chauhan et al. 2019). Still, whether these nanoformulations will be more effective in the clinic compared to relatively inexpensive generic TME-normalizing drugs is unclear.

5.2 Combination with TME Normalization

RT relies on oxygen to kill cancer cells. TME normalization increases oxygen delivery to tumors. Accordingly, TME-normalizing therapies may act as radiosensitizers when administered before RT by alleviating hypoxia and improving outcomes in preclinical and clinical studies (Jain 2014; Batchelor et al. 2013; Winkler et al. 2004). In mice, AAT transiently normalizes vessels thereby enhancing their function and providing a window of reduced hypoxia in which RT is effective (Winkler et al. 2004). In patients, AAT is used with radiation and the patients that have increased tumor oxygenation after AAT have increased survival (Batchelor et al. 2013). Similarly, losartan enhanced tumor shrinkage by chemoradiation in patients with locally advanced PDAC thereby enabling more tumor resections (Murphy et al. 2019). Besides effects on hypoxia, TME normalization could facilitate RT-induced abscopal effects by altering the distribution and phenotype of immune cells. VEGF and TGFβ signaling pathways act directly on immune cells suppressing their function and also construct barriers to immune-cell migration within the TME (Vanpouille-Box et al. 2015). Thus, at various stages TME normalization could facilitate progression through the cancer-immunity cycle that is initiated when RT induces ICD causing the release of tumor-associated antigens (Fig. 12.4).

5.3   Combination with Chemotherapy

Systemic chemotherapy can synergize with local RT by acting against distant metastases that RT cannot affect (independent of inducing a systemic antitumor immune response). Additionally, chemotherapy and RT may cooperate through at least five mechanisms (Nishimura 2004). First, certain chemotherapies that incorporate into DNA enhance radiation damage. Halgenated pyrimidines and cisplatin, through different mechanisms, interact with DNA to enhance RT (Vokes and Weichselbaum 1990). Second, while some cancer cells can repair themselves after RT (particularly sublethal doses), certain chemotherapies (e.g., halogenated pyrimidines, nucleoside analogs, and cisplatin) reduce this capacity. This could be particularly important in fractionated RT so as to induce the abscopal effect because lower sublethal doses are used (Grégoire et al. 1996; Milas 2009). Third, certain chemotherapies can help accumulate cells in a proliferative radiosensitive phase while other chemotherapies can eliminate radioresistant cells that are in a non-proliferative phase. Taxanes arrest cells in proliferative phases of the cell cycle (Mason et al. 1997; Milas et al. 1995; Suzuki et al. 2003), while nucleoside analogs affect non-proliferative cancer cells (Milas 2009). Fourth, chemotherapies can affect hypoxic cells. For example, paclitaxel increases tumor oxygenation (Milas et al. 1995) in part by decompressing vessels thereby increasing blood flow and killing cancer cells thereby reducing oxygen consumption. Alternatively, certain chemotherapies become toxic in hypoxic conditions thereby selectively killing hypoxic cells so that RT will primarily act on normoxic cancer cells (Milas 2009). Fifth, chemotherapies combined with fractionated RT can inhibit repopulation of cancer cells thereby improving the effectiveness of the subsequent fraction of RT (Nishimura 2004). One downside of these combinations is the chemotherapy could increase the toxicity of RT to normal tissues.

On the other hand, cytotoxic nanomedicines might benefit when used after RT. Specifically, RT increases the penetration of nanomedicines in murine tumors by normalizing the TME and modulating immune cells (Stapleton et al. 2018; Miller et al. 2017). However, in murine studies the TME-normalizing effects of RT are dependent on the dose and vary across tumor types (Clément-Colmou et al. 2020), so this approach might require personalization. Alternatively, the delivery of nanomedicines targeting P-selectin can be improved by RT-induced expression of P-selectin (Shamay et al. 2016). Whether the successful outcome seen in these murine studies will translate into human cancer is an outstanding question.

5.4 Combination with Immunotherapy

Immunotherapy promotes TME normalization and ameliorates hypoxia (Munn and Jain 2019), which causes resistance to radiation. Thus, in settings where immunotherapy enhances oxygen delivery, it is radiosensitizing and could precede RT (Sharabi et al. 2015). Alternatively, RT modulates the TME to promote subsequent immunotherapy through several mechanisms. First, RT normalizes the TME and ameliorates hypoxia (Clément-Colmou et al. 2020; Netti et al. 1999; Stapleton et al. 2018). While radiation immediately kills normoxic cancer cells and therefore increases the fraction of hypoxic cells, the depletion of cancer cells reduces solid stress and decompresses vessels (Stylianopoulos et al. 2012) thereby increasing perfusion and ameliorating hypoxia by increasing supply and also reducing consumption (Bussink et al. 2000). Meanwhile, reduced cancer cell density reduces the expression of pro-angiogenic factors, and RT might directly kill proliferating ECs, so RT could have an anti-angiogenic effect that drastically prunes tumor vessels and eventually results in regrowth of the vasculature (Kozin et al. 2012). In this case, care must be taken to confirm that RT is not inducing hypoxia through excessive pruning. Reduced solid stress, in this case caused by RT-induced cancer cell killing, also decompresses lymphatic vessels (Stylianopoulos et al. 2012). Thus, RT modulates IFP transiently, which can be exploited to increase delivery of macromolecules and nanomedicines including immunotherapies and radiosensitizers (Stapleton et al. 2018; Netti et al. 1999).

The RT-induced abscopal effect involves inducing ICD in one or more lesions, which can then induce a systemic immune response against distant metastases (Min et al. 2017; Peng et al. 2018; Chen et al. 2019b, 2018; He et al. 2016). RT-induced ICD increases the diversity of the TCR repertoire in tumors (Twyman-Saint Victor et al. 2015). However, radiation dose and fractionation affect the induction of abscopal effects. Fractionated rather than single-dose RT seems to induce ICD (Dewan et al. 2009; Demaria et al. 2005). High-dose RT may limit immunogenicity because it causes enzymatic digestion of cytosolic DNA, which eliminates one mechanism of immune recognition, though more research is likely needed to determine the dose dependency in different tumors (Vanpouille-Box et al. 2017). Indeed, EMA-approved NBTXR3 with RT stimulates an antitumor immune response (Thariat et al. 2019), underscoring the potential of this approach.

5.5   Treatment with Three or Four Modalities

There is potential to combine these various sensitizers. Nano-based high atomic number metal radiosensitizers, whether administered systemically or locally, could have increased intratumor distribution with TME normalization (Jain and Stylianopoulos 2010; Martin et al. 2020). Vascular normalization increases the delivery of smaller nanomedicines (Chauhan et al. 2012; Martin et al. 2019a; Chauhan and Jain 2013). Mechanotherapeutics enhance the delivery of systemically administered (Panagi et al. 2020; Chauhan et al. 2013; Papageorgis et al. 2017) and locally administered nanomedicines (Diop-Frimpong et al. 2011; Liu et al. 2012). Increased accumulation and intratumor distribution could increase the number of cancer cells undergoing ICD. Similarly, TME normalization could increase the accumulation and intratumor delivery of small-molecule chemotherapy towards inducing more ICD. As discussed, antitumor T cells can normalize the vasculature in some types of tumors, so both immunotherapy and TME normalization could alleviate hypoxia towards potentiating RT. Thus, through multiple mechanisms, TME normalization might be able to increase the amount of antitumor T cells in the tumor, thereby further reducing hypoxia.

In addition, various immunotherapies can benefit from TME normalization (Fukumura et al. 2018; Munn and Jain 2019), which helps to overcomes each barrier posed in the cancer-immunity cycle (Martin et al. 2020). As mentioned, TME normalization might increase the ability of chemotherapy and/or RT to induce ICD, which could then enhance efficacy of ICB. Also, TME normalization could limit amounts of immunosuppressive cytokines originating in the tumor and collecting in the draining lymph nodes. T cells move through the circulatory system and infiltrate tumors, eventually penetrating the parenchyma. Although tumors limit chemotaxis of T cells (Harlin et al. 2009), vascular normalization pushes TAMs towards an M1-like antitumor phenotype secreting chemokines that bind T cells (Rolny et al. 2011) and modulates T cells to express receptors to facilitate chemotaxis (Wallin et al. 2016). Once reaching tumors, T cells must penetrate from blood supply to cancer cells. Vascular normalization might increase T cell infiltration and activity (Huang et al. 2012), in part by increasing the number of perfused vessels with TME normalization, which reduces the distance T cells must migrate because they initially flow closer to cancer cells (Huang et al. 2012; Chauhan et al. 2019; Chen et al. 2019a). Nonetheless, T cells (Taggart et al. 2018) and natural killer (NK) cells (Melder et al. 1996) both are inhibited from passing through the wall of immature vessels because of low levels of adhesion molecules. By inducing maturation, vascular normalization with AATs enhances the steps of T cell penetration (Shrimali et al. 2010; Hamzah et al. 2008; Wallin et al. 2016). Afterwards, vascular normalization increases T cell recognition of cancer cells by (a) reducing hypoxia-induced shedding of MHC I molecules (Siemens et al. 2008) and (b) increasing expression of MHC I molecules by limiting nitric oxide (Siemens et al. 2008) and VEGF (Wallin et al. 2016). Accordingly, vascular normalization increases antigen-specific migration of T cells (Wallin et al. 2016).

6 Challenges

6.1 Rigorous Preclinical Models

Genetically engineered mouse models (GEMMs) are often considered ideal because they form tumors without implantation and have mutations reflecting clinical disease. They can often recapitulate the physiology of the TME, such as hypoperfusion in PDAC (Olive et al. 2009). Cell lines isolated from such GEMMs, which are then grown in mice and can be transplanted as a solid chunk into the recipient mice, can recapitulate hypoperfusion (Chauhan et al. 2013). One advantage of this solid passage technique is that cancer cells are introduced along with their co-opted TME. In cancer initiation, mutations occur in single cells gradually and the physiology TME is affected in the earliest stages of malignant transformation (Hagendoorn et al. 2006). In contrast, GEMMs have mutations in many cells before there are any changes to the TME. Similar to solid passage, there is value of implanting tumor spheroids rather than inoculating with single cell suspensions to better reflect the growth and spread of cancer in patients (Aktar et al. 2019).

Orthotopic models are useful to recapitulate the TME. Subcutaneous models have different TME properties than orthotopic tumors (Olive et al. 2009; Netti et al. 2000; Yuan et al. 1994). Another consideration is syngeneic versus human xenografts, but the latter have mixed human cancer cells and murine host cells in the TME, so testing TME modulating radiosensitizers is suboptimal in these models especially when the importance of the immune system is considered (Bristow et al. 2018). Nonetheless, by using human stromal cells with murine cancer cells in immunocompromised mice, it is possible to deplete the human cells selectively with diphtheria toxin to isolate the effects of specific cells in the TME (Padera et al. 2004; Duda et al. 2010; Stylianopoulos et al. 2012).

There should be standard operating procedures in the use of preclinical models to determine optimal combinations of drugs. Indeed, comparing data across studies is complicated by suboptimal experimental design, execution, and reporting (Stone et al. 2016). When testing radiosensitizers, they should be tested in combination with the standard of care, which is often chemoradiation (Coleman et al. 2016). Appropriate primary endpoints such as local tumor control or tumor regrowth delay should be carefully selected (Coleman et al. 2016).

6.2 Treatment Windows

Over long courses of treatment, TME normalization might lose its effectiveness. Tumors can develop resistance pathways (Goel et al. 2011) and excessive doses and/ or treatment lengths could excessively deplete the stroma leading to treatment resistance (Winkler et al. 2004; Huang et al. 2012). Thus, strategies that fortify vessels by reinvesting them of pericytes and reprograms CAFs towards quiescence should be prioritized to avoid facing a limited window of TME normalization efficacy (Martin et al. 2019b). If stroma destruction could be avoided with TME normalization, then the normalization window may be lengthened.

If the TME normalization window is known, then RT and/or chemotherapy towards inducing ICD should be administered in this window. However, it is not clear when immunotherapy should be administered after ICD-inducing chemotherapy and/or RT. Furthermore, it is not clear whether these cytotoxic therapies should be continued during the course of ICB. The answers to these questions might be further complicated by the long circulation time of nano- and macromolecule-based therapies.

6.3   *Imaging Biomarkers*

Imaging could be used to measure predictive biomarkers of response to RT (Kirsch et al. 2017) and to radiosensitizers. As we proposed above, hypoxia is a critical biomarker of treatment resistance and response. Low hypoxia leads to better responses to RT. Thus, imaging hypoxia in patients could be useful in developing radiosensitizers, predicting patient response to RT and determining windows to administer radiosensitizers and RT.

Many radiosensitizers are nanomedicines or macromolecules, which could have heterogeneous distribution in the various metastases within patients and spatially within a single lesion (Martin et al. 2020). Thus, drug tracing of radiosensitizers could help serve as predictive biomarkers, biomarkers of response and tools to investigate mechanisms of resistance.

Imaging of probes sized similar to nanomedicines and macromolecules that emit PET or MRI signals have demonstrated heterogeneous distribution in patients with solid tumors (Lee et al. 2017; Ramanathan et al. 2017). Advances in imaging approaches could help probe the TME (Mi et al. 2016) and the effects of immunotherapies in patients (Kulkarni et al. 2016). These probes could be used to evaluate TME-normalizing strategies that reduce heterogeneity of small-molecule, oxygen, nanomedicine, and macromolecule distribution. Thus, they might serve as predictive markers of delivery and response. While current predictive biomarker strategies, including tumor histology, flow cytometry, and whole-genome sequencing, provide a small window of the TME characteristics that affect RT response, imaging of drugs could facilitate visualization of dynamic events that could complement or replace other biomarker methods. With such an approach, TME normalization could help advance nanomedicine development and vice-versa.

7   Perspectives

More research will help to effectively combine RT with radiosensitizers, including identifying and validating predictive biomarkers and biomarkers of response. Additionally, developing an understanding of the temporal effects of the various radiosensitizers will allow more effective drug combinations that have fewer toxicities and possibly personalization of therapeutic strategies. Here, we propose that alleviating hypoxia is the critical biomarker for radiosensitizers and RT.

Indeed, hypoxia is a biomarker of worse outcomes for patients, induces tumor progression through multiple mechanisms, and promotes resistance to most cancer treatment modalities, including RT and TME-targeting radiosensitizers. Hypoxia is caused by poor tumor vessel function. Pathological angiogenesis and desmoplasia impair vessels causing hypoperfusion and resulting in hypoxia, acidity, and immunosuppression. Here, we described how normalizing the TME will reverse these pathologies, thereby potentiating the effectiveness of RT. Thus, TME-normalizing strategies can be considered radiosensitizers. Furthermore, we describe how TME-normalizing strategies benefit immunotherapy and particularly ICB, which has revolutionized cancer treatment yet is estimated to currently only benefit 13% of cancer patients (Haslam and Prasad 2019). The limited percentage of patients who currently benefit from ICB alone indicates an urgent need for novel combination strategies, so we highlight the mutually beneficial combinations of RT with ICB and how TME normalization can improve the efficacy of this combination. Various nanotechnologies and chemotherapies can be integrated rationally to further enhance efficacy and limit the toxicity of RT, immunotherapy, and TME-normalizing combination regimens.

Given the various mechanisms of synergies between these cancer therapies, future research will elucidate how to optimally combine these drugs. Unfortunately, preclinical studies are often limited by suboptimal model choices, inconsistent reporting and protocols, and a lack of proper controls and study endpoints. These challenges limit researchers' ability to determine optimal treatment windows for each therapy, as has been done for TME normalization. One solution is the use of imaging biomarkers in patients. Recently, imaging of perfusion, oxygen, and drug delivery in tumors has improved, and these biomarkers are central to determining how to best combine RT with radiosensitizers that target the TME including chemotherapy, immunotherapy, AATs, and mechanotherapeutics.

Acknowledgements This book chapter is based on our recent review articles (Martin et al. 2020, Martin et al. 2019b). The research leading to these results has received funding from the National Foundation for Cancer Research; the Ludwig Center at Harvard; the Jane's Trust Foundation; the Advanced Medical Research Foundation, the U.S. National Cancer Institute grants R35-CA197743, R01-CA208205, and U01-CA224348 and the U.S. Department of Defense Breast Cancer Research Program Innovator Award W81XWH-10-1-0016 (to R.K.J.).

Competing Interests R.K.J. has received honoraria from Amgen, has acted as a consultant of Chugai, Merck, Ophthotech, Pfizer, SPARC, SynDevRx, and XTuit, owns equity in Enlight, Ophthotech, and SynDevRx, and serves on the Boards of Trustees of Tekla Healthcare Investors, Tekla Life Sciences Investors, Tekla Healthcare Opportunities Fund, and Tekla World Healthcare Fund. J.D.M is an employee of NanoCarrier Co.

References

Aicher A, Rentsch M, Sasaki K, Ellwart JW, Fandrich F, Siebert R, Cooke JP, Dimmeler S, Heeschen C (2007) Nonbone marrow-derived circulating progenitor cells contribute to postnatal neovascularization following tissue ischemia. Circ Res 100(4):581–589. https://doi.org/10.1161/01.RES.0000259562.63718.35

Aktar R, Dietrich A, Tillner F, Kotb S, Löck S, Willers H, Baumann M, Krause M, Bütof R (2019) Pre-clinical imaging for establishment and comparison of orthotopic non-small cell lung carcinoma: in search for models reflecting clinical scenarios. Br J Radiol 92(1095):20180539

Algire GH, Chalkley HW (1945) Vascular reactions of normal and malignant tissues in vivo. I. Vascular reactions of mice to wounds and to normal and neoplastic transplants. J Natl Cancer Inst 6:73–85

Allen E, Jabouille A, Rivera LB, Lodewijckx I, Missiaen R, Steri V, Feyen K, Tawney J, Hanahan D, Michael IP (2017) Combined antiangiogenic and anti–PD-L1 therapy stimulates tumor immunity through HEV formation. Sci Transl Med 9(385):eaak9679

Arvanitis CD, Ferraro GB, Jain RK (2020) The blood–brain barrier and blood–tumour barrier in brain tumours and metastases. Nat Rev Cancer 20:26–41

Baine MK, Turcu G, Zito CR, Adeniran AJ, Camp RL, Chen L, Kluger HM, Jilaveanu LB (2015) Characterization of tumor infiltrating lymphocytes in paired primary and metastatic renal cell carcinoma specimens. Oncotarget 6(28):24990–25002

Baish JW, Stylianopoulos T, Lanning RM, Kamoun WS, Fukumura D, Munn LL, Jain RK (2011) Scaling rules for diffusive drug delivery in tumor and normal tissues. Proc Natl Acad Sci U S A 108(5):1799–1803. https://doi.org/10.1073/pnas.1018154108

Baluk P, Morikawa S, Haskell A, Mancuso M, McDonald DM (2003) Abnormalities of basement membrane on blood vessels and endothelial sprouts in tumors. Am J Pathol 163(5):1801–1815

Batchelor TT, Gerstner ER, Emblem KD, Duda DG, Kalpathy-Cramer J, Snuderl M, Ancukiewicz M, Polaskova P, Pinho MC, Jennings D, Plotkin SR, Chi AS, Eichler AF, Dietrich J, Hochberg FH, Lu-Emerson C, Iafrate AJ, Ivy SP, Rosen BR, Loeffler JS, Wen PY, Sorensen AG, Jain RK (2013) Improved tumor oxygenation and survival in glioblastoma patients who show increased blood perfusion after cediranib and chemoradiation. Proc Natl Acad Sci U S A 110(47):19059–19064

Batchelor TT, Sorensen AG, di Tomaso E, Zhang WT, Duda DG, Cohen KS, Kozak KR, Cahill DP, Chen PJ, Zhu M, Ancukiewicz M, Mrugala MM, Plotkin S, Drappatz J, Louis DN, Ivy P, Scadden DT, Benner T, Loeffler JS, Wen PY, Jain RK (2007) AZD2171, a pan-VEGF receptor tyrosine kinase inhibitor, normalizes tumor vasculature and alleviates edema in glioblastoma patients. Cancer Cell 11(1):83–95. https://doi.org/10.1016/j.ccr.2006.11.021

Bonvalot S, Rutkowski PL, Thariat J, Carrère S, Ducassou A, Sunyach M-P, Agoston P, Hong A, Mervoyer A, Rastrelli M (2019) NBTXR3, a first-in-class radioenhancer hafnium oxide nanoparticle, plus radiotherapy versus radiotherapy alone in patients with locally advanced soft-tissue sarcoma (Act. In. Sarc): a multicentre, phase 2–3, randomised, controlled trial. Lancet Oncol 20(8):1148–1159

Bristow RG, Alexander B, Baumann M, Bratman SV, Brown JM, Camphausen K, Choyke P, Citrin D, Contessa JN, Dicker A (2018) Combining precision radiotherapy with molecular targeting and immunomodulatory agents: a guideline by the American Society for Radiation Oncology. Lancet Oncol 19(5):e240–e251

Bussink J, Kaanders JHA, Rijken PFJ, Raleigh JA, Van der Kogel AJ (2000) Changes in blood perfusion and hypoxia after irradiation of a human squamous cell carcinoma xenograft tumor line. Radiat Res 153(4):398–404

Calcinotto A, Filipazzi P, Grioni M, Iero M, De Milito A, Ricupito A, Cova A, Canese R, Jachetti E, Rossetti M (2012) Modulation of microenvironment acidity reverses anergy in human and murine tumor-infiltrating T lymphocytes. Cancer Res 72(11):2746–2756

Carmeliet P, Dor Y, Herbert JM, Fukumura D, Brusselmans K, Dewerchin M, Neeman M, Bono F, Abramovitch R, Maxwell P, Koch CJ, Ratcliffe P, Moons L, Jain RK, Collen D, Keshert E, Keshet E (1998) Role of HIF-1alpha in hypoxia-mediated apoptosis, cell proliferation and tumour angiogenesis. Nature 394(6692):485–490

Carmeliet P, Jain RK (2011a) Molecular mechanisms and clinical applications of angiogenesis. Nature 473(7347):298–307. https://doi.org/10.1038/nature10144

Carmeliet P, Jain RK (2011b) Principles and mechanisms of vessel normalization for cancer and other angiogenic diseases. Nat Rev Drug Discov 10(6):417–427. https://doi.org/10.1038/nrd3455

Chakravarthy A, Khan L, Bensler NP, Bose P, De Carvalho DD (2018) TGF-β-associated extracellular matrix genes link cancer-associated fibroblasts to immune evasion and immunotherapy failure. Nat Commun 9(1):4692

Chang YS, di Tomaso E, McDonald DM, Jones R, Jain RK, Munn LL (2000) Mosaic blood vessels in tumors: frequency of cancer cells in contact with flowing blood. Proc Natl Acad Sci U S A 97(26):14608–14613

Chauhan VP, Chen IX, Tong RT, Ng MR, Martin JD, Naxerova K, Wu MW, Huang P, Boucher Y, Kohane DS, Langer R, Jain RK (2019) Reprogramming the microenvironment with tumor-selective angiotensin blockers enhances cancer immunotherapy. Proc Natl Acad Sci U S A 116(22):10674–10680. https://doi.org/10.1073/pnas.1819889116/

Chauhan VP, Jain RK (2013) Strategies for advancing cancer nanomedicine. Nat Mater 12(11):958–962. https://doi.org/10.1038/nmat3792

Chauhan VP, Martin JD, Liu H, Lacorre DA, Jain SR, Kozin SV, Stylianopoulos T, Mousa AS, Han X, Adstamongkonkul P, Popovic Z, Huang P, Bawendi MG, Boucher Y, Jain RK (2013) Angiotensin inhibition enhances drug delivery and potentiates chemotherapy by decompressing tumour blood vessels. Nat Commun 4:2516. https://doi.org/10.1038/ncomms3516

Chauhan VP, Stylianopoulos T, Boucher Y, Jain RK (2011) Delivery of molecular and nanoscale medicine to tumors: transport barriers and strategies. Annu Rev Chem Biomol Eng 2:281–298. https://doi.org/10.1146/annurev-chembioeng-061010-114300

Chauhan VP, Stylianopoulos T, Martin JD, Popovic Z, Chen O, Kamoun WS, Bawendi MG, Fukumura D, Jain RK (2012) Normalization of tumour blood vessels improves the delivery of nanomedicines in a size-dependent manner. Nat Nanotechnol 7(6):383–388. https://doi.org/10.1038/nnano.2012.45

Chen DS, Mellman I (2017) Elements of cancer immunity and the cancer–immune set point. Nature 541(7637):321–330

Chen IX, Chauhan VP, Posada J, Ng MR, Wu MW, Adstamongkonkul P, Huang P, Lindeman N, Langer R, Jain RK (2019a) Blocking CXCR4 alleviates desmoplasia, increases T-lymphocyte infiltration, and improves immunotherapy in metastatic breast cancer. Proc Natl Acad Sci U S A 116(10):4558–4566

Chen Q, Chen J, Yang Z, Xu J, Xu L, Liang C, Han X, Liu Z (2019b) Nanoparticle-enhanced radiotherapy to trigger robust cancer immunotherapy. Adv Mater 31(10):1802228

Chen Y, Huang Y, Reiberger T, Duyverman AM, Huang P, Samuel R, Hiddingh L, Roberge S, Koppel C, Lauwers GY, Zhu AX, Jain RK, Duda DG (2014) Differential effects of sorafenib on liver versus tumor fibrosis mediated by stromal-derived factor 1 alpha/C-X-C receptor type 4 axis and myeloid differentiation antigen-positive myeloid cell infiltration in mice. Hepatology 59(4):1435–1447. https://doi.org/10.1002/hep.26790

Chen Y, Ramjiawan RR, Reiberger T, Ng MR, Hato T, Huang Y, Ochiai H, Kitahara S, Unan EC, Reddy TP, Fan C, Huang P, Bardeesy N, Zhu AX, Jain RK, Duda DG (2015) CXCR4 inhibition in tumor microenvironment facilitates anti-programmed death receptor-1 immunotherapy in sorafenib-treated hepatocellular carcinoma in mice. Hepatology 61(5):1591–1602. https://doi.org/10.1002/hep.27665

Chen Z, Liu L, Liang R, Luo Z, He H, Wu Z, Tian H, Zheng M, Ma Y, Cai L (2018) Bioinspired hybrid protein oxygen nanocarrier amplified photodynamic therapy for eliciting anti-tumor immunity and abscopal effect. ACS Nano 12(8):8633–8645

Clément-Colmou K, Potiron V, Pietri M, Guillonneau M, Jouglar E, Chiavassa S, Delpon G, Paris F, Supiot S (2020) Influence of radiotherapy fractionation schedule on the tumor vascular microenvironment in prostate and lung cancer models. Cancers 12(1):121

Coleman CN, Higgins GS, Brown JM, Baumann M, Kirsch DG, Willers H, Prasanna PG, Dewhirst MW, Bernhard EJ, Ahmed MM (2016) Improving the predictive value of preclinical studies in support of radiotherapy clinical trials. Clin Cancer Res 22(13):3138–3147

Costa A, Kieffer Y, Scholer-Dahirel A, Pelon F, Bourachot B, Cardon M, Sirven P, Magagna I, Fuhrmann L, Bernard C (2018) Fibroblast heterogeneity and immunosuppressive environment in human breast cancer. Cancer Cell 33(3):463–479. e410

Datta M, Coussens LM, Nishikawa H, Hodi FS, Jain RK (2019) Reprogramming the tumor micro-environment to improve immunotherapy: emerging strategies and combination therapies. Am Soc Clin Oncol Educ Book 39:165–174

Demaria S, Kawashima N, Yang AM, Devitt ML, Babb JS, Allison JP, Formenti SC (2005) Immune-mediated inhibition of metastases after treatment with local radiation and CTLA-4 blockade in a mouse model of breast cancer. Clin Cancer Res 11(2):728–734

Dewan MZ, Galloway AE, Kawashima N, Dewyngaert JK, Babb JS, Formenti SC, Demaria S (2009) Fractionated but not single-dose radiotherapy induces an immune-mediated abscopal effect when combined with anti–CTLA-4 antibody. Clin Cancer Res 15(17):5379–5388

Diop-Frimpong B, Chauhan VP, Krane S, Boucher Y, Jain RK (2011) Losartan inhibits collagen I synthesis and improves the distribution and efficacy of nanotherapeutics in tumors. Proc Natl Acad Sci U S A 108(7):2909–2914. https://doi.org/10.1073/pnas.1018892108

Duda DG, Cohen KS, Kozin SV, Perentes JY, Fukumura D, Scadden DT, Jain RK (2006) Evidence for incorporation of bone marrow-derived endothelial cells into perfused blood vessels in tumors. Blood 107(7):2774–2776. https://doi.org/10.1182/blood-2005-08-3210

Duda DG, Duyverman AM, Kohno M, Snuderl M, Steller EJ, Fukumura D, Jain RK (2010) Malignant cells facilitate lung metastasis by bringing their own soil. Proc Natl Acad Sci U S A 107(50):21677–21682

Dvorak HF (2002) Vascular permeability factor/vascular endothelial growth factor: a critical cytokine in tumor angiogenesis and a potential target for diagnosis and therapy. J Clin Oncol 20(21):4368–4380

Eguchi D, Ikenaga N, Ohuchida K, Kozono S, Cui L, Fujiwara K, Fujino M, Ohtsuka T, Mizumoto K, Tanaka M (2013) Hypoxia enhances the interaction between pancreatic stellate cells and can-cer cells via increased secretion of connective tissue growth factor. J Surg Res 181(2):225–233

Emblem KE, Gerstner ER, Sorensen G, Rosen BR, Wen PY, Batchelor TT, Jain RK (2016) Matrix-depleting anti-hypertensives decompress tumor blood vessels and improve perfu-sion in patients with glioblastomas receiving anti-angiogenic therapy. Cancer Res 76(14 Supplement):3975–3975

Emblem KE, Mouridsen K, Bjornerud A, Farrar CT, Jennings D, Borra RJ, Wen PY, Ivy P, Batchelor TT, Rosen BR, Jain RK, Sorensen AG (2013) Vessel architectural imaging identifies cancer patient responders to anti-angiogenic therapy. Nat Med 19(9):1178–1183. https://doi.org/10.1038/nm.3289

Ergun S, Hohn HP, Kilic N, Singer BB, Tilki D (2008) Endothelial and hematopoietic progenitor cells (EPCs and HPCs): hand in hand fate determining partners for cancer cells. Stem Cell Rev 4(3):169–177. https://doi.org/10.1007/s12015-008-9028-y

Estrella V, Chen T, Lloyd M, Wojtkowiak J, Cornnell HH, Ibrahim-Hashim A, Bailey K, Balagurunathan Y, Rothberg JM, Sloane BF, Johnson J, Gatenby RA, Gillies RJ (2013) Acidity generated by the tumor microenvironment drives local invasion. Cancer Res 73(5):1524–1535. https://doi.org/10.1158/0008-5472.CAN-12-2796

Facciabene A, Peng X, Hagemann IS, Balint K, Barchetti A, Wang L-P, Gimotty PA, Gilks CB, Lal P, Zhang L (2011) Tumour hypoxia promotes tolerance and angiogenesis via CCL28 and Treg cells. Nature 475(7355):226–230

Feng D, Nagy JA, Hipp J, Dvorak HF, Dvorak AM (1996) Vesiculo-vacuolar organelles and the regulation of venule permeability to macromolecules by vascular permeability factor, histamine, and serotonin. J Exp Med 183(5):1981–1986

Fernández-Sánchez ME, Barbier S, Whitehead J, Béalle G, Michel A, Latorre-Ossa H, Rey C, Fouassier L, Claperon A, Brullé L (2015) Mechanical induction of the tumorigenic β-catenin pathway by tumour growth pressure. Nature 523:92–95

Folkman J (1971) Tumor angiogenesis: therapeutic implications. N Engl J Med 285(21):1182–1186

Fukumura D, Kloepper J, Amoozgar Z, Duda DG, Jain RK (2018) Enhancing cancer immunotherapy using antiangiogenics: opportunities and challenges. Nat Rev Clin Oncol 15:325–340

Fukumura D, Salehi HA, Witwer B, Tuma RF, Melder RJ, Jain RK (1995) Tumor necrosis factor α-induced leukocyte adhesion in normal and tumor vessels: effect of tumor type, transplantation site, and host strain. Cancer Res 55(21):4824–4829

Fukumura D, Xavier R, Sugiura T, Chen Y, Park EC, Lu N, Selig M, Nielsen G, Taksir T, Jain RK, Seed B (1998) Tumor induction of VEGF promoter activity in stromal cells. Cell 94(6):715–725

Garcia-Foncillas J, Martinez P, Lahuerta A, Cussac AL, Gonzalez MG, Sanchez Gomez RM, Alvarez I, Anton A, Illarramendi JJ, De Juan A, Galve Calvo E, Plazaola A, Morales S, Hernando B, Lao J, Boni V, Puertolas T, Sherer S, Palacios G, Lopez-Vega JM (2012) Dynamic contrast-enhanced MRI versus 18F-misonidazol-PET/CT to predict pathologic response in bevacizumab-based neoadjuvant therapy in breast cancer. J Clin Oncol 30. (suppl; abstr 10512)

Gerlowski LE, Jain RK (1986) Microvascular permeability of normal and neoplastic tissues. Microvasc Res 31(3):288–305

Goel S, Duda DG, Xu L, Munn LL, Boucher Y, Fukumura D, Jain RK (2011) Normalization of the vasculature for treatment of cancer and other diseases. Physiol Rev 91(3):1071–1121. https://doi.org/10.1152/physrev.00038.2010

Goldman E (1907) The growth of malignant disease in man and the lower animals with special reference to the vascular system. Lancet 2:1236–1240

Greenberg JI, Shields DJ, Barillas SG, Acevedo LM, Murphy E, Huang J, Scheppke L, Stockmann C, Johnson RS, Angle N (2008) A role for VEGF as a negative regulator of pericyte function and vessel maturation. Nature 456(7223):809

Greenblatt M, Philippe SK (1968) Tumor angiogenesis: transfilter diffusion studies in the hamster by the transparent chamber technique. J Natl Cancer Inst 41(1):111–124

Grégoire V, Hunter NR, Brock WA, Hittelman WN, Plunkett W, Milas L (1996) Improvement in the therapeutic ratio of radiotherapy for a murine sarcoma by indomethacin plus fludarabine. Radiat Res 146(5):548–553

Griffon-Etienne G, Boucher Y, Brekken C, Suit HD, Jain RK (1999) Taxane-induced apoptosis decompresses blood vessels and lowers interstitial fluid pressure in solid tumors: clinical implications. Cancer Res 59(15):3776–3782

Gullino PM (1978) Angiogenesis and oncogenesis. J Natl Cancer Inst 61(3):639–643

Hagendoorn J, Tong R, Fukumura D, Lin Q, Lobo J, Padera TP, Xu L, Kucherlapati R, Jain RK (2006) Onset of abnormal blood and lymphatic vessel function and interstitial hypertension in early stages of carcinogenesis. Cancer Res 66(7):3360–3364

Hamzah J, Jugold M, Kiessling F, Rigby P, Manzur M, Marti HH, Rabie T, Kaden S, Gröne H-J, Hämmerling GJ (2008) Vascular normalization in Rgs5-deficient tumours promotes immune destruction. Nature 453(7193):410–414

Harlin H, Meng Y, Peterson AC, Zha Y, Tretiakova M, Slingluff C, McKee M, Gajewski TF (2009) Chemokine expression in melanoma metastases associated with CD8+ T-cell recruitment. Cancer Res 69(7):3077–3085

Hashizume H, Baluk P, Morikawa S, McLean JW, Thurston G, Roberge S, Jain RK, McDonald DM (2000) Openings between defective endothelial cells explain tumor vessel leakiness. Am J Pathol 156(4):1363–1380

Haslam A, Prasad V (2019) Estimation of the percentage of US patients with cancer who are eligible for and respond to checkpoint inhibitor immunotherapy drugs. JAMA Netw Open 2(5):e192535–e192535

Hatfield SM, Kjaergaard J, Lukashev D, Schreiber TH, Belikoff B, Abbott R, Sethumadhavan S, Philbrook P, Ko K, Cannici R (2015) Immunological mechanisms of the antitumor effects of supplemental oxygenation. Sci Transl Med 7(277):277ra230

He C, Duan X, Guo N, Chan C, Poon C, Weichselbaum RR, Lin W (2016) Core-shell nanoscale coordination polymers combine chemotherapy and photodynamic therapy to potentiate checkpoint blockade cancer immunotherapy. Nat Commun 7:12499

Heist RS, Duda DG, Sahani DV, Ancukiewicz M, Fidias P, Sequist LV, Temel JS, Shaw AT, Pennell NA, Neal JW, Gandhi L, Lynch TJ, Engelman JA, Jain RK (2015) Improved tumor vascularization after anti-VEGF therapy with carboplatin and nab-paclitaxel associates with survival in lung cancer. Proc Natl Acad Sci U S A 112(5):1547–1552

Helmlinger G, Netti PA, Lichtenbeld HC, Melder RJ, Jain RK (1997) Solid stress inhibits the growth of multicellular tumor spheroids. Nat Biotechnol 15(8):778–783. https://doi.org/10.1038/nbt0897-778

Huang Y, Kim BY, Chan CK, Hahn SM, Weissman IL, Jiang W (2018) Improving immune–vascular crosstalk for cancer immunotherapy. Nat Rev Immunol 18(3):195–203

Huang Y, Yuan J, Righi E, Kamoun WS, Ancukiewicz M, Nezivar J, Santosuosso M, Martin JD, Martin MR, Vianello F, Leblanc P, Munn LL, Huang P, Duda DG, Fukumura D, Jain RK, Poznansky MC (2012) Vascular normalizing doses of antiangiogenic treatment reprogram the immunosuppressive tumor microenvironment and enhance immunotherapy. Proc Natl Acad Sci U S A 109(43):17561–17566. https://doi.org/10.1073/pnas.1215397109

Hurwitz H, Fehrenbacher L, Novotny W, Cartwright T, Hainsworth J, Heim W, Berlin J, Baron A, Griffing S, Holmgren E, Ferrara N, Fyfe G, Rogers B, Ross R, Kabbinavar F (2004) Bevacizumab plus irinotecan, fluorouracil, and leucovorin for metastatic colorectal cancer. N Engl J Med 350(23):2335–2342

Ide AG, Baker NH, Warren SL (1939) Vascularization of the Brown-Pearce rabbit epithelioma transplant as seen in the transplant ear chamber. Am J Radiol 42:891–899

Isner JM (2002) Myocardial gene therapy. Nature 415:234

Jain RK (1988) Determinants of tumor blood flow: a review. Cancer Res 48(10):2641–2658

Jain RK (2001) Normalizing tumor vasculature with anti-angiogenic therapy: a new paradigm for combination therapy. Nat Med 7(9):987–989. https://doi.org/10.1038/nm0901-987

Jain RK (2003) Molecular regulation of vessel maturation. Nat Med 9(6):685–693. https://doi.org/10.1038/nm0603-685

Jain RK (2005) Normalization of tumor vasculature: an emerging concept in antiangiogenic therapy. Science 307(5706):58–62. https://doi.org/10.1126/science.1104819

Jain RK (2008) Taming vessels to treat cancer. Sci Am 298(1):56–63

Jain RK (2013) Normalizing tumor microenvironment to treat cancer: bench to bedside to biomarkers. J Clin Oncol 31(17):2205–2218

Jain RK (2014) Antiangiogenesis strategies revisited: from starving tumors to alleviating hypoxia. Cancer Cell 26(5):605–622. https://doi.org/10.1016/j.ccell.2014.10.006

Jain RK, Carmeliet PF (2001) Vessels of death or life. Sci Am 285(6):38–45

Jain RK, Martin JD, Stylianopoulos T (2014) The role of mechanical forces in tumor growth and therapy. Annu Rev Biomed Eng 16:321–346. https://doi.org/10.1146/annurev-bioeng-071813-105259

Jain RK, Munn LL, Fukumura D (2002) Dissecting tumour pathophysiology using intravital microscopy. Nat Rev Cancer 2(4):266–276. https://doi.org/10.1038/nrc778

Jain RK, Schlenger K, Hockel M, Yuan F (1997) Quantitative angiogenesis assays: progress and problems. Nat Med 3(11):1203–1208

Jain RK, Stylianopoulos T (2010) Delivering nanomedicine to solid tumors. Nat Rev Clin Oncol 7(11):653–664

Jayson GC, Kerbel R, Ellis LM, Harris AL (2016) Antiangiogenic therapy in oncology: current status and future directions. Lancet 388(10043):518–529. https://doi.org/10.1016/S0140-6736(15)01088-0

Jin J, Hu C, Xiao Y, Zhang H, Ellsworth S, Schild S, Bogart J, Dobelbower M, Kavadi V, Narayan S (2017) Higher radiation dose to immune system is correlated with poorer survival in patients with stage III non-small cell lung cancer: a secondary study of a phase 3 cooperative group trial (NRG Oncology RTOG 0617). Int J Radiat Oncol Biol Phys 99(2):S151–S152

Kamoun WS, Ley CD, Farrar CT, Duyverman AM, Lahdenranta J, Lacorre DA, Batchelor TT, di Tomaso E, Duda DG, Munn LL, Fukumura D, Sorensen AG, Jain RK (2009) Edema control by cediranib, a vascular endothelial growth factor receptor-targeted kinase inhibitor, prolongs survival despite persistent brain tumor growth in mice. J Clin Oncol 27(15):2542–2552

Kirsch DG, Diehn M, Kesarwala AH, Maity A, Morgan MA, Schwarz JK, Bristow R, Demaria S, Eke I, Griffin RJ (2017) The future of radiobiology. J Natl Cancer Inst 110(4):329–340

Ko EC, Raben D, Formenti SC (2018) The integration of radiotherapy with immunotherapy for the treatment of non-small cell lung cancer. Clin Cancer Res 24(23):5792–5806

Kozin SV, Duda DG, Munn LL, Jain RK (2011) Is vasculogenesis crucial for the regrowth of irradiated tumours? Nat Rev Cancer 11(7):532. https://doi.org/10.1038/nrc2007-c1

Kozin SV, Duda DG, Munn LL, Jain RK (2012) Neovascularization after irradiation: what is the source of newly formed vessels in recurring tumors? J Natl Cancer Inst 104(12):899–905. https://doi.org/10.1093/jnci/djs239

Kuczek DE, Larsen AMH, Thorseth M-L, Carretta M, Kalvisa A, Siersbæk MS, Simões AMC, Roslind A, Engelholm LH, Noessner E (2019) Collagen density regulates the activity of tumor-infiltrating T cells. J Immunother Cancer 7(1):68

Kulkarni A, Rao P, Natarajan S, Goldman A, Sabbisetti VS, Khater Y, Korimerla N, Chandrasekar V, Mashelkar RA, Sengupta S (2016) Reporter nanoparticle that monitors its anticancer efficacy in real time. Proc Natl Acad Sci U S A 113(15):E2104–E2113

Lee DC, Sohn HA, Park Z-Y, Oh S, Kang YK, Lee K-m, Kang M, Jang YJ, Yang S-J, Hong YK (2015) A lactate-induced response to hypoxia. Cell 161(3):595–609

Lee H, Shields AF, Siegel BA, Miller KD, Krop I, Ma CX, LoRusso PM, Munster PN, Campbell K, Gaddy DF (2017) 64Cu-MM-302 positron emission tomography quantifies variability of enhanced permeability and retention of nanoparticles in relation to treatment response in patients with metastatic breast cancer. Clin Cancer Res 23(15):4190–4202

Less JR, Posner MC, Skalak TC, Wolmark N, Jain RK (1997) Geometric resistance and microvascular network architecture of human colorectal carcinoma. Microcirculation 4(1):25–33

Less JR, Skalak TC, Sevick EM, Jain RK (1991) Microvascular architecture in a mammary carcinoma: branching patterns and vessel dimensions. Cancer Res 51(1):265–273

Levin VA, Chan J, Datta M, Yee JL, Jain RK (2017) Effect of angiotensin system inhibitors on survival in newly diagnosed glioma patients and recurrent glioblastoma patients receiving chemotherapy and/or bevacizumab. J Neuro-Oncol 134(2):325–330

Liu H, Naxerova K, Pinter M, Incio J, Lee H, Shigeta K, Ho WW, Crain JA, Jacobson A, Michelakos T, Dias-Santos D, Zanconato A, Hong TS, Clark JW, Murphy JE, Ryan DP, Deshpande V, Lillemoe KD, Fernandez-del Castillo C, Downes M, Evans RM, Michaelson J, Ferrone CR, Boucher Y, Jain RK (2017) Use of angiotensin system inhibitors is associated with immune activation and longer survival in nonmetastatic pancreatic ductal adenocarcinoma. Clin Cancer Res 23(19):5959–5969

Liu J, Liao S, Diop-Frimpong B, Chen W, Goel S, Naxerova K, Ancukiewicz M, Boucher Y, Jain RK, Xu L (2012) TGF-β blockade improves the distribution and efficacy of therapeutics in breast carcinoma by normalizing the tumor stroma. Proc Natl Acad Sci U S A:201117610

Liu Y, Zhang P, Li F, Jin X, Li J, Chen W, Li Q (2018) Metal-based nanoenhancers for future radiotherapy: radiosensitizing and synergistic effects on tumor cells. Theranostics 8(7):1824

Maenhout SK, Thielemans K, Aerts JL (2014) Location, location, location: functional and phenotypic heterogeneity between tumor-infiltrating and non-infiltrating myeloid-derived suppressor cells. Onco Targets Ther 3(10):e956579

Mariathasan S, Turley SJ, Nickles D, Castiglioni A, Yuen K, Wang Y, Kadel EE III, Koeppen H, Astarita JL, Cubas R, Jhunjhunwala S, Banchereau R, Yang Y, Guan Y, Chalouni C, Ziai J, Sęnbabaogĺu Y, Santoro SP, Sheinson D, Hung J, Giltnane JM, Pierce AA, Mesh K, Lianoglou S, Riegler J, Carano RAD, Eriksson P, Höglund M, Somarriba L, Halligan DL, van der Heijden MS, Loriot Y, Rosenberg JE, Fong L, Mellman I, Chen DS, Green M, Derleth C, Fine GD, Hegde PS, Bourgon R, Powles T (2018) TGFβ attenuates tumour response to PD-L1 blockade by contributing to exclusion of T cells. Nature 554(7693):544–548

Martin JD, Cabral H, Stylianopoulos T, Jain RK (2020) Improving cancer immunotherapy using nanomedicine: progress, opportunities and challenges. Nat Rev Clin Oncol 17:251–266

Martin JD, Panagi M, Wang C, Khan TT, Martin MR, Voutouri C, Toh K, Papageorgis P, Mpekris F, Polydorou C, Ishii G, Takahashi S, Gotohda N, Suzuki T, Wilhelm ME, Melo VA, Quader S, Norimatsu J, Lanning RM, Kojima M, Stuber MD, Stylianopoulos T, Kataoka K, Cabral H (2019a) Dexamethasone increases Cisplatin-loaded Nanocarrier delivery and efficacy in meta-static breast cancer by normalizing the tumor microenvironment. ACS Nano 13(6):6396–6408

Martin JD, Seano G, Jain RK (2019b) Normalizing function of tumor vessels: Progress, opportuni-ties and challenges. Annu Rev Physiol 81:505–534

Martin JD, Fukumura D, Duda DG, Boucher Y, Jain RK (2016) Reengineering the tumor microen-vironment to alleviate hypoxia and overcome cancer heterogeneity. Cold Spring Harb Perspect Med 6(12):a027094

Mason K, Hunter N, Terry N, Patel N, Harada S, Jibu T, Seong J, Milas L (1997) Enhanced radio-response of paclitaxel-sensitive and-resistant tumours in vivo. Eur J Cancer 33(8):1299–1308

Matsumura Y, Maeda H (1986) A new concept for macromolecular therapeutics in cancer chemo-therapy: mechanism of tumoritropic accumulation of proteins and the antitumor agent smancs. Cancer Res 46(12 Part 1):6387–6392

Mazzone M, Bergers G (2019) Regulation of blood and lymphatic vessels by immune cells in tumors and metastasis. Annu Rev Physiol 81:535–560

Mazzone M, Dettori D, Leite de Oliveira R, Loges S, Schmidt T, Jonckx B, Tian YM, Lanahan AA, Pollard P, Ruiz de Almodovar C, De Smet F, Vinckier S, Aragones J, Debackere K, Luttun A, Wyns S, Jordan B, Pisacane A, Gallez B, Lampugnani MG, Dejana E, Simons M, Ratcliffe P, Maxwell P, Carmeliet P (2009) Heterozygous deficiency of PHD2 restores tumor oxygen-ation and inhibits metastasis via endothelial normalization. Cell 136(5):839–851. https://doi.org/10.1016/j.cell.2009.01.020

Meijer TW, Kaanders JH, Span PN, Bussink J (2012) Targeting hypoxia, HIF-1, and tumor glucose metabolism to improve radiotherapy efficacy. AACR

Melder RJ, Koenig GC, Witwer BP, Safabakhsh N, Munn LL, Jain RK (1996) During angiogen-esis, vascular endothelial growth factor and basic fibroblast growth factor regulate natural killer cell adhesion to tumor endothelium. Nat Med 2(9):992–997

Mi P, Kokuryo D, Cabral H, Wu H, Terada Y, Saga T, Aoki I, Nishiyama N, Kataoka K (2016) A pH-activatable nanoparticle with signal-amplification capabilities for non-invasive imaging of tumour malignancy. Nat Nanotechnol 11(8):724–730

Milas L (2009) Principles of combining radiation therapy and chemotherapy, chap 4. In: Radiation oncolgy: rationale, technique, results, pp 102–117. https://www.amazon.com/Radiation-Oncology-Rationale-Technique-Results/dp/0323049710

Milas L, Hunter N, Mason KA, Milross C, Peters LJ (1995) Tumor reoxygenation as a mechanism of taxol-induced enhancement of tumor radioresponse. Acta Oncol 34(3):409–412

Miller MA, Chandra R, Cuccarese MF, Pfirschke C, Engblom C, Stapleton S, Adhikary U, Kohler RH, Mohan JF, Pittet MJ (2017) Radiation therapy primes tumors for nanotherapeutic delivery via macrophage-mediated vascular bursts. Sci Transl Med 9(392):eaal0225

Min Y, Roche KC, Tian S, Eblan MJ, McKinnon KP, Caster JM, Chai S, Herring LE, Zhang L, Zhang T (2017) Antigen-capturing nanoparticles improve the abscopal effect and cancer immunotherapy. Nat Nanotechnol 12(9):877–882

Morikawa S, Baluk P, Kaidoh T, Haskell A, Jain RK, McDonald DM (2002) Abnormalities in pericytes on blood vessels and endothelial sprouts in tumors. Am J Pathol 160(3):985–1000

Motzer RJ, Penkov K, Haanen J, Rini B, Albiges L, Campbell MT, Venugopal B, Kollmannsberger C, Negrier S, Uemura M (2019) Avelumab plus axitinib versus sunitinib for advanced renal-cell carcinoma. N Engl J Med 380(12):1103–1115

Mpekris F, Baish JW, Stylianopoulos T, Jain RK (2017) Role of vascular normalization in benefit from metronomic chemotherapy. Proc Natl Acad Sci U S A 114(8):1994–1999

Mpekris F, Voutouri C, Baish JW, Duda DG, Munn LL, Stylianopoulos T, Jain RK (2020) Combining microenvironment normalization strategies to improve cancer immunotherapy. Proc Natl Acad Sci U S A 117:3728–3737

Müller P, Rothschild SI, Arnold W, Hirschmann P, Horvath L, Bubendorf L, Savic S, Zippelius A (2016) Metastatic spread in patients with non-small cell lung cancer is associated with a reduced density of tumor-infiltrating T cells. Cancer Immunol Immunother 65(1):1–11

Munn LL, Jain RK (2019) Vascular regulation of anti-tumor immunity. Science 365(6453):544–555

Murphy JE, Wo JY-L, Ryan DP, Clark JW, Jiang W, Yeap BY, Drapek LC, Ly L, Baglini CV, Blaszkowsky L, Ferrone C, Parikh AR, Weekes C, Nipp RD, Kwak EL, Allen JN, Corcoran RB, Ting DT, Faris JE, Zhu AX, Goyal L, Berger DL, Qadan M, Lillemoe KD, Talele N, Jain RK, Delaney TF, Duda DG, Boucher Y, Fernandez-del Castillo C, Hong TS (2019) A phase II study of neoadjuvant FOLFIRINOX in combination with losartan followed by chemoradiotherapy in locally advanced pancreatic cancer: R0 resection rate and clinical outcomes. JAMA Oncol 5(7):1020–1027

Netti PA, Berk DA, Swartz MA, Grodzinsky AJ, Jain RK (2000) Role of extracellular matrix assembly in interstitial transport in solid tumors. Cancer Res 60(9):2497–2503

Netti PA, Hamberg LM, Babich JW, Kierstead D, Graham W, Hunter GJ, Wolf GL, Fischman A, Boucher Y, Jain RK (1999) Enhancement of fluid filtration across tumor vessels: implication for delivery of macromolecules. Proc Natl Acad Sci U S A 96(6):3137–3142

Netti PA, Roberge S, Boucher Y, Baxter LT, Jain RK (1996) Effect of transvascular fluid exchange on pressure-flow relationship in tumors: a proposed mechanism for tumor blood flow heterogeneity. Microvasc Res 52(1):27–46. https://doi.org/10.1006/mvrc.1996.0041

Nishimura Y (2004) Rationale for chemoradiotherapy. Int J Clin Oncol 9(6):414–420

Noman MZ, Desantis G, Janji B, Hasmim M, Karray S, Dessen P, Bronte V, Chouaib S (2014) PD-L1 is a novel direct target of HIF-1α, and its blockade under hypoxia enhanced MDSC-mediated T cell activation. J Exp Med 211(5):781–790

Noman MZ, Hasmim M, Messai Y, Terry S, Kieda C, Janji B, Chouaib S (2015) Hypoxia: a key player in antitumor immune response. A review in the theme: cellular responses to hypoxia. Am J Phys Cell Phys 309(9):C569–C579

Öhlund D, Handly-Santana A, Biffi G, Elyada E, Almeida AS, Ponz-Sarvise M, Corbo V, Oni TE, Hearn SA, Lee EJ (2017) Distinct populations of inflammatory fibroblasts and myofibroblasts in pancreatic cancer. J Exp Med 214(3):579–596

Olive KP, Jacobetz MA, Davidson CJ, Gopinathan A, McIntyre D, Honess D, Madhu B, Goldgraben MA, Caldwell ME, Allard D (2009) Inhibition of hedgehog signaling enhances delivery of chemotherapy in a mouse model of pancreatic cancer. Science 324(5933):1457–1461

Padera TP, Stoll BR, Tooredman JB, Capen D, di Tomaso E, Jain RK (2004) Pathology: cancer cells compress intratumour vessels. Nature 427(6976):695. https://doi.org/10.1038/427695a

Palazon A, Tyrakis PA, Macias D, Veliça P, Rundqvist H, Fitzpatrick S, Vojnovic N, Phan AT, Loman N, Hedenfalk I (2017) An HIF-1α/VEGF-A Axis in cytotoxic T cells regulates tumor progression. Cancer Cell 32(5):669–683. e665

Panagi M, Voutouri C, Mpekris F, Papageorgis P, Martin MR, Martin JD, Polydorou C, Louca M, Kataoka K, Cabral H, Stylianopoulos T (2020) TGF-β inhibition combined with cytotoxic nanomedicine normalizes triple negative breast cancer microenvironment towards anti-tumor immunity. Theranostics 10:1910–1922

Papageorgis P, Polydorou C, Mpekris F, Voutouri C, Agathokleous E, Kapnissi-Christodoulou CP, Stylianopoulos T (2017) Tranilast-induced stress alleviation in solid tumors improves the efficacy of chemo-and nanotherapeutics in a size-independent manner. Sci Rep:7, 46140

Patan S, Munn LL, Jain RK (1996) Intussusceptive microvascular growth in a human colon adenocarcinoma xenograft: a novel mechanism of tumor angiogenesis. Microvasc Res 51(2):260–
272. https://doi.org/10.1006/mvre.1996.0025

Patan S, Munn LL, Tanda S, Roberge S, Jain RK, Jones RC (2001a) Vascular morphogenesis
and remodeling in a model of tissue repair: blood vessel formation and growth in the ovarian
pedicle after ovariectomy. Circ Res 89(8):723–731

Patan S, Tanda S, Roberge S, Jones RC, Jain RK, Munn LL (2001b) Vascular morphogenesis and
remodeling in a human tumor xenograft: blood vessel formation and growth after ovariectomy
and tumor implantation. Circ Res 89(8):732–739

Peng J, Xiao Y, Li W, Yang Q, Tan L, Jia Y, Qu Y, Qian Z (2018) Photosensitizer micelles together
with IDO inhibitor enhance cancer photothermal therapy and immunotherapy. Advanced
Science 5(5):1700891

Philip B, Ito K, Moreno-Sanchez R, Ralph SJ (2013) HIF expression and the role of hypoxic
microenvironments within primary tumours as protective sites driving cancer stem cell renewal
and metastatic progression. Carcinogenesis 34(8):1699–1707. https://doi.org/10.1093/carcin/
bgt209

Pinter M, Jain RK (2017) Targeting the renin-angiotensin system to improve cancer treatment:
implications for immunotherapy. Sci Transl Med 9(410):eaan5616

Pitroda SP, Chmura SJ, Weichselbaum RR (2019) Integration of radiotherapy and immunotherapy
for treatment of oligometastases. Lancet Oncol 20(8):e434–e442

Postow MA, Sidlow R, Hellmann MD (2018) Immune-related adverse events associated with
immune checkpoint blockade. N Engl J Med 378(2):158–168

Quintela-Fandino M, Lluch A, Manso LM, Calvo I, Cortes J, García-Saenz JA, Gil JM, Martinez-
Jañez N, González-Martín A, Adrover E (2016) 18F-fluoromisonidazole PET and activity of
neoadjuvant nintedanib in early HER2-negative breast cancer: a window-of-opportunity randomized trial.. American Association for Cancer Research:clincanres. 0738.2016

Rafii S, Lyden D, Benezra R, Hattori K, Heissig B (2002) Vascular and haematopoietic stem cells:
novel targets for anti-angiogenesis therapy? Nat Rev Cancer 2(11):826–835

Rahbari NN, Kedrin D, Incio J, Liu H, Ho WW, Nia HT, Edrich CM, Jung K, Daubriac J, Chen
I, Heishi T, Martin JD, Huang Y, Maimon N, Reissfelder C, Weitz J, Boucher Y, Clark JW,
Grodzinsky AJ, Duda DG, Jain RK, Fukumura D (2016) Anti-VEGF therapy induces ECM
remodeling and mechanical barriers to therapy in colorectal cancer liver metastases. Sci Transl
Med 8(360):360ra135–360ra135

Ramanathan RK, Korn R, Raghunand N, Sachdev JC, Newbold RG, Jameson G, Fetterly GJ, Prey
J, Klinz SG, Kim J (2017) Correlation between ferumoxytol uptake in tumor lesions by MRI
and response to nanoliposomal irinotecan in patients with advanced solid tumors: a pilot study.
Clin Cancer Res 23(14):3638–3648

Regan DP, Coy JW, Chahal KK, Chow L, Kurihara JN, Guth AM, Kufareva I, Dow SW (2019)
The angiotensin receptor blocker losartan suppresses growth of pulmonary metastases via
AT1R-independent inhibition of CCR2 Signaling and monocyte recruitment. J Immunol
202(10):3087–3102

Ricci-Vitiani L, Pallini R, Biffoni M, Todaro M, Invernici G, Cenci T, Maira G, Parati EA, Stassi
G, Larocca LM, De Maria R (2010) Tumour vascularization via endothelial differentiation of
glioblastoma stem-like cells. Nature 468(7325):824–828. https://doi.org/10.1038/nature09557

Rini BI, Plimack ER, Stus V, Gafanov R, Hawkins R, Nosov D, Pouliot F, Alekseev B, Soulières
D, Melichar B (2019) Pembrolizumab plus axitinib versus sunitinib for advanced renal-cell
carcinoma. N Engl J Med 380(12):1116–1127

Rockwell S, Dobrucki IT, Kim EY, Marrison ST, Vu VT (2009) Hypoxia and radiation therapy:
past history, ongoing research, and future promise. Curr Mol Med 9(4):442–458

Rodríguez-Ruiz ME, Vanpouille-Box C, Melero I, Formenti SC, Demaria S (2018) Immunological mechanisms responsible for radiation-induced abscopal effect. Trends Immunol
39(8):644–655

Rolny C, Mazzone M, Tugues S, Laoui D, Johansson I, Coulon C, Squadrito ML, Segura I, Li X, Knevels E (2011) HRG inhibits tumor growth and metastasis by inducing macrophage polarization and vessel normalization through downregulation of PlGF. Cancer Cell 19(1):31–44

Rytelewski M, Haryutyunan K, Nwajei F, Shanmugasundaram M, Wspanialy P, Zal MA, Chen C-H, El Khatib M, Plunkett S, Vinogradov SA (2019) Merger of dynamic two-photon and phosphorescence lifetime microscopy reveals dependence of lymphocyte motility on oxygen in solid and hematological tumors. J Immunother Cancer 7(1):78

Sahai E, Astsaturov I, Cukierman E, DeNardo DG, Egeblad M, Evans RM, Fearon DT, Greten FR, Hingorani SR, Hunter T, Hynes RO, Jain RK, Janowitz T, Jorgensen C, Kimmelman AC, Kolonin M, Maki RG, Powers S, Pure E, Ramirez D, Scherz-Shouval R, Sherman MH, Stewart S, Tlsty TD, Tuveson DA, Watt FM, Weaver VM, Weeraratna A, Werb Z (2020) A framework for advancing our understanding of cancer-associated fibroblasts. Nat Rev Cancer 20:174–186

Sajithlal GB, McGuire TF, Lu J, Beer-Stolz D, Prochownik EV (2010) Endothelial-like cells derived directly from human tumor xenografts. Int J Cancer 127(10):2268–2278. https://doi.org/10.1002/ijc.25251

Salmon H, Franciszkiewicz K, Damotte D, Dieu-Nosjean M-C, Validire P, Trautmann A, Mami-Chouaib F, Donnadieu E (2012) Matrix architecture defines the preferential localization and migration of T cells into the stroma of human lung tumors. J Clin Invest 122(3):899

Schito L, Semenza GL (2016) Hypoxia-inducible factors: master regulators of cancer progression. Trends Cancer 2(12):758–770

Schmittnaegel M, Rigamonti N, Kadioglu E, Cassará A, Rmili CW, Kiialainen A, Kienast Y, Mueller H-J, Ooi C-H, Laoui D (2017) Dual angiopoietin-2 and VEGFA inhibition elicits antitumor immunity that is enhanced by PD-1 checkpoint blockade. Sci Transl Med 9(385):eaak9670

Seano G, Jain RK (2020) Vessel co-option in glioblastoma: emerging insights and opportunities. Angiogenesis 23:9–16

Semenza GL (2016) Dynamic regulation of stem cell specification and maintenance by hypoxia-inducible factors. Mol Asp Med 47-48:15–23. https://doi.org/10.1016/j.mam.2015.09.004

Sevick EM, Jain RK (1989a) Geometric resistance to blood flow in solid tumors perfused ex vivo: effects of tumor size and perfusion pressure. Cancer Res 49(13):3506–3512

Sevick EM, Jain RK (1989b) Viscous resistance to blood flow in solid tumors: effect of hematocrit on intratumor blood viscosity. Cancer Res 49(13):3513–3519

Shamay Y, Elkabets M, Li H, Shah J, Brook S, Wang F, Adler K, Baut E, Scaltriti M, Jena PV (2016) P-selectin is a nanotherapeutic delivery target in the tumor microenvironment. Sci Transl Med 8(345):345ra387-345ra387

Sharabi AB, Lim M, DeWeese TL, Drake CG (2015) Radiation and checkpoint blockade immunotherapy: radiosensitisation and potential mechanisms of synergy. Lancet Oncol 16(13):e498–e509

Sheridan C (2019) Pancreatic cancer provides testbed for first mechanotherapeutics. Nat Biotechnol 37(8):829

Sherman MH, Yu RT, Engle DD, Ding N, Atkins AR, Tiriac H, Collisson EA, Connor F, Van Dyke T, Kozlov S, Martin P, Tseng TW, Dawson DW, Donahue TR, Masamune A, Shimosegawa T, Apte MV, Wilson JS, Ng B, Lau SL, Gunton JE, Wahl GM, Hunter T, Drebin JA, O'Dwyer PJ, Liddle C, Tuveson DA, Downes M, Evans RM (2014) Vitamin D receptor-mediated stromal reprogramming suppresses pancreatitis and enhances pancreatic cancer therapy. Cell 159(1):80–93. https://doi.org/10.1016/j.cell.2014.08.007

Shigeta K, Datta M, Hato T, Kitahara S, Chen IX, Matsui A, Kikuchi H, Mamessier E, Aoki S, Ramjiawan RR, Ochiai H, Bardeesy N, Huang P, Cobbold M, Zhu AX, Jain RK, Duda DG (2019) Dual Programmed Death Receptor-1 and Vascular Endothelial Growth Factor Receptor-2 Blockade Promotes Vascular Normalization and Enhances Antitumor Immune Responses in Hepatocellular Carcinoma. Hepatology 71:1247–1261

Shrimali RK, Yu Z, Theoret MR, Chinnasamy D, Restifo NP, Rosenberg SA (2010) Antiangiogenic agents can increase lymphocyte infiltration into tumor and enhance the effectiveness of adoptive immunotherapy of cancer. Cancer Res 70(15):6171–6180

Siemens DR, Hu N, Sheikhi AK, Chung E, Frederiksen LJ, Pross H, Graham CH (2008) Hypoxia increases tumor cell shedding of MHC class I chain-related molecule: role of nitric oxide. Cancer Res 68(12):4746–4753

Socinski MA, Jotte RM, Cappuzzo F, Orlandi F, Stroyakovskiy D, Nogami N, Rodríguez-Abreu D, Moro-Sibilot D, Thomas CA, Barlesi F (2018) Atezolizumab for first-line treatment of metastatic nonsquamous NSCLC. N Engl J Med 378:2288–2301

Soda Y, Marumoto T, Friedmann-Morvinski D, Soda M, Liu F, Michiue H, Pastorino S, Yang M, Hoffman RM, Kesari S, Verma IM (2011) Feature article: transdifferentiation of glioblastoma cells into vascular endothelial cells. Proc Natl Acad Sci U S A 108(11):4274–4280. https://doi.org/10.1073/pnas.1016030108

Sorensen AG, Batchelor TT, Zhang WT, Chen PJ, Yeo P, Wang M, Jennings D, Wen PY, Lahdenranta J, Ancukiewicz M, di Tomaso E, Duda DG, Jain RK (2009) A "vascular normalization index" as potential mechanistic biomarker to predict survival after a single dose of cediranib in recurrent glioblastoma patients. Cancer Res 69(13):5296–5300. https://doi.org/10.1158/0008-5472.CAN-09-0814

Sorensen AG, Emblem KE, Polaskova P, Jennings D, Kim H, Ancukiewicz M, Wang M, Wen PY, Ivy P, Batchelor TT (2012) Increased survival of glioblastoma patients who respond to antiangiogenic therapy with elevated blood perfusion. Cancer Res 72(2):402–407

Spivak-Kroizman TR, Hostetter G, Posner R, Aziz M, Hu C, Demeure MJ, Von Hoff D, Hingorani SR, Palculict TB, Izzo J (2013) Hypoxia triggers hedgehog-mediated tumor–stromal interactions in pancreatic cancer. Cancer Res 73(11):3235–3247

Stapleton S, Allen C, Pintilie M, Jaffray DA (2013) Tumor perfusion imaging predicts the intratumoral accumulation of liposomes. J Control Release 172(1):351–357

Stapleton S, Dunne M, Milosevic M, Tran CW, Gold MJ, Vedadi A, McKee T, Ohashi PS, Allen C, Jaffray DA (2018) Radiation and heat improve the delivery and efficacy of nanotherapeutics by modulating intra-tumoral fluid dynamics. ACS Nano 12(8):7583–7600

Stone HB, Bernhard EJ, Coleman CN, Deye J, Capala J, Mitchell JB, Brown JM (2016) Preclinical data on efficacy of 10 drug-radiation combinations: evaluations, concerns, and recommendations. Transl Oncol 9(1):46–56

Stylianopoulos T, Jain RK (2013) Combining two strategies to improve perfusion and drug delivery in solid tumors. Proc Natl Acad Sci U S A 110(46):18632–18637. https://doi.org/10.1073/pnas.1318415110

Stylianopoulos T, Martin JD, Chauhan VP, Jain SR, Diop-Frimpong B, Bardeesy N, Smith BL, Ferrone CR, Hornicek FJ, Boucher Y, Munn LL, Jain RK (2012) Causes, consequences, and remedies for growth-induced solid stress in murine and human tumors. Proc Natl Acad Sci U S A 109(38):15101–15108. https://doi.org/10.1073/pnas.1213353109

Stylianopoulos T, Martin JD, Snuderl M, Mpekris F, Jain SR, Jain RK (2013) Coevolution of solid stress and interstitial fluid pressure in tumors during progression: implications for vascular collapse. Cancer Res 73(13):3833–3841. https://doi.org/10.1158/0008-5472.CAN-12-4521

Stylianopoulos T, Munn LL, Jain RK (2018) Reengineering the physical microenvironment of tumors to improve drug delivery and efficacy: from mathematical modeling to bench to bedside. Trends Cancer 4(4):292–319

Sun C, Jain RK, Munn LL (2007) Non-uniform plasma leakage affects local hematocrit and blood flow: implications for inflammation and tumor perfusion. Ann Biomed Eng 35(12):2121–2129

Suzuki M, Nakamatsu K, Kanamori S, Masunaga S-I, Nishimura Y (2003) Additive effects of radiation and docetaxel on murine SCCVII tumors in vivo: special reference to changes in the cell cycle. Radiat Res 159(6):799–804

Taggart D, Andreou T, Scott KJ, Williams J, Rippaus N, Brownlie RJ, Ilett EJ, Salmond RJ, Melcher A, Lorger M (2018) Anti–PD-1/anti–CTLA-4 efficacy in melanoma brain metastases depends on extracranial disease and augmentation of CD8+ T cell trafficking. Proc Natl Acad Sci U S A 115(7):E1540–E1549

Tauriello DV, Palomo-Ponce S, Stork D, Berenguer-Llergo A, Badia-Ramentol J, Iglesias M, Sevillano M, Ibiza S, Cañellas A, Hernando-Momblona X (2018) TGFβ drives immune evasion in genetically reconstituted colon cancer metastasis. Nature 554(7693):538–543

Thariat J, Laé M, Carrère S, Papai Z, Ducassou A, Rochaix P, Sapi Z, Birtwisle-Peyrottes I, Shen CJ, Fernando NH (2019) Antitumor immune response induced by NBTXR3 activated by radiotherapy. ASCO Annual Meeting 2019

Thienpont B, Steinbacher J, Zhao H, D'Anna F, Kuchnio A, Ploumakis A, Ghesquière B, Van Dyck L, Boeckx B, Schoonjans L (2016) Tumour hypoxia causes DNA hypermethylation by reducing TET activity. Nature 537:63

Tian L, Goldstein A, Wang H, Lo HC, Kim IS, Welte T, Sheng K, Dobrolecki LE, Zhang X, Putluri N (2017) Mutual regulation of tumour vessel normalization and immunostimulatory reprogramming. Nature 544(7649):250–254

Togashi Y, Shitara K, Nishikawa H (2019) Regulatory T cells in cancer immunosuppression—implications for anticancer therapy. Nat Rev Clin Oncol 16:356–371

Tolaney SM, Boucher Y, Duda DG, Martin JD, Seano G, Ancukiewicz M, Barry WT, Goel S, 1430 Lahdenrata J, Isakoff SJ, Yeh ED, Jain SR, Golshan M, Brock J, Snuderl M, Winer EP, Krop IE, Jain RK (2015) Role of vascular density and normalization in response to 1431 neoadjuvant bevacizumab and chemotherapy in breast cancer patients. Proc Natl Acad Sci U S 1432 A 112(46):14325–14330

Tse JM, Cheng G, Tyrrell JA, Wilcox-Adelman SA, Boucher Y, Jain RK, Munn LL (2012) Mechanical compression drives cancer cells toward invasive phenotype. Proc Natl Acad Sci U S A 109(3):911–916. https://doi.org/10.1073/pnas.1118910109

Tumeh PC, Harview CL, Yearley JH, Shintaku IP, Taylor EJ, Robert L, Chmielowski B, Spasic M, Henry G, Ciobanu V (2014) PD-1 blockade induces responses by inhibiting adaptive immune resistance. Nature 515(7528):568–571

Twyman-Saint Victor C, Rech AJ, Maity A, Rengan R, Pauken KE, Stelekati E, Benci JL, Xu B, Dada H, Odorizzi PM (2015) Radiation and dual checkpoint blockade activate non-redundant immune mechanisms in cancer. Nature 520(7547):373–377

Ueda S, Kuji I, Shigekawa T, Takeuchi H, Sano H, Hirokawa E, Shimada H, Suzuki H, Oda M, Osaki A (2014) Optical imaging for monitoring tumor oxygenation response after initiation of single-agent bevacizumab followed by cytotoxic chemotherapy in breast cancer patients. PLoS One 9(6):e98715

Ueda S, Saeki T, Osaki A, Yamane T, Kuji I (2017) Bevacizumab induces acute hypoxia and cancer progression in patients with refractory breast cancer: multimodal functional imaging and multiplex cytokine analysis. Clin Cancer Res 23(19):5769–5778

Ueda S, Saeki T, Takeuchi H, Shigekawa T, Yamane T, Kuji I, Osaki A (2016) In vivo imaging of eribulin-induced reoxygenation in advanced breast cancer patients: a comparison to bevacizumab. Br J Cancer 114:1212

Vanpouille-Box C, Alard A, Aryankalayil MJ, Sarfraz Y, Diamond JM, Schneider RJ, Inghirami G, Coleman CN, Formenti SC, Demaria S (2017) DNA exonuclease Trex1 regulates radiotherapy-induced tumour immunogenicity. Nat Commun 8:15618

Vanpouille-Box C, Diamond JM, Pilones KA, Zavadil J, Babb JS, Formenti SC, Barcellos-Hoff MH, Demaria S (2015) TGFβ is a master regulator of radiation therapy-induced antitumor immunity. Cancer Res 75(11):2232–2242

Vasudev NS, Reynolds AR (2014) Anti-angiogenic therapy for cancer: current progress, unresolved questions and future directions. Angiogenesis 17(3):471–494. https://doi.org/10.1007/s10456-014-9420-y

Veglia F, Gabrilovich DI (2017) Dendritic cells in cancer: the role revisited. Curr Opin Immunol 45:43–51

Viallard C, Larrivée B (2017) Tumor angiogenesis and vascular normalization: alternative therapeutic targets. Angiogenesis 20(4):409–426

Vokes EE, Weichselbaum RR (1990) Concomitant chemoradiotherapy: rationale and clinical experience in patients with solid tumors. J Clin Oncol 8(5):911–934

Voron T, Colussi O, Marcheteau E, Pernot S, Nizard M, Pointet A-L, Latreche S, Bergaya S, Benhamouda N, Tanchot C (2015) VEGF-A modulates expression of inhibitory checkpoints on CD8+ T cells in tumors. J Exp Med 212(2):139–148

Voutouri C, Kirkpatrick ND, Chung E, Mpekris F, Baish JW, Munn LL, Fukumura D, Stylianopoulos T, Jain RK (2019) Experimental and computational analyses reveal dynamics of tumor vessel cooption and optimal treatment strategies. Proc Natl Acad Sci U S A:201818322

Wallin JJ, Bendell JC, Funke R, Sznol M, Korski K, Jones S, Hernandez G, Mier J, He X, Hodi FS (2016) Atezolizumab in combination with bevacizumab enhances antigen-specific T-cell migration in metastatic renal cell carcinoma. Nat Commun 7:12624

Wang R, Chadalavada K, Wilshire J, Kowalik U, Hovinga KE, Geber A, Fligelman B, Leversha M, Brennan C, Tabar V (2010) Glioblastoma stem-like cells give rise to tumour endothelium. Nature 468(7325):829–833. https://doi.org/10.1038/nature09624

Weidner N, Folkman J, Pozza F, Bevilacqua P, Allred EN, Moore DH, Meli S, Gasparini G (1992) Tumor angiogenesis: a new significant and independent prognostic indicator in early-stage breast carcinoma. J Natl Cancer Inst 84(24):1875–1887. https://doi.org/10.1093/jnci/84.24.1875

Wilson WR, Hay MP (2011) Targeting hypoxia in cancer therapy. Nat Rev Cancer 11(6):393–410. https://doi.org/10.1038/nrc3064

Winkler F, Kozin SV, Tong RT, Chae SS, Booth MF, Garkavtsev I, Xu L, Hicklin DJ, Fukumura D, di Tomaso E, Munn LL, Jain RK (2004) Kinetics of vascular normalization by VEGFR2 blockade governs brain tumor response to radiation: role of oxygenation, angiopoietin-1, and matrix metalloproteinases. Cancer Cell 6(6):553–563. https://doi.org/10.1016/j.ccr.2004.10.011

Yuan F, Salehi HA, Boucher Y, Vasthare US, Tuma RF, Jain RK (1994) Vascular permeability and microcirculation of gliomas and mammary carcinomas transplanted in rat and mouse cranial windows. Cancer Res 54(17):4564–4568

Zheng X, Fang Z, Liu X, Deng S, Zhou P, Wang X, Zhang C, Yin R, Hu H, Chen X (2018) Increased vessel perfusion predicts the efficacy of immune checkpoint blockade. J Clin Invest 128(5):2104–2115

Chapter 13
Radiosensitizers in the Era of Immuno-Oncology

Jonathan E. Leeman and Jonathan D. Schoenfeld

Abstract Radiation treatment is known to have immunomodulatory effects that contribute to its therapeutic efficacy. With the introduction and approval of immune checkpoint inhibitors in recent years, interest in combinatorial approaches has grown, as there is a strong scientific rationale that may account for synergy between radiation and immunotherapies. This includes enhancement of local effects of radiation via immune activation as well as the potential for abscopal effects that have been observed in unirradiated lesions. The optimal radiation dose and fractionation, timing and sequencing with immunotherapy and treatment volumes are important practical questions that are currently being explored. Combination of radiation with immunotherapies as well as additional molecular targeted agents with immunomodulatory activity are just beginning to be explored. This chapter summarizes the use of immunotherapies as radiosensitizers or agents to enhance systemic responses in combination with optimized local therapy.

Keywords Abscopal effect · Clinical trials · CTLA-4 · Cytosolic DNA · Immune checkpoint blockade · Immuno-oncology · Immunotherapy · PD-1 · PD-L1 · Radiosensitization · STING

1 The Immunotherapy Era

Immunotherapy has become a central pillar of modern oncologic care. Multiple immunomodulatory agents have been approved in the last 10 years—most prominently immune checkpoint blockade agents (ICB). ICBs are antibodies

J. E. Leeman (✉) · J. D. Schoenfeld
Department of Radiation Oncology, Dana Farber Cancer Institute/Brigham and Women's Hospital, Boston, MA, USA
e-mail: jonathane_leeman@dfci.harvard.edu

© Springer Nature Switzerland AG 2020
H. Willers, I. Eke (eds.), *Molecular Targeted Radiosensitizers*, Cancer Drug Discovery and Development, https://doi.org/10.1007/978-3-030-49701-9_13

directed at T-cell receptors or their ligands that suppress inhibitory immune signaling. The most success has been achieved with antibodies directed at cytotoxic T-lymphocyte-associated antigen 4 (CTLA-4), programmed death 1 (PD-1), and programmed death ligand 1 (PD-L1). Multiple agents have demonstrated activity in a variety of cancer types in the recurrent and metastatic setting, with some patients achieving durable responses. Emerging data is beginning to demonstrate a role in the treatment of localized disease as well (Antonia et al. 2017; Antonia et al. 2018). Due to the known immunomodulatory effects of ionizing radiation, clinical and laboratory research has been directed at attempting to elucidate synergistic mechanism between these two therapies and methods for maximizing clinical efficacy and safety.

2 Pre-Clinical Rationale for Combining Radiation with Immunotherapies

Classical radiation biology describes the 4 R's that govern the response of tumors and tissues to radiation therapy: recovery, reassortment, repopulation, and reoxygenation (Willers et al. 2019). In addition to these factors, it is clear that the immune response plays a key role in clinical radiation sensitivity. This has been observed both clinically and in preclinical models. In a mouse model of fibrosarcoma, the radiation dose required to achieve tumor control was found to be significantly higher following immune suppression with thymectomy or whole animal irradiation (Stone et al. 1979). In a syngeneic mouse model of head and neck cancer, the efficacy of cisplatin and radiation in clearing tumors was blunted by immune suppression (Spanos et al. 2009). This is in line with the clinical observation that immunosuppression in patients results in lower rates of tumor control following radiation therapy (Arbab et al. 2019; Chera et al. 2017). Importantly, following radiation to ablative doses in animal models, reduction of tumor burden has been found to be dependent on T-cell responses (Lee et al. 2009). Tumors that have been irradiated also show more robust infiltration of tumor infiltrating lymphocytes and immune activation in draining lymph nodes (Lugade et al. 2005). Furthermore, irradiated cells more readily present tumor antigens and incur a T-cell response with release of IFN-gamma in draining lymphatics (Lugade et al. 2005).

Ionizing radiation has been shown to induce immunogenic cell death in a manner that is dose dependent and contributes to a pro-immunogenic phenotype that counters the immunosuppressive environment which characterizes many solid tumors (Golden et al. 2014). This process leads to release and uptake of tumor antigens with cross presentation by activated dendritic cells which traffic to tumor draining lymphatics (Ngwa et al. 2018). In addition, the type 1 interferon pathway in dendritic cells has been shown to play a critical role in radiation sensitivity. Cross-priming is enhanced in tumor infiltrating dendritic cells of wild-type mice but lacking in type I interferon-deficient mice (Burnette et al. 2011). Growing evidence supports a central role for the cGAS-STING intracellular DNA sensing system in the radiation response (Deng et al. 2014a; Woo et al. 2014). This, in turn leads to downstream effects including expression of MHC class 1 and cytokines that promote T-cell trafficking to the tumor microenvironment including CCL5 and CXCL10 and activation of NK cells (Li et al. 2019; Sokolowska and Nowis 2018).

However, radiation has also been shown to have immunosuppressive effects and sequelae that may hinder the anti-tumor immune response. Radiation has been shown to promote TGF-beta signaling which promotes cell survival. Furthermore, irradiation of tumor-associated macrophages results in cellular changes that lead to increases in tumor cell invasion and angiogenesis (Teresa Pinto et al. 2016) and promotes an M2 macrophage response (Chiang et al. 2012). These negative effects are compounded by the inherent radiosensitivity of tumor infiltrating lymphocytes which may be depleted during radiation therapy and blunt the adaptive immune response. Therefore, because tumor irradiation results in both immunosuppressive and immunogenic effects, the addition of appropriate immunomodulatory agents to therapy may be necessary to tip the balance in favor of promoting pro-immunogenic and anti-tumor processes.

Preclinical studies have demonstrated substantial synergistic effects with the combined administration of radiation therapy and clinically available immune modulating agents, including immune checkpoint blockade with anti-PD-1/PD-L1 and anti-CTLA4 agents. Twyman-Saint Victor et al. evaluated the immune response underlying radiation therapy combined with dual anti-PD-1/PD-L1 and anti-CTLA4 blockade. It was found that radiation diversified the T-cell repertoire in tumor-associated lymphocytes. Meanwhile, blockade of CTLA4 primarily inhibited T-regulatory cells (Tregs), which resulted in an increase in the CD8/Treg ratio. Importantly, the combination of radiation and anti-CTLA4 and anti-PD-1 blockade resulted in improved outcomes compared to radiation with either anti-CTLA4 or anti-PD-1 agents alone across a variety of models (Twyman-Saint Victor et al. 2015). Synergy has also been identified in multiple other preclinical studies (Chae et al. 2018).

With the recognition that the immune microenvironment plays a key role in the response following radiation, newer agents are being explored in combination with radiation therapy to alter the microenvironment to result in a favorable immune response. Secondary mitochondrial-derived activators of caspase (SMAC) mimetics are a class of drugs that inhibit caspase function and alter innate and adaptive immunity through NFKb signaling. In a syngeneic mouse model, the combination of the SMAC mimetic Debio 1143 significantly enhanced the efficacy of 30 Gy of radiation via augmentation of a tumor-specific adaptive immune response and inhibition of cellular infiltrates that lead to immunosuppression (Tao et al. 2019). In head and neck cancer cell lines and xenografts, the addition of the SMAC mimetic birinapant to radiation has been shown to result in inhibition of tumor growth in a manner that is dependent on FADD amplification, a frequent genomic alteration in head and neck squamous cell carcinoma (HNSCC) (Eytan et al. 2016). SMAC mimetics are one example of newer classes of immune modulating agents demonstrating synergy with radiation therapy that are entering development pipelines. Interest is also growing in combinations of ICB with agents targeting the DNA damage response. This includes PARP inhibitors and ATM inhibitors which are demonstrating combinatorial effects when given with immunotherapies (Konstantinopoulos et al. 2019; Zhang et al. 2019), which are discussed in Chap. 9.

Taken together, this body of preclinical literature has demonstrated that combinations of radiation therapy and immunotherapies can result both in enhancement of local effects (radiosensitization) as well as the potential for systemic effects in non-irradiated lesions. However, these findings are not readily extrapolated to human disease for multiple reasons including differences in tumor size between mice and humans as well as inherent differences between human and murine immunity. Therefore, the radiosensitizing effects of ICB as well as potential abscopal effects require clinical validation, which is presently an active area of current study.

In these ways, it has become increasing clear that radiosensitivity is more than a product of intrinsic cellular responses and that both innate and adaptive immune responses play a central role determining the radiation sensitivity and resistance of human cancers. In the present era of immuno-oncology, where immune modulatory agents have entered the armamentarium, consideration and understanding of the immune response is all the more important. In the modern practice of oncology, many patients will receive both radiation therapies with immune modulating agents and so it is critical that we determine the safety profile of such combinations as well as potential areas where synergy can be achieved.

3 Abscopal Effects of Radiation Treatment

Much of the promise surrounding radiation and ICB combinations is related to observations of "abscopal" effects which mirror a phenomenon observed in preclinical models—specifically, an observed tumor response in a non-irradiated lesion presumably due to an incited systemic immune response resulting from local radiation treatment. Anecdotally, multiple case series have demonstrated regression of non-irradiated disease, when radiation has been combined with ICB or when radiation was initiated during ICB administration. These reports have been most frequent in cases of melanoma (Abuodeh et al. 2016; Chandra et al. 2015; Golden et al. 2013; Hiniker et al. 2012; Postow et al. 2012; Schoenfeld et al. 2015; Stamell et al. 2013).

In an effort to provide formal evidence of the abscopal effect, two prospective studies have been conducted to evaluate systemic response after randomizing patients to receive PD-1 blockade with or without stereotactic body radiation therapy (SBRT). The PEMBRO-RT study randomized patients with advanced non-small cell lung carcinoma (NSCLC) to receive pembrolizumab (200 mg/kg every 3 weeks) either alone or after SBRT (8 Gy x 3). SBRT was delivered to a single tumor site. Ninety-two patients were enrolled and 76 were randomized. The primary endpoint of ORR at 12 weeks was 18% in the pembrolizumab alone arm and 36%

in the pembrolizumab + SBRT arm ($p = 0.07$). Median progression-free survival (PFS) was 1.9 months in the pembrolizumab and 6.6 months in the pembrolizumab + SBRT arm ($p = 0.19$). Interestingly, patients who seemed to benefit most from the addition of radiation therapy were those with PD-L1-negative tumors. In this subgroup, PFS and overall survival (OS) were significantly improved with radiation therapy (Theelen et al. 2019). In a separate study of patients with metastatic HNSCC, patients were randomized to receive nivolumab 3 mg/kg every 2 weeks with or without SBRT to a single site of disease (59% lung tumors, 27 Gy in 3 fractions). SBRT was delivered between cycles 1 and 2 of nivolumab. Forty-eight patients have been enrolled and no difference was seen in the primary endpoint of ORR in non-irradiated lesions (25.9% with SBRT, 30.8% without SBRT). Of interest is the observation that HPV-negative and EBV-negative tumors demonstrated higher response rates as did tumors with high mutational burden (McBride et al. 2018).

In summary, despite multiple anecdotal reports, the present evidence supporting the abscopal effect is limited (Table 13.1). Studies point to specific subpopulations who may benefit from the addition of radiation to PD-1 blockade such as patients with PD-L1-negative tumors or high tumor mutational burden. The PEMRBO-RT study does indicate the potential for harnessing the abscopal effect. Presently, however, results have been borderline significant or non-significant. Ultimately, larger studies will be needed.

4 Safety of Immunotherapy and Radiation in the Definitive Treatment Setting

The vast majority of data evaluating toxicity with immunotherapy and radiation delivered to palliative doses do not demonstrate a substantial risk of adverse events. One exception may be a possible increase in risk in radionecrosis following cranial radiation therapy in combination with ICB (Martin et al. 2018). However, radiation doses that are delivered in the definitive setting, with curative intent, are higher as are rates of radiation-associated toxicities. In this setting, increasing the risk of treatment-associated toxicity has the potential to limit therapy and prevent patients from receiving potentially curative treatment. In addition, the phenomenon of "hyperprogression" or rapid progression of disease following initiation of ICB has been reported in 9–17% of patients undergoing treatment for metastatic disease (Champiat et al. 2017; Kato et al. 2017; Kim et al. 2018). The mechanisms underlying hyperprogression are poorly understood but the possibility for introducing this risk to patients with potentially curable disease is a concern. Lastly, as these therapies and combinations are relatively new, the long-term effects remain to be characterized and are of importance for patients who may be cured of their disease and have long life expectancy. For these reasons, the safety of ICB and radiation combinations require careful assessment independently of studies that have been conducted for patients with metastatic disease.

Table 13.1 Randomized prospective trials evaluating abscopal effects from combining immune checkpoint blockade with radiation therapy

Study	Cancer histology/ population	Primary endpoint	Immune checkpoint inhibitor	ICB dose/ schedule	Radiation regimen	Response data
McBride et al., ASCO 2018 NCT02684253 (McBride et al. 2018)	Metastatic HNSCC $N = 53$	ORR in unirradiated lesions	Nivolumab Anti-PD1	3 mg/kg q2 weeks	27 Gy in 3 fractions (SBRT) delivered between cycles 1 and 2 of nivolumab	Nivolumab vs Nivolumab + SBRT: ORR: 30.8% vs 25.9%, $p = 0.93$ (trend towards improved ORR with SBRT and nivolumab in virus-negative cohort) 1-year PFS: 28% vs 16%, $p = 0.89$ 1-year OS: 46% vs 54%, $p = 0.46$
"PEMBRO-RT", JAMA oncology 2019 NCT02492568 (Theelen et al. 2019)	Advanced NSCLC (second line or more treatment) $N = 92$ enrolled, $N = 76$ randomized	ORR	Pembrolizumab Anti-PD1	200 mg q3 weeks	24 Gy in 3 fractions (SBRT) delivered within 7 days prior to first cycle of pembrolizumab	Pembrolizumab vs Pembrolizumab + SBRT: ORR at 12 weeks: 18% vs 36%, $p = 0.07$ (more responders in PD-L1-negative group with SBRT) Median PFS: 1.9 m vs 6.6 m, $p = 0.08$ Median OS: 7.6 m vs 15.9 m, $p = 0.16$

The results of currently published or presented prospective studies that have evaluated combinations of ICB and radiotherapy in the definitive setting are summarized in Table 13.2. The DETERRED trial reported safety and efficacy results at the American Society of Clinical Oncology 2019 Annual Meeting in the treatment of locally advanced NSCLC using the addition of atezolizumab in combination with chemoradiation. The study enrolled patients in two phases: In the first phase ($N = 10$), patients were treated with chemoradiation (conventionally fractionated to 60–66 Gy in 30–33 fractions with weekly low-dose carboplatin and paclitaxel) followed by carboplatin/paclitaxel with atezolizumab followed by maintenance atezolizumab. The second phase ($N = 30$) treated patients with chemoradiation with concurrent atezolizumab followed by carboplatin/paclitaxel with atezolizumab followed by maintenance atezolizumab. Grade (G) 3+ atezolizumab-related adverse events were experienced by 40% (4/10) of patients in part 1 and 23% of patients in part 2. In part 1, the 1-year PFS and OS rates were 50% and 79%, respectively. In part 2, the 1-year PFS and OS rates were 57% and 79%, respectively (Lin et al. 2019). In the future, it will be important for this regimen of chemoradiation with concurrent immunotherapy to be tested against the PACIFIC regimen of chemoradiation followed adjuvant immunotherapy which has become standard of care.

A phase 1b study of 27 patients who underwent concurrent and adjuvant pembrolizumab with cisplatin-based chemoradiotherapy for locally advanced HNSCC importantly found that the addition of pembrolizumab did not compromise delivery of chemoradiation to full dose. All patients received the prescribed dose of radiation (70 Gy), and 85% received the target dose of cisplatin (≥ 200 mg/m^2). Seventy-eight percent of patients completed the prescribed dosage of pembrolizumab, and only three patients discontinued due immune-related adverse events (Powell et al. 2017).

A phase II randomized trial (GORTEC 2015-01, "PembroRad") is enrolling cisplatin-ineligible patients to receive radiation therapy in combination with either cetuximab or pembrolizumab. The most recent report at the American Society of Clinical Oncology 2018 Annual Meeting evaluated 133 patients who had been randomized. Compliance with treatment was high; 92% of patients received the full prescribed radiation dose and 87% received the prescribed three administrations of pembrolizumab. Rates of G3+ adverse events were lower in the pembrolizumab arm compared to the cetuximab arm including mucositis, dermatitis, and rash. Notably, higher rates of dysthyroidism were seen with pembrolizumab (18% vs 6%) (Sun et al. 2018).

The GORTEC 2017-01 study (REACH trial) is a phase III randomized trial for patients with locally advanced HSNCC to receive cisplatin-based chemoradiation or cetuximab-based radiation (if ineligible for cisplatin) versus radiation with cetuximab and concurrent plus adjuvant avelumab (anti-PD-L1) for a total of 1 year. Of the first 14 patients evaluated, three patients developed grade 4 toxicities including mucositis, dermatitis, and lymphopenia (Tao et al. 2018).

Table 13.2 Prospective safety data evaluating radiotherapy and immune checkpoint blockade combinations in the definitive setting

Study	Cancer histology	Population	Primary endpoint(s)	Immune checkpoint inhibitor	ICB dose/schedule	Other concurrent systemic therapy	Radiation dose	Toxicity data	Response data
Powell et al., ASCO 2017 NCT02586207 (Powell et al. 2017)	Head and neck squamous cell carcinoma $N = 27$ safety cohort (expansion cohort $N = 57$ planned)	Cisplatin eligible Stage III-IVB	Dose limiting AEs Complete response rate at day 150	Pembrolizumab Anti-PD1	200 mg q3w × 8 doses	Cisplatin 40 mg/m² × 6 doses	70 Gy/35 fx	3 ICB discontinuations due irAEs (AST elevation, peripheral motor neuropathy, Lhermitte-like syndrome) 44% grade 3 dysphagia 30% grade 3 mucositis 15% grade 3 radiation dermatitis 15% grade 3 weight loss	78% with CR at day 150 −85% for HPV+ −57%forHPV-
RTOG 3504, ASCO 2018, IJROBP 2018 NCT02764593 (Ferris et al. 2018; Gillison et al. 2018)	Head and neck squamous cell carcinoma $N = 29$	Intermediate-high risk (based on stage, smoking history, and p16 status)	Dose limiting toxicity	Nivolumab Anti-PD1	240 mg q14d × 10 concurrent (360 mg q21d for arm 2), 480 mg q28d × 7 adjuvant	Arm 1: Cisplatin 40 mg/m² qweek × 7 doses Arm 2: Cisplatin 100 mg/m² q21d × 3 doses Arm 3: Cetuximab 250/400 mg/m² qweek × 7 doses	70 Gy/35 fx	Arm 1: 0/10 DLT Arm 2: 0/10 DLT Arm 3: 1/9 DLT (grade 3 mucositis)	Arm 1: 0 events (median f/u 11.5 months) Arm 2: 1 death (median f/u 10.4 months) Arm 3: 1 disease progression (median f/u 8.0 months)

GORTEC 2015-01 "PembroRad", ASCO 2018 **NCT02707588** (Sun et al. 2018)	Head and neck squamous cell carcinoma $N = 133$	Cisplatin ineligible Stage III-IVB	Locoregional control at 15 months	Pembrolizumab Anti-PD1	200 mg q3w during RT	Arm 1: Pembro-RT Arm 2: Cetuximab-RT	69.96 Gy/33 fx	Grade 3+ AEs (pembrolizumab vs cetuximab): *Dermatitis 19% vs 59% Mucositis 31% vs 59% Rash 0% vs 15% Dysthyroidism 18% vs 6%*	N/A
GORTEC 2017-01 REACH trial, ASCO 2017 **NCT02999087** (Tao et al. 2018)	Head and neck squamous cell carcinoma $N = 29$ (total $n = 688$ planned)	High dose cisplatin eligible of ineligible	Progression-free survival	Avelumab Anti-PDL1	10 mg/kg q2 weeks	Cetuximab 400 mg/m² loading dose, 250 mg/m² weekly	69.96 Gy/33 fx	3 patients with grade 4 AEs (dermatitis, lymphopenia, oral mucositis)	N/A
Weiss et al., ASCO 2018 **NCT02609503** (Weiss et al. 2018)	Head and neck squamous cell carcinoma $N = 16$ ($N = 29$ planned)	Cisplatin ineligible Stage III-IVA	Progression-free survival	Pembrolizumab Anti-PD1	200 mg q3w × 6 doses	N/A	7 weeks IMRT	Grade 3 AEs: 7 lymphopenia 5 mucositis 1 nausea 1 anorexia	N/A

(continued)

Table 13.2 (continued)

Study	Cancer histology	Population	Primary endpoint(s)	Immune checkpoint inhibitor	ICB dose/schedule	Other concurrent systemic therapy	Radiation dose	Toxicity data	Response data
DUART trial, ASCO 2018 NCT02891161 (Joshi et al. 2018)	Bladder cancer $N = 6$ ($n = 42$ planned)	Unresectable or unfit for surgery, T3-4, N0-2, post-neoadjuvant chemotherapy	Safety	Durvalumab Anti-PDL1	1500 mg d1, d28 and adjuvantly q4weeks for 12 months	N/A	64.8 Gy/36 fx	No DLTs observed in the 5/6 patients that have completed durvaRT, no grade 3 irAEs. Most common toxicity fatigue (3/6, 50%)	3/4 patients with ongoing response after durvaRT, 1 with progression
ETOP NICOLAS, ASCO 2018, NCT02434081 (Peters et al. 2018)	Non-small cell lung cancer ($n = 58$ safety cohort)	Stage III (N2/3)	Primary safety endpoint: Grade 3 pneumonitis	Nivolumab Anti-PD1	360 mg q4weeks, followed by 480 mg q4weeks for up to one year	Platinum based (with etoposide, vinorelbine or pemetrexed)	66 Gy/33 fx	13 grade 1/2 pneumonitis events (22.4%) 6 grade 3 pneumonitis events (10.3%) 3 grade 5 events (5.2%, 2 stroke, 1 esophageal fistula)	N/A
LUN 14-179, ASCO 2018, NCT02343952 (Durm et al. 2018)	Non-small cell lung cancer $N = 93$	Stage III unresectable	Time to metastatic disease or death	Pembrolizumab Anti-PD1	200 mg q3weeks for up to 1 year (consolidation 4–8 weeks after CRT if no progression)	N/A	59–66.6 Gy	Grade 3+ toxicities: Pneumonitis 6.5% Fatigue 4.3% Cough 1.1% Dyspnea 5.4% Diarrhea 4.3% Other 4.3%	Median time to metastatic disease or death: 22.4 months Median PFS 17.0 months Median OS: Not reached 12-months OS: 81.0% 24-month OS: 61.9%

PACIFIC trial, Antonia et al. 2017, NEJM **NCT02125461** (Antonia et al. 2017)	Non-small cell lung cancer $N = 713$ (2:1 randomization to receive durvalumab)	Stage III unresectable	Progression-free survival and overall survival	Durvalumab Anti-PDL1	10 mg/kg q2 weeks for up to 12 months (consolidation beginning 1–42 days after completion of RT)	N/A	54–66 Gy	Durvalumab vs placebo: Any grade 3–4: 29.9% vs 26.1% Pneumonitis: 3.4% vs 2.6% Grade 5 toxicity: 4.4% vs 5.6% Grade 5 pneumonitis: 0.8% vs 1.3% Dyspnea 1.5% vs 2.6% Pneumonia 4.4% vs 3.8%	Durvalumab vs. placebo: Median time to death or distant metastasis: 23.2 vs 14.6 months 18-month PFS: 44.2% 27.0%
DETERRED trial, Lin et al., ASCO 2019, **NCT02525757** (Lin et al. 2019)	NSCLC $N = 40$	Locally advanced	PFS	Atezolizumab Anti-PDL1	1200 mg q3 weeks	Carboplatin/ paclitaxel	60–66 Gy/30–33 fx	23% with atezolizumab related SAEs (diarrhea, nephritis, dyspnea, fatigue and heart failure). Radiation pneumonitis was seen in 4 patients: 3 grade 2 and 1 grade 3.	1 year PFS 50%, OS 79%

A multi-center phase II trial of pembrolizumab with definitive dose radiation in cisplatin-ineligible patients has reported early toxicity data (NCT02609503) in the treatment of HNSCC. Fifteen of 16 patients were able to complete the prescribed 6 cycles of pembrolizumab and all patients completed 70 Gy of radiation. Fourteen G3+ toxicities have been observed thus far (7 lymphopenia, 5 mucositis, 1 nausea, 1 anorexia). Three treatment failures have been reported (Weiss et al. 2018).

5   Efficacy of Radiation Therapy and ICB in the Definitive Treatment Setting

Upon careful inspection of survival curves of multiple immunotherapy trials, it is found that the curves tend to overlap initially and separate only later. This is opposed to typical Kaplan–Meier curves that are associated with proportional hazards and show continuous separation over time. An analysis of several landmark immunotherapy trials has shown that there appears to be significant deviation from proportional hazards in these trials and that there appears to be a more substantial benefit from immunotherapy when the first 20% of events are excluded (Alexander et al. 2018). This suggest that patients who experience early disease progression may be less likely to benefit from immunotherapy. While cytotoxic chemotherapies have a relatively immediate onset of effect, immune checkpoint blockade depends on the generation of an adaptive immune response that may take longer to generate immune effector cells. Therefore, patients with rapidly progressive disease or a large tumor burden may be less likely to benefit from ICB and therapies may be discontinued early due to lack of immediate response. Consistent with this, in a trial testing ipilimumab after radiation therapy for bone metastasis in prostate cancer, patients with higher alkaline phosphatase, lower hemoglobin, and the presence of visceral metastases were less likely to benefit from ipilimumab (Kwon et al. 2014). Similarly, patients with visceral metastasis and higher LDH seem to be less responsive to immunotherapies with anti-CTLA4 or anti-PD-1 blockade (Sen et al. 2018). Therefore, it may be that there is an important role for radiation therapy in reducing burden of disease and delaying progression, in order to allow time for an adaptive immune response to mature. These findings also support a role for immunotherapy in the locally advanced or adjuvant setting where the disease burden is limited or minimal and so the efficacy of ICB can be maximized.

6 Clinical Data on Radiation Therapy and ICB in the Definitive Setting

The PACIFIC trial is a landmark study that demonstrated a significant benefit to the addition of adjuvant durvalumab (anti-PD-L1) following platinum-based chemoradiation for the treatment of locally advanced NSCLC. Seven hundred and thirteen patients were enrolled and randomized in a 2:1 fashion to receive either durvalumab or placebo adjuvantly for 12 months. The addition of durvalumab resulted in significant improvement in PFS and OS. Importantly, essentially all subgroups were found to benefit from durvalumab, even patients with minimal tumor expression of PD-L1. This study has provided some of the strongest clinical evidence supporting the use of ICB in the definitive setting in combination with chemoradiation (Antonia et al. 2017; Antonia et al. 2018).

An additional trial evaluating the role of nivolumab in locally advanced NSCLC has reported similar findings. Ninety-three patients were evaluated after platinum-based chemoradiation for Stage III NSCLC and nivolumab was administered adjuvantly for 12 months. The median PFS was 17 months and median survival was not reached. Grade 3+ pneumonitis only occurred in 6.5% of patients (Durm et al. 2018). A post hoc analysis of the KEYNOTE-001 study of patients with recurrent/metastatic NSCLC interestingly found that patients who had received prior radiation as part of their initial therapy seemed to experience longer PFS and OS (Shaverdian et al. 2017). Taken together, the above data have provided concordant results demonstrating a substantial clinical benefit to the addition of ICB following chemoradiation for locally advanced NSCLC and treatment appears to be well tolerated.

Lastly, a retrospective analysis of a cohort of patients from four centers who underwent brain radiation therapy for brain metastases from NSCLC, melanoma, or renal cell carcinoma in combination with ICB found positive outcomes with a median survival of 634 days, which compared favorably with historical controls (Pike et al. 2017). This is in keeping with multiple other studies that have found favorable outcomes with combinations of brain radiation and ICB (Ahmed et al. 2016; Qian et al. 2016) and suggests that patients responding to ICB who have isolated intracranial progression may be amenable to salvage with radiation and continued ICB treatment.

7 Practical Questions Related to Combining Radiation with ICB

How to optimally sequence and time radiation therapy with ICB is an important and relevant question. Whether radiation should be given prior to, during, or following ICB for maximal effect and safety remains unknown. Radiation is known to have immunosuppressive effects which in theory could hinder the adaptive immune response generated from ICB. Clinical evidence seems to suggest that abscopal effects tend to occur when radiation is given concurrently or immediately following ICB. This may be due to immune priming that is initiated by ICB allowing for recognition of radiation-induced tumor antigens that may be released and recognized. In the PACIFIC trial, timing of immunotherapy following radiation was found to be important. Patients who started adjuvant durvalumab within 14 days of completing chemoradiation were found to have improved PFS compared to patients who started 14–42 days after chemoradiation (hazard ratio 0.39 vs 0.63) though this could also reflect selection bias (Antonia et al. 2017). Analysis of 750 patients who received radiation and ICB (either anti-PD-1/PD-L1 or anti-CTLA4) found that overall survival was improved when radiation was given concurrently with ICB rather than before or after (20 months vs 6–7 months) (Samstein et al. 2017). A study of 75 patients with brain metastases from melanoma who received both stereotactic radiosurgery (SRS) and ICB found that patients who received radiation within 4 weeks of ICB experienced a more significant reduction in lesion size (Qian et al. 2016). Preclinical data has suggested that radiation (10 Gy in 2 fractions) showed enhanced activity when delivered with anti-PDL1 antibody concurrently at either the start or end of RT but not when given 7 days after radiation has been completed (Dovedi et al. 2014). The most appropriate sequencing and timing of ICB and radiation may also be dependent on the agent and ICB target. A study of tumor bearing mice found that optimal timing of radiation (20 Gy) with ICB was different with anti-CTLA4 blockade versus anti-OX40 blockade. With anti-CTLA4, ICB was more effective when given prior to radiation while anti-OX40 therapy was optimally given 1 day following radiation (Young et al. 2016).

In clinical practice, a wide range of radiation doses and fractionation schedules in use are dependent on the cancer type and context. This includes conventionally fractionated radiation (1.8–2 Gy per fraction), moderately hypofractionated radiation (2–6 Gy per fraction), high dose per fraction treatment typically given with SRS or SBRT (>6 Gy per fraction) and hyperfractionated treatment sometimes given twice per day. The mechanism of cell death induced by radiation likely differs depending on the dose per fraction that is delivered. However, the paradigms that govern most effective radiation doses for cytotoxic effects may need to be reconsidered when the goal of treatment is synergy with immunotherapy and immunomodulation. It is possible that prolonged courses of daily radiation may be counterproductive because tumor infiltrating lymphocytes are known to be highly radiosensitive and may therefore be continually killed by conventional schedules of radiation (Marciscano et al. 2018). Indeed, in a series of patients treated with radiation and ICB, more prolonged fractionation regimens were associated with significant lymphopenia and worse outcomes on ICB therapy (Pike et al. 2019).

A mouse model of the abscopal effect was developed by Camphausen et al. and involved measurement of lung carcinoma or fibrosarcoma tumor growth in the dorsum of the animal following irradiation of the leg. They found that higher dose per fraction treatment (10 Gy x 5 versus 2 Gy x 12) resulted in more evidence of an abscopal effect with inhibition of unirradiated tumor growth and in a p53-dependent fashion (Camphausen et al. 2003). In a murine model of melanoma, it was found that single fractions of radiation (15 Gy x 1 versus 5 Gy x 3) resulted in a more pronounced immune response with more immune activation in draining lymphatics as well as increase in tumor infiltrating lymphocytes and cell kill (Lugade et al. 2005). Similarly, another study found that 20 Gy given in single fraction was found to be more effective than 20 Gy in four fractions. The improvement found with single fraction treatment was reversed by inhibition of CD8+ lymphocytes suggesting that cytotoxic T-cells play an important role in the response to single fraction high dose treatment. Consistent with the findings of the above preclinical studies, a review of patients treated with both ICB and radiation found that the use of larger dose per fraction treatment (>4 Gy per fraction) was associated with longer survival. Therefore, prospective trials will be needed to assess the true clinical benefit of combining high dose per fraction treatment with immunotherapies (see Table 13.1).

While the above presented studies point to increased immune synergy with high dose per fraction radiation therapy, there is also compelling evidence for anti-tumor immunomodulation when radiation is given in multiple fractions as opposed to a single fraction combined with anti-CTLA4 blockade (Dewan et al. 2009; Vanpouille-Box et al. 2015). This may be because single fraction high dose treatment inhibits cGAS-STING activation and the ensuing cytosolic DNA immunogenic response (Vanpouille-Box et al. 2015). Delivery of 10 Gy of radiation has been found to activate expression of cellular immune response proteins and release of inflammatory damage-associated molecular pattern molecules when radiation was given in ten consecutive fractions as opposed to a single high dose fraction (John-Aryankalayil et al. 2010). Presently, prospective comparative clinical data are needed to better define the optimal radiation dose and schedule for induction of an abscopal effect.

Radiation field design may have an important effect on synergistic efficacy with ICB. In the treatment of many head and neck cancers, the draining cervical lymphatics are treated electively with radiation to eliminate potential deposits of microscopic disease as the initial pattern of spread. This approach is often applied in radiation treatment to other cancer types including prostate cancer, breast cancer, anorectal cancer, and gynecologic cancers. In a preclinical model, the addition of lymphatic irradiation to tumor irradiation resulted in a blunting of the effect of ICB due to reductions in adaptive immune response, chemokine expression, and immune infiltration (Marciscano et al. 2018). In this way, it is possible that classical approaches to radiation field design may need rethinking in the era of immunotherapy to maximize synergy and avoid unnecessary irradiation of lymphoid tissue which may be of importance. It is worth noting that in the treatment of locally advanced lung cancer, radiation is nowadays typically limited to areas of gross tumor or nodal stations which are radiographically or pathologically involved with tumor while other lymphatic stations are spared. This may have contributed to some of the success of radiation and ICB achieved in the PACIFIC trial and other studies in NSCLC described above.

8   Future Directions

As of now, the largest clinical experience and body of evidence surrounds the use of radiation with anti-CTLA4 and anti-PD-1/PD-L1 blocking agents, which have now entered routine clinical practice in the management of many different cancer types. However, there are newer ICB agents in the pipeline include drugs targeting OX40, TIM3, GITR, and LAG3 (Mahoney et al. 2015). It remains to be seen whether the existing knowledge of radiosensitization and immunomodulation with currently used agents can be extrapolated to new types of ICB. Furthermore, other types of immunotherapies are currently being explored in combination with radiation. Early evidence has demonstrated a role for radiation as part of conditioning for treatment with chimeric antigen receptor (CAR) T-cells (DeSelm et al. 2018) which have shown significant promise in hematologic malignancies as well as solid tumors.

As an experimental approach, partial tumor irradiation is beginning to be explored. As previously discussed, tumor infiltrating lymphocytes are highly sensitive to radiation which has known immunosuppressive effects. Irradiation of only a portion of the gross tumor volume as opposed to the entirety of the tumor may allow sparing of essential immune components that may potentiate the immune response of radiation. The use of more conformal techniques such as proton therapy remains to be explored in this context. Additionally, there is reason to believe that the use of brachytherapy may enhance immune activation through multiple mechanisms related to radiation dose heterogeneity and gradient (Patel et al. 2018). The question of whether to irradiate draining lymphatics and to what dose for optimal immunomodulation is an important one that requires exploration (Marciscano et al. 2018).

As our understanding of the molecular underpinnings of the abscopal effect improve, delivery of pharmacologic adjuvant agents may enhance immune responses achieved with radiation therapy. Immunotherapies have been shown to allow for improved systemic control that for some patients can be highly durable. In this setting, locoregional control of disease becomes even more important and therefore there exists a rationale for radiation plus targeted radiosensitizers for local therapy in combination with ICB for systemic control. However, these benefits must be weighed against potentially toxicity concerns associated with these combinations.

STING agonists may assist with potentiating optimal systemic responses (Deng et al. 2014b; Vanpouille-Box et al. 2015; Woo et al. 2014). There may also be a role for more classical radiosensitizing agents (platinum, 5-fluorouracil, temozolomide) which may potentially enhance tumor antigen release. However, benefits must also be weighed against immunosuppressive effects of these regimens which may hamper the effects of ICB. A growing body of evidence supports the use of PARP inhibitors in combination with ICB. PARP inhibition has been shown to upregulate PD-L1 expression (Jiao et al. 2017; Sato et al. 2017). Furthermore, niraparib has been shown to have immunomodulatory effects such as increase in tumor infiltrating T-cells and interferon pathways (Shen et al. 2019; Wang et al. 2019). The TOPACIO/ KEYNOTE-162 study has shown promising results with the combination of niraparib and pembrolizumab in the treatment of recurrent ovarian cancer or metastatic triple-negative breast cancer (Konstantinopoulos et al. 2019). It will be important to determine how radiation treatment can be introduced into these developing treatment paradigms with the goal of enhancing immune synergy with this newer generation of systemic therapy.

In these ways, the era of immunotherapy has opened up new and exciting possibilities in multidisciplinary oncologic care and pressed clinicians and researchers to rethink classical concepts and mechanisms of radiosensitization. As immunotherapies have entered the standard of care in the management of multiple cancer types, evidence is expanding that demonstrates renewed importance for radiation therapy as a way to maximize synergy and improve patient outcomes.

References

Abuodeh Y, Venkat P, Kim S (2016) Systematic review of case reports on the abscopal effect. Curr Probl Cancer 40:25–37. https://doi.org/10.1016/j.currproblcancer.2015.10.001

Ahmed KA, Stallworth DG, Kim Y, Johnstone PAS, Harrison LB, Caudell JJ, Yu HHM, Etame AB, Weber JS, Gibney GT (2016) Clinical outcomes of melanoma brain metastases treated with stereotactic radiation and anti-PD-1 therapy. Ann Oncol 27:434–441. https://doi.org/10.1093/annonc/mdv622

Alexander BM, Schoenfeld JD, Trippa L (2018) Hazards of hazard ratios—deviations from model assumptions in immunotherapy. N Engl J Med 378:1158–1159. https://doi.org/10.1056/NEJMc1716612

Antonia SJ, Villegas A, Daniel D, Vicente D, Murakami S, Hui R, Kurata T, Chiappori A, Lee KH, de Wit M, Cho BC, Bourhaba M, Quantin X, Tokito T, Mekhail T, Planchard D, Kim YC, Karapetis CS, Hiret S, Ostoros G, Kubota K, Gray JE, Paz-Ares L, de Castro CJ, Faivre-Finn C, Reck M, Vansteenkiste J, Spigel DR, Wadsworth C, Melillo G, Taboada M, Dennis PA, Ozguroglu M, Investigators P (2018) Overall survival with durvalumab after chemoradiotherapy in Stage III NSCLC. N Engl J Med 379(24):2342–2350. https://doi.org/10.1056/NEJMoa1809697

Antonia SJ, Villegas A, Daniel D, Vicente D, Murakami S, Hui R, Yokoi T, Chiappori A, Lee KH, de Wit M, Cho BC, Bourhaba M, Quantin X, Tokito T, Mekhail T, Planchard D, Kim Y-C, Karapetis CS, Hiret S, Ostoros G, Kubota K, Gray JE, Paz-Ares L, de Castro Carpeño J, Wadsworth C, Melillo G, Jiang H, Huang Y, Dennis PA, Özgüroğlu M, Investigators PACIFIC (2017) Durvalumab after chemoradiotherapy in Stage III Non-Small-Cell Lung Cancer. N Engl J Med 377:1919–1929. https://doi.org/10.1056/NEJMoa1709937

Arbab M, Margalit DN, Tishler RB, Rabinowits G, Pashtan IM, Borgelt BB, Powlis W, Holdsworth CH, Warren LE, Schoenfeld JD (2019) Outcomes following radiation for cutaneous squamous cell carcinoma of the head and neck: associations between immune suppression and recurrence. Head Neck 41:2111–2115. https://doi.org/10.1002/hed.25663

Burnette BC, Liang H, Lee Y, Chlewicki L, Khodarev NN, Weichselbaum RR, Fu Y-X, Auh SL (2011) The efficacy of radiotherapy relies upon induction of type i interferon-dependent innate and adaptive immunity. Cancer Res 71:2488–2496. https://doi.org/10.1158/0008-5472.CAN-10-2820

Camphausen K, Moses MA, Ménard C, Sproull M, Beecken W-D, Folkman J, O'Reilly MS (2003) Radiation abscopal antitumor effect is mediated through p53. Cancer Res 63:1990–1993

Chae YK, Arya A, Iams W, Cruz MR, Chandra S, Choi J, Giles F (2018) Current landscape and future of dual anti-CTLA4 and PD-1/PD-L1 blockade immunotherapy in cancer; lessons learned from clinical trials with melanoma and non-small cell lung cancer (NSCLC). J Immunother Cancer 6:39. https://doi.org/10.1186/s40425-018-0349-3

Champiat S, Dercle L, Ammari S, Massard C, Hollebecque A, Postel-Vinay S, Chaput N, Eggermont A, Marabelle A, Soria J-C, Ferté C (2017) Hyperprogressive disease is a new pattern of progression in cancer patients treated by Anti-PD-1/PD-L1. Clin Cancer Res 23:1920–1928. https://doi.org/10.1158/1078-0432.CCR-16-1741

Chandra RA, Wilhite TJ, Balboni TA, Alexander BM, Spektor A, Ott PA, Ng AK, Hodi FS, Schoenfeld JD (2015) A systematic evaluation of abscopal responses following radiotherapy in patients with metastatic melanoma treated with ipilimumab. Onco Targets Ther 4:e1046028. https://doi.org/10.1080/2162402X.2015.1046028

Chera BS, Amdur RJ, Mendenhall W, Zevallos J, Hayes DN (2017) Beware of deintensification of radiation therapy in patients with p16-positive oropharynx cancer and rheumatological diseases. Pract Radiat Oncol 7:e261–e262. https://doi.org/10.1016/j.prro.2016.12.004

Chiang C-S, Fu SY, Wang S-C, Yu C-F, Chen F-H, Lin C-M, Hong J-H (2012) Irradiation promotes an m2 macrophage phenotype in tumor hypoxia. Front Oncol 2:89. https://doi.org/10.3389/fonc.2012.00089

Deng L, Liang H, Burnette B, Beckett M, Darga T, Weichselbaum RR, Fu Y-X (2014a) Irradiation and anti-PD-L1 treatment synergistically promote antitumor immunity in mice. J Clin Invest 124:687–695. https://doi.org/10.1172/JCI67313

Deng L, Liang H, Xu M, Yang X, Burnette B, Arina A, Li X-D, Mauceri H, Beckett M, Darga T, Huang X, Gajewski TF, Chen ZJ, Fu Y-X, Weichselbaum RR (2014b) STING-dependent cytosolic DNA sensing promotes radiation-induced type I interferon-dependent antitumor immunity in immunogenic tumors. Immunity 41:843–852. https://doi.org/10.1016/j.immuni.2014.10.019

DeSelm C, Palomba ML, Yahalom J, Hamieh M, Eyquem J, Rajasekhar VK, Sadelain M (2018) Low-dose radiation conditioning enables CAR T cells to mitigate antigen escape. Mol Ther 26:2542–2552. https://doi.org/10.1016/j.ymthe.2018.09.008

Dewan MZ, Galloway AE, Kawashima N, Dewyngaert JK, Babb JS, Formenti SC, Demaria S (2009) Fractionated but not single-dose radiotherapy induces an immune-mediated abscopal effect when combined with anti-CTLA-4 antibody. Clin Cancer Res 15:5379–5388. https://doi.org/10.1158/1078-0432.CCR-09-0265

Dovedi SJ, Adlard AL, Lipowska-Bhalla G, McKenna C, Jones S, Cheadle EJ, Stratford IJ, Poon E, Morrow M, Stewart R, Jones H, Wilkinson RW, Honeychurch J, Illidge TM (2014) Acquired resistance to fractionated radiotherapy can be overcome by concurrent PD-L1 blockade. Cancer Res 74:5458–5468. https://doi.org/10.1158/0008-5472.CAN-14-1258

Durm GA, Althouse SK, Sadiq AA, Jalal SI, Jabbour S, Zon R, Kloecker GH, Fisher WB, Reckamp KL, Kio EA, Langdon RM, Adesunloye B, Gentzler RD, Hanna NH (2018) Phase II trial of concurrent chemoradiation with consolidation pembrolizumab in patients with unresectable stage III non-small cell lung cancer: Hoosier Cancer Research Network LUN 14-179. J Clin Oncol 36:8500–8500. https://doi.org/10.1200/JCO.2018.36.15_suppl.8500

Eytan DF, Snow GE, Carlson S, Derakhshan A, Saleh A, Schiltz S, Cheng H, Mohan S, Cornelius S, Coupar J, Sowers AL, Hernandez L, Mitchell JB, Annunziata CM, Chen Z, Van Waes C (2016) SMAC mimetic birinapant plus radiation eradicates human head and neck cancers with genomic amplifications of cell death genes FADD and BIRC2. Cancer Res 76:5442–5454. https://doi.org/10.1158/0008-5472.CAN-15-3317

Ferris RL, Gillison ML, Harris J, Colevas AD, Mell LK, Kong C, Jordan R, Moore K, Truong MT, Kirsch C, Clump DA, Ohr J, He K, Blakaj D, Deeken JF, Machtay M, Curran WJ, Le Q-T (2018) Safety evaluation of nivolumab (Nivo) concomitant with cetuximab-radiotherapy for intermediate (IR) and high-risk (HR) local-regionally advanced head and neck squamous cell carcinoma (HNSCC): RTOG 3504. J Clin Oncol 36:6010–6010. https://doi.org/10.1200/JCO.2018.36.15_suppl.6010

Gillison M, Ferris RL, Zhang Q, Colevas AD, Mell LK, Kirsch C, Moore KL, Truong MT, Kong CS, Jordan R, Clump DA II, Ohr J, He K, Blakaj D, Deeken J, Machtay M, Curran WJ Jr, Harris J, Le QT (2018) Safety evaluation of nivolumab concomitant with platinum-based chemoradiation therapy for intermediate and high-risk local-regionally advanced head and neck squamous cell carcinoma: RTOG Foundation 3504. Int J Radiat Oncol Biol Phys 100:1307–1308. https://doi.org/10.1016/j.ijrobp.2017.12.022

Golden EB, Demaria S, Schiff PB, Chachoua A, Formenti SC (2013) An abscopal response to radiation and ipilimumab in a patient with metastatic non-small cell lung cancer. Cancer Immunol Res 1:365–372. https://doi.org/10.1158/2326-6066.CIR-13-0115

Golden EB, Frances D, Pellicciotta I, Demaria S, Helen Barcellos-Hoff M, Formenti SC (2014) Radiation fosters dose-dependent and chemotherapy-induced immunogenic cell death. Onco Targets Ther 3:e28518. https://doi.org/10.4161/onci.28518

Hiniker SM, Chen DS, Reddy S, Chang DT, Jones JC, Mollick JA, Swetter SM, Knox SJ (2012) A systemic complete response of metastatic melanoma to local radiation and immunotherapy. Transl Oncol 5:404–407

Jiao S, Xia W, Yamaguchi H, Wei Y, Chen M-K, Hsu J-M, Hsu JL, Yu W-H, Du Y, Lee H-H, Li C-W, Chou C-K, Lim S-O, Chang S-S, Litton J, Arun B, Hortobagyi GN, Hung M-C (2017) PARP inhibitor upregulates PD-L1 expression and enhances cancer-associated immunosuppression. Clin Cancer Res 23:3711–3720. https://doi.org/10.1158/1078-0432.CCR-16-3215

John-Aryankalayil M, Palayoor ST, Cerna D, Simone CB, Falduto MT, Magnuson SR, Coleman CN (2010) Fractionated radiation therapy can induce a molecular profile for therapeutic targeting. Radiat Res 174:446–458. https://doi.org/10.1667/RR2105.1

Joshi M, Tuanquin L, Kaag M, Zakharia Y, Liao J, Merrill S, Musapatika D, DeGraff D, Zheng H, Warrick J, Holder SL, Stein M, Drabick JJ (2018) Phase Ib study of concurrent durvalumab and radiation therapy (DUART) followed by adjuvant durvalumab in patients with urothelial cancer of the bladder: BTCRC-GU15-023 study. J Clin Oncol 36:455–455. https://doi.org/10.1200/JCO.2018.36.6_suppl.455

Kato S, Goodman A, Walavalkar V, Barkauskas DA, Sharabi A, Kurzrock R (2017) Hyperprogressors after immunotherapy: analysis of genomic alterations associated with accelerated growth rate. Clin Cancer Res 23:4242–4250. https://doi.org/10.1158/1078-0432.CCR-16-3133

Kim Y, Kim CH, Kim HS, Sun J-M, Ahn JS, Ahn M-J, Lee S-H, Lee HY, Park K (2018) Hyperprogression after immunotherapy: clinical implication and genomic alterations in advanced non-small cell lung cancer patients (NSCLC). J Clin Oncol 36:9075–9075. https://doi.org/10.1200/JCO.2018.36.15_suppl.9075

Konstantinopoulos PA, Waggoner S, Vidal GA, Mita M, Moroney JW, Holloway R, Van Le L, Sachdev JC, Chapman-Davis E, Colon-Otero G, Penson RT, Matulonis UA, Kim YB, Moore KN, Swisher EM, Färkkilä A, D'Andrea A, Stringer-Reasor E, Wang J, Buerstatte N, Arora S, Graham JR, Bobilev D, Dezube BJ, Munster P (2019) Single-arm phases 1 and 2 trial of niraparib in combination with pembrolizumab in patients with recurrent platinum-resistant ovarian carcinoma. JAMA Oncol. https://doi.org/10.1001/jamaoncol.2019.1048

Kwon ED, Drake CG, Scher HI, Fizazi K, Bossi A, van den Eertwegh AJM, Krainer M, Houede N, Santos R, Mahammedi H, Ng S, Maio M, Franke FA, Sundar S, Agarwal N, Bergman AM, Ciuleanu TE, Korbenfeld E, Sengeløv L, Hansen S, Logothetis C, Beer TM, McHenry MB, Gagnier P, Liu D, Gerritsen WR, CA184-043 Investigators (2014) Ipilimumab versus placebo after radiotherapy in patients with metastatic castration-resistant prostate cancer that had progressed after docetaxel chemotherapy (CA184-043): a multicentre, randomised, double-blind, phase 3 trial. Lancet Oncol 15:700–712. https://doi.org/10.1016/S1470-2045(14)70189-5

Lee Y, Auh SL, Wang Y, Burnette B, Wang Y, Meng Y, Beckett M, Sharma R, Chin R, Tu T, Weichselbaum RR, Fu Y-X (2009) Therapeutic effects of ablative radiation on local tumor require CD8+ T cells: changing strategies for cancer treatment. Blood 114:589–595. https://doi.org/10.1182/blood-2009-02-206870

Li A, Yi M, Qin S, Song Y, Chu Q, Wu K (2019) Activating cGAS-STING pathway for the optimal effect of cancer immunotherapy. J Hematol Oncol 12:35. https://doi.org/10.1186/s13045-019-0721-x

Lin SH, Lin Y, Mok I, Young JA, Phan S, Sandler A, Papadimitrakopoulou V, Heymach J, Tsao AS (2019) Phase II trial combining atezolizumab concurrently with chemoradiation therapy in locally advanced non-small cell lung cancer. J Clin Oncol 37:8512–8512. https://doi.org/10.1200/JCO.2019.37.15_suppl.8512

Lugade AA, Moran JP, Gerber SA, Rose RC, Frelinger JG, Lord EM (2005) Local radiation therapy of B16 melanoma tumors increases the generation of tumor antigen-specific effector cells that traffic to the tumor. J Immunol 174:7516–7523

Mahoney KM, Rennert PD, Freeman GJ (2015) Combination cancer immunotherapy and new immunomodulatory targets. Nat Rev Drug Discov 14:561–584. https://doi.org/10.1038/nrd4591

Marciscano AE, Ghasemzadeh A, Nirschl TR, Theodros D, Kochel CM, Francica BJ, Muroyama Y, Anders RA, Sharabi AB, Velarde E, Mao W, Chaudhary KR, Chaimowitz MG, Wong J, Selby MJ, Thudium KB, Korman AJ, Ulmert D, Thorek DLJ, DeWeese TL, Drake CG (2018) Elective nodal irradiation attenuates the combinatorial efficacy of stereotactic radiation therapy and immunotherapy. Clin Cancer Res. https://doi.org/10.1158/1078-0432.CCR-17-3427

Martin AM, Cagney DN, Catalano PJ, Alexander BM, Redig AJ, Schoenfeld JD, Aizer AA (2018) Immunotherapy and symptomatic radiation necrosis in patients with brain metastases treated with stereotactic radiation. JAMA Oncol 4:1123–1124. https://doi.org/10.1001/jamaoncol.2017.3993

McBride SM, Sherman EJ, Tsai CJ, Baxi SS, Aghalar J, Eng J, Zhi WI, McFarland DC, Michel LS, Spielsinger D, Zhang Z, Flynn J, Dunn L, Ho AL, Riaz N, Pfister DG, Lee NY (2018) A phase II randomized trial of nivolumab with stereotactic body radiotherapy (SBRT) versus nivolumab alone in metastatic (M1) head and neck squamous cell carcinoma (HNSCC). J Clin Oncol 36:6009–6009. https://doi.org/10.1200/JCO.2018.36.15_suppl.6009

Ngwa W, Irabor OC, Schoenfeld JD, Hesser J, Demaria S, Formenti SC (2018) Using immunotherapy to boost the abscopal effect. Nat Rev Cancer 18:313–322. https://doi.org/10.1038/nrc.2018.6

Patel RB, Baniel CC, Sriramaneni RN, Bradley K, Markovina S, Morris ZS (2018) Combining brachytherapy and immunotherapy to achieve in situ tumor vaccination: a review of cooperative mechanisms and clinical opportunities. Brachytherapy 17:995–1003. https://doi.org/10.1016/j.brachy.2018.07.004

Peters S, De Ruysscher D, Dafni U, Felip E, Guckenberger M, Vansteenkiste JF, Huber RM, Nadal-Alforja E, Irigoyen A, Becker A, Piguet A-C, Kassapian M, Gasca-Ruchti A, Martinez Marti A, Andratschke N, Lambrecht M, Belka C, Roschitzki-Voser H, Stahel RA (2018) Safety evaluation of nivolumab added concurrently to radiotherapy in a standard first line chemo-RT regimen in unresectable locally advanced NSCLC: the ETOP NICOLAS phase II trial. J Clin Oncol 36:8510–8510. https://doi.org/10.1200/JCO.2018.36.15_suppl.8510

Pike LRG, Bang A, Mahal BA, Taylor A, Krishnan M, Spektor A, Cagney DN, Aizer AA, Alexander BM, Rahma O, Balboni T, Ott PA, Hodi FS, Schoenfeld JD (2019) The impact of radiation therapy on lymphocyte count and survival in metastatic cancer patients receiving PD-1 immune checkpoint inhibitors. Int J Radiat Oncol Biol Phys 103:142–151. https://doi.org/10.1016/j.ijrobp.2018.09.010

Pike LRG, Bang A, Ott P, Balboni T, Taylor A, Catalano P, Rawal B, Spektor A, Krishnan M, Cagney D, Alexander B, Aizer AA, Buchbinder E, Awad M, Gandhi L, Hodi FS, Schoenfeld JD (2017) Radiation and PD-1 inhibition: Favorable outcomes after brain-directed radiation. Radiother Oncol 124:98–103. https://doi.org/10.1016/j.radonc.2017.06.006

Postow MA, Callahan MK, Barker CA, Yamada Y, Yuan J, Kitano S, Mu Z, Rasalan T, Adamow M, Ritter E, Sedrak C, Jungbluth AA, Chua R, Yang AS, Roman R-A, Rosner S, Benson B, Allison JP, Lesokhin AM, Gnjatic S, Wolchok JD (2012) Immunologic correlates of the abscopal effect in a patient with melanoma. N Engl J Med 366:925–931. https://doi.org/10.1056/NEJMoa1112824

Powell SF, Gitau MM, Sumey CJ, Reynolds JT, Lohr M, McGraw S, Nowak RK, Terrell AM, Jensen AW, Blanchard MJ, Ellison C, Black LJ, Thompson PA, Gold KA, Cohen EEW, Lee JH, Spanos WC (2017) Safety of pembrolizumab with chemoradiation (CRT) in locally advanced squamous cell carcinoma of the head and neck (LA-SCCHN). J Clin Oncol 35:6011–6011. https://doi.org/10.1200/JCO.2017.35.15_suppl.6011

Qian JM, Yu JB, Kluger HM, Chiang VLS (2016) Timing and type of immune checkpoint therapy affect the early radiographic response of melanoma brain metastases to stereotactic radiosurgery. Cancer 122:3051–3058. https://doi.org/10.1002/cncr.30138

Samstein R, Rimner A, Barker CA, Yamada Y (2017) Combined immune checkpoint blockade and radiation therapy: timing and dose fractionation associated with greatest survival duration among over 750 treated patients. Int J Radiat Oncol Biol Phys 99:S129–S130. https://doi.org/10.1016/j.ijrobp.2017.06.303

Sato H, Niimi A, Yasuhara T, Permata TBM, Hagiwara Y, Isono M, Nuryadi E, Sekine R, Oike T, Kakoti S, Yoshimoto Y, Held KD, Suzuki Y, Kono K, Miyagawa K, Nakano T, Shibata A (2017) DNA double-strand break repair pathway regulates PD-L1 expression in cancer cells. Nat Commun 8:1751. https://doi.org/10.1038/s41467-017-01883-9

Schoenfeld JD, Mahadevan A, Floyd SR, Dyer MA, Catalano PJ, Alexander BM, McDermott DF, Kaplan ID (2015) Ipilmumab and cranial radiation in metastatic melanoma patients: a case series and review. J Immunother Cancer 3:50. https://doi.org/10.1186/s40425-015-0095-8

Sen S, Hess K, Hong DS, Naing A, Piha-Paul S, Janku F, Fu S, Subbiah IM, Liu H, Khanji R, Huang L, Moorthy S, Karp DD, Tsimberidou A, Meric-Bernstam F, Subbiah V (2018) Development of a prognostic scoring system for patients with advanced cancer enrolled in immune checkpoint inhibitor phase 1 clinical trials. Br J Cancer 118:763–769. https://doi.org/10.1038/bjc.2017.480

Shaverdian N, Lisberg AE, Bornazyan K, Veruttipong D, Goldman JW, Formenti SC, Garon EB, Lee P (2017) Previous radiotherapy and the clinical activity and toxicity of pembrolizumab in the treatment of non-small-cell lung cancer: a secondary analysis of the KEYNOTE-001 phase 1 trial. Lancet Oncol 18:895–903. https://doi.org/10.1016/S1470-2045(17)30380-7

Shen J, Zhao W, Ju Z, Wang L, Peng Y, Labrie M, Yap TA, Mills GB, Peng G (2019) PARPi triggers the STING-dependent immune response and enhances the therapeutic efficacy of immune checkpoint blockade independent of BRCAness. Cancer Res 79:311–319. https://doi.org/10.1158/0008-5472.CAN-18-1003

Sokolowska O, Nowis D (2018) STING signaling in cancer cells: important or not? Arch Immunol Ther Exp 66:125–132. https://doi.org/10.1007/s00005-017-0481-7

Spanos WC, Nowicki P, Lee DW, Hoover A, Hostager B, Gupta A, Anderson ME, Lee JH (2009) Immune response during therapy with cisplatin or radiation for human papillomavirus-related head and neck cancer. Arch Otolaryngol Head Neck Surg 135:1137–1146. https://doi.org/10.1001/archoto.2009.159

Stamell EF, Wolchok JD, Gnjatic S, Lee NY, Brownell I (2013) The abscopal effect associated with a systemic anti-melanoma immune response. Int J Radiat Oncol Biol Phys 85:293–295. https://doi.org/10.1016/j.ijrobp.2012.03.017

Stone HB, Peters LJ, Milas L (1979) Effect of host immune capability on radiocurability and subsequent transplantability of a murine fibrosarcoma. J Natl Cancer Inst 63:1229–1235

Sun XS, Sire C, Tao Y, Martin L, Alfonsi M, Prevost JB, Rives M, Lafond C, Tourani J-M, Biau J, Geoffrois L, Coutte A, Liem X, Vauleon E, Drouet F, Ramee J-F, Waksi G, Sinigaglia L, Auperin A, Bourhis J (2018) A phase II randomized trial of pembrolizumab versus cetuximab, concomitant with radiotherapy (RT) in locally advanced (LA) squamous cell carcinoma of the head and neck (SCCHN): first results of the GORTEC 2015-01 "PembroRad" trial. J Clin Oncol 36:6018–6018. https://doi.org/10.1200/JCO.2018.36.15_suppl.6018

Tao Y, Auperin A, Sun XS, Sire C, Martin L, Bera G, Coutte A, Miroir J, Lafond C, Colin-Batailhou N, Maillard A, Gibel L, Michel C, Guigay J, Bourhis J (2018) Avelumab-cetuximab-radiotherapy (RT) versus standards of care (SoC) in locally advanced squamous cell carcinoma of the head and neck (SCCHN): safety phase of the randomized trial GORTEC 2017-01 (REACH). J Clin Oncol 36:6076–6076. https://doi.org/10.1200/JCO.2018.36.15_suppl.6076

Tao Z, McCall NS, Wiedemann N, Vuagniaux G, Yuan Z, Lu B (2019) SMAC mimetic Debio 1143 and ablative radiation therapy synergize to enhance antitumor immunity against lung cancer. Clin Cancer Res 25:1113–1124. https://doi.org/10.1158/1078-0432.CCR-17-3852

Teresa Pinto A, Laranjeiro Pinto M, Patrícia Cardoso A, Monteiro C, Teixeira Pinto M, Filipe Maia A, Castro P, Figueira R, Monteiro A, Marques M, Mareel M, Dos Santos SG, Seruca

R, Adolfo Barbosa M, Rocha S, José Oliveira M (2016) Ionizing radiation modulates human macrophages towards a pro-inflammatory phenotype preserving their pro-invasive and pro-angiogenic capacities. Sci Rep 6:18765. https://doi.org/10.1038/srep18765

Theelen WSME, Peulen HMU, Lalezari F, van der Noort V, de Vries JF, Aerts JGJV, Dumoulin DW, Bahce I, Niemeijer A-LN, de Langen AJ, Monkhorst K, Baas P (2019) Effect of pembrolizumab after stereotactic body radiotherapy vs pembrolizumab alone on tumor response in patients with advanced non-small cell lung cancer: results of the PEMBRO-RT phase 2 randomized clinical trial. JAMA Oncol. https://doi.org/10.1001/jamaoncol.2019.1478

Twyman-Saint Victor C, Rech AJ, Maity A, Rengan R, Pauken KE, Stelekati E, Benci JL, Xu B, Dada H, Odorizzi PM, Herati RS, Mansfield KD, Patsch D, Amaravadi RK, Schuchter LM, Ishwaran H, Mick R, Pryma DA, Xu X, Feldman MD, Gangadhar TC, Hahn SM, Wherry EJ, Vonderheide RH, Minn AJ (2015) Radiation and dual checkpoint blockade activate non-redundant immune mechanisms in cancer. Nature 520:373–377. https://doi.org/10.1038/nature14292

Vanpouille-Box C, Diamond JM, Pilones KA, Zavadil J, Babb JS, Formenti SC, Barcellos-Hoff MH, Demaria S (2015) TGFβ is a master regulator of radiation therapy-induced antitumor immunity. Cancer Res 75:2232–2242. https://doi.org/10.1158/0008-5472.CAN-14-3511

Wang Z, Sun K, Xiao Y, Feng B, Mikule K, Ma X, Feng N, Vellano CP, Federico L, Marszalek JR, Mills GB, Hanke J, Ramaswamy S, Wang J (2019) Niraparib activates interferon signaling and potentiates anti-PD-1 antibody efficacy in tumor models. Sci Rep 9:1853. https://doi.org/10.1038/s41598-019-38534-6

Weiss J, Bauman JR, Deal AM, Sheth S, Chera BS, Shen C, Hilliard C, Seiwert TY, Mehra R, Grilley-Olson JE (2018) Preliminary toxicity data from the combination of pembrolizumab and definitive-dose radiotherapy for locally advanced head and neck cancer with contraindication to cisplatin therapy. J Clin Oncol 36:6069–6069. https://doi.org/10.1200/JCO.2018.36.15_suppl.6069

Willers H, Keane FK, Kamran SC (2019) Toward a new framework for clinical radiation biology. Hematol Oncol Clin North Am 33(6):929–945. https://doi.org/10.1016/j.hoc.2019.07.001

Woo S-R, Fuertes MB, Corrales L, Spranger S, Furdyna MJ, Leung MYK, Duggan R, Wang Y, Barber GN, Fitzgerald KA, Alegre M-L, Gajewski TF (2014) STING-dependent cytosolic DNA sensing mediates innate immune recognition of immunogenic tumors. Immunity 41:830–842. https://doi.org/10.1016/j.immuni.2014.10.017

Young KH, Baird JR, Savage T, Cottam B, Friedman D, Bambina S, Messenheimer DJ, Fox B, Newell P, Bahjat KS, Gough MJ, Crittenden MR (2016) Optimizing timing of immunotherapy improves control of tumors by hypofractionated radiation therapy. PLoS One 11:e0157164. https://doi.org/10.1371/journal.pone.0157164

Zhang Q, Green MD, Lang X, Lazarus J, Parsels JD, Wei S, Parsels LA, Shi J, Ramnath N, Wahl DR, Pasca di Magliano M, Frankel TL, Kryczek I, Lei YL, Lawrence TS, Zou W, Morgan MA (2019) Inhibition of ATM increases interferon signaling and sensitizes pancreatic cancer to immune checkpoint blockade therapy. Cancer Res 79:3940–3951. https://doi.org/10.1158/0008-5472.CAN-19-0761

Index

© Springer Nature Switzerland AG 2020
H. Willers, I. Eke (eds.), *Molecular Targeted Radiosensitizers*, Cancer Drug Discovery and Development, https://doi.org/10.1007/978-3-030-49701-9

Printed in the United States
by Baker & Taylor Publisher Services